Iron Metabolism

Iron Metabolism – From Molecular Mechanisms to Clinical Consequences

Fourth Edition

ROBERT CRICHTON

Université Catholique de Louvain, Belgium

WILEY

Library of Congress Cataloging-in-Publication data applied for

ISBN 9781118925614

A catalogue record for this book is available from the British Library.

Set in 10/12pt Times by SPi Global, Pondicherry, India
Printed and bound in Singapore by Markono Print Media Pte Ltd

Cover image: Protein Structure of hepcidin courtesy of Brad Jordan, Discovery Attribute Sciences, Amgen, Inc., Thousand Oaks, CA, USA (*J. Biol. Chem.*, **284**, 24155–24167 (2009); http://dx.doi.org/10.1074/jbc.M109.017764.)
Schematic of regulation of hepatic hepcidin production courtesy of Dr Andrea Steinbicker, Universitätsklinikum Münster, Germany (*Nutrients*, **5** (8), 3034–3061 (2013); doi: 10.3390/nu5083034.)

Contents

Preface

It is astonishing to realise that a slim volume of some 260 pages (Crichton, 1991), first conceived in the course of a discussion with the egregious Ellis Horwood at the Christmas buffet of the Royal Society of Chemistry Inorganic Biochemistry Discussion Group, has grown to such a size. Ellis Horwood had established his own scientific publishing house, Ellis Horwood Limited, based in the charming old Market Cross House in the West Sussex town of Chichester and, with his usual inimitable enthusiasm, he persuaded me – rather easily as it turned out – to contribute to his series of *Inorganic Chemistry* books. The outcome was *Inorganic Biochemistry of Iron Metabolism*, and any thoughts of subsequent editions had certainly not crossed my mind.

I say rather easily, because since the publication of the proceedings of the second meeting on proteins of iron storage and transport (Crichton, 1975), there had been a void which was crying out to be filled for a definitive work which would bring together an overview of the dramatic developments which had been taking place in the field of iron metabolism since then. All of the manuscripts of the presentations at that meeting in Louvain-la-Neuve were incorporated into the book *Proteins of Iron Storage and Transport in Biochemistry and Medicine*, produced by North Holland/American Elsevier in record time – the meeting was held from 2nd–5th April, 1975 and the book (all 454 pages) appeared in July of that year! They included the contribution by Jean Montreuil and Genevieve Spik from Lille, who arrived without a manuscript, but after being closeted in an office with an English-speaking secretary, duly produced the goods before the end of the meeting, as well as Clem Finch's Concluding Remarks recorded on a Dictaphone at the end of the meeting, typed that evening during the concluding Banquet, and duly dispatched, corrected, the following morning along with all of the other camera-ready texts. This volume, which represented the first time that all of the major figures on the iron scene had published jointly what was a sort of 'state of the art of iron metabolism, 1975', sold over 600 copies, and was still being cited more than a decade after the meeting itself. However, despite intermittent efforts after the New York meeting in 1977, the Sapporo meeting in 1983 and the Lille meeting in 1985 (Brown *et al.*, 1977; Uroshizaki *et al.*, 1983; Spik *et al.*, 1985), there was a real potential for a book that would bring together all aspects of iron metabolism.

My decision to undertake this ambitious project was greatly facilitated by the fact that I was in line for a sabbatical – in reality six rather than 12 months – which I spent at the invitation of Professor Robert Freedman in the Biology Department of the University of Kent in Canterbury. Ironically (no pun intended) for the author of a book on inorganic chemistry, my office was in the Chemistry Department. In those prehistoric times one hunted down references on the shelves of the University library overlooking the majestic and historical Cathedral, photocopied them (a new innovation), and then read them, highlighting the important sections. When the references (hunted down in *Chemical Abstracts*) were not available in Canterbury, one undertook a day trip to London to consult the Science Library there. Then, with reams of fluorescent highlighted papers, one sat down to write one's own text, mostly in my flat on the Canterbury Road in the agreeable seaside town of Whitstable, with its beach and bracing sea air.

The outcome, in 12 chapters, is quite similar to this 4th edition, dealing with iron chemistry, the importance of iron in biology, microbial, plant and fungal iron uptake, transferrin and its receptor (a relatively recent discovery), intracellular iron, iron homeostasis, iron absorption, iron deficiency and overload, iron and oxidative damage and finally, iron and infection. There were some 800 references in all, regrouped at the end of the book, in the classical chemical presentation without title, but with the final page number. I would think that, with the resources then available, I had read the abstracts of all of the articles (in *Chemical Abstracts*) and read the better part of 50–60% of the most important articles. The figures were entirely in black and white!

When, ten years later, I undertook a 2nd edition (Crichton, 2001), the title – now *Inorganic Biochemistry of Iron Metabolism. From Molecular Mechanisms to Clinical Consequences* – had been transferred to John Wiley & Sons, and the 326-page outcome even had a central glossy page insert which included 16 'Plates' of coloured figures (all of the others were black and white). For this edition I enlisted the help of six colleagues, Volkmar Braun and Klaus Hantke for microbial iron uptake, Jo Marx and Manuela Santos for the pathophysiology of iron deficiency and iron overload, Roberta Ward for the chapter on oxidative stress, and Johann Boelaert for iron and infection. There were some 1500 references, this time regrouped at the end of each chapter, but again without titles. Once again, it is probable (I cannot speak for my colleagues) that at least the abstracts of the papers cited had been read as well as most of the key articles.

By the time of the 3rd edition (Crichton, 2009), I had returned to the essentially single author format, with two chapters being entrusted to my long-term collaborator, Roberta Ward. Reflecting the way the field was growing, the microbial iron chapter included a view of intracellular iron metabolism, while the plant and fungal chapter highlighted the extraordinary developments in our understanding of yeast iron uptake systems. Although discovered just after the 2nd edition, hepcidin was relegated to the iron absorption chapter in which systemic iron balance was reviewed. The chapter on iron and infection was replaced by a new chapter on brain iron homeostasis and its perturbation in neurodegenerative diseases. Virtually all of the figures were in colour, and the 2200 references this time included titles (which makes for a lot more work – as a colleague remarked, "you can always invent the final page number, but the title......?", yet I think it is more useful in deciding if the reader really wants to hunt it down).

This 4th edition has reached even larger dimensions, with the number of references soaring to over 3500. As in the previous edition, we begin with a chapter on the solution chemistry of iron in biological media, the biologically very important interactions of iron with dioxygen, followed by a short review of hydrolysis of iron salts, the characterisation of ferrihydrite and its ageing to more crystalline products. The chapter concludes with a section on biomineralisation, with particular emphasis on magnetite formation by magnetotactic bacteria. The essential role of iron in biology is once again reviewed in Chapter 2, illustrated by examples drawn where possible from the recent literature.

The section on microbial iron has been subdivided this time into two chapters to take account of the important role of iron acquisition in the virulence of microbial pathogens and, in particular, as potential antimicrobial therapeutic targets. Chapter 3 discusses iron uptake from ferric siderophores in Gram-negative and Gram-positive bacteria, as well as the systems used by both classes of bacteria to take up Fe^{2+}. Iron release from siderophores and intracellular iron metabolism are then reviewed, and the chapter concludes with a discussion of the mechanisms involved in the regulation of gene expression by iron.

Iron sequestration provides the innate host defence, known as nutritional immunity, which leads bacterial and fungal pathogens to scavenge iron from their hosts. Chapter 4 is devoted to iron assimilation by pathogens, beginning with an overview of host defence mechanisms and nutritional immunity. The importance of pathogenicity islands, horizontally transferred mobile genetic elements involved in the dissemination of antibiotic resistance and virulence genes in pathogenic organisms, which frequently also encode iron uptake systems, specific to pathogenic strains (Gyles and Boerlin, 2014) is then outlined. Pathogen-specific iron uptake systems, involving pathogen-specific siderophores, host sources of iron such as transferrin, lactoferrin and haem, ferrous iron and ferric citrate, are then analysed. The structural basis of iron piracy by pathogenic *Neisseria* from human transferrin has been elucidated (Noinaj *et al.*, 2012). These studies establish a rational basis for the host specificity of TbpA, the TonB-dependent outer membrane transporter for human transferrin, show how TbpA promotes iron release from transferrin, and elucidate how TbpB, the lipoprotein coreceptor, facilitates this process. Recent cloning and sequencing of transferrin orthologues from 21 hominoid monkey species (Barber and Elde, 2014) revealed that hominoid transferrin has undergone recurrent positive selection at the binding interface with bacterial TbpA, providing a mechanism to counteract bacterial iron piracy. The regulation of pathogen iron uptake by Fur and Fur homologues, and by pathogen ECF sigma factors, are discussed, and we conclude with a brief outline of the strategies employed by opportunistic fungal pathogens, which represent a growing health threat, to acquire iron from their host.

Our understanding of iron uptake by plants and fungi has been greatly influenced by the fulgurant progress in genome sequencing, and Chapter 5 presents our current views on this area, with its important consequences for agriculture. Iron is the most commonly deficient micronutrient in the human diet, with iron deficiency affecting around 1.6 billion people (Chapter 11), and plants represent one of the principal sources of our dietary iron. However, while iron plays a key role among minerals in improving plant product quality, and is an important determinant in photosynthetic efficiency in algae and higher plants (Briat *et al.*, 2015), Fe deficiency – notably in calcareous soils – is very common. As our understanding of iron assimilation and distribution pathways in plants evolves, this information will assist in the development of strategies to improve both iron content and bioavailability of the edible parts of crops, in order to better improve our diet. Chapter 5 begins with a review of iron uptake by plant root systems, together with long distance iron transport in graminaceous and non-graminaceous plants, followed by a review of new tools in plant research, including integrative-omic analyses, and a discussion of intracellular plant iron metabolism and homeostasis. The final part of the chapter gives an account of iron uptake, metabolism and regulation in fungi.

Chapter 6 deals with mammalian cellular iron uptake and export, as in previous editions, beginning with the transferrin superfamily. Most transferrin family members have a familiar bilobal structure, resulting from an ancient gene duplication, with an iron-binding site in each of two homologous lobes. However, in the course of evolution transferrin homologues with a variety of domain architectures are found, including monolobals, bilobals with one or both iron-binding sites abrogated, bilobals with long insertions or with membrane anchors, and even trilobals (Gaffney and Valentine, 2012). Indeed, quite a number of the members do not appear to play any role in iron binding or transport. A discussion of the detailed structure of transferrins is then followed by an analysis of the binding not only of iron, but also of other metal ions, to the transferrin molecule. The structure of the transferrin receptor and its central role in cellular iron uptake from transferrin precedes a summary of other potential sources of cellular iron uptake, and the chapter concludes with an account of ferroportin and its role in iron export.

In Chapter 7 an overview of mammalian iron metabolism is presented, including an account of the diverse ways in which different cells of the body handle iron. The erythrocyte-forming cells of the bone marrow are the main iron *importers*, consuming most of the plasma iron for haem synthesis and its incorporation into the oxygen transport protein haemoglobin. In contrast, both the enterocytes of the gastrointestinal tract and the macrophages of the spleen and liver (Kupffer cells) are involved in the *import* and *export* of iron. The former capture dietary iron and then export it to the rest of the body. In contrast, splenic macrophages acquire iron from the phagocytosis of effete red blood cells, and then export it through transferrin for the requirements of other cells of the body, with the bulk going to the erythroid bone marrow. Dietary iron absorption from the intestinal mucosa in mammals concludes the Chapter, with an assessment of dietary sources of iron, and a review of the mechanisms of mucosal iron absorption.

Chapter 8 regroups a detailed analysis of our present understanding of intracellular iron utilisation in mammals, opening with a description of intracellular iron pools. Most of the iron taken up by the cell enters the kinetically labile iron pool (LIP) in the cytosol, the functional attributes of which were first presciently described by Allan Jacobs in 1977 (Jacobs, 1977), although its precise nature still seems to be uncertain (Cabantchik, 2014). While most of the iron in the LIP is destined for the mitochondria, there are increasing indications that members of the poly C binding protein (PCBP) family have iron chaperone activity, supplying iron both to ferritin and to enzymes of the family of iron and α-ketoglutarate-dependent dioxygenases (Shi *et al.*, 2008; Nandal *et al.*, 2011). Mitochondrial iron uptake and storage are briefly discussed before a detailed account of the current views on Fe–S cluster biosynthesis, Fe–S protein biogenesis and the maturation of cytosolic and nuclear Fe–S proteins (Stehling *et al.*, 2014). The chapter concludes with a discussion of haem biosynthesis and catabolism, the latter focusing on haem oxygenase and its activation.

Chapter 9 is devoted to iron storage proteins, beginning with a presentation of the ferritin superfamily, made up of at least 12 'subfamilies' (see Figure 9.1), of which the ferritins are the most abundant. Within the superfamily there are three distinct types of iron storing and detoxifying proteins which constitute the ferritin subfamily: the classical 24-meric ferritins; the haem-containing 24-meric bacterioferritins of prokaryotes; and the prokaryotic 12-meric Dps proteins, which bind to and protect DNA. All three are derived from far more simplistic rubrerythrin-like molecules, which play roles in defence against toxic oxygen species (Andrews, 2010). The extensive structural studies on the ferritins, Dps proteins and rubrerythrins are then reviewed, and this first section concludes with an account of the mineral core and the lysosomal degradation product of ferritin, haemosiderin. The second part of the chapter includes a detailed discussion of mechanisms involved in the uptake and release of iron by ferritins and Dps proteins. While there is considerable agreement on how iron enters the protein shell, and on the role of the ferroxidase centre in iron oxidation, there is still some controversy concerning the mechanism of iron storage by ferritins (Honarmand Ebrahimi *et al.*, 2014; Bradley *et al.*, 2014), although the opposing views may end up being reconciled. The chapter concludes with a brief overview of recent biotechnological applications of ferritins.

The exciting recent developments in our understanding of cellular and systemic iron homeostasis and their regulation are outlined in Chapter 10. The role of the IRE/IRP system in the regulation of cellular iron metabolism has undergone much refinement in detail, but the overarching picture of elegance in regulating mRNA translation remains. That is, when iron is scarce the uptake pathways are turned on and the storage and utilisation pathways are turned off, with the reverse happening in iron abundance (Kühn, 2014). Since the serendipitous discovery of its involvement in iron metabolism (Nicolas *et al.*, 2001; Pigeon *et al.*, 2001), the key role of hepcidin in regulating systemic iron homeostasis has become the brightest beacon on the iron scene. As Tom Ganz has elegantly put it, "The iron hormone hepcidin and its receptor and cellular iron exporter ferroportin control the major fluxes of iron into blood plasma: intestinal iron absorption, the delivery of recycled iron from macrophages, and the release of stored iron from hepatocytes" (Ganz, 2013). Finally, over the last few years the role of hypoxia-inducible factors (HIFs), notably HIF-2, in iron homeostasis has emerged. These transcription factors regulate responses to hypoxia but also regulate key proteins of iron metabolism (Simpson and McKie, 2015). The way in which the activity of hepcidin, the master regulator of systemic iron homeostasis, the cellular IRE/IRP system, and HIF-2 are coordinated will no doubt gradually begin to be better understood. The interplay between the three regulatory systems – the IRE/IRP system, the HIF system and the ultimate key orchestrator of systemic iron homeostasis, the hepcidin/ferroportin system – is slowly beginning to be understood.

Important questions concerning the integration of these regulatory systems remain, some of which are addressed in Chapter 11, which reviews our current understanding of human iron deficiency and iron overload (both hereditary and acquired), together with an assessment of their therapy. The mainstay of iron-deficiency anaemia (IDA) treatment and prevention remains iron fortification of staple foodstuffs, which is considered to be the most cost-effective method for providing additional iron for populations with a high prevalence of IDA (Lynch, 2011). This in turn underlines the importance of developing agronomic, plant breeding and transgenic approaches to increase the Fe content and the bioavailability of the edible parts of crops in order to improve the human diet (Briat *et al*., 2015). Introduction of the orally active chelator deferasirox (DFX, Exjade®; Novartis Pharma AG, Basel, Switzerland) has allowed a greater diversity of therapeutic strategies for the treatment of acquired iron overload (Saliba *et al*., 2015). However, as has been pointed out by Ioav Cabantchik (Cabantchik *et al*., 2013), these chelation regimens might not be suitable for treating disorders of iron maldistribution, as those are characterised by toxic islands of siderosis appearing in a background of normal or subnormal iron levels (e.g. sideroblastic anaemias, neurosiderosis and cardiosiderosis in Friedreich's ataxia and neurosiderosis in Parkinson's disease). New therapeutic approaches involving the normalisation of hepcidin levels in order to lower serum iron levels are being pursued in animal models of haemochromatosis and of acquired iron overload (Ganz, 2013; Schmidt and Fleming, 2014), with particularly promising results in animal models, notably of additive effects when combined with chelation therapy (Schmidt *et al*., 2015).

Chapter 12 is a new addition, penned by my long-suffering collaborator of many years, Professor Roberta Ward, on the relationship between iron and the body's defence against inflammation and infection, the immune system. Iron and immunity are closely linked. Iron withholding by many of the proteins involved in iron metabolism is a major strategy in preventing bacteria from utilising iron for growth. The monocytes, macrophages, microglia and lymphocytes of the innate immune system are able to combat bacterial insults by carefully controlling their iron fluxes, while a variety of effector molecules, including hypoxia factor-1 and haem oxygenase orchestrate the inflammatory response by mobilising cytokines, neurotrophic factors, chemokines and reactive oxygen species (ROS) and reactive nitrogen species (RNS). Both iron excess or deficiency can adversely affect the ability of these cells to respond to the bacterial insult.

Chapter 13, as in previous editions, examines the dark side of iron's interactions with molecular oxygen. After a brief introduction, the physiological context in which the different ROS and RNS are formed are reviewed, as are the cellular defence mechanisms against ROS and RNS. Particular emphasis is placed on the thioredoxin/peroxiredoxin system (Lu and Holmgren, 2014). We are all familiar with signalling pathways, which involve conformational changes induced by altering the charge of proteins, either by phosphorylation/dephosphorylation via kinases/phosphatases, or by Ca^{2+}-binding. However, we have become increasingly aware during the past few decades that, whereas high levels of ROS and RNS have deleterious effects, at low concentrations they can play an important signalling role in the control of cellular function by responding to changes in the intracellular redox potential. The chapter ends with an overview of the role of ROS and RNS in causing oxidative damage, by catalysing pathways which result in essentially irreversible modifications of amino acid residues in proteins.

Since the 2nd edition, a chapter has been devoted to the interactions between iron and other metals, and the 4th edition is no exception. Both experimental data and clinical findings have indicated that diseases of iron metabolism can be associated with alterations in the metabolism of other essential metal ions, particularly divalent cations (Loréal *et al.*, 2014). Chapter 14 first deals with the interactions of iron with the essential metal ions copper, zinc, cobalt, manganese and, for the first time, despite its quite different coordination chemistry, calcium. Exactly how Ca^{2+} interferes with iron transport is not clear, although voltage dependence or intracellular Ca^{2+} signalling seems to be ruled out (Shawki and MacKenzie, 2010). There are many toxic 'heavy' metals, some of which have gained access to the human population as a result of our own activities, such as the leaching of aluminium, the most abundant metal in the Earth's crust, into our environment as a consequence of the acid rain generated by emissions of sulphur dioxide and nitrogen oxide; in some regions of Eastern Europe the soil pH values fell below 3. We discuss the interference of the nonessential, toxic metals lead, cadmium and aluminium with iron.

The final chapter, also written in collaboration with Roberta Ward, addresses a subject which has been of particular interest to both of us over the past decade (Crichton and Ward, 2006, 2014; Ward *et al.*, 2013), namely the role of iron in neurodegenerative diseases. When we first advanced the idea that many neurodegenerative diseases involved dysfunction of brain homeostasis of essential metal ions – notably iron, copper and zinc (Crichton and Ward, 2006) – the evidence was not nearly as convincing as it is today. Sadly, our understanding of brain iron homeostasis is still in its infancy, but neurodegeneration with brain iron accumulation now covers – as the reader can see in Chapter 15 – a wide range of neurodegenerative diseases, including Parkinson's, Alzheimer's and Huntington's diseases and multiple sclerosis.

So, there have been many developments in iron metabolism since the last edition, and I assume the entire responsibility for any omissions or errors that have undoubtedly crept into my text, if only on account of the length and breadth of its subject matter. I would also like to thank Roberta Ward for her important contributions to Chapters 12 and 15, and to the many colleagues, who have given me useful advice.

Robert Crichton
January, 2016

References

Andrews, S.C. (2010) The Ferritin-like superfamily: Evolution of the biological iron storeman from a rubrerythrin-like ancestor. *Biochim. Biophys. Acta*, **1800**, 691–705.

Barber, M.F. and Elde, N.C. (2014) Nutritional immunity. Escape from bacterial iron piracy through rapid evolution of transferrin. *Science*, **346**, 1362–1366.

Bradley, J.M., Moore, G.R. and Le Brun, N.E. (2014) Mechanisms of iron mineralization in ferritins: one size does not fit all. *J. Biol. Inorg. Chem.*, **19**, 775–785.

Briat, J.F., Dubos, C. and Gaymard, F. (2015) Iron nutrition, biomass production, and plant product quality. *Trends Plant Sci.*, **20**, 33–40.

Brown, E.B., Aisen, P., Fielding, J. and Crichton, R.R. (1977) *Proteins of Iron Metabolism*. Grune & Stratton, New York, 443 pp.

Cabantchik, Z.I. (2014) Labile iron in cells and body fluids: physiology, pathology, and pharmacology. *Front. Pharmacol.*, **5**, 45.

Cabantchik, Z.I., Munnich, A., Youdim, M.B. and Devos, D. (2013) Regional siderosis: a new challenge for iron chelation therapy. *Front. Pharmacol.*, **4**, 167.

Crichton, R.R. (ed.) (1975) *Proteins of Iron Storage and Transport in Biochemistry and Medicine*. North-Holland/American Elsevier, Amsterdam, New York, 454 pp.

Crichton, R.R. (1991) *Inorganic Biochemistry of Iron Metabolism*. Ellis Horwood, Chichester, 263 pp.

Crichton, R.R. (2001) *Inorganic Biochemistry of Iron Metabolism: From Molecular Mechanisms to Clinical Consequences*, 2nd edn. John Wiley & Sons Ltd, Chichester, 326 pp.

Crichton, R.R. (2009) *Inorganic Biochemistry of Iron Metabolism: From Molecular Mechanisms to Clinical Consequences*, 3rd edn. John Wiley & Sons Ltd, Chichester, 461 pp.

Crichton, R.R. and Ward, R.J. (2006) *Metal-based Neurodegeneration: From Molecular Mechanisms to Therapeutic Strategies*. John Wiley & Sons Ltd, Chichester, 227 pp.

Crichton, R.R. and Ward, R.J. (2014) *Metal-based Neurodegeneration*. John Wiley & Sons Ltd, Chichester, 423 pp.

Gaffney, J.P. and Valentine, A.M. (2012) Beyond bilobal: transferrin homologs having unusual domain architectures. *Biochim. Biophys. Acta*, **1820**, 212–217.

Ganz, T. (2013) Systemic iron homeostasis. *Physiol. Rev.*, **93**, 1721–1741.

Gyles, C. and Boerlin, P. (2014) Horizontally transferred genetic elements and their role in pathogenesis of bacterial disease. *Vet. Pathol.*, **51**, 328–340.

Honarmand Ebrahimi, K.H., Hagedoorn, P.L. and Hagen, W.R. (2014) Unity in the biochemistry of the iron-storage proteins ferritin and bacterioferritin. *Chem. Rev.*, **115**, 295–326.

Jacobs, A. (1977) Low molecular weight intracellular iron transport compounds. *Blood*, **50**, 433–439.

Kühn, L.C. (2014) Iron regulatory proteins and their role in controlling iron metabolism. *Metallomics*, **7**, 232–243.

Loréal, O., Cavey, T., Bardou-Jacquet, E., *et al.* (2014) Iron, hepcidin and the metal connection. *Front. Pharmacol.*, **5**, 128.

Lu, J. and Holmgren, A. (2014) The thioredoxin antioxidant system. *Free Radic. Biol. Med.*, **66**, 75–87.

Lynch, S.R. (2011) Why nutritional iron deficiency persists as a worldwide problem. *J. Nutr.*, **141**, 763S–768S.

Nandal, A., Ruiz, J.C., Subramanian, P., *et al.* (2011) Activation of the HIF prolyl hydroxylase by the iron chaperones PCBP1 and PCBP2. *Cell Metab.*, **14**, 647–657.

Nicolas, G., Bennoun, M., Devaux, I., *et al.* (2001) Lack of hepcidin gene expression and severe tissue iron overload in upstream stimulatory factor 2 (USF2) knockout mice. *Proc. Natl Acad. Sci. USA*, **98**, 8780–8785.

Noinaj, N., Easley, N.C., Oke, M., *et al.* (2012) Structural basis for iron piracy by pathogenic *Neisseria*. *Nature*, **483**, 53–58.

Pigeon, C., Ilyin, G., Courselaud, B., *et al.* (2001) A new mouse liver-specific gene, encoding a protein homologous to human antimicrobial peptide hepcidin, is overexpressed during iron overload. *J. Biol. Chem.*, **276**, 7811–7819.

Saliba, A.N., Harb, A.R. and Taher, A.T. (2015) Iron chelation therapy in transfusion-dependent thalassemia patients: current strategies and future directions. *J. Blood Med.*, **6**, 197–209.

Schmidt, P.J. and Fleming, M.D. (2014) Modulation of hepcidin as therapy for primary and secondary iron overload disorders: preclinical models and approaches. *Hematol. Oncol. Clin. North Am.*, **28**, 387–401.

Schmidt, P.J., Racie, T., Westerman, M., *et al.* (2015) Combination therapy with a Tmprss6 RNAi-therapeutic and the oral iron chelator deferiprone additively diminishes secondary iron overload in a mouse model of β-thalassemia intermedia. *Am. J. Hematol.*, **90**, 310–313.

Shawki, A. and Mackenzie, B. (2010) Interaction of calcium with the human divalent metal-ion transporter-1. *Biochem. Biophys. Res. Commun.*, **393**, 471–475.

Shi, H., Bencze, K.Z., Stemmler, T.L. and Philpott, C.C. (2008) A cytosolic iron chaperone that delivers iron to ferritin. *Science*, **320** 1207–1210.

Simpson, R.J. and McKie, A.T. (2015) Iron and oxygen sensing: a tale of 2 interacting elements? *Metallomics*, **7**, 223–231.

Spik, G., Montreuil, J., Crichton, R.R. and Mazurier, J. (eds) (1985) *Proteins of Iron Storage and Transport*. Elsevier, Amsterdam, 380 pp.

Stehling, O., Wilbrecht, C. and Lill, R. (2014) Mitochondrial iron-sulfur protein biogenesis and human disease. *Biochimie*, **100**, 61–77.

Uroshizaki, I., Aisen, P., Listowsky, I. and Drysdale, J.W. (eds) (1983) *Structure and Function of Iron Storage and Transport Proteins*. Elsevier, Amsterdam, 546 pp.

Ward, R., Crichton, R. and Dexter, D. (eds) (2013) *Mechanisms and Metal Involvement in Neurodegenerative Diseases*. Royal Society of Chemistry, Metallobiology Series, 226 pp.

1

Solution Chemistry of Iron

1.1 Iron Chemistry

In the Earth's crust, iron is the fourth most abundant element and the second most abundant metal (the most abundant is aluminium). Situated in the Periodic Table in the middle of the first transition series (characterised by having incompletely filled d orbitals), iron has access to a number of oxidation states (from –II to +VI), the principal being II (d^6) and III (d^5). A number of iron-dependent monooxygenases are able to generate high-valent Fe(IV) or Fe(V) reactive intermediates during their catalytic cycle. Whereas, Fe^{2+} is extremely water-soluble, Fe^{3+} is quite insoluble in water ($K_{sp} = 10^{-39}$ M and at pH 7.0, $[Fe^{3+}] = 10^{-18}$ M) and significant concentrations of water-soluble Fe^{3+} species can be attained only by strong complex formation with appropriate ligands.

The interaction between Fe^{2+} and Fe^{3+} and ligand donor atoms will depend on the strength of the chemical bond formed between them. An idea of the strength of such bonds can be found in the concept of 'hard' and 'soft' acids and bases (HSAB) (Pearson, 1963). 'Soft' bases have donor atoms of high polarisability with empty, low-energy orbitals; they usually have low electronegativity and are easily oxidised. In contrast, 'hard' bases have donor atoms of low polarisability, and only have vacant orbitals of high energy; they have high electronegativity and are difficult to oxidise. Metal ions are 'soft' acids if they are of low charge density, have a large ionic radius. and have easily excited outer electrons. 'Hard' acid metal ions have high charge density, a small ionic radius, and no easily excited outer electrons. In general, 'hard' acids prefer 'hard' bases and 'soft' acids form more stable complexes with 'soft' bases (Pearson, 1963). Fe(III) with an ionic radius of 0.067 nm and a charge of 3^+ is a 'hard' acid and will prefer 'hard' oxygen ligands such as phenolate and carboxylate, compared to imidazole or thiolate. In contrast, Fe(II) with an ionic radius of

Iron Metabolism – From Molecular Mechanisms to Clinical Consequences, Fourth Edition. Robert Crichton.
© 2016 John Wiley & Sons, Ltd. Published 2016 by John Wiley & Sons, Ltd.

0.083 nm and a charge of only 2^+ is on the borderline between 'hard' and 'soft,' favouring nitrogen (imidazole and pyrrole) and sulphur ligands (thiolate and methionine) over oxygen ligands.

The coordination number of 6 is the most frequently found for both Fe(II) and Fe(III) giving octahedral stereochemistry, although four-coordinate (tetrahedral) and particularly five-coordinate complexes (trigonal bipyramidal or square pyrimidal) are also found. For octahedral complexes, two different spin states[1] can be observed. Strong-field ligands (e.g. Fe^{3+} OH^-), where the crystal field splitting is high and hence electrons are paired, give low-spin complexes, while weak-field ligands (e.g. CO, CN^-), where crystal field splitting is low, favour a maximum number of unpaired electrons and give high-spin complexes Changes of spin state affect the ion size of both Fe(II) and Fe(III), the high-spin ion being significantly larger than the low-spin ion. As we will see in Chapter 2, this is put to good use as a trigger for the cooperative binding of dioxygen to haemoglobin. High-spin complexes are kinetically labile, while low-spin complexes are exchange-inert. For both oxidation states only high-spin tetrahedral complexes are formed, and both oxidation states are Lewis acids, particularly the ferric state.

The unique biological role of iron comes from the extreme variability of the Fe^{2+}/Fe^{3+} redox potential, which can be fine-tuned by well-chosen ligands, so that iron sites can encompass almost the entire biologically significant range of redox potentials, from about -0.5 V to about $+0.6$ V. However, as we will see in Chapter 13, copper allows access to an even higher range of redox potentials (0 V to $+0.8$ V), which turned out to be of crucial importance in the Earth's rapidly evolving aerobic environment, following the arrival of water-splitting, oxygen-generating photosynthetic organisms.

1.2   Interactions of Iron with Dioxygen and Chemistry of Oxygen Free Radicals

Molecular oxygen was not present when life began on Earth, with its essentially reducing atmosphere, and both the natural abundance of iron and its redox properties predisposed it to play a crucial role in the first stages of life on Earth. About one billion (10^9) years ago, photosynthetic prokaryotes (Cyanobacteria) appeared and dioxygen was evolved into the Earth's atmosphere. It probably required 200–300 million years – a relatively short time on a geological time scale – for oxygen to attain a significant concentration in the atmosphere, since at the outset the oxygen produced by photosynthesis would have been consumed by the oxidation of ferrous ions in the oceans. Once dioxygen had become a dominant chemical entity, iron hydroxides precipitated, as the Precambrian deposits of red ferric oxides laid down in the geological strata at that time bear witness. Concomitant with the loss of iron bioavailability, the oxidation of Cu(I) led to soluble Cu(II). While enzymes active in anaerobic metabolism were designed to be active in the lower portion of the redox potential spectrum, the presence of dioxygen created the need for a new redox active metal with $E_o M^{n+1}/M^n$ from 0 to 0.8 V. Copper, now bioavailable (Crichton and Pierre, 2001), was ideally suited for this role and began to be used in enzymes with higher redox potentials (as a di-copper centre in laccase and a mixed iron-copper centre in cytochrome oxidase) to take advantage of the oxidizing power of dioxygen. Some typical redox potentials for iron and copper proteins and chelates are given in Figure 1.1.

Although oxygen must ultimately completely oxidise all biological matter, its propensity for biological oxidation is considerably slowed by the fact that in its ground state (lowest energy state)

---

[1] The spin state is defined as the orientation in a strong magnetic field of an unpaired electron (or a nuclear spin), i.e. either parallel or antiparallel to the direction of the magnetic field.

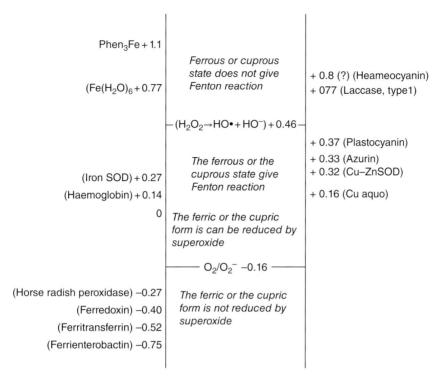

Phen$_3$Fe + 1.1

(Fe(H$_2$O)$_6$ + 0.77

Ferrous or cuprous state does not give Fenton reaction

+ 0.8 (?) (Heameocyanin)
+ 077 (Laccase, type1)

—(H$_2$O$_2$→HO• + HO$^-$) + 0.46—

+ 0.37 (Plastocyanin)
+ 0.33 (Azurin)
+ 0.32 (Cu–ZnSOD)

(Iron SOD) + 0.27

The ferrous or the cuprous state give Fenton reaction

(Haemoglobin) + 0.14

+ 0.16 (Cu aquo)

0

The ferric or the cupric form is can be reduced by superoxide

—— O$_2$/O$_2$$^-$ −0.16 ——

(Horse radish peroxidase) −0.27

The ferric or the cupric form is not reduced by superoxide

(Ferredoxin) −0.40
(Ferritransferrin) −0.52
(Ferrienterobactin) −0.75

Figure 1.1   *Some redox potentials (in Volts) of iron and copper enzymes and chelates at pH 7 relative to the standard hydrogen electrode. Figure reproduced with permission from Crichton and Pierre (2001)*

it exists as a triplet spin state, whereas most biological molecules are in the singlet state as their lowest energy level. Spin inversion is relatively slow, so that oxygen reacts much more easily with other triplet state molecules or with free radicals than with singlet state molecules.

The arrangement of electrons in most atoms and molecules is such that they occur in pairs, each of which have opposite intrinsic spin angular momentum. Molecules which have one or more unpaired electrons are termed free-radicals: these are generally very reactive and will act as chain carriers in chemical reactions. Thus, the hydrogen atom, with one unpaired electron, is a free radical, as are most transition metals and the oxygen molecule itself. The dioxygen molecule has two unpaired electrons, each located in a different π* anti-bonding orbital. Since these two electrons have the same spin quantum number, if the oxygen molecule attempts to oxidise another atom or molecule by accepting a pair of electrons from it, both new electrons must have parallel spins in order to fit into the vacant spaces in the π* orbitals. A pair of electrons in an atomic or molecular orbital would have anti-parallel spins (of +½ and −½) in accordance with Pauli's principle. This imposes a restriction on oxidation by O$_2$, which means that dioxygen tends to accept its electrons one at a time and slows its reaction with non-radical species (Halliwell and Gutteridge, 1984). Transition metals can overcome this spin restriction on account of their ability to accept and donate single electrons. The interaction of iron centres and oxygen is of paramount importance in biological inorganic chemistry, and some of the main features have been summarised in Figure 1.2.

The reactivity of O$_2$ can be increased in another way, by moving one of the unpaired electrons in a way that alleviates the spin restriction to give the two singlet states of O$_2$. The most important of the two forms of singlet O$^1_2$δ$_g$ in biological systems has no unpaired electrons, is not a radical,

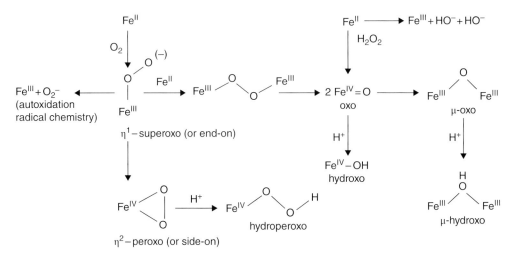

Figure 1.2 *Iron–oxygen chemistry. Multibridged species have been omitted. Figure reproduced with permission from Crichton and Pierre (2001)*

and can be obtained when a number of biological pigments such as chlorophylls, retinal, flavins or porphyrins are illuminated in the presence of O_2. When a single electron is accepted by the ground-state O_2 molecule, it must enter one of the π^* anti-bonding orbitals, to form the superoxide radical, O_2^-. The addition of a second electron to O_2^- gives the peroxide ion O_2^{2-} with no unpaired electrons. At physiological pH, O_2^{2-} will immediately protonate to give hydrogen peroxide, H_2O_2. The third reactive oxygen species found in biological system is the hydroxyl free radical. Two hydroxyl radicals, ·OH can be formed by homolytic fission of the O–O bond in H_2O_2, either by heating or by irradiation. However, as Fenton first observed in 1894 (Fenton, 1894), a simple mixture of H_2O_2 and an Fe(II) salt also produces the ·OH radical (Eq. 1.1):

$$Fe^{2+} + H_2O_2 \rightarrow \quad Fe^{3+} + \bullet OH + OH^- \tag{1.1}$$

In the presence of trace amounts of iron, superoxide can then reduce Fe^{3+} to molecular oxygen and Fe^{2+}. The sum of this reaction (Eq. 1.2), plus the Fenton reaction (Eq. 1.1), produces molecular oxygen, hydroxyl radical and hydroxyl anion from superoxide and hydrogen peroxide, in the presence of catalytic amounts of iron – the so-called Haber–Weiss[2] reaction (Eq. 1.3) (Haber and Weiss, 1934).

$$Fe^{3+} + O_2^- \rightarrow \quad Fe^{2+} + O_2 \tag{1.2}$$

$$O_2^- + H_2O_2 \rightarrow \quad O_2 + \bullet OH + OH^- \tag{1.3}$$

Iron or copper complexes will catalyse Fenton chemistry only if two conditions are met simultaneously, namely that the ferric complex can be reduced and that the ferrous complex has an oxidation potential such that it can transfer an electron to H_2O_2. However, it must also be added that this reasoning supposes that standard conditions are present and at equilibrium, which is rarely the case

---

[2] The reaction was originally described by Haber and Wilstätter (1931), but the original paper was published in German! The more frequently cited Haber and Weiss paper does cite the original, but in neither is a reference to Fenton given.

for biological systems. A simple example will illustrate the problem: whereas, under standard conditions reaction (1.2) has a redox potential of -330 mV (at an O_2 concentration of 1 atmosphere), *in vivo* with $[O_2] = 3.5 \times 10^{-5}$ M and $[O_2^-] = 10^{-11}$ M the redox potential is $+230$ mV (Pierre and Fontecave, 1999).

In aqueous solution in the absence of oxygen, iron is present as the hydrated hexa-aqua ferrous II ion, $Fe(H_2O)_6^{2+}$. In the early stages of evolution the atmosphere was thought to be essentially reducing with a very low oxygen pressure, and thus a high concentration of reduced iron would have been present. The appearance of molecular oxygen, which accompanied the arrival of photosynthetic organisms capable of the fixation of atmospheric carbon dioxide with concomitant water splitting to yield electrons, protons and oxygen, changed the situation dramatically, since the following reaction (Eq. 1.4) (here simplified by neglecting the hydration of the ferrous ion) would result:

$$Fe(II)aq + O_2 \rightarrow Fe(III)aq + O_{2-} \qquad (1.4)$$

Except at very low pH values, the hexa-aqua ferric ion, $Fe(H_2O)_6^{3+}$, would then undergo a series of hydrolysis and polymerisation reactions leading progressively to more and more insoluble ferric polynuclears. These would then precipitate to provide geologic evidence of the oxygenation of the atmosphere by the presence around the mid Precambrian of intense red deposits of ferric oxides. The inorganic chemistry involved in these processes is becoming better understood (Jolivet *et al.*, 2004), and the remainder of this chapter is concerned with the pathways of iron hydrolysis and polymerisation, and concludes with some thoughts on biomineralisation.

1.3   Hydrolysis of Iron Salts

Iron salts have a strong predisposition to hydrolyze in aqueous solutions, in a complex process involving the following steps (Flynn, 1984): (i) an initial hydrolysis with the formation of soluble low-molecular-weight complexes; (ii) the formation and ageing of polynuclear clusters; and finally (iii) the precipitation of insoluble Fe(III) oxides and hydroxides. At low pH, iron typically forms hexacoordinated aquo complexes, $[Fe(H_2O)_6]^{z+}$, in which polarisation of the coordinated water molecules will depend on the oxidation state and the size of the cation. Ferric aquo complexes are more acidic than ferrous, and hydroxylation of the cations occurs in very distinct ranges of pH, as can be seen from the speciation diagram (Figure 1.3).

Hydrolysis originates from the loss of protons from the aqua metal ion – going from $[Fe(OH)_h Fe(H_2O)_{6-h}]^{(z-h)+}$, where $h = 0$, with progressively increasing values of h, with each step accompanied by the release of H^+. The first step for ferric iron is shown in the reaction (Eq. 1.5):

$$\left[Fe(H_2O)_6 \right]^{3+} \rightleftharpoons \left[Fe(H_2O)_5 (OH) \right]^{2+} + H^+ \qquad (1.5)$$

Between pH 5 and pH 9, which is clearly of relevance to living organisms as well as aquatic systems, ferric salts hydrolyze immediately whereas ferrous salts, in the absence of oxygen or other oxidizing agents, give solutions of ferrous aqua ions, $Fe(H_2O)_6^{2+}$. Thus, in biological media the hydrated ferrous ion is a real species (Figure 1.3), whereas the hydrated ferric ion is relatively rare (Jolivet *et al.*, 2004), although significant concentrations of $Fe(H_2O)_6^{3+}$ are present at very low pH values. In most lakes, estuaries, streams and rivers, iron levels are high and Fe^{2+} is produced by the photolysis of inner-sphere complexes of particulate and colloidal iron(III) hydroxides with biogenic organic ligands. Since the photic zones in which this takes place are aerobic, there is continuous

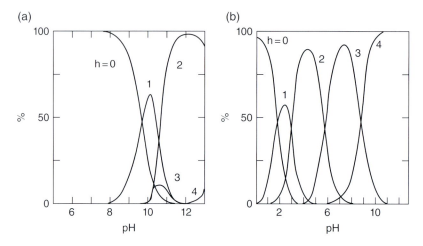

Figure 1.3 *Speciation of [Fe(OH)$_h$(H$_2$O)$_{6-h}$]$^{(z-h)+}$ complexes of (a) Fe(II); (b) Fe(III). From Jolivet* et al. *(2004)*

reoxidation of iron, producing secondary colloidal iron(III) hydroxides. In deeper waters, settling organic matter can supply reducing equivalents to convert FeO·OH to Fe^{2+}. In contrast, iron levels in surface seawater are extremely low, ranging from 0.02 to 1 nM (Wu and Luther, 1996).

Hydroxylated complexes can condense by the elimination of water and formation of μ-hydroxo bridges (olation) (Eq. 1.6), whereas oxohydroxy complexes – where there is no water molecule – condense in a two-step mechanism leading to the formation of μ-oxo bridges (oxolation) (Eq. 1.7):

$$H_2O - \overset{|}{\underset{|}{M}} - OH + - \overset{|}{\underset{|}{M}} - OH_2 \longrightarrow H_2O - \overset{|}{\underset{|}{M}} - OH - \overset{|}{\underset{|}{M}} - OH_2 + H_2O \qquad (1.6)$$

$$- \overset{|}{\underset{|}{M}} - OH + - \overset{|}{\underset{|}{M}} - OH \longrightarrow - \overset{|}{\underset{|}{M}} - O - \overset{|}{\underset{|}{M}} - OH \longrightarrow - \overset{|}{\underset{|}{M}} - O - \overset{|}{\underset{|}{M}} - + H_2O \qquad (1.7)$$

For ferric complexes, condensation occurs from strongly acidic media (pH ~1), whereas ferrous complexes condense only above pH 6, and the formation of polycationic ferrous species is poorly documented. Ferrous ions under anaerobic conditions can be hydroxylated from the [Fe(OH)$_2$Fe(H$_2$O)$_4$]^0 stage at pH > 6–7, leading to the precipitation of Fe(OH)$_2$. The reaction pathway for the formation of Fe(OH)$_2$, as shown in Figure 1.4, involves the olation of [Fe$_2$(OH)$_2$(H$_2$O)$_8$]$^{2+}$ dimers to planar tetramers [Fe$_4$(OH)$_8$(H$_2$O)$_8$]^0, followed by the rapid growth of nuclei in the same plane and resulting in the layered brucite structure [typical of hydroxides of divalent metal ions – brucite is the mineral form of magnesium hydroxide, Mg(OH)$_2$]. Both, in the solid state or in aqueous solutions, ferrous phases are extremely sensitive to oxidation, forming mixed ferric–ferrous products (green rusts, magnetite, goethite, lepidocrocite). The rapid oxidation of Fe(OH)$_2$ at pH 7 represents a unique way to form lepidocrocite, γ-FeO·OH, which is isostructural with the aluminium oxide hydroxide, boehmite, γ-AlO·OH.

The hydrolysis of ferric solutions is readily induced by the addition of base. Upon the addition of base at a rather acid pH, the purple ferric aqua-ion Fe(H$_2$O)$_6$$^{3+}$ initially undergoes a first

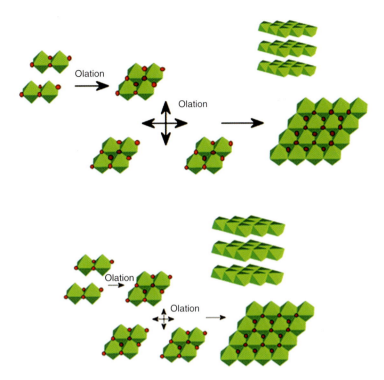

Figure 1.4   *A possible reaction pathway for the formation of Fe(OH)$_2$. From Jolivet* et al. *(2004)*

deprotonation step, which is followed by reversible dimerisation, giving a yellow solution of mono-and dinuclear species. The equilibria leading to mono- and dinuclear hydrolysis products such as [FeOH]$^{2+}$, [Fe(OH)$_2$]$^+$ and [Fe$_2$(OH)$_2$]$^{4+}$ are established rapidly and are well understood (Cornell *et al.*, 1989). These low-molecular species interact to produce hydrolytic polymers such as [Fe$_p$(OH)$_r$(H$_2$O)$_s$]$^{(3-r)+}$, or [Fe$_p$O$_r$(OH)$_s$]$^{(3p-2r-s)+}$ and precipitated oxides such as Fe(OH)$_3$, FeO·OH and Fe$_2$O$_3$ (Feng and Nansheng, 2000; Flynn, 1984; Schwertmann *et al.*, 1999).

On account of their high reactivity, ferric complexes condense very rapidly, and the process is difficult to stop without the use of very strongly complexing polydentate ligands. However, a range of species containing polynuclear Fe(III) cores have been characterised using a number of polycarboxylate or amino ligands (Lippard, 1988; Taft and Lippard, 1990; Taft *et al.*, 1993; Schmitt *et al.*, 2001; Jones *et al.*, 2002; Hellman *et al.*, 2006), two of which are illustrated in Figure 1.5.

1.4   Formation and Characterisation of Ferrihydrite

The addition of base to solutions of ferric ions at pH values >3 immediately leads to the precipitation of a poorly ordered, amorphous, red-brown ferric hydroxide precipitate. This synthetic precipitate resembles ferrihydrite, a hydrous ferric oxyhydroxide mineral found in many near-surface soils and sediments (Rancourt *et al.*, 2001; Schwertmann *et al.*, 1987), and is also present in the iron oxyhydroxide core of the iron storage protein, ferritin (see Chapter 6). Ferrihydrite can be considered as the least stable but most reactive form of iron(III), the group name for amorphous phases with large specific surface areas (>340 m^2 g^{-1}). The presence of ferrihydrite is often

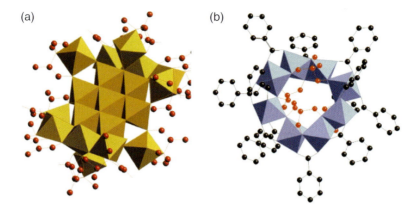

Figure 1.5 *Examples of polycationic structures formed by ferric ions in the presence of strongly complexing ligands. (a) [Fe$_{19}$O$_6$(OH)$_{14}$(L)^{10}(H$_2$O)$_{12}$]$^+$ L = N(CH$_2$COOH)$_2$(CH$_2$CH$_2$OH); (b) Fe$_8$(PhCOO)$_{12}$(thme)$_4$.2Et$_2$O (thme: tris-hydroxymethylethane). From Jolivet et al. (2004)*

underestimated because of difficulties in its definitive identification and also because of its common designation (covering a range of poorly ordered compounds), such as amorphous iron hydroxide, colloidal ferric hydroxide, Fe(OH)$_3$.

Ferrihydrite has been identified as a preterrestrial component of meteorites, and may be a constituent of the soils of Mars (Bishop *et al.*, 1995). On Earth, ferrihydrite is ubiquitous in natural waters, in the sediments derived from these waters, and is a constituent of a wide variety of soils, particularly those formed under cool and moist conditions as the precursor of hematite. It is also abundantly present in the precipitates resulting from acid mine drainage. Its high surface area and reactivity enable it to sequester a number of species through absorption, coprecipitation and redox reactions (Fortin and Langley, 2005). Because of its extremely high surface area and reactivity, ferrihydrite is manufactured for a variety of industrial applications (Li *et al.*, 2011), including coal liquefaction and metallurgical processing (Huffman *et al.*, 1993; Riveros *et al.*, 2001), and as an effective heavy metal scavenger in wastewater treatments (Ford *et al.*, 1997).

The conventional classification of ferrihydrite is based on the number of X-ray diffraction (XRD) peaks. Normally, a distinction is drawn between two types of ferrihydrite, referred to as '2-line ferrihydrite,' which describes a material that exhibits little crystallinity, and '6-line ferrihydrite,' which has the best crystallinity. In a typical XRD pattern of these materials, the 2-line form displays two broad peaks at 1.5 and 2.5 Å, while the more crystalline 6-line form displays six peaks at 1.5 (a doublet), 1.7, 2.0, 2.2, and 2.5 Å (Jambor and Dutrizac, 1998). The degree of order found in synthetic ferrihydrite depends on the method of preparation and the time of its ageing, which requires careful control of pH, temperature and concentration. The brief heating of Fe(III) solutions to about 80 °C typically produces '6-line ferrihydrite,' whereas the 2-line variety is typically produced at ambient temperatures by the addition of alkali to raise the pH to about 7. It seems to be agreed that ferrihydrite is not amorphous and has at least some degree of crystallinity. Despite the ease of its synthesis in the laboratory, no single formula is widely accepted, and compositions ranging from Fe$_5$HO$_8$·4H$_2$O (Towe and Bradley, 1967), through 5Fe$_2$O$_3$·9H$_2$O (Towe, 1981) and Fe$_{10}$O$_{14}$(OH)$_2$ (Michel *et al.*, 2007a) to the recent Fe$_{8.2}$O$_{8.5}$(OH)$_{7.4}$ + 3H$_2$O (Michel *et al.*, 2010) have been proposed. It has been demonstrated that almost all of the water can be replaced by adsorbed species in quantities that cannot be accommodated within the crystal structure, and it was proposed that the bulk structural unit for ferrihydrite is an Fe(O,OH)$_6$ octahedron, where the surface

(a)   (b)

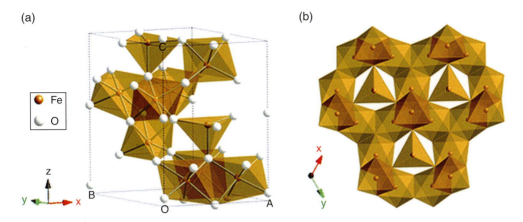

Figure 1.6 *Ferrihydrite structure. (a) Unit cell and (b) basic motif of the ferrihydrite model proposed by Michel et al., 2007. From Smith et al. (2012)*

structure is a mixture of octahedrally and tetrahedrally coordinated Fe (Jambor and Dutrizac, 1998). These 'coordination–unsaturated' surface sites are readily accessible to the adsorption of foreign species and, together with the large surface area referred to above, most likely account for the high adsorptive capacity of ferrihydrite.

While it is considered to be a good example of a nanomineral (Hochella *et al.*, 2008), the crystal structure (Jambor and Dutrizac, 1998; Manceau, 2009; Michel *et al.*, 2007a; Rancourt and Meunier, 2008), physical (Rancourt and Meunier, 2008; Hiemstra and Van Rielsdijk, 2009) and magnetic (Coey and Readman, 1973; Pankhurst and Pollard, 1992; Pannalai *et al.*, 2005; Berquo *et al.*, 2007, 2009; Cabello *et al.*, 2009) properties of ferrihydrite remain controversial. Over the years, a number of structural models have been proposed for ferrihydrite (reviewed in Jambor and Dutrizac, 1998). Towe and Bradley (1967) and Chukrov *et al.* (1974) both proposed what were essentially defective hematite structures, whereas Drits *et al.* (1993) proposed a multicomponent model consisting of defective and defect-free ferrihydrite phases mixed with ultradisperse hematite. Unlike other iron hydroxides which have been studied, the exact structure and chemical composition of ferrihydrite has remained a matter of considerable debate, and until recently there has been no consensus on its crystal structure. Most of the disagreement has centred around the presence of multiple structural phases and the local environment of the iron (Drits *et al.*, 1993; Janney *et al.*, 2000, 2001; Jansen *et al.*, 2002).

Recent X-ray scattering studies from both 2-line and 6-line ferrihydrite suggest that the coherent scattering domains share a common structure, despite the fact that the average crystallite size and water content were different (Michel *et al.*, 2007b). An atomic arrangement of ferrihydrite (Figure 1.6) has been proposed (Michel *et al.*, 2007a) using the pair-distribution function (PDF) method for structural analysis, which involves a comparison between PDFs generated from the experimental X-ray scattering data with those calculated from structural models (Billinge and Kanatzidis, 2004). On the basis of their results, these authors concluded that in its ideal form, the structure contains 20% tetrahedrally and 80% octahedrally coordinated iron, and has a basic structural motif closely related to the Baker–Figgis–δ-Keggin cluster[3] (Casey, 2006).

---

[3] The Baker–Figgis–Keggin isomers (of which there are five, from α to ε) are aluminium hydroxide clusters which have central metals tetrahedrally coordinated to oxygen [M(O)$_4$] sites, and are familiar structures among scientists who study polyoxometalates. They form aluminium clusters with the stoichiometry $MO_4Al_{12}(OH)_{24}(H_2O)_{12}^{7+}$(aq) [M = Ge(IV), Ga(III), or Al(III)].

The compositional, structural, and magnetic changes that occur upon aging of '2-line' ferrihydrite in the presence of adsorbed citrate at elevated temperature has been studied more recently (Michel *et al.*, 2010). Whereas, aging under these conditions ultimately results in the formation of hematite, analysis of the atomic pair distribution function and complementary physico-chemical and magnetic data indicate the formation of an intermediate ferrihydrite phase of larger particle size with few defects, more structural relaxation and electron spin ordering, and pronounced ferrimagnetism relative to its disordered ferrihydrite precursor. The results validate the previously proposed structural model (Michel *et al.*, 2007a) and identify a pathway for forming ferrimagnetic ferrihydrite which might explain the magnetic enhancement that typically precedes the formation of hematite in aerobic soil and weathering environments. The 20:80 ratio of tetrahedral to octahedral Fe sites proposed is supported by XANES/EXAFS studies (Carta *et al.*, 2009; Maillot *et al.*, 2011), and a new synthetic route to chemically pure 2-line ferrihydrite (Smith *et al.*, 2012) confirms that the structure of ferrihydrite is consistent, repeatable, regardless of the synthetic method used, the water content or particle size of the crystallites, and is adequately described by the hexagonal model.

1.5   Ageing of Amorphous Ferrihydrite to more Crystalline Products

Ferrihydrite is thermodynamically unstable and transforms with time into the more stable crystalline oxides hematite and goethite (Figure 1.7). Between pH 5 and 8, on account of the poor solubility of ferrihydrite ($\sim 10^{-10}$ M), the transformation can only proceed by *in situ* dehydration and local rearrangement, resulting in very small crystallites of hematite, α-Fe_2O_3. When the solubility of ferrihydrite is higher (pH <4 or >8), transformation can proceed by a dissolution/crystallisation pathway, leading to goethite, α-FeOOH (Figure 1.7). The thermolysis of acidic solutions (pH <3) of ferrihydrite at 90–100 °C leads to hematite (Jolivet, 2000). The presence of adsorbed species can drastically increase the transformation temperature, as illustrated by the observation that an Si/Fe ratio of 0.25 in ferrihydrite increases the temperature required to convert ferrihydrite to hematite to 800 °C. This effect of complexing ligands such as silicate, and particularly phosphate, in delaying or preventing the transformation of ferrihydrite into crystalline mineral phases, may explain the presence of ferrihydrite both in very old soils and in the mineral core of mammalian ferritins (Jolivet *et al.*, 2004).

The presence of both ferrous and ferric ions in solutions orients the condensation presence to the formation of specific phases, namely green rusts and spinel-type magnetite (or maghemite). The type of product formed depends on many factors, including pH, and particularly the composition of the system, defined as $x = Fe^{3+}(Fe^{2+} + Fe^{3+})$ (Figure 1.8). For $x < 0.66$ and $OH^-/Fe_{total} = 2$ (pH 8), hydroxylation of the mixture gives green rusts, in which the Fe^{2+} and Fe^{3+} ions occupy octahedral sites giving a positive charge to the sheet-like structure, which is balanced by the intercalation of anions. When tetrahedral anions such as sulphate are present, the 'green rust SO_4' has the unique composition, Fe(II)/Fe(III) = 2 (Refait *et al.*, 1998; Géhin *et al.*, 2002).

In contrast, magnetite Fe_3O_4 can be easily obtained (Figure 1.8) by coprecipitating aqueous Fe^{2+} and Fe^{3+} ions with $x = 0.66$. The iron atoms are distributed in the octahedral (Oh) and tetrahedral (Td) sites of the face-centred cube of oxygen according to ($[Fe^{3+}]_{Td}[Fe^{2+}Fe^{3+}]_{Oh}O_4$). Magnetite is characterised by rapid electron hopping between the iron cations in the octahedral sublattice, and during the quasi-immediate crystallisation of the spinel at room temperature, electron transfer between Fe^{2+} and Fe^{3+} ions plays a fundamental role in the process (Jolivet *et al.*, 2004).

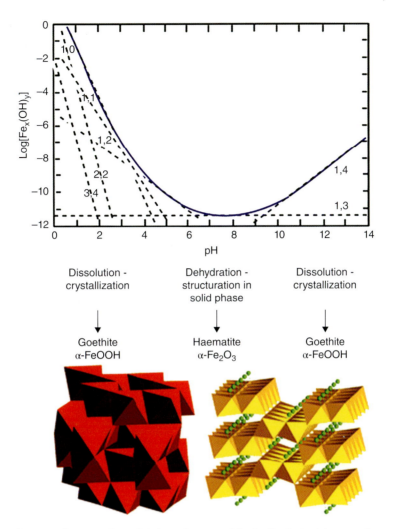

Figure 1.7 *Influence of pH on the solubility of iron and ferric (hydro)oxide crystal structures. From Jolivet et al. (2004)*

1.6 Biomineralisation

The most obvious product of biomineralisation is the calcium phosphate of vertebrate teeth and bones, but others include calcium in the shells of marine organisms, silicon in grasses, and the calcium carbonate shells of molluscs. Biomineralisation involves the formation of these inorganic materials under the influence of proteins, carbohydrates and lipids. The way in which biominerals grow is intimately linked to the problem of morphology, and it is difficult to think of a better introduction to this field than the pioneering work of D'Arcy Thompson.

D'Arcy Wentworth Thompson (1860–1948) was a polymath, equally well qualified to occupy chairs of Zoology, Mathematics and Physics, but chose the former in Dundee and then St Andrews, and was a pioneer of bio-mathematics. His classic book '*On growth and form*' is essentially about

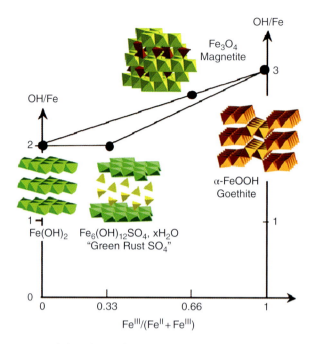

Figure 1.8 *Representation of the phases formed in solution as a function of the composition and hydroxylation ratio in the ferrous–ferric system. From Jolivet* et al. *(2004)*

biominerals (Thompson, 1917). This fascinating problem includes the initiation of nucleation, growth of the inorganic crystalline phases, and definition of the volume and shape of the inorganic material, which is determined by the organic mould (lipid, protein, carbohydrate) within which the inorganic mineral structure is deposited (reviewed in Mann, 2007; Bäuerlein, 2000; Wilt 2005; Nudelman and Sommerdijk, 2012).

There are 14 iron oxides, hydroxides and oxyhydroxides that have been more or less well-defined, 10 of which are known to occur in Nature (Table 1.1). Of these, goethite, hematite and

Table 1.1 *Oxides, hydroxides and oxyhydroxides of iron*

Mineral	Nominal formula	Phase	Nominal formula
Goethite	α-FeOOH	synthetic	$Fe(OH)_2$
Akaganéite	β-FeOOH	synthetic	β-Fe_2O_3
Lepidocrocite	γ-FeOOH	synthetic	ε-Fe_2O_3
Feroxyhite	δ-FeOOH	synthetic	FeOOH
Hematite	α-Fe_2O_3		
Maghemite	γ-Fe_2O_3		
Magnetite	Fe_3O_4		
Wüstite	FeO		
Bernalite	$Fe(OH)_3$		
Ferrihydrite	$Fe_5HO_8 \cdot 4H_2O/\ 5Fe_2O_3 \cdot 9H_2O/\ Fe_{10}O_{14}(OH)_2$		

Adapted with permission from Jambor, J.L. and Dutrizac, J.E. (1998) Occurrence and constitution of natural and synthetic ferrihydrite, a widespread iron oxyhydroxide. *Chem. Rev.,* **98**, 2549–2585; © 1998, American Chemical Society.

Table 1.2   *Diagnostic criteria for iron oxide minerals*

Mineral	Colour	Most intense X-ray lines (Å)	IR bands (cm⁻¹)	Magnetic hyperfine field (T)		
				295 °K	77 °K	4 °K
Ferrihydrite	Reddish brown	2.54, 2.24, 1.97, 1.73, 1.47		–	–	47–50
Hematite	Bright red	2.70, 3.68, 2.52	345, 470, 540	51.8	54.2/53.5	54.2/53.5
Maghemite	Red to brown	2.52, 2.95	400, 450, 570, 590, 630	50	–	52.6
Magnetite	Black	2.53, 2.97		49.1/46.0	–	–
Goethite	Yellowish brown	4.18, 2.45, 2.69	400, 590	38.2	50.3	
Lepidocrocite	Orange	6.26, 3.29, 2.47, 1.937	890, 797 1026, 1161, 753	–	–	45.8
Akaganéite	Yellowish brown	3.33, 2.55, 7.47	840, 640	–	47.1, 46.7, 45.3	48.9, 47.8, 47.3
Feroxyhyte	Reddish brown	2.54, 2.22, 1.69, 1.47	1110, 920, 790, 670	42.0	53.0	53.5
Bernalite	Dark green	3.784, 1.682, 2.393, 2.676, 1.892		42.0		55.7

Adapted with permission from Jambor, J.L. and Dutrizac, J.E. (1998) Occurrence and constitution of natural and synthetic ferrihydrite, a widespread iron oxyhydroxide. *Chem. Rev.*, **98**, 2549–2585; ©1998, American Chemical Society.

magnetite occur in sufficient abundance to be considered as rock-forming minerals. Lepidocrocite, ferrihydrite and maghemite are found in sediments from many localities, but they all occur much less frequently and in much lower abundance than goethite, hematite and magnetite. The diagnostic criteria for each of these iron oxides are listed in Table 1.2.

The biomineralisation of a number of iron oxide minerals has been studied. The oxy-hydroxide phase ferrihydrite (as discussed above) constitutes the central core of the iron storage protein ferritin, and its biomineralisation will be considered in greater detail in Chapter 6. Goethite (α-FeOOH) is biomineralised by limpets, and lepidocrocite (γ-FeOOH) by chitons (Mann, 1988), while magnetite (Fe_3O_4) is found in the magnetosomes of magnetotactic bacteria (Blakemore, 1975) and also in vertebrates (Kirschvink *et al.*, 2001).

1.7   Magnetite Biomineralisation by Magnetotactic Bacteria

Aquatic bacteria exhibiting magnetotaxis – that is, orienting and migrating along geomagnetic field lines – were discovered serendipitously in the mid 1970s.[4] This ability is dependent on the formation of intracellular magnetic structures, magnetosomes, which allow magnetotactic bacteria to orient in external magnetic fields. The magnetosome consists of a chain of nanometre-sized,

---

[4] At the Marine Station at Woods Hole, Massachusetts, Richard Blakemore observed that bacteria from marine and freshwater muds accumulated at the North side of drops of water and sediment, when placed upon a microscope slide, and that these bacteria swam towards and away from the south and north pole of a bar magnet, respectively (Blakemore, 1975). He subsequently showed that such magnetotactic bacteria behave like self-propelled, permanent magnetic dipole moments. Magnetotactic bacteria use magnetite (Fe_3O_4) as an internal compass with which to navigate, and in the Northern hemisphere their magnetic dipole is oriented northward, whereas magnetotactic bacteria from the Southern hemisphere have their dipole oriented southward. These microorganisms, isolated in the Northern hemisphere, swim northwards and downwards along the Earth's magnetic field lines, to avoid the higher oxygen concentrations of surface water, which are toxic to them. If transferred to the Southern hemisphere they '*perd leur Nord*', and swim upward!

membrane-bound crystals of the magnetic iron minerals magnetite (Fe_3O_4) or, less frequently, greignite (Fe_3S_4) (Figure 1.9). Magnetotactic bacteria (MTB) are found in a variety of freshwater and marine aquatic environments and belong to a wide range of phylogenetic groups. The most commonly studied MTB have a single magnetosome chain consisting of 15–20 crystals of magnetite each ~50 nm in diameter, although a considerable diversity in magnetosome morphologies has been found within the rich diversity of MTB. For an historical perspective of the discovery and early studies on the ecological distribution of MTB the reader is referred to the article by Blakemore (1982), while more recent reviews can be found in Faivre and Schüler (2008), Jogler and Schüler (2009), Komeili (2012), Lower and Bazylinski (2013), and Rahn-Lee and Komeili (2013).

Magnetosome-like structures and magnetic minerals have been demonstrated in eukaryotes, including algae, fish, termites, honey-bees, pigeons, and even in humans, and in some cases they appear to be used for orientation purposes (Kirschvink *et al.*, 2001; Walker *et al.*, 2002). The strict control over the biomineralisation in magnetosomes is reminiscent of that found in the formation of silica shells by diatoms and of tooth and bone formation in animals. Further, magnetosome-like chains of magnetite survive over long periods of geological time in sediments, enabling geobiologists to use bacterial magnetite as 'magnetofossils' to follow the evolution of the history of life in ancient rocks. This led to the hypothesis that magnetosomes may represent one of the most ancient biomineralisation systems, which has been progressively adapted to accommodate the formation of the biominerals found in eukaryotic organisms (Kirschvink and Hagedorn, 2000).

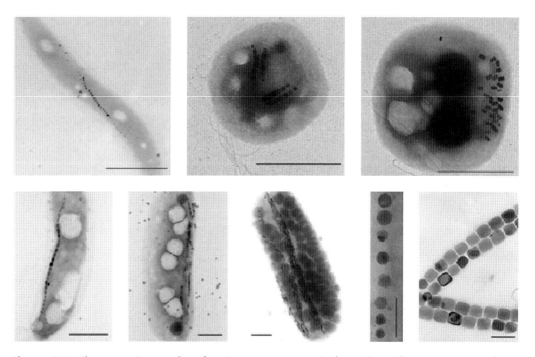

Figure 1.9 *Electron micrographs of various magnetotactic bacteria and magnetosome chains, illustrating the diversity of the cell morphology, of the magnetosome, and of the arrangement of magnetosomes in bacteria. From Faivre, D. and Schüler, D. (2008)*

Comparative genomic analyses have shown that the genes encoding most of the magnetosome-specific proteins, termed *mam* (magnetosome membrane) genes, are organised within a discrete region of the bacterial genome, termed the magnetosome island (MAI), with many of the characteristics of genomic islands often associated with pathogenic organisms (see section on pathogenicity islands in Chapter 4). These genes appear to be involved in the formation of the magnetosome membrane, the biomineralisation of magnetite, and organisation of the magnetosome chain.

The number of MTBs which have been isolated and cultivated in axenic culture has increased considerably during the past few years (for a review, see Lefèvre and Wu, 2013), resulting in a great increase in DNA sequences. Currently, 13 genomic regions which contain the genes responsible for magnetosome production have been sequenced, including the genomes of six cultured MTB and magnetosome gene clusters from seven cultured MTBs (Lefèvre and Wu, 2013). All MTBs have in common a set of genes within the *mamAB* operon (Lefèvre *et al.*, 2013; Richter *et al.*, 2007), which have recently been shown to be crucial for magnetite biomineralisation (Lohsse *et al.*, 2011; Murat *et al.*, 2010; Ullrich and Schüler, 2010). Ten of these genes (*mamABEIKLMOPQ*) are conserved in all magnetite-producing MTB, whereas only nine of them – the exception being *mamL* – seem to be conserved in the two greigite-producing MTB (Lefèvre *et al.*, 2013).

The functions of several of these genes and their associated proteins in magnetosome synthesis and construction of the magnetosome chain have begun to be elucidated through bioinformatics and/or experimental evidence (Komeili, 2012; Lohsse *et al.*, 2011; Murat *et al.*, 2010), and will be discussed below. As proposed by Komeili (2012), in which more details can be found, magnetosome formation has been divided into four stages: (i) biogenesis of the magnetosome membrane; (ii) magnetosome protein sorting; (iii) magnetosome chain formation; and (iv) biomineralisation. A model for magnetosome formation is finally presented.

1.7.1 Biogenesis of the Magnetosome Membrane

It has been clear for some time that the magnetosome membrane originates from the inner cell membrane, and four proteins have been identified from comprehensive genetic analysis to be involved in the formation of the magnetosome membrane (Murat *et al.*, 2010). These are MamI and MamL, which are MTB-specific proteins (Richter *et al.*, 2007) involved in invagination of the magnetosome membrane (Murat *et al.*, 2010), and MamB and MamQ, which are part of large families conserved beyond MTBs. MamB is a member of the cation diffusion facilitator (CDF) family which may be involved in iron transport as well as in magnetosome membrane assembly (Uebe *et al.*, 2011). MamQ has a LemA domain, a ~40-residue helix-loop-helix fold conserved in prokaryotic DNA/RNA-binding proteins (Lin *et al.*, 2000), and also appears to be involved in invagination of the magnetosome membrane (Lohsse *et al.*, 2011; Murat *et al.*, 2010). Other factors are likely to be involved, including possibley MamY (Tanaka *et al.*, 2006).

1.7.2 Protein Sorting

Approximately 20-40 proteins are localised or enriched in the magnetosome membrane (Grünberg *et al.*, 2001, 2004), and the surface of the membrane seems to be covered in a layer of magnetosome proteins (Yamamota *et al.*, 2010), including Mam A, which has a tetratricopeptide repeat (TPR) and is required for vesicle activation (Komeili *et al.*, 2004; Zeytuni *et al.*, 2011; Yamamoto *et al.*, 2010). The X-ray structure of MamA (Zeytuni *et al.*, 2011) sheds light on the way in which it self-assembles and may provide surfaces for binding of other proteins to the magnetosome membrane. Mam E – like MamA and MamP – has a PDZ domain (a common structural domain of 80–90 amino acids found in signalling proteins), which could mediate protein–protein interactions.

This would be compatible with the proposition that it recruits other proteins to the magnetosome membrane (Lohsse *et al*., 2011; Murat *et al*., 2010; Quinlan *et al*., 2011).

1.7.3 Chain Formation

Individual magnetosomes need to be organised into chains in order to orient the cell in a magnetic field. The presence of filaments with dimensions similar to actin filaments alongside the magnetosome chain (Scheffel *et al*., 2006; Komeili *et al*., 2006; Katzmann *et al*., 2010), together with the presence of MamK, an actin-like filamentous protein encoded by one of the genes of the MAI (Grünberg *et al*., 2001), suggested that MamK might provide a structural scaffold for the organisation of the magnetome chain (Scheffel *et al*., 2006; Komeili *et al*., 2006; Taoka *et al*., 2007), probably as the structural component of its cytoskeleton. Like traditional actins, MamK forms dynamic filaments that require an intact NTPase motif for their turnover *in vivo*. Two acidic proteins, MamJ and LimJ, are thought to function as regulators of the dynamic behaviour of MamK filaments (Scheffel *et al*., 2006; Komeili *et al*., 2006; Draper *et al*., 2011).

1.7.4 Biomineralisation

Despite tremendous advances in the present understanding of the genes involved and the possible roles of the proteins encoded by these genes, the current understanding of iron chemistry involved in biomineralisation lags behind. Magnetite formation is achieved by a process of mineralisation which involves: (i) a reductive uptake of iron from the external environment of the bacterial cell, and its transport (perhaps as ferritin) across the magnetosome membrane; (ii) an accumulation of iron within the precursor of the vesicular structure of the magnetosome; (iii) transformation of the initial iron deposit (most likely in the form of ferrihydrite) into magnetite; and (iv) crystallisation of the magnetite mineral to give a particle within the vesicle of a specific size and orientation. The MamP, MamE and MamT proteins have a double MTB-specific *c*-type cytochrome domain that possibly ensures redox control and Fe^{2+}/Fe^{3+} stoichiometry, and may contribute to the process of biocrystallisation (Siponen *et al*., 2012).

 The results of initial studies by Frankel *et al*. (1983), using Mössbauer spectroscopy, suggested three different phases in the biomineralisation step: a low-density-hydrous ferric oxide, followed by a high-density-hydrous ferric oxide (namely ferrihydrite [Fh]), which on partial reduction transforms to magnetite. A subsequent Mössbauer study implied a pathway from membrane-bound ferritin, which together with ferrous iron led to the coprecipitation of magnetite (Faivre *et al*., 2007). In a real-time *in vivo* study of *Magnetospirillum gryphiswaldense* magnetosome formation using X-ray magnetic circular dichroism, it was concluded that haematite (α-Fe_2O_3) was a precursor to magnetite (Staniland *et al*., 2007). A more recent study using Fe K-edge X-ray absorption near-edge structure (XANES) and high-resolution transmission electron microscopy (TEM) confirmed ferrihydrite, in the form of bacterial ferritin cores characterised by a poorly crystalline structure and high phosphorus content, as the source of iron for magnetite formation (Fdez-Gubieda *et al*., 2013). Magnetite formation through phase transformation from a highly disordered phosphate-rich ferric hydroxide phase, consistent with prokaryotic ferritins, via transient nanometric ferric (oxyhydr)oxide intermediates within the magnetosome organelle, has been confirmed using X-ray absorption spectroscopy at cryogenic temperatures and TEM imaging techniques (Baumgartner *et al*., 2013a). These results bear a remarkable resemblance to recent findings of synthetic magnetite formation in solution (Baumgartner *et al*., 2013b).

 A small subset of magnetosome membrane proteins, encoded by genes of the *mamCD* and *mms6* gene clusters, which are adjacent to one another in the MAI, are tightly associated with the magnetite crystal. These proteins – Mms5, Mms6, Mms7 (MamC), and Mms13 (MamD) – have common features in their amino acid sequences, including hydrophobic N-terminal and hydrophilic C-terminal regions which contain dense carboxyl and hydroxyl groups that bind iron ions (Arakaki *et al.*, 2003). It has been proposed that Mms6 is involved in the regulation of crystal morphology during magnetite mineralisation (Tanaka *et al.*, 2010), and that the proteins MamGFDC, while not required for magnetite crystallisation, regulate the size of the magnetosome crystals (Scheffel *et al.*, 2008).

1.7.5 A Model for Magnetosome Formation

A possible model for magnetosome formation has been proposed recently (Figure 1.10), which incorporates much of the information described above (Komeili, 2012). In the first step, reshaping

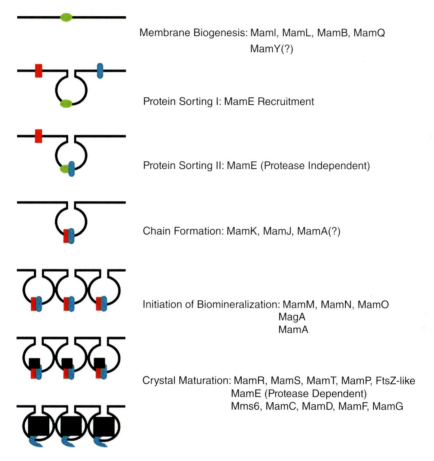

Membrane Biogenesis: MamI, MamL, MamB, MamQ
MamY(?)

Protein Sorting I: MamE Recruitment

Protein Sorting II: MamE (Protease Independent)

Chain Formation: MamK, MamJ, MamA(?)

Initiation of Biomineralization: MamM, MamN, MamO
MagA
MamA

Crystal Maturation: MamR, MamS, MamT, MamP, FtsZ-like
MamE (Protease Dependent)
Mms6, MamC, MamD, MamF, MamG

Figure 1.10   *A model for magnetosome formation. Based on numerous studies, one possible model for magnetosome formation is proposed here. First, the reshaping of the inner cell membrane by MamI, MamL, MamQ, MamB and other factors (green) creates the magnetosome membrane. Second, MamE is recruited to the nascent magnetosome. Third, MamE (in blue), independent of its protease activity, recruits other proteins (red) to the magnetosome. Fourth, MamK and MamJ help to organise magnetosomes into chains. Note that this step is independent of biomineralisation and may occur before or after crystal formation. Fifth, biomineralisation is initiated and small crystals of magnetite are formed. Finally, these small crystals are matured into large crystals in a step that requires the proteolytic activity of MamE. From Komeili (2012)*

of the inner cell membrane by MamI, MamL, MamQ, MamB and other factors creates the magnetosome membrane. In the second step, MamE is recruited to the nascent magnetosome, and in a third step MamE (independent of its protease activity) recruits other proteins to the magnetosome. In step four, MamK and MamJ help to organise magnetosomes into chains (this step is independent of biomineralisation, and may occur before or after crystal formation), while in step five biomineralisation is initiated and small crystals of magnetite are formed. In the final step, these small crystals mature into large crystals in a process that requires not only the proteolytic activity of MamE but also a number of other factors, including the Mms proteins.

References

Arakaki, A., Webb, J. and Matsunaga, T. (2003) A novel protein tightly bound to bacterial magnetic particles in *Magnetospirillum magneticum* strain AMB-1. *J. Biol. Chem.*, **278**, 8745–8750.

Bäuerlein, E. (ed.) (2000) *The Biomineralization of Nano- and Micro-Structures*. Wiley-VCH, Weinheim.

Baumgartner, J., Morin, G., Menguy, N., Perez Gonzalez, T., *et al.* (2013a) Magnetotactic bacteria form magnetite from a phosphate-rich ferric hydroxide via nanometric ferric (oxyhydr)oxide intermediates. *Proc. Natl Acad. Sci. USA*, **110**, 14883–14888.

Baumgartner, J., Dey, A., Bomans, P.H., Le Coadou, C., *et al.* (2013b) Nucleation and growth of magnetite from solution. *Nat. Mater.*, **12**, 310–314.

Berquo, T.S., Banerjee, S.K., Ford, R.G., Penn, R.L. and Pichler, T. (2007) High crystallinity Si-ferrihydrite: an insight into its Neel temperature and size dependence of magnetic properties. *J. Geophys. Res.-Sol. Ea.*, **112**, B02.

Berquo, T.S., Erbs, J.J., Lindquist, A., Penn, R.L. and Banerjee, S.K. (2009) Effects of magnetic interactions in antiferromagnetic ferrihydrite particles. *J. Phys. Condens. Matter*, **21**, 176005.

Billinge, S.J.L. and Kanatzidis, M.G. (2004) Beyond crystallography: the study of disorder, nanocrystallinity and crystallographically challenged materials with pair distribution functions. *Chem. Commun.*, **7**, 749–760.

Bishop, J.L., Pieters, C.M., Burns, R.G., Edwards, J.O., *et al.* (1995) Reflectance spectroscopy of ferric sulfate-bearing montmorillonites as Mars soil analog materials. *Icarus*, **117**, 101–119.

Blakemore, R. (1975) Magnetotactic bacteria. *Science*, **190**, 377–379.

Blakemore, R.P. (1982) Magnetotactic bacteria. *Annu. Rev. Microbiol.*, **36**, 217–238.

Cabello, E., Morales, M.P., Serna, C.J., Barron, V. and Torrent, J. (2009) Magnetic enhancement during the crystallization of ferrihydrite at 25° and 30°C. *Clays Clay Miner.*, **57**, 46–53.

Carta, D., Casula, M.F., Carrias, A., Falqui, A., *et al.* (2009) Structural and magnetic characterization of synthetic ferrihydrite nanoparticles. *Mater. Chem. Phys.*, **113**, 349–355.

Casey, W.H. (2006) Large aqueous aluminium hydroxide molecules. *Chem. Rev.*, **106**, 1–16.

Chukrov, F.V., Zvyagin, B.B., Gorshkov, A.I., Yermilova, L.P. and Balashova, V.V. (1974) Ferrihydrite. *Int. Geol. Rev.*, **16**, 1131–1143.

Coey, J.M.D. and Readman, P.W. (1973) New spin structure in an amorphous ferric gel. *Nature*, **246**, 476–478.

Cornell, R.M., Giovanoli, R. and Schneider, W. (1989) Review of the hydrolysis of iron(III) and the crystallization of amorphous iron(III) hydroxide hydrate. *J. Chem. Tech. Biotech.*, **46**, 115–134.

Crichton, R.R. and Pierre, J.-L. (2001) Old iron, young copper: from Mars to Venus. *Biometals*, **14**, 99–112.

Draper, O., Byrne, M.E., Li, Z., Keyhani, S., *et al.* (2011) MamK, a bacterial actin, forms dynamic filaments in vivo that are regulated by the acidic proteins MamJ and LimJ. *Mol. Microbiol.*, **82**, 342–354.

Drits, V.A., Sakharov, B.A., Salyn, A.L. and Manceau, A. (1993) The structure of six-line ferrihydrite, *Clay Miner.*, **28**, 185.

Faivre, D. and Schüler, D. (2008) Lagnetetactic bacteria and magnetosomes. *Chem. Rev.*, **108**, 4875–4898.

Faivre, D., Böttger, L.H., Matzanke, B.F. and Schüler, D. (2007) Intracellular magnetite biomineralization in bacteria proceeds by a distinct pathway involving membrane-bound ferritin and an iron(II) species. *Angew. Chem. Int. Ed. Engl.*, **46**, 8495–8499.

Fdez-Gubieda, M.L., Muela, A., Alonso, J., García-Prieto, A., *et al.* (2013) Magnetite biomineralization in *Magnetospirillum gryphiswaldense*: time-resolved magnetic and structural studies. *ACS Nano.*, **7**, 3297–3305.

Feng, W. and Nansheng, D. (2000) Photochemistry of hydrolytic iron(III) species and photoinduced degradation of organic compounds. A minireview. *Chemosphere*, **41**, 1137–1147.

Fenton, H.J.H. (1894) The oxidation of tartaric acid in presence of iron. *J. Chem. Soc. Trans.*, **10**, 157–158.

Flynn, C.M., Jr (1984) Hydrolysis of inorganic iron (III) salts. *Chem. Rev.*, **84**, 31–41.

Ford R.G., Bertsch, P.M. and Farley, K.J. (1997) Changes in transition and heavy metal partitioning during hydrous iron oxide ageing. *Environ. Sci. Technol.*, **31**, 2028–2033.

Fortin, D. and Langley, S. (2005) Formation and occurrence of biogenic iron-rich minerals. *Earth Sci. Rev.*, **72**, 1–19.

Frankel, R.B., Papaefthymiou, G.C., Blakemore, R.P. and O'Brien, W. (1983) Fe_3O_4 precipitation in magnetotactic bacteria. *Biochim. Biophys. Acta*, **763**, 147–159.

Géhin, A., Ruby, C., Abdelmoula, M., Benali, O., *et al.* (2002) Synthesis of Fe(II-III) hydroxysulphate green rust by coprecipitation *Solid State Sci.*, **4**, 61–66.

Grünberg, K., Wawer, C., Tebo, B.M. and Schüler, D. (2001) A large gene cluster encoding several magnetosome proteins is conserved in different species of magnetotactic bacteria. *Appl. Environ. Microbiol.*, **67**, 4573–4582.

Grünberg, K., Müller, E.C., Otto, A., Reszka, R, *et al.* (2004) Biochemical and proteomic analysis of the magnetosome membrane in *Magnetospirillum gryphiswaldense*. *Appl. Environ. Microbiol.*, **70**, 1040–1050.

Haber, F. and Weiss, J. (1934) The catalytic decomposition of hydrogen peroxide by iron salts. *Proc. Roy. Soc. Ser. A*, **147**, 332–351.

Haber, F. and Willstätter, R. (1931) Unpaarigheit und Radikalketten in Reaktion-Mechanismus organischer und enzymatitischer Vorgänge. *Chem. Ber.*, **64**, 2844–2856.

Halliwell, B. and Gutteridge, J.M.C. (1984) Oxygen toxicity, oxygen radicals, transition metals and disease. *Biochem. J.*, **219**, 1–14.

Hellman, H., Laitinen, R.S., Kaila, L, Jalonen, J., *et al.* (2006) Identification of hydrolysis products of $FeCl_3.6H_2O$ by ESI-MS. *J. Mass Spectrom.* **41**, 1421–1429.

Hiemstra, T. and Van Riemsdijk, W.H. (2009) A surface structural model for ferrihydrite I: Sites related to primary charge, molar mass, and mass density. *Geochim. Cosmochim. Acta*, **73**, 4423–4436.

Hochella, M.F., Jr, Lower, S.K., Maurice, P.A., Penn, R.L., *et al.* (2008) Nanominerals, mineral nanoparticles, and Earth systems. *Science*, **319**, 1631–1635.

Huffman, G.P., Ganguly, B., Zhao, J., Rao, K R.P.M., *et al.* (1993) Structure and dispersion of iron-based catalysts for direct coal liquefaction. *Energy Fuels*, **7**, 285–296.

Jambor, J.L. and Dutrizac, J.E. (1998) Occurrence and constitution of natural and synthetic ferrihydrite, a widespread iron oxyhydroxide. *Chem. Rev.*, **98**, 2549–2585.

Janney, D.E., Cowley, J.M. and Buseck, P.R. (2000) Structure of synthetic 2-line ferrihydrite by electron nanodiffraction. *Am. Miner.*, **85**, 1180–1187.

Janney, D.E., Cowley, J.M. and Buseck, P.R. (2001) Structure of synthetic 6-line ferrihydrite by electron nanodiffraction. *Am. Miner.*, **86**, 327–335.

Jansen, E., Kyek, A., Schafer, W. and Schwertmann, U. (2002) The structure of six-line ferrihydrite, *Appl. Phys. Mater. Sci. Process.*, **74**, S1004–S1006.

Jogler, C. and Schüler, D. (2009) Genomics, genetics, and cell biology of magnetosome formation. *Annu. Rev. Microbiol.*, **63**, 501–521.

Jolivet, J.-P. (2000) *Metal Oxide Chemistry and Synthesis. From Solution to Solid State*. John Wiley & Sons, Chichester.

Jolivet, J.-P., Chanéac, C. and Trone, E. (2004) Iron oxide chemistry. From molecular clusters to extended solid networks. *Chem. Commun.*, 481–487.

Jones, L.F., Batsanov, A., Brechin, E.C., Collison, D., *et al.* (2002) Octametallic and hexadecametallic ferric wheels. *Angew. Chem., Int. Ed. Engl.*, **41**, 4318–4321.

Katzmann, E, Scheffel, A., Gruska, M., Plitzko, J.M. and Schüler, D. (2010) Loss of the actin-like protein MamK has pleiotropic effects on magnetosome formation and chain assembly in *Magnetospirillum gryphiswaldense*. *Mol. Microbiol.*, **77**, 208–224.

Kirschvink, J.L. and Hagedorn, J.W. (2000) in *The Biomineralization of Nano- and Micro-Structures* (ed. E. Bäuerlein), Wiley-VCH, Weinheim, pp. 1139–1150.

Kirschvink, J.L., Walker, M.M. and Diebel, C.E. (2001) Magnetite-based magnetoreception. *Curr. Opin. Neurobiol.*, **11**, 462–467.

Komeili, A. (2012) Molecular mechanisms of compartmentalization and biomineralization in magnetotactic bacteria. *FEMS Microbiol. Rev.*, **36**, 232–255.

Komeili, A., Vali, H., Beveridge, T.J. and Newman, D.K. (2004) Magnetosome vesicles are present before magnetite formation, and MamA is required for their activation. *Proc. Natl Acad. Sci. USA*, **101**, 3839–3844.

Komeili, A., Li, Z., Newman, D.K. and Jensen, G.J. (2006) Magnetosomes are cell membrane invaginations organized by the actin-like protein MamK. *Science*, **311**, 242–245.

Lefèvre, C.T. and Wu, L.-F. (2013) Evolution of the bacterial organelle responsible for magnetotaxis. *Trends Microbiol.*, **21**, 534–543.

Lefèvre, C.T., Trubitsyn, D., Abreu, F., Kolinko, S., *et al.* (2013) Comparative genomic analysis of magnetotactic bacteria from the Deltaproteobacteria provides new insights into magnetite and greigite magnetosome genes required for magnetotaxis. *Environ. Microbiol.*, **15**, 2712–2735.

Li, Z., Zhang, T. and Li, K. (2011) One-step synthesis of mesoporous two-line ferrihydrite for effective elimination of arsenic contaminants from natural water. *Dalton Trans.*, **40**, 2062–2066.

Lin, F., Blake, D.L., Callebaut, I. and Skerjanc, I.S. (2000). MAN1, an inner nuclear membrane protein that shares the LEM domain with lamina-associated polypeptide 2 and emerin. *J. Biol. Chem.*, **275**, 4840–4847.

Lippard, S.J. (1988) Oxo-bridged polyiron centers in biology and chemistry. *Angew. Chem., Int. Ed. Engl.*, **27**, 344–361.

Lohsse, A., Ullrich, S., Katzmann, E., Borg, S., *et al.* (2011) Functional analysis of the magnetosome island in *Magnetospirillum gryphiswaldense*: the mamAB operon is sufficient for magnetite biomineralization. *PLoS ONE*, **6**, e25561.

Lower, B.H. and Bazylinski, D.A. (2013) The bacterial magnetosome: a unique prokaryotic organelle. *J. Mol. Microbiol. Biotechnol.*, **23**, 63–80.

Maillot, F., Morin, G., Wang, Y., Bonnin, D., *et al.* (2011) New insight into the structure of nanocrystalline ferrihydrite: EXAFS evidence for tetrahedrally coordinated iron(III). *Geochim. Cosmochim. Acta*, **75**, 2708–2720.

Manceau, A. (2009) Evaluation of the structural model for ferrihydrite derived from real-space modelling of high-energy X-ray diffraction data. *Clay Miner.*, **44**, 19–34.

Mann, S. (1988) Molecular recognition in biomineralization. *Nature*, **332**, 119–124.

Mann, S. (2007) in *Biominerals and Biomineralization* (eds I. Bertini, H.B. Gray, E.I. Stiefel and J.S. Valentine), University Science Books, Sausalito, California, pp. 79–94.

Michel, F.M., Ehm, L., Antao, S.M., Lee, P.L., *et al.* (2007a) The structure of ferrihydrite, a nanocrystalline material. *Science*, **316**, 1726–1729.

Michel, F.M., Ehm, L., Liu, G., Han, W.Q., *et al.* (2007b) Similarities in 2- and 6-line ferrihydrite based on pair distribution function analysis of X-ray total scattering. *Chem. Mater.*, **19**, 1489–1496.

Michel, F.M., Barrón, V., Torrent, J., Morales, M.P., *et al.* (2010) Ordered ferrimagnetic form of ferrihydrite reveals links among structure, composition, and magnetism. *Proc. Natl Acad. Sci. USA*, **107**, 2787–2792.

Murat, D., Quinlan, A., Vali, H. and Komeili, A. (2010) Comprehensive genetic dissection of the magnetosome gene island reveals the step-wise assembly of a prokaryotic organelle. *Proc. Natl Acad. Sci. USA*, **107**, 5593–5598.

Nudelman, F. and Sommerdijk, N.A. (2012) Biomineralization as an inspiration for materials chemistry. *Angew. Chem.*, **51**, 6582–6596.

Pannalai, S.J., Crowe, S.A., Cioppa, M.T., Symons, D.T.A., *et al.* (2005) Room-temperature magnetic properties of ferrihydrite: A potential magnetic remanence carrier? *Earth Planet Sci. Lett.*, **236**, 856–870.

Pankhurst, Q.A. and Pollard, R.J. (1992) Structural and magnetic properties of ferrihydrite. *Clays Clay Miner.*, **40**, 268–272.

Pearson, R.G. (1963) Hard and soft acids and bases. *J. Am. Chem. Soc.*, **85**, 3533–3539.

Pierre, J.-L. and Fontecave, M. (1999) Iron and activated oxygen species in biology: the basic chemistry. *Biometals*, **12**, 195–199.

Quinlan, A., Murat, D., Vali, H. and Komeili, A. (2011) The HtrA/DegP family protease MamE is a bifunctional protein with roles in magnetosome protein localization and magnetite biomineralization. *Mol. Microbiol.*, **80**, 1075–1087.

Rahn-Lee, L. and Komeili, A. (2013) The magnetosome model: insights into the mechanisms of bacterial biomineralization. *Front. Microbiol.*, **4**, Article 352.

Rancourt, D.G. and Meunier, J.F. (2008) Constraints on structural models of ferrihydrite as a nanocrystalline material. *Am. Miner.*, **93**, 1412–1417.

Rancourt, D.G., Fortin, D., Pichler, T., Thibault, P.-J., *et al.* (2001) Mineralogy of a natural As-rich hydrous ferric oxide coprecipitate formed by mixing of hydrothermal fluid and seawater: Implications regarding surface complexation and color banding in ferrihydrite deposits. *Am. Miner.*, **86**, 834–851.

Refait, P.H., Abdelmoula, M. and Géhin, J.-M.R. (1998) Mechanisms of formation and structure of green rust one in aqueous corrosion of iron in the presence of chloride ions. *Corros. Sci.*, **40**, 1547–1560.

Richter, M., Kube, M., Bazylinski, D.A., Lombardot, T., *et al.* (2007) Comparative genome analysis of four magnetotactic bacteria reveals a complex set of group-specific genes implicated in magnetosome biomineralization and function. *J. Bacteriol.*, **13**. 4899–4910.

Riveros, P.A., Dutrizac, J.E. and Spencer, P. (2001) Arsenic disposal practices in the metallurgical industry. *Can. Metall. Q.*, **40**, 395–420.

Scheffel, A., Gruska, M., Faivre, D., Linaroudis, A., *et al.* (2006) An acidic protein aligns magnetosomes along a filamentous structure in magnetotactic bacteria. *Nature*, **440**, 110–114.

Scheffel, A., Gärdes, A., Grünberg, K., Wanner, G. and Schüler D. (2008) The major magnetosome proteins MamGFDC are not essential for magnetite biomineralization in *Magnetospirillum gryphiswaldense* but regulate the size of magnetosome crystals. *J. Bacteriol.*, **190**, 377–386.

Schmitt, W., Murugesu, M., Goodwin, J.C., Hill, J.P., *et al.* (2001) Strategies for producing cluster-based magnetic arrays. *Polyhedron*, **20**, 1687–1697.

Schwertmann, U., Carlson, L. and Murad, E. (1987) Properties of iron oxides in two Finnish lakes in relation to the environment of their formation. *Clays Clay Miner.*, **35**, 297–304.

Schwertmann, U., Friedl, J. and Stanjek, H. (1999) From Fe(III) ions to ferrihydrite and then to hematite. *J. Colloid Interface Sci.*, **209**, 215–223.

Siponen, M.I., Adryanczyk, G., Ginet, N., Arnoux, P. and Pignol, D. (2012) Magnetochrome: a c-type cytochrome domain specific to magnetotactic bacteria. *Biochem. Soc. Trans.*, **40**, 1319–1323.

Smith, S.J., Page, K., Kim, H., Campbell, B.J., *et al.* (2012) Novel synthesis and structural analysis of ferrihydrite. *Inorg. Chem.*, **51**, 6421–6424.

Staniland, S., Ward, B., Harrison, A., van der Laan, G. and Telling, N. (2007) Rapid magnetosome formation shown by real-time X-ray magnetic circular dichroism. *Proc. Natl Acad. Sci. USA*, **104**, 19524–19528.

Taft, K.L. and Lippard, S.J. (1990) Synthesis and structure of $[Fe(OMe)_2(O_2CCH_2Cl)]_{10}$: a molecular ferric wheel. *J. Am. Chem. Soc.*, **112**, 9629–9630.

Taft, K.L., Papaefthymiou, G.C. and Lippard, S.J. (1993) A mixed-valent polyiron oxo complex that models the biomineralization of the ferritin core. *Science*, **259**, 1302–1305.

Tanaka, M., Okamura, Y., Arakali, A., Tanaka, T., *et al.* (2006) Origin of magnetosome membrane: proteomic analysis of magnetosome membrane and comparison with cytoplasmic membrane. *Proteomics*, **6**, 5234–5247.

Tanaka, M., Mazuyama, E., Arakaki, A. and Matsunaga, T. (2010) MMS6 protein regulates crystal morphology during nano-sized magnetite biomineralization in vivo. *J. Biol. Chem.*, **286**, 6386–6392.

Taoka, A., Asada, R., Wu, L.F. and Fukumori, Y. (2007) Polymerization of the actin-like protein MamK, which is associated with magnetosomes. *J. Bacteriol.*, **189**, 8737–8740.

Thompson, D.W. (1917) *On growth and form.* Cambridge University Press, Cambridge, pp. 793.

Towe, K.M. (1981) Structural distinction between ferritin and iron-dextran (imferon). An electron diffraction comparison. *J. Biol. Chem.*, **256**, 9377–9378.

Towe, K.M. and Bradley, W.F. (1967) Mineralogical constitution of colloidal 'hydrous ferric oxides'. *J. Colloid Interface Sci.*, **24**, 384–392.

Uebe, R., Henn, V. and Schüler, D. (2011) The MagA protein of *Magnetospirilla* is not involved in bacterial magnetite biomineralization. *J. Bacteriol.*, **194**, 1018–1023.

Ullrich, S. and Schüler, D. (2010) Cre-lox-based method for generation of large deletions within the genomic magnetosome island of *Magnetospirillum gryphiswaldense. Appl. Environ. Microbiol.*, **76**, 2439–2444.

Walker, M.M., Dennis, T.E. and Kirschvink, J.L. (2002) The magnetic sense and its use in long-distance navigation by animals. *Curr. Opin. Neurobiol.*, **12**, 735–744.

Wilt, F.H. (2005) Developmental biology meets materials science: Morphogenesis of biomineralized structures. *Dev. Biol.*, **280**, 15–25.

Wu, J. and Luther, G.W., III (1996) Spatial and temporal distribution of iron in the surface water of the north-western Atlantic Ocean. *Geochim. Cosmochim. Acta*, **60**, 2729–2741.

Yamamoto, D., Taoka, A., Uchihashi, T., Sasaki, H., *et al.* (2010) Visualization and structural analysis of the bacterial magnetic organelle magnetosome using atomic force microscopy. *Proc. Natl Acad. Sci. USA*, **107**, 9382–9387.

Zeytuni, N., Ozyamak, E., Ben-Harush, K., Davidov, G., *et al.* (2011) Self-recognition mechanism of MamA, a magnetosome-associated TPR-containing protein, promotes complex assembly. *Proc. Natl Acad. Sci. USA*, **108**, E480–E487.

2

The Essential Role of Iron in Biology

2.1 Introduction: Iron an Essential Element in Biology

In the National Gallery of Scotland hangs a celebrated painting by Titian depicting the three ages of man. In the description of the prehistory of human technology, there are also three ages, namely the Stone Age, the Bronze Age and the Iron Age, defined by the materials out of which cutting tools and weapons were manufactured. The Stone Age, which began about two million years ago, is defined broadly as the period during which stone was widely used to make implements with a sharp edge, a point, or a percussion surface. It lasted roughly 3.4 billion years and ended between 6000 BC and 2000 BC, and was superseded by the Bronze Age, during which metals – initially copper – began to be used for the manufacture of weapons. The use of copper spread from Anatolia through Mesopotamia and the Middle East from 4000–3000 BC. True bronze (an alloy of copper and tin) was used only rarely initially, but during the second millennium BC the use of true bronze increased greatly. The Bronze Age was also marked by important inventions, such as the wheel and the ox-drawn plough and the development of viable systems of writing. However, by around 1200 BC the ability to heat and forge another metal, iron, brought the Bronze Age to an end. The Iron Age began when iron began to replace bronze in implements and weapons, despite requiring the use of much higher temperatures than bronze. In its natural form, iron is barely harder than bronze and is not useful for tools unless it is combined with carbon to make steel, with the percentage of carbon determining many important characteristics of the final product, notably its hardness. The shift away from bronze occurred because iron, when alloyed with a small amount of carbon (0.2–0.8%, absorbed from the charcoal used in its extraction from iron ores), is harder, more durable, and maintains a sharper edge than bronze. For over three thousand years, until its replacement by even more hardened steel in the middle of the 19th century, iron formed the material basis of

Iron Metabolism – From Molecular Mechanisms to Clinical Consequences, Fourth Edition. Robert Crichton.
© 2016 John Wiley & Sons, Ltd. Published 2016 by John Wiley & Sons, Ltd.

human civilisation in Europe, Asia, and Africa. However, while we have many relics from both the Stone and the Bronze Ages, little remains of the Iron Age on account of the poor stability of iron in the face of oxygen and water (rust is not a very practical way of preserving historical relics!).

We are of course interested here in the importance of iron for biological systems, and before taking an overview of the diversity of its role illustrated by the different classes of iron proteins, we begin by noting a few simple examples.

Bacteria of the Enterobacteriaceae, a group of Gram-negative, facultative anaerobes, which include the major human pathogens *Shigella* sp., *Salmonella* sp., *Yersinia* sp. and pathogenic *Escherichia coli*, require iron in micromolar concentrations. In order to achieve this, from environments which may range from the completely anaerobic conditions of the human large intestine to situations in the external environment with very high oxygen levels, they devote a not inconsiderable part of their genome (Table 2.1) to iron-uptake systems (Carpenter and Payne, 2014). And, as we will see in Chapter 3, many pathogenic bacteria can also acquire iron, in the form of haem, transferrin or lactoferrin, from their mammalian hosts.

Iron (Fe) is also essential for plants and animals. In humans, Fe deficiency affects an estimated 30% of the world population, particularly in developing countries, causing around 0.8 million deaths annually (World Health Organization, 2002). Rice is one of the most important staple crops in these regions, but in calcareous soils with a high pH, which represent approximately 30% of the world's cultivated soil, iron is present as poorly bioavailable ferric complexes. However, introduction of the yeast ferric reductase gene into rice plants can increase crop yields eightfold (Ishimaru *et al.*, 2007), and enriching iron adsorption not only improves rice yield, but also globally increases iron in rice grains, enhancing their dietary potential (Bashir *et al.*, 2013).

Despite its ubiquitous expression at low levels in most normal human tissues, the transferrin receptor (TfR) is expressed on malignant cells at levels many times higher than those on normal cells, and its expression can be correlated with tumour stage or cancer progression. This makes TfR a potential vector for drug delivery to malignant cells and thus, an attractive therapeutic agent for cancer chemotherapy (reviewed in Daniels *et al.*, 2013).

Table 2.1 *Genes encoding iron transport systems in the Enterobacteriaceae*

Gene	Role in iron transport
tonB, exbB, exbD	Provides energy for siderophore or haem transport across the outer membrane
entABCDEF	Enterobactin production
ahpC	Enhances enterobactin production
fepABCDE	Enterobactin transport
iroB	Glucosylates enterobactin
iroCDEN	Salmochelin transport
iucABCD	Aerobactin production
iutA	Aerobactin outer membrane receptor
fhuCDB	Aerobactin periplasmic ABC permease
ybtE, HMWP1, HMWP1, ybtU	Yersiniabactin production
feoABC	Ferrous iron transport
sitABCD	Ferrous iron and manganese transport
yfe	Ferrous iron and manganese transport

Reproduced with permission from Elsevier from Carpenter, C. and Payne, S.M. (2014) Regulation of iron transport systems in Enterobacteriaceae in response to oxygen and iron availability. *J. Inorg. Biochem.*, **133**, 110–117.

Why then is iron such an essential element for almost all life forms? The answer most probably lies in the capacity of iron to participate in one-electron transfer (i.e. free radical) reactions, notably one specific free radical reaction which is essential for DNA synthesis – the reduction of ribonucleotides to the corresponding deoxyribonucleotides, catalysed by ribonucleotide reductases (RNRs), all of which are radical metalloenzymes (Stubbe and Riggs-Gelasco, 1998; Stubbe *et al.*, 2001; Nordlund and Reichard, 2006). Since all known cellular life forms store their genetic information in DNA, RNRs are ubiquitous in living organisms. They all share a common catalytic mechanism involving activation of the ribonucleotide by abstraction of the 3'-hydrogen atom of the ribose by a transient thiyl radical of the enzyme (Figure 2.1). Ribonucleotide reductases can be divided into three classes, largely based on their interaction with oxygen and the way in which they generate the thiyl radical required for ribonucleotide reduction (Figure 2.2) (Jordan and Reichard, 1998). Class I RNRs contain two non-identical dimeric subunits (R1 and R2), and require oxygen to generate a stable tyrosyl radical through a dimetallic M–O–M centre in the smaller R2 subunit. The cofactor can be either di-iron (class Ia), dimanganese (class Ib), or manganese–iron (class Ic) (Högbom, 2011; Cotruvo and Stubbe, 2011). During catalysis, the radical is continuously shuttled to a cysteine residue, some 30 Å away in the larger R1 subunit, where it generates the thiyl radical. With the exception of *Euglena gracilis* (Hamilton, 1974), all eukaryotes, from yeast to man have class I RNRs, as do some eubacteria, including *E. coli*, and a few archaebacteria. Class II RNRs are indifferent to oxygen, contain a single subunit and generate their thiyl radical using the Co(III)-containing cofactor adenosylcobalamine, probably via the formation of a deoxyadenosyl radical. Class III RNRs are anaerobic enzymes, inactivated by oxygen, which generate a glycyl radical, the counterpoint to the tyrosyl radical in class I RNRs, through an FeS cluster and *S*-adenosylmethionine. Whereas RNRs of class I and II use electrons from redox-active cysteines of small proteins (e.g. thioredoxin or glutaredoxin), class III enzymes use formate as electron donor. We discuss the mechanism of class I RNRs later in the chapter.

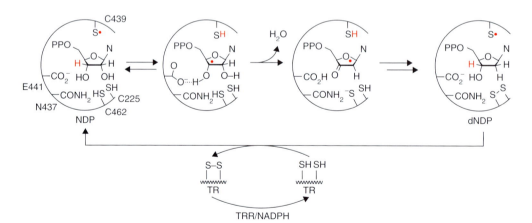

Figure 2.1 *Mechanism of NDP reduction by RNR. The S• shown on C$_{439}$ of α2 in the first reaction step is reversibly generated by Y$_{122}$• in β2 by the mechanism described later in the chapter. Reprinted with permission from Minnihan, E.C., Nocera, D.G. and Stubbe, J. (2013) Reversible, long-range radical transfer in E. coli class Ia ribonucleotide reductase. Acc. Chem. Res.,* **46***, 2524–2535; © 2013, American Chemical Society*

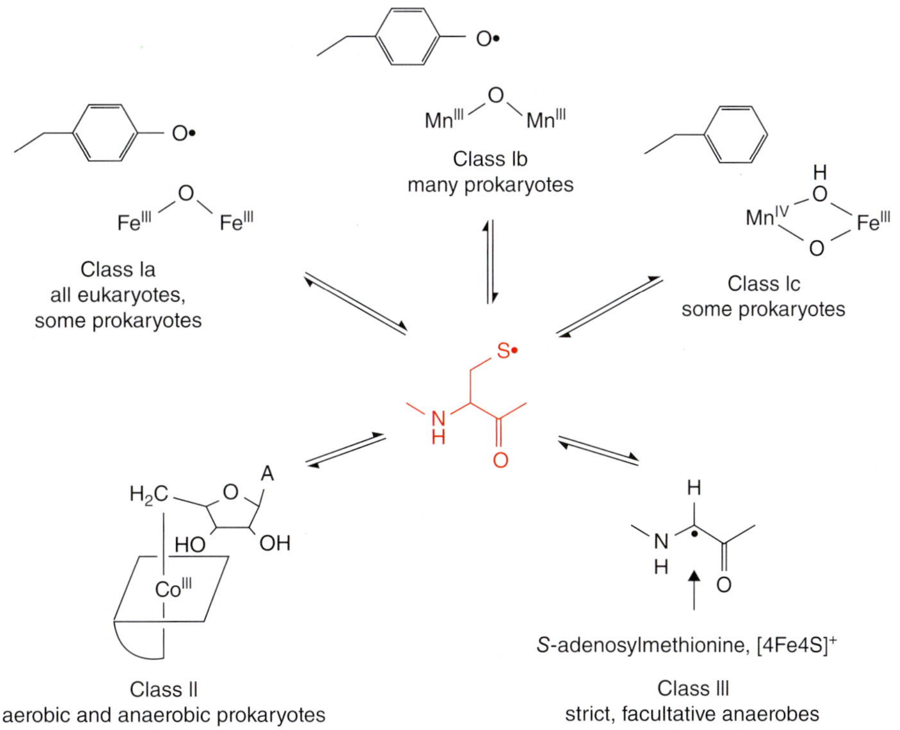

Figure 2.2 *Classes of RNRs. RNRs are classified on the basis of the metallocofactor used to reversibly generate the cysteine thiyl radical (red) essential for catalysis. Class Ia RNRs use a diferric-Y• cofactor, class Ib RNRs use a dimanganese(III)-Y• cofactor, class Ic RNRs use a Mn(IV)Fe(III) cofactor, class II RNRs use adenosylcobalamin, and class III RNRs use a glycyl radical generated by an activating enzyme requiring S-adenosylmethionine and a [4Fe–4S]⁺ cluster. Reprinted with permission from Cotruvo and Stubbe (2012); © Royal Society of Chemistry*

2.2   Physical Techniques for the Study of Iron in Biological Systems

There are a considerable number of techniques available for the study of iron in biological systems, some of them highly specific, some of a more general applicability. It is not the intention to describe these techniques in any detail, but rather to indicate what information can be derived from the application of the method in question to an iron-containing sample. Several important practical generalisations should be made at the outset. The first is that, in general, the more techniques that can be used on a biological sample the better, since there are virtually no situations in which one single method will give all of the information required, and the information derived from one technique will often prove complementary to that given by a second. Second, there is little sense in using sophisticated physico-chemical techniques to analyze impure samples, and vice-versa, highly purified biological materials should not be subjected to poor analytical techniques. The final – and perhaps most important – point was very clearly expressed in a recent publication (Crichton and Louro, 2013): "…above all recognise that the key to metalloprotein characterisation is collaboration – do not think that you can simply phagocytise a technique from a colleague who knows the technique inside-out – it will be much richer to collaborate, incorporating his or her research into your research". So, it is hoped that what follows will be a helpful guide to which techniques might be appropriate for any iron-containing protein. For much more detailed information on a large number of these techniques, we refer the reader to Crichton and Louro (2013). Some of the techniques which can be utilised for the study of iron-containing metalloproteins are summarised in the following paragraphs.

Whereas in what now seems a truly distant past, proteins were isolated directly from an appropriate biological source, today it is standard practice to produce proteins by overexpressing them in an expression vector, often with an appropriate 'tag' to aid in the purification. This means that the amino acid sequence of the protein can be deduced directly from the cloned DNA, opening the door for a series of bioinformatic approaches which may be mined to find if the protein belongs to an already known family, perhaps to deduce information concerning its fold and eventual domain structure (Robson, 2012). While *in-silico* research can never replace good old-fashioned biochemical methods to establish the functional characteristics of a protein, much useful information can often be gleaned prior to applying spectroscopic and other techniques.

Transitions between different electronic states result in absorption of energy in the ultraviolet, visible and, for many transition metal complexes the near- infrared region of the electromagnetic spectrum. Spectroscopic methods which probe these electronic transitions can, under favourable conditions, provide detailed information on the electronic and magnetic properties of both the metal ion and its ligands. Electronic spectra of metalloproteins find their origins in: (i) internal ligand absorption bands, such as $\pi \rightarrow \pi^*$ electronic transitions in porphyrins; (ii) transitions associated entirely with metal orbitals (d-d transitions); and (iii) charge transfer bands between the ligand and the metal, such as the $S \rightarrow Fe(II)$ charge transfer bands seen in the optical spectra of Fe/S proteins.

For studying the magnetic properties of paramagnetic iron proteins, electron paramagnetic resonance (EPR) spectroscopy is a particularly useful tool (Hagen, 2006, 2009, 2013) that can be used with frozen dilute solutions of proteins, and is quite sensitive (high-spin ferric ions can be detected in the μM range). EPR spectra are usually represented as the first derivative of the measured absorption spectrum, and are characterised by the four main parameters; intensity; linewidth; *g*-value (which defines position); and multiplet structure. In principle, this can give information on the type of bonding involved, the oxidation state of the metal ion, and possibly the type of metalloligand centre, quantification of the concentration of the paramagnetic species, identification of ligands in the first coordination sphere, and functional characterisation.

The theory underlying a nuclear magnetic resonance (NMR) experiment is very similar to that for EPR, but the set-up is very different for technical reasons. In EPR, the promotion of molecules from their ground state to an excited state by microwave radiation is detected by the corresponding *absorption* of energy. In contrast, NMR relies on a *relaxation* process – the radiofrequency radiation raises molecules to their excited state, and the experiment then monitors their return (relaxation) to the ground state (Louro, 2013). The most frequently used method in NMR is to apply a pulse of radiofrequency to the sample and then detect the transient signal as the nuclear spins return to their ground state. The transient signal then undergoes a Fourier transformation to give the NMR spectrum. From NMR experiments, four parameters can be derived: the chemical shift (δ) which, like the *g*-value in EPR, defines the field position of the NMR signal (in this case with respect to a reference marker added to the sample); the intensity (I); the relaxation times; and the coupling constant. The full assignment of the hundreds of different resonances in the NMR spectrum and the measurement of a great number of interproton distances and torsional angles can allow the complete three-dimensional structures of medium-sized proteins to be determined in solution.

Until a decade ago, metalloproteins containing paramagnetic metal ions were not thought to be suitable for the application of NMR techniques because the presence of paramagnetic centres destroys the resolution of the spectrum. However, the loss of resolution is less severe when the paramagnetic centre exhibits fast electronic relaxation, and with the application of advanced pulse techniques and data handling methods the limitations that paramagnetism presented previously can be overcome (Bertini *et al.*, 2005; Banci *et al.*, 2010; Louro, 2013). The presence of paramagnetism in a protein allows structural and mechanistic information by means of NMR that have no equivalent in the NMR study of diamagnetic proteins.

Mössbauer spectroscopy, or nuclear gamma resonance absorption, represents an absolutely iron-specific method because ^{57}Fe is unique among biological metals in that it manifests the Mössbauer effect. Mössbauer spectroscopy probes high-energy transitions in the atomic nucleus and is based on the phenomenon of recoil-free γ-ray resonance absorption. Under normal conditions, atomic nuclei recoil when they emit or absorb gamma rays, and the wavelength varies with the amount of recoil. However, during the course of his PhD thesis at the Technical University of Munich, Rudolf Mössbauer found that, at a sufficiently low temperature, a significant fraction of the nuclei of ^{191}In embedded in a crystal lattice may emit or absorb gamma rays without any recoil (Mössbauer, 1958a,b). The strictly monochromatic γ-radiation emitted from the excited nucleus of a suitable isotope during a radioactive decay pathway can therefore be absorbed by the same isotope in the sample. Biological applications (Bill, 2013) are essentially restricted to ^{57}Fe, the natural abundance of which is 2.2%, although its content can be increased by isotope supplementation. The interest of the method lies in the fact that, if the energy transitions occur within the nucleus itself, their magnitude depends on the density and arrangement of extranuclear electrons – that is, on the chemical state of the atoms. The extremely small perturbation (10^{-8} eV) caused by the difference of chemical state between emitter and absorber can be easily offset and measured by Doppler modulation. The Mössbauer signal is influenced by the nuclear charge, the nature of the surrounding ligands, and the symmetry of the ligand field. The observed isomer shift, δ (in mm s^{-1}) gives information about the metal oxidation and spin states and the nature of the ligands coordinated to the iron, while the quadrupole splitting, ΔE_Q, is dependent on electric field gradients at the nucleus and reflects the asymmetry of the electric field surrounding the metal centre.

Because proteins are made up of chiral amino acids they can discriminate between right and left circularly polarised light (lcp and rcp, respectively). The different absorption of lcp and rcp light (reflected by different extinction coefficients) is termed circular dichroism (CD). CD is particularly useful for detecting metals bound within proteins, and can often detect and resolve electronic transitions that are not easily accessible by classical absorption spectroscopy. In addition, CD is a useful tool for obtaining information about the secondary structure of proteins. In the presence of a magnetic field, even non-chiral molecules exhibit CD spectra, which can be measured by the technique called magnetic circular dichroism (MCD). The intensity developed by spin–orbit coupling between excited states and between ground states and excited states can be exploited, particularly at low temperature, which generates more intense metal-centred d-d transitions in low-temperature MCD relative to absorption spectra. Although the theoretical analysis of MCD spectra is usually complex, it can be a powerful fingerprint for the identification of bound ligands. MCD has provided significant insight into the nature of the axial donors at haem centres and has had a major impact on the study of the electronic structures of the ground states of a range of non-haem iron proteins (McMaster and Oganesyan, 2010).

Resonance Raman spectroscopy gives information about molecular vibrational frequencies, typically in the range of 10^{12} to 10^{14} Hz, corresponding to radiation in the infrared region of the electromagnetic spectrum. In resonance Raman spectroscopy, the energy of an incoming laser beam is tuned to be near to an electronic transition (in resonance), while vibrational modes associated with the particular transition exhibit a greatly increased Raman scattering intensity, usually overwhelming Raman signals from all other transitions In haemoproteins (e.g. haemoglobin), tuning the laser to near the charge transfer electronic transition of the iron centre yields a spectrum which only reflects the stretching and bending modes associated with the tetrapyrrole iron. Resonance Raman spectroscopy reduces the complexity of the spectrum, allowing only a few vibrational modes to be examined at a time (Loehr and Sanders-Loehr, 1993). The main advantage of resonance Raman spectroscopy over classical Raman spectroscopy is the large increase in the intensity of the peaks (by a factor of as much as 10^6), allowing spectra to be obtained with sample concentrations as low as 10^{-8} M. Surface-enhanced Raman scattering, in which the metalloprotein molecules are in contact with a roughened metallic surface, provides enhancements of the order of 10^6 and even as high as 10^{14}, allowing the study of single molecules (Millo *et al.*, 2011).

The availability of easily tuneable high-flux X-ray beams from synchrotron radiation has led to the development of new types of X-ray spectroscopy. The absorption of X-rays by a solid or liquid sample is measured as a function of wavelength at energies around the absorption edge – that is, around the energy that is required to liberate an electron from the metal, giving rise to two forms of X-ray absorption spectroscopy:

- X-ray absorption near-edge structure (XANES) at or near the edge yields information on the valence and coordination of the metal ion.
- The extended X-ray absorption fine structure (EXAFS), measured just above the edge, gives a pattern of rapid oscillations, which represents an interference effect from the neighbouring atoms of the meta ion (Strange and Feiters, 2008; Feiters and Mayer-Klauke, 2013).

A Fourier transform of the oscillations can be analyzed to give, in favourable cases, information on the number, types and distances of neighbouring atoms. This usually requires parallel studies on model compounds of known structure, and for many metal centres in proteins, and can give extremely accurate structural information without the requirement for an ordered sample, as is required for X-ray diffraction. Geometric information derived from fitting EXAFS data to a model structure can be reliable to ±0.01 Å.

Protein crystallography is the most important technique for the structure determination of macromolecules, with thousands of structures being determined every year (Brito and Archer, 2013). Structure determination of proteins requires the availability of an ordered sample in the form of a single crystal, but more coherent protocols for protein crystallisation have greatly improved what used to be something of a 'black art'. The other reasons for this explosion of X-ray crystallographic prowess are the use of cryo-crystallography, the use of brighter and tuneable synchrotron-generated X-ray beams (which can enable reliable data collection on crystals which would have been considered too small for study some years ago), better data collection facilities, and finally the quasi-generalised use of multiple anomalous dispersion (notably by replacement of methionine residues in the protein by selenomethionine residues) to resolve the 'phase problem'.

Since many iron proteins have at least one surface-exposed redox centre, which can serve as an entry point for electrons from an electrode, they can be studied by electrochemical methods using equipment which is relatively inexpensive, and available in most chemistry laboratories (Armstrong, 2005; Léger, 2013). In favourable situations a series of experiments can be carried out using the same 'film' of protein adsorbed onto the electrode.

Spectroscopic methods have the advantage over protein crystallography in that they can allow time-resolved measurements to be made which can detect short-lived intermediates. However, to obtain structural information, the observed spectroscopic data must be fitted to molecular structures. This can be done with reference structures which model the spectroscopic properties of the metalloprotein site, which could be synthetic low-molecular-weight complexes of known molecular structure, or high-resolution metalloprotein structures obtained by X-ray crystallography or high-field NMR. Yet another promising approach is the use of quantum chemical calculations of spectroscopic properties of metalloproteins and model compounds to elucidate their geometrical and electronic structures (Neese, 2003; Kirchner *et al.*, 2007).

2.3   Classes of Iron Proteins

As was pointed out in Chapter 1, Fe^{3+} can be considered as a 'hard' acid, with a preference for ligands which are 'hard' bases, notably those which contain oxygen as a donor atom, such as hydroxyl, carboxyl, and other oxygen-containing groups. In contrast, Fe^{2+} is intermediate between a 'hard' acid and a ' soft' acid, and can accommodate both the 'hard' oxygen-based ligands and the 'soft' ligands such as those containing nitrogen and sulphur: examples are histidine, protoporphyrin, cysteine, and inorganic sulphur. The distribution of the donor atoms which ligate the metal, and their geometry, will thus determine the functional properties of the metal centre. In the case where one of the coordination spheres is unoccupied, the possibility exists of binding a sixth non-protein ligand. As we saw in Chapter 1, the aqueous solution chemistry of iron is dominated by forms of Fe^{2+} and Fe^{3+}, whose complexes readily undergo electron transfer and acid–base reactions. This explains the wide range and variety of catalytic and other functions of which the element is capable, and underlines the importance of iron in biological systems. Another feature of iron which makes it so important is its abundance although, as was pointed out before, since the advent of oxygen into the Earth's atmosphere iron bioavailability has been seriously compromised. When we invoke the extensive range of redox potentials available to the metal by varying its interaction with coordinating ligands, to which is added its capacity to participate in one-electron transfer (i.e. free radical) reactions, it is easy to see why iron is virtually indispensable for life.

Iron-containing proteins could be classified according to a number of criteria – for example the functional role of the metal ion, defined as: (i) structural; (ii) metal storage and transport; (iii) electron transport; (iv) dioxygen binding; and (v) catalytic – the latter being extremely large and diverse. As in previous editions, a presentation has been chosen which is based essentially on the coordination chemistry of the metal. This has the advantage of allowing the reader to more easily appreciate the diversity of biochemical functions which iron can play, viewed through the ligands which bind it to the protein. We consider first haemoproteins into which an iron protoporphyrin is incorporated in different apo-proteins to produce O_2 carriers, O_2 activators or electron-transfer proteins. Second, we consider proteins containing iron–sulphur clusters, many of which are involved in electron transfer, although catalytic iron–sulphur clusters are also known (as will be seen later). The final consideration is the non-haem, non-iron–sulphur, iron-containing proteins which include, in addition to enzymes, proteins of iron storage and transport. The incorporation of iron into porphyrins and Fe–S clusters is discussed in Chapter 8.

2.4   Haemoproteins

The first class of iron-containing proteins that we consider are those in which the iron is bound to four ring nitrogen atoms of a porphyrin molecule (haem) and to one or two axial ligands from the protein. The porphyrin consists of four pyrrole rings, linked by methene bridges; in most haemoproteins it has four methyl, two vinyl and two propionyl substituents, known as protoporphyrin IX. The enzyme ferrochelatase, located on the matrice face of the inner mitochondrial membrane, incorporates ferrous iron into protoporphyrin IX to form haem (as described in Chapter 8), which is subsequently incorporated into different haemoproteins. Three types of haemoprotein have been identified:

- Oxygen carriers
- Activators of molecular oxygen
- Electron transport proteins (cytochromes)

2.4.1 Oxygen Carriers

Oxygen transport and storage in many higher eukaryotes, is assured by haemoglobins and myoglobins. These were the first proteins to have their X-ray crystal structures determined by John Kendrew and Max Perutz, for which they received the Nobel Prize for Chemistry in 1962. When the structures of insect and lamprey haemoglobins were determined some years later (Hendrickson and Love, 1971; Huber *et al.*, 1969, 1971), it became clear that all these oxygen-binding proteins share a common tertiary structure, known as the globin fold, an example of which is sperm whale myoglobin[1] (Figure 2.3a). However, whereas the monomeric myoglobin with a single haem has a hyperbolic oxygen-binding curve, the tetrameric haemoglobin with four haem groups has a sigmoidal oxygen-binding curve (Figure 2.3b). This reflects the cooperativity of oxygen binding – the fourth O_2 molecule binds with 100-fold greater affinity than the first. We know that, like other allosteric proteins, haemoglobin exists in two distinct and different conformations, corresponding to the T (deoxy) and R (oxy) states. Indeed, the conformations of oxy- and deoxy-haemoglobins are so different that crystals of deoxyhaemoglobin break when oxygen is introduced (Haurowitz, 1938), as described briefly below. Since, in the haemoglobin structure the haem groups are so far apart, this positive cooperativity must be transmitted by the protein itself, but what might be the trigger that would signal to a neighbouring subunit that oxygenation had taken place?

Max Perutz left Vienna in September 1936 to undertake a doctoral thesis on protein crystallography under the direction of the legendary J. D. Bernal, in Cambridge. A year later he had still not settled on a thesis subject and was beginning to have concerns about his future (Perutz, 1980). In the summer of 1937, he returned to Austria on vacation and, remembering that one of his cousins in Prague had married a biochemist, Felix Haurowitz, Perutz called on him for advice (Perutz, 1980). Haurowitz had recently shown that as oxygen enters the hexagonal plates of horse deoxyhaemoglobin crystals the plates become disordered and monoclinic needles of oxyhaemoglobin form in their place (Haurowitz, 1938). So, Haurowitz suggested that Perutz take as the subject of his thesis the structure of haemoglobin, as he wanted to see how oxygen could change haemoglobin's shape. Subsequently, Perutz set to work, not knowing that it would take him 22 years to even make a start (Eisenberg, 1994).

In haemoglobins and myoglobins the haem is tightly bound to the protein through a large number of hydrophobic interactions and by a single coordinate bond between the imidazole of a 'proximal histidine' and the ferrous iron (Figure 2.4). Whether these molecules bind molecular oxygen in a cooperative or a non-cooperative way, they are monomers, dimers or tetramers, and they come from mammals, insects, worms or even the nodules of leguminous plants, they all have the common globin tertiary fold. They possess an unoccupied sixth coordination site,

---

[1] If the structures of these two haemoglobins had not been initially determined at low resolution, their similarity to the corresponding fold of myoglobin and haemoglobin might have gone undetected.

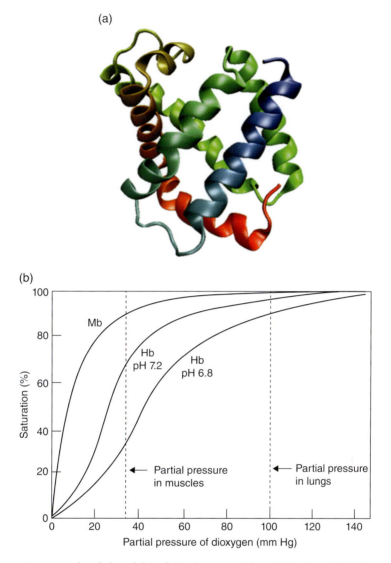

Figure 2.3 *(a) An example of the globin fold, the myoglobin (PDB ID 1MBA) from the mollusc Aplysia limacine at a resolution of 0.16 nm. From Wikipedia. (b) The oxygen-binding curves of myoglobin and haemoglobin. Reprinted with permission from Collman, J.P., Boulatov, R., Sunderland, C.J. and Fu, L. (2004) Functional analogues of cytochrome c oxidase, myoglobin, and hemoglobin.* Chem. Rev., ***104**, 561–588; © 2004, American Chemical Society*

situated within a hydrophobic pocket, sterically hindered by the presence of a distal histidine residue, and are capable of reversibly binding molecular oxygen. In contrast, simple ferrous porphyrins are irreversibly oxidised by molecular oxygen, leading ultimately to stable (μ-oxo)-di-iron(III) species. Reversible oxygenation at room temperature can be achieved with synthetic ferrous porphyrins by using sterically encumbered ligands to protect the O_2-binding site and thus preventing the approach of two iron–porphyrin moieties. The dioxygen molecule is bound

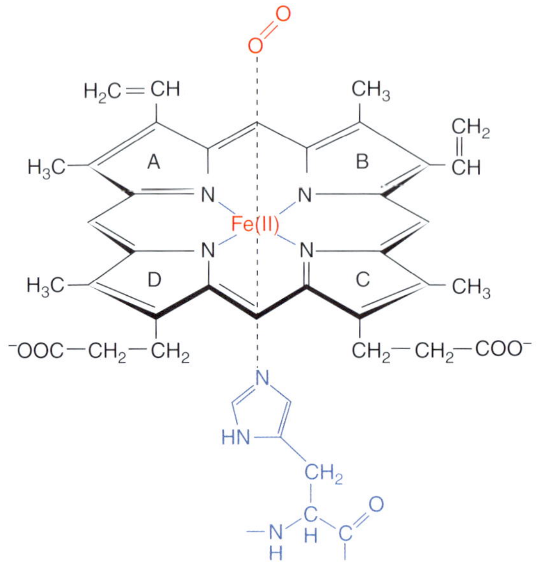

Figure 2.4 *A detailed picture of the haem group. The haem group, Fe(II)-protoporphyrin IX is shown liganded to His and O₂, as in the oxygenated state in oxy-myoglobin or oxy-hemoglobin (© 2004, John Wiley & Sons, Ltd)*

end-on to the iron, both in model complexes, in haemoglobin and in myoglobin. There is good evidence from resonance Raman spectroscopy for electron transfer to dioxygen, such that we could consider oxy-haemoglobin and oxy-myoglobin as ferric-superoxo complexes, in which the superoxo is stabilised by hydrogen bonding to the distal histidine proton (Figure 2.4), which is essentially equivalent to the ferric-superoxo 'compound III' in cytochrome P450s and peroxidases (these are discussed later).

The most important difference between monomeric and oligomeric haemoglobins is of course the cooperativity of the oxygen binding by the latter (Figure 2.3b) (tetrameric mammalian haemoglobins fix the fourth oxygen molecule with a 100-fold greater affinity than the first). Before the high-resolution structural refinements of myoglobin and haemoglobin it had been suggested that the size of the iron atom might be the key factor in triggering the subunit transition from the low-affinity (deoxy, or T) to the high-affinity (oxy, or R) state. The first to draw attention to this potential 'trigger' was Bob Williams (Williams, 1961). Ferrous porphyrins have six d electrons and can occupy three spin states. High-spin iron(II) porphyrins are invariably five-coordinate with the iron atom well displaced out of the haem plane towards the single axial ligand. Six-coordinate ferrous porphyrins with two axial ligands, one on either side of the haem plane, are invariably diamagnetic and low-spin ($S = 0$). The covalent radius is such that low-spin iron(II) fits into the porphyrin core with minimum disruption and lies almost in the plane of the haem. Iron(II) porphyrins can also assume an intermediate spin state ($S = 1$) which has no biological counterpart. Model X-ray studies with porphyrin model compounds had shown that the five-coordinate high-spin Fe(II) sits a small distance out of the haem plane, whereas in the presence of a sixth coordinating ligand the low-spin Fe(II) is pulled into the haem plane (reviewed in Perutz, 1979). Perutz developed a 'stereochemical mechanism' of how haemoglobin worked, based on the observation that a number of salt bridges at subunit interfaces that are present in deoxyhaemoglobin are absent in the oxy form (Perutz, 1970; Perutz *et al.*, 1998). It was proposed that, upon binding of O_2 to haem in the T quaternary structure, the spin-state transition would force the iron atom into the haem plane, pushing the haem closer to His F8, the axial fifth ligand of the haem iron, causing movement of the F-helix (Figure 2.5). This would result in the breaking of a salt bridge, the release of a proton and destabilisation of the structure at the subunit interface between αβ dimers of the tetramer, thereby pushing the quaternary structure equilibrium towards the R-state. In this mechanism the salt bridges play three roles: (i) they stabilise the T quaternary structure relative to R; (ii) they lower the oxygen affinity in the T state because of the energy required to break them on oxygen binding; and (iii) they release protons when they are broken, which explains the almost century-old effect discovered by the physiologist father of the atomic physicist Niels Bohr, Christian, namely that the affinity of haemoglobin for oxygen is lowered when the pH decreases (Bohr *et al.*, 1904).

In myoglobin (and by homology, also in haemoglobin), the N–H proton of the distal histidine E7 in the O_2 binding pocket (Figure 2.4) forms a hydrogen bond with the iron-coordinated dioxygen molecule, and imposes an angular bend on the oxygen molecule. In carbon monoxide (CO) adducts of myoglobin and haemoglobin, the steric hindrance caused by the distal histidine results in a less favourable binding geometry (CO prefers a linear coordination). Thus, CO, a poison which is present both in tobacco smoke and in automobile exhausts, but which is also produced in the normal biological degradation of haem, binds only about 250-fold more tightly than O_2 to both myoglobin and haemoglobin, whereas the affinity of free haem for CO much greater. This tailoring of the iron porphyrin centres to bind O_2 rather than its toxic surrogate CO, means that endogenously produced CO has not proved lethal to humans, long before the discovery of means for its exogenous production. Nonetheless, the progressive irritation of the gendarme on traffic duty on the Place de l'Etoile at rush hour still reflects the greater affinity of haemoglobin for CO rather than O_2!

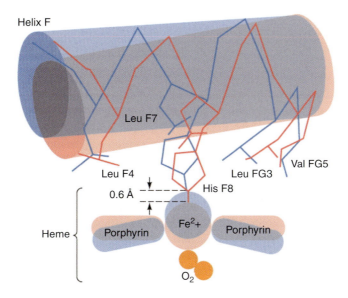

Figure 2.5 *The triggering mechanism for the T to R transition in haemoglobin (© 2004, John Wiley & Sons, Ltd)*

2.4.2 Activators of Molecular Oxygen

These haem enzymes include cytochrome oxidases, catalases and peroxidases, and cytochrome P-450s. They are characterised by a penta-coordinate geometry in which the sixth site of the metal centre can bind either molecular oxygen, hydrogen peroxide or, in the case of cytochrome P-450s, even form iron–carbon bonds with the substrate. Substrate specificity and oxygen activation is determined by the interaction between haem iron and ligands and the control of the spin state (Smith and Williams, 1970). For all of these the high-spin iron–porphyrin system can go to the radical cation state at a redox potential close enough to that of the couple Fe(IV)/Fe(III) to allow a ferryl type of iron to participate in chemical reactions such as the activation of oxygen or oxidation of molecules at the expense of hydrogen peroxide.

Mitochondrial cytochrome *c* oxidases (mtCcOs) are haem–copper oxidases, which catalyse the reduction of molecular oxygen to water, at the rate of up to 250 molecules of O_2 per second, with electrons from cytochrome *c* and protons from the mitochondrial matrix (Eq. 2.1).

$$O_2 + 4H^+ + 4e^- \rightarrow 2H_2O \tag{2.1}$$

The energy released in this process is coupled to the translocation of an additional four protons across the membrane, which in turn contributes to the chemiosmotic gradient required for ATP synthesis. Since the electrons and protons are taken up from opposite sides of the membrane, the reaction results in a net charge separation across the membrane which, together with the coupled proton pumping, corresponds to the overall translocation of two positive charges across the membrane per electron transferred to O_2.

Over the past two decades it has become clear that CcOs are members of a large and quite diverse superfamily of enzymes, the respiratory haem–copper oxidases (Pereira *et al.*, 2001; Hemp and Gennis, 2008; Sousa *et al.*, 2012). The haem–copper oxidases are responsible for more than 90% of the O_2 consumed by biological reactions on Earth, and are related to one another not only by their haem–copper active site with a low-spin haem located next to it, but also by their capacity to conserve part of the free energy of the O_2 reduction reaction in the form of a proton motive force across the mitochondrial or bacterial membrane (Wikstrom, 2004).

The crystal structures of aa_3-type CcOs from bovine heart mitochondria and bacteria (*Rhodobacter sphaeroides* and *Paracoccus denitrificans*) have been determined (Iwata *et al.*, 1995; Tsukihara *et al.*, 1996, 2003; Ostermeir *et al.*, 1997; Yoshikawa *et al.*, 1998; Svensson-Ek *et al.*, 2002), culminating in the structure at a resolution of 2.0 Å of CcO from *Rhodobacter sphaeroides* which contains only the two catalytic subunits and a number of alkyl chains of lipids and detergent (Qin *et al.*, 2006). The structure of the CcO from *R. sphaeroides* is presented in Figure 2.6a, while a more detailed view of the redox-active cofactors and amino acid residues on the proton transfer pathways is given in Figure 2.6b (Brzezinski and Johansson, 2010).

Electrons from cytochrome *c* are donated via the dinuclear copper centre (Cu_A) in the hydrophilic domain of subunit II to haem *a* in subunit I, which contains the catalytic centre. Subunit III has no metal centres; subunit III may prevent, or decrease, the probability of side reactions during O_2 reduction that cause irreversible inactivation of CcO (Bratton *et al.*, 1999). Haem *a* reduces haem a_3, part of the dinuclear haem a_3-Cu_A centre (DNC), where oxygen binds and is subsequently reduced. The tyrosine residue, Y(I-288), which is covalently crosslinked to His240, one of the Cu_B ligands, is redox active and is also part of the active site.

The current concept of the mechanism of O_2 reduction by CcO is summarised in Figure 2.7 (Wikström, 2012). Starting with the catalytically active oxidised O state (ferric haem a_3, cupric Cu_B), the first and second electron transfers are charge-compensated by substrate-proton uptake

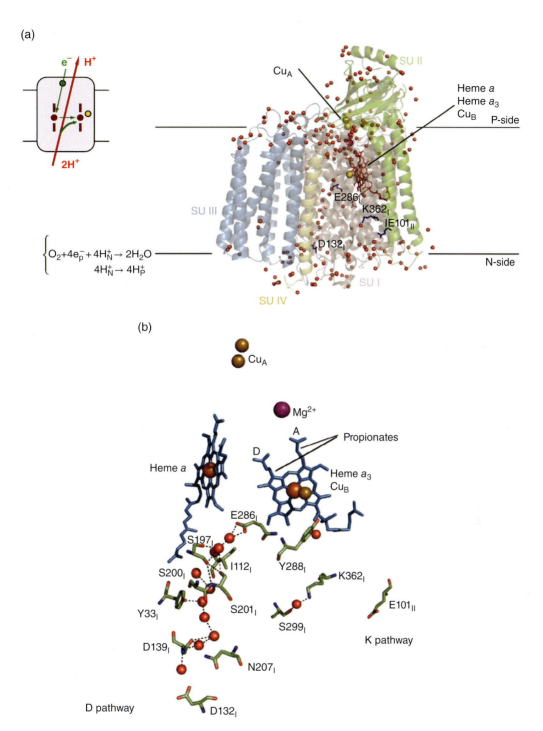

(a)

e⁻ H⁺

2H⁺

SU II

Cuₐ

Heme a
Heme a_3
Cuᵦ P-side

$$O_2 + 4e_p^- + 4H_N^+ \rightarrow 2H_2O$$
$$4H_N^+ \rightarrow 4H_P^+$$

SU III

E286ᵢ
K362ᵢ
IE101ᵢᵢ
D132ᵢ

N-side

SU I

SU IV

(b)

Cuₐ

Mg²⁺

A
D Propionates

Heme a

Heme a_3
Cuᵦ

E286ᵢ
S197ᵢ
I112ᵢ Y288ᵢ
S200ᵢ K362ᵢ
Y33ᵢ S201ᵢ E101ᵢᵢ
S299ᵢ
D139ᵢ K pathway
N207ᵢ
D pathway D132ᵢ

Figure 2.6 (a) The structure of cytochrome c oxidase from R. sphaeroides (PDB code 1M56). The four subunits of the enzyme are coloured as indicated in the figure. Haems a and a₃ are shown in red, and the copper centres Cuₐ and Cuᵦ in yellow. The red spheres are water molecules resolved in the structure. Residues Glu286, Asp132, Lys362, all in subunit I, and Glu101 in subunit II, are shown in the figure (the subscript indicates the subunit number). The approximate position of the membrane is indicated by the solid lines, where the p- and n-sides are the more positively and negatively charged sides of the membrane, respectively. The purple sphere is a non-redox-active Mg²⁺ ion found in the structure. (b) The D and K proton pathways shown in more detail. The haem a₃ propionates are also indicated. Reprinted with permission from Elsevier from Brzezinski, P. and Johansson, A.L. (2010) Variable proton-pumping stoichiometry in structural variants of cytochrome c oxidase. Biochim. Biophys. Acta, **1797**, 710–723

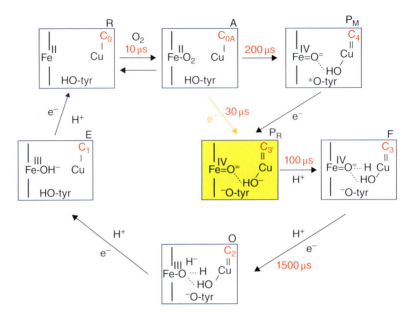

Figure 2.7 *Catalytic cycle of cytochrome c oxidase. The rectangle represents the binuclear site, which includes haem a_3 (Fe), Cu_B, and the crosslinked tyrosine (HO-tyr). Bonds are not shown between oxygen and hydrogen in water, hydroxide and phenolic OH, and dotted lines indicate hydrogen bonds. Approximate time constants (1/k; room temperature) are given in red for the reaction of COX with ~1 mM O_2; these vary somewhat depending on the source of COX. The fully reduced enzyme (Cu_A and haem a reduced) takes the path indicated by the yellow arrow, where an electron from haem a is transferred to the binuclear site in conjunction with scission of the O–O bond, yielding state P_R marked in yellow. If only the binuclear site is reduced, the reaction with O_2 goes instead to state P_M, where the fourth electron has been taken from the tyrosine. The protons indicated at reaction arrows are 'substrate' protons to be consumed in the formation of water from reduced dioxygen. The steps where water leaves the site are not known exactly, but the scheme implies the steps O → E and E → R. Proton pumping is not depicted. Hydrogen bonding from a hydroxide (P_M, P_R) or water ligand (F, O) of Cu_B to the oxo or hydroxy ligand of the haem is depicted schematically (dotted). Note also that the strong hydrogen bonding to the hydroxide-ligated haem in O keeps the ferric iron in a high spin state, slightly proximally displaced from the porphyrin plane. Reproduced with permission from Elsevier from Wikström, M. (2012) Active site intermediates in the reduction of O(2) by cytochrome oxidase, and their derivatives.* Biochim. Biophys. Acta, **1817**, 468–475

and produce the one-electron-reduced E state (ferric haem a_3, cuprous Cu_B) and the two-electron-reduced R state (ferrous haem a_3, cuprous Cu_B). These steps constitute the 'reductive' steps of the cycle. In the R state, ferrous haem a_3 binds O_2 within 10 μs, forming the unstable oxyferrous A state (Fe^{II}–O_2 Cu^I), formally equivalent to the oxyferrous state in oxyhaemoglobin or oxymyoglobin. In this oxygen adduct there is considerable charge transfer from the haem iron to the dioxygen ligand, and once again a ferric-superoxide structure may be a more appropriate description (Wikström, 2012). If further electrons are not available from haem a, only the dinuclear site is reduced and the reaction with O_2 goes on from A to the P_M state[2] (Figure 2.7), where

---

[2] Although the P states were initially thought to be ferric–cupric-peroxy states (hence the P nomenclature) of the haem–copper site (Wikstrom, 1981), it was subsequently suggested that in the P state, the O–O bond is already broken with the heme in the ferryl form (Weng and Baker, 1991).

the fourth electron has been taken from the tyrosine generating the neutral tyrosine radical. However, if an electron is supplied (yellow arrow in Figure 2.7), A is rapidly transformed to the P_R state, which is isoelectronic with the intermediate state F. This latter has been assigned to a ferryl-cupric state of the dinuclear centre (Wikström, 1981). Interestingly, states P_M and P_R have identical optical spectra, considering the additional electron in the latter, and resonance Raman shows that the F=O signature of P_M is the same as P_R, establishing the ferryl structure of the haem in both (Kitigawa and Ogura, 1998; Proshlyakov *et al.*, 1998; Ogura and Kitigawa, 2004).

Part of the energy released in the redox reaction is conserved by a vectorial transfer of protons across the membrane from the *N*-side to the *P*-side, thereby maintaining an electrochemical proton gradient that is used for the synthesis of ATP. Two proton-transfer pathways leading from the *N*-side surface towards the binuclear centre have been identified and are indicated in Figure 2.6b.

Catalases and peroxidases both promote H_2O_2 reduction by mechanisms that involve ferryl intermediates. Catalases differ from peroxidases by their use of H_2O_2 both as electron acceptor and donor, catalysing the disproportionate reaction (catalytic activity) (Eq. 2.2), whereas both catalases and peroxidases can oxidise a variety of organic substrates (peroxidatic activity) (Eq. 2.3):

$$H_2O_2 + H_2O_2 \rightarrow 2H_2O + O_2 \tag{2.2}$$

$$AH_2 + H_2O_2 \rightarrow A + 2H_2O \tag{2.3}$$

In peroxidases and catalases the enzyme extracts one electron from haem iron in the active site, and a second electron from an organic moiety to reduce H_2O_2 in one step to O^{2-} and OH^-. The immediate product of this chemistry is Compound I, which contains a ferryl-oxo-species and an organic radical, analogous to the a_3^{4+}= O/radical found in intermediate *P* in cytochrome oxidase. The organic radical in Compound I is reduced in a subsequent step to produce Compound II, which maintains the ferryl-oxo structure, and exactly the same chemistry is found in the oxidase to produce the *F* intermediate (Figure 2.7). This similarity in the chemistry catalysed by these oxygen-activating haem proteins may extend further to other enzymes involved in activating and reducing oxygen and peroxides.

Enzymes that incorporate oxygen atoms from molecular oxygen into their substrates can be classified into two categories, monooxygenases (Eq. 2.4) and dioxygenases (Eq. 2.5), depending on whether one or both oxygen atoms from dioxygen are incorporated into the substrate, where XH and AH_2 represent substrate and an electron donor, respectively:

$$XH + {}^*O_2 + AH_2 \rightarrow X({}^*O)H + H_2{}^*O + A \tag{2.4}$$

$$XH + {}^*O_2 \rightarrow X({}^*O_2)H \tag{2.5}$$

Cytochrome P450 monooxygenases (P450 or CYP) constitute a superfamily of structurally diverse and functionally versatile haem-containing enzymes, with more than 15 000 known genes distributed across all biological kingdoms (Ortiz de Montellano, 2005). Cytochrome P450s play important roles in the hydroxylation of endogenous physiological substrates as well as a vast range of drugs and other compounds foreign to the organism (xenobiotics).[3] When cytochrome P450 functions as a monooxygenase it requires a two-electron donor, which transfers electrons. Most CYPs require two electrons, delivered by a flavin- or [2Fe–2S]-cluster-containing redox partner, in addition to substrate and molecular oxygen (Eq. 2.6):

---

[3] Xenos, as Michael Flanders remarked in the Flanders and Swann recording 'At the Drop of a Hat', is the Greek word for stranger or guest; as in xenophobia – fear and hatred of guests!

$$RH + O_2 + 2e^- + 2H^+ \rightarrow ROH + H_2O \qquad (2.6)$$

They also catalyse a panoply of other reactions, the most common of which are heteroatom oxygenation and heteroatom release (dealkylation), epoxide formation and group migration (reviewed in Lamb and Waterman, 2014). In the resting state, the P450 haem iron atom is the ferric (III) low-spin state, six-coordinated by the four nitrogen atoms of the haem, the anionic thiolate sulphur atom from a cysteine residue (the only conserved amino acid in all 15 000 P450 sequences), and a water molecule in the distal position. The linkage of the haem Fe to the cysteine thiolate generates the characteristic Soret absorption band at 450 nm in the ferrous CO complex.

The X-ray crystal structure of the soluble cytochrome P-450 from *Pseudomonas putida* grown on camphor (P-450-CAM) has been determined (Poulos *et al.*, 1985), and reveals that the haem group with its cysteine ligand is deeply embedded in the hydrophobic interior of the protein (Figure 2.8a). The general P450 monooxygenation cycle is shown schematically in Figure 2.9. The binding of a substrate to the low-spin ferric enzyme leads to a displacement of water and a shift to the high-spin state. The substrate-bound complex has a greater reduction potential and more easily accepts an electron from an ancillary redox partner. After the first reduction, the haem iron binds oxygen, forming an oxy–haem complex which then receives the second electron from the redox partner. After two subsequent protonations and heterolysis of the O–O bond an oxygenated product is formed and the haem returns to the resting low-spin state (Sevrioukova and Poulos, 2013).

The interaction between P450 and its redox partners is not so well established. For rapid turnover, the redox partner must bind, deliver an electron, and then dissociate, which precludes the formation of stable long-lived complexes, making protein cocrystallisation difficult. To date, there is only one known crystal structure of a P450-redox partner complex, between the haem- and FMN-domains of P450BM3 (Sevrioukova and Poulos, 1999). In this structure, the FMN module docks on the proximal side of the haem (Figure 2.8b). The redox partner of P450cam is the 2Fe2S ferredoxin, putidaredoxin (Pdx), of *Thermus thermophilus* CYP175A1 a ferredoxin that contains one 3Fe4S and one 4Fe4S cluster; for *Sulfolobus acidocaldarius* CYP119 it is also thought to be a 3Fe4S and a 4Fe4S cluster. The structures of these three CYPs, based on computer docking and modelling, are presented in Figure 2.8 a, c, and d (Sevrioukova and Poulos, 1999).

2.4.3 Electron Transport Proteins

The third class of haemoproteins, the cytochromes, have iron in a hexa-coordinate low-spin system and were first discovered by McMunn in 1884, who called them 'histohaematins'. However. the editor and chemist Hoppe Seyler[4] declined to publish this discovery and the work remained unnoticed until 1925 when David Keilin, using a hand spectroscope, rediscovered the characteristic absorption (Soret) bands of the three cytochromes *a*, *b* and *c* in respiring cells, and correctly concluded that they transferred electrons from substrate oxidation to the terminal oxidase that is known today as cytochrome *c* oxidase (Keilin, 1925). The three principal classes of cytochromes *a*, *b* and *c* have a distinctive three-banded absorption spectrum in the reduced state, and also differ by the nature of the side chains to their basic protoporphyrin IX core (Figure 2.10a). The *b*-type haems

---

[4] These were the days of the modest 'Herausgeber' of scientific journals – Justus von Liebigs Annalen der Chimie, Naunyn Schmiedebergs Archiv für Physiologie, Hoppe Seylers Zeitschrift für Physiologische Chemie. It is recorded that when Freidrich Meischer submitted his publication on the discovery of DNA (from pus-saturated surgical bandages) Hoppe Seyler delayed publication for a year, and accompanied Meischer's article with a confirmatory note of his own and a couple of research papers on the subject from his own laboratory. Apropos McMunn, one of my favourite textbook errors is the description of McMunn as a German biochemist!

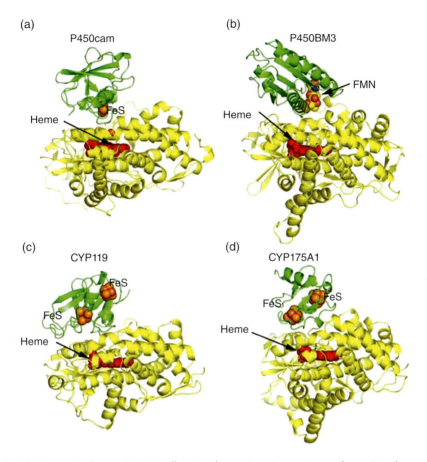

Figure 2.8 *Various cytochrome P450 (yellow)-redox partner (green) complexes. Panels a, c and d are based on computer docking and modelling, while panel b represents the crystal structure. Reproduced with permission from Elsevier from Sevrioukova, I.F. and Poulos, T.L. (1999) Structural biology of redox partner interactions in P450cam monooxygenase: a fresh look at an old system.* Arch. Biochem. Biophys., ***507***, *66–74*

have protoporphyrin IX (as in haemoglobin), whereas *a*-type haems contain a long hydrophobic tail of isoprene units attached to the porphyrin, as well as a formyl group in place of a methyl substituent. In typical *c*-type cytochromes the vinyl groups of the protoporphyrin IX form covalent thioether bonds with cysteine thiols that occur in a Cys-Xxx-Xxx-Cys-His motif (Figure 2.10b). The axial ligands of haem iron vary with cytochrome type. In cytochromes *a* and *b*, both ligands are usually His residues, whereas in cytochrome *c* the histidine adjacent to the CXXCH motif is a ligand to the haem iron atom, and the sixth ligand is the sulphur of a methionine residue located distant from the CXXCH motif in the primary structure of the protein (Figure 2.10c). In bacterial *c*-type cytochromes, histidine (rather than methionine) is often the sixth iron ligand, and there are examples with cysteine, an N-terminal amino group, asparagine, lysine or a vacant coordination site. There are few restrictions on the nature of the Xxx-Xxx residues (reviewed in Allen *et al.*, 2008).

Cytochromes are widely distributed and serve as electron-carrier proteins in the mitochondria, endoplasmic reticulum and photosynthetic organelles, as well as in bacterial redox chains. The

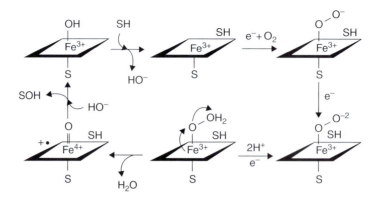

Figure 2.9 *Cytochrome P450 catalytic cycle. Reproduced with permission from Elsevier from Sevrioukova, I.F. and Poulos, T.L. (2013) Understanding the mechanism of cytochrome P450 3A4: recent advances and remaining problems.* Dalton Trans., **42**, 3116–3126

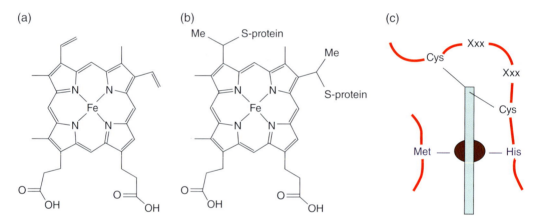

Figure 2.10 *Structures of (a) haem (Fe-protoporphyrin IX) and (b) haem bound to a polypeptide chain as in a typical c-type cytochrome, in which the vinyl groups of the haem are saturated by the addition of cysteine thiols that occur in a Cys-Xxx-Xxx-Cys-His motif (only the sulphur atoms of the cysteines are shown), forming covalent bonds between haem and protein. (c) Cartoon representation of haem attachment to protein in mitochondrial cytochrome c. The porphyrin ring is shown in blue, and the haem iron atom in brown. The cysteines of the CXXCH motif form covalent bonds to the haem, and the histidine acts as a ligand to the haem iron atom via a nitrogen atom. The sixth ligand to the iron atom is the sulphur of a methionine residue located distantly from the CXXCH motif in the primary structure of the protein. Reproduced with permission from Elsevier from Allen, J.W., Jackson, A.P., Rigden, D.J., Willis, A.C., et al. (2008) Order within a mosaic distribution of mitochondrial c-type cytochrome biogenesis systems?* FEBS J., **275**, 2385–2402

iron in all cytochromes can alternate between an oxidised Fe(III) low-spin state with a single unpaired electron and a formal charge for the haem of +1, and a reduced Fe(II) low-spin form with no unpaired electrons and a net charge of zero. Since the iron remains low spin, electron transfer is greatly facilitated.

Cytochrome *c*, which serves as a mobile transporter of electrons between complex III and IV (cytochrome *c* oxidase) of the respiratory chain, is by far the best-characterised cytochrome, and the

X-ray structures of many eukaryotic and prokaryotic cytochromes c reveal them to have the same overall molecular fold. Whereas mitochondrial cytochrome c is exclusively involved in electron transfer there are many members of the cytochrome c family which have multiple haems, with redox potentials covering the range -290 to $+400\,mV$ and are often involved in proton-coupled electron transfer (PCET) that involves electron transfer/proton transfer in which electrons and protons transfer together.

Bacterial multihaem cytochromes c (MCCs) contain at least two (but often many more) haem groups that are covalently bound to the characteristic haem c-binding motifs (Sharma *et al.*, 2010). MCCs carry out a diverse range of functions in bacterial energy metabolism, and play an important role in reactions that contribute significantly to global nitrogen, sulphur and iron cycling. These include nitrification, respiratory nitrate and nitrite reductases, which generate ammonia, anaerobic ammonium oxidation, iron(III) reduction and the conversion of sulphur compounds such as sulphite, thiosulphate and tetrathionate (Simon *et al.*, 2011). Many MCCs are redox mediators which facilitate electron transport between the membrane quinone/quinol pool and primary dehydrogenases, or terminal reductases organised in bacterial respiratory chains.

Characteristic of MCCs are the bacterial cytochrome c nitrite reductases (NrfAs). Octahaem cytochrome c nitrite reductase from *Thioalkalivibrio nitratireducens* (TvNiR), like the previously characterised pentahaem nitrite reductases (NrfAs), catalyses the six-electron reductions of nitrite to ammonia and of sulphite to sulphide, and its structure is presented in Figure 2.11. Both, in the crystalline state and in solution, TvNiR exists as a stable hexamer containing 48 haems (Polyakov *et al.*, 2009). All of the haems are covalently attached to the protein, and all but haem 1 have bis-His axial ligands. Haem 1, the active site, has the characteristic lysine residue as axial ligand at the proximal position of the catalytic haem, leaving the sixth coordination position free for nitrite binding, together with the catalytic triad of tyrosine, histidine, and arginine at the distal side.

The cytochrome bc_1 complex (coenzyme Q cytochrome c reductase) couples electron transfer from hydroquinone to cytochrome c (cyt c) with the translocation of protons across the membrane in a mechanism called the Q cycle (Figure 2.12), making an important contribution to the proton motive force used for ATP synthesis. Cytochrome bc_1 has three redox-active subunits: cytochrome b, which contains both b_H and b_L haems; cytochrome c_1 with a single c-type haem; and the iron–sulphur protein (ISP) with a [Fe_2–S_2] Rieske cluster. X-ray structures of mitochondrial complexes from vertebrates and yeast, and of bacterial complexes from several bacteria, have been determined, and the crystal structure of the dimeric *Paracoccus denitrificans* cytochrome bc_1 complex is presented in Figure 2.13 (Kleinschroth *et al.*, 2011). The ISP connects two functional units to an obligate dimer, as its transmembrane helix (TMH) is anchored to one monomer and the catalytic head domain interacts with the other. In addition, the movement of the ISP head domain is essential for the mechanism. The [2Fe–S] cluster receives an electron when the head domain docks onto cyt b in the so-called b-position, and it is reoxidised by cyt c_1 after the domain reorients towards the latter into its c-position.

2.5 Iron–Sulphur Proteins

Fe–S proteins are presumed to be among the first catalysts that Nature had to work with (Huber and Wächtershäuser, 2006).[5] This second class of iron-containing proteins contain iron atoms bound to sulphur, either forming a cluster linked to the polypeptide chain uniquely by the thiol groups of

---

[5]While a passionate enthusiast for evolutionary theories, and their experimental testing, Günther Wächtershäuser is in his professional life a patent lawyer.

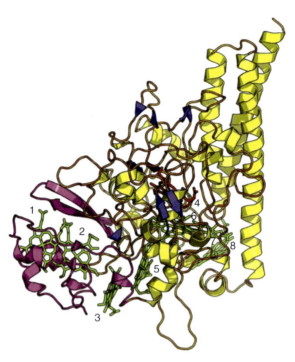

Figure 2.11 *Structure of the TvNiR monomer. The N-terminal domain is shown in pink. In the catalytic domain, the α-helices are shown in yellow and the β-sheets in blue. The haems, labelled sequentially from the N terminus, are green and the catalytic haem is red. Reproduced with permission from Elsevier from Polyakov, K.M., Boyko, K.M., Tikhonova, T.V., Slutsky, A., et al. (2009) High-resolution structural analysis of a novel octaheme cytochrome c nitrite reductase from the haloalkaliphilic bacterium* Thioalkalivibrio nitratireducens. *J. Mol. Biol.,* **389**, *846–862*

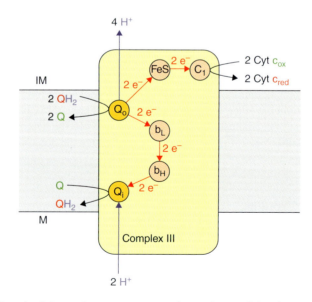

Figure 2.12 *The Q cycle. Schematic representation of complex III of the electron transport chain. The gray area is the inner mitochondrial membrane. Q represents the ubiquinone form of CoQ10, and QH2 represents the ubiquinol form (From Wikipedia)*

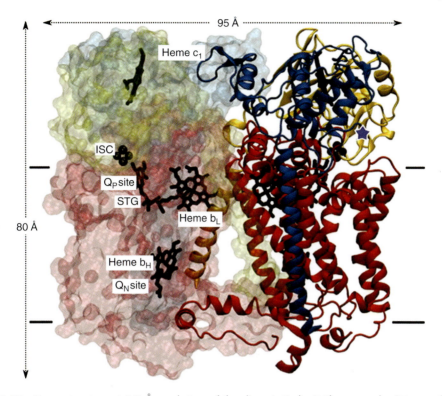

Figure 2.13 *X-ray structure at 2.7 Å resolution of the dimeric P. denitrificans cyt bc$_1$$^{\Delta ac}$ complex. The left monomer of the complex is shown in a transparent surface representation. The right monomer is depicted as Cα trace with secondary structure elements. Cofactors and the inhibitor stigmatellin (STG) are shown in stick-and-ball representation. The colour code is cyt b in red, cyt c$_1$ in blue and iron–sulphur protein (ISP) in yellow. The cofactors and the bound stigmatellin are shown in black. The position of the membrane is indicated with black horizontal lines. The molecule is viewed parallel to the membrane with the cytoplasmic side at the bottom. Labelling for cofactors, inhibitor and Q sites are given for one monomer only. The resolved N terminus of cyt c$_1$$^{\Delta ac}$ is marked with a blue asterisk. Reproduced with permission from Elsevier from Kleinschroth, T., Castellani, M., Trinh, C.H., Morgner, N., et al. (2011) X-ray structure of the dimeric cytochrome bc(1) complex from the soil bacterium Paracoccus denitrificans at 2.7-Å resolution. Biochim. Biophys. Acta, **1807**, 1606–1615*

cysteine residues (rubredoxins), or else with both inorganic sulphide and cysteine thiols as ligands. Although they have a very widespread distribution in all living organisms, their recognition as a distinct class of metalloproteins took place only in the 1960s after the discovery of their characteristic EPR spectra in the oxidised state. Iron–sulphur proteins can be classified as either *simple* or *complex*, with the latter containing in addition to the iron–sulphur clusters, flavins, molybdenum and haem. Within the protein to which they are bound, Fe–S clusters can adopt redox potentials from −500 mV to +300 mV (Meyer, 2008), and hence they can serve as excellent donors and acceptors of electrons in a variety of biological reactions (Lill, 2009). Examples are bacterial and mitochondrial respiratory complexes I–III, photosystem I, ferredoxins and hydrogenases. However, as we will see, they can also function in enzymes which catalyse a series of important reactions.

Simple iron–sulphur proteins contain a number of basic core structures which have been characterised crystallographically both in model compounds and in iron–sulphur proteins. Schematic representations of crystallographically demonstrated protein sites in FeS proteins are presented in Figure 2.14 (Venkateswara Rao and Holm, 2004). Low-molecular-weight proteins containing the first and the next five types are generically referred to as rubredoxins (Rd) and ferredoxins (Fd), respectively. In some cases, electron and proton transfer are coupled, so that the potentials are pH-dependent. In addition to discrete Rd and Fd proteins as components of electron-transfer pathways, the Fe–S clusters are also found within the enzyme molecules themselves.

Rubredoxins, found only in bacteria, are small proteins (some contain only 50 amino acids) with an [Fe–S] cluster consisting of a single Fe atom in a typical mercaptide coordination (Figure 2.14; **1**),

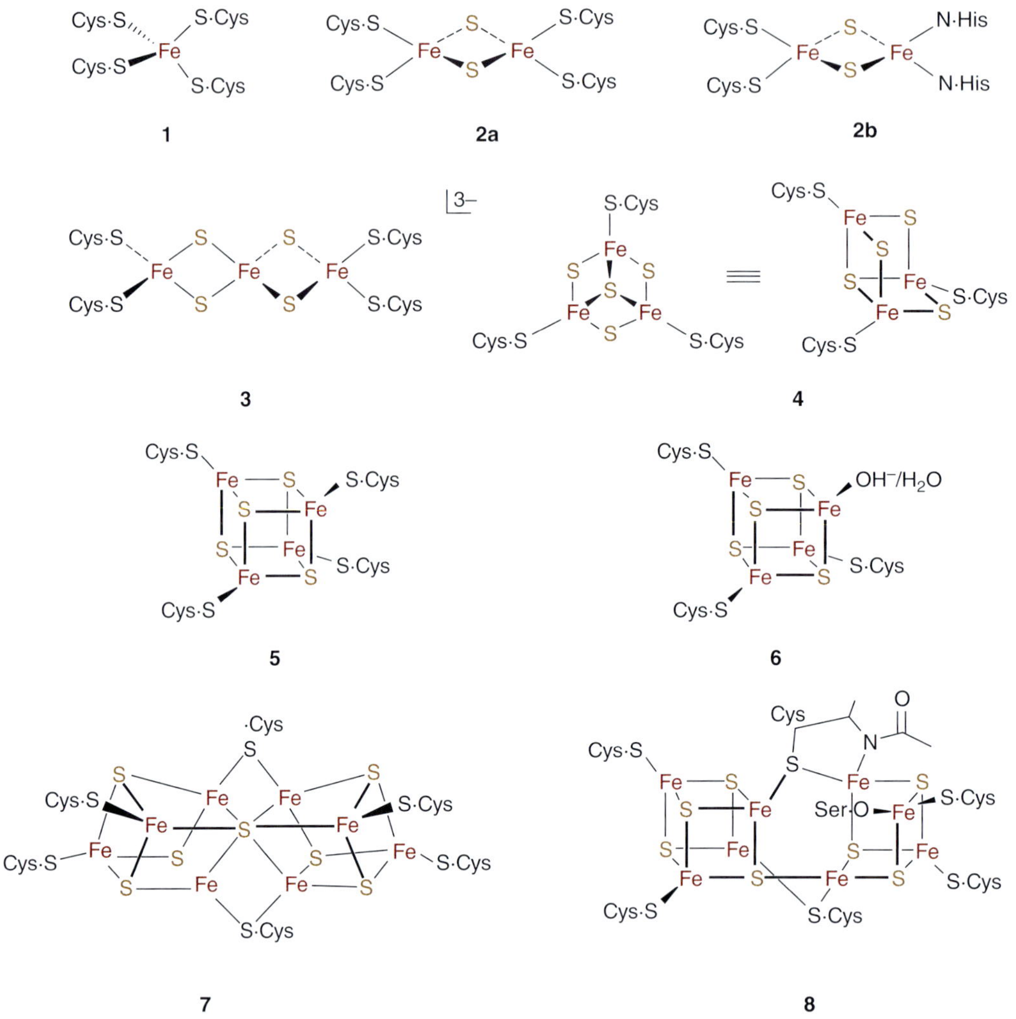

Figure 2.14 *Schematic representations of crystallographically demonstrated protein sites containing one (**1**), two (**2**), three (**3**, **4**), four (**5**, **6**), and eight (**7**, **8**) iron atoms. Formulas **7** and **8** describe the P cluster of nitrogenase as the as-isolated (P^N) and two-electron oxidised (P^{OX}) states, respectively. Reprinted with permission from Venkateswara Rao, P. and Holm, R.H. (2004) Synthetic analogues of the active sites of iron–sulfur proteins. Chem. Rev., **104**, 1135–1158; © 2004, American Chemical Society*

that is, with an iron centre liganded to four Cys residues. The valence state of the iron atom can be +2 or +3, and both oxidised and reduced forms are high spin.

Ferredoxins containing rhombic two iron–two sulphide [Fe_2–S_2] clusters (Figure 2.14; **2**) have typical oxidation states of +1 or +2 (the charges of the coordinating ligand residues are not considered), and can undergo a one-electron transfer to generate a valence-trapped $Fe^{III}Fe^{II}$ species. In proteins of known structure, one iron atom is closer to the surface (by about 0.5 nm), and this is the Fe atom on which the added electron resides. Ferredoxins with [Fe_2–S_2] clusters do not appear to participate in two-electron transfers. In addition to the conventional [Fe_2–S_2] ferredoxins with four cysteine ligands (Figure 2.14, **2a**), the electron-transfer chains of mitochondria and photosynthetic bacteria contain Rieske proteins which have a cluster in which two imidazole groups are bound to the same iron atom (Figure 2.14; **2b**). This is the iron atom which is reduced, and the presence of two neutral ligands increases the redox potential to more positive values than conventional [Fe_2–S_2] ferredoxins.

[Fe_3–S_4] clusters are found on both linear and cuboidal forms (Figure 2.14; **3, 4**). The initial observation of a protein-bound linear cluster occurred in 1984, with a partially unfolded form of aconitase, a linear cluster is the only cluster present in recombinant human iron regulatory protein 1. Structures of cuboidal [Fe_3–S_4] protein clusters (Figure 2.14; **4**) consist of three edge-shared Fe_2S_2 rhombuses which form a cuboidal cluster; that is, a cubane cluster missing an iron atom (Venkateswara Rao and Holm, 2004).

The cubane-type [Fe_4–S_4] clusters are by far the most frequently encountered in biology; the stable oxidation states are +1 and +2 for ferredoxins (Fds), and +2 and +3 for high potential iron (HPs) clusters. Their core oxidation states and formal iron valence states are shown in Figure 2.15. Fd_{ox} and HP_{red} are isoelectronic with a spin-paired ($S = 0$) ground state. HP_{ox} and Fd_{red} are then one electron more oxidised and reduced, respectively, The three oxidation states have not been observed in one protein unless its tertiary structure has been seriously perturbed.

The first recognised occurrence of a protein-bound, site-differentiated cluster was with the enzyme aconitase, which converts citrate to isocitrate in the tricarboxylic acid cycle. The resting form of the active enzyme contains the 3:1 site-differentiated cluster (Figure 2.14; **6**) whose unique iron atom, as shown by crystallography of the mitochondrial enzyme (Lloyd *et al.*, 1999) is the site of substrate binding and catalysis. Aconitase was the first iron–sulphur *enzyme* to be recognised. The inactive form of aconitase contains the cuboidal cluster (Figure 2.14; **4**), derived from **6** by a reversible iron insertion reaction with very little change in structure (Robbins and Stout, 1989). The cluster interconversion reaction is an essential paradigm for other protein-bound clusters

Core oxidation state:	$[Fe_4S_4]^0$	$[Fe_4S_4]^{1+}$	$[Fe_4S_4]^{2+}$	$[Fe_4S_4]^{3+}$	
	4Fe(II)	3Fe(II) + Fe(III)	2Fe(II) + 2Fe(III)	Fe(II) + 3Fe(III)	
Proteins:	Fe protein† $\xleftarrow{}$	$\underset{-0.8\,V}{\overset{-0.3\ to}{\rightleftharpoons}}$ Fd$_{red}$	$\underset{-0.8\,V}{\rightleftharpoons}$ Fd$_{ox}$/HP$_{red}$	$\underset{+0.5\,V}{\overset{+0.1\ to}{\rightleftharpoons}}$ HP$_{ox}$	(29)
Analogues:	$[Fe_4S_4(SR)_4]^{4-} \rightleftharpoons$	$^+[Fe_4S_4(SR)_4]^{3-} \rightleftharpoons$	$^+[Fe_4S_4(SR)_4]^{2-} \rightleftharpoons$	$^+[Fe_4S_4(SR)_4]^{1-}$	(30)

Fd = ferredoxin, HP = "high-potential" protein, $^+$Isolated, †Nitrogenase.

Figure 2.15 *Electron-transfer series of Fe_4S_4 protein sites **5** and analogues **13a**, showing core oxidation states and formal iron valence states. Isoelectronic species are arranged vertically. Reprinted with permission from Venkateswara Rao, P. and Holm, R.H. (2004) Synthetic analogues of the active sites of iron–sulfur proteins. Chem. Rev., **104**, 1135–1158; © 2004, American Chemical Society*

which, in the cubane form, lack a fourth Cys residue for binding to an iron site. It is the iron atom at the differentiated site that is labile.

There are a number of more complex Fe–S clusters including the electron-transfer P cluster of nitrogenase, as shown in Figure 2.14 in its crystallographically defined P^N (**7**) and P^{OX} (**8**) states. The P clusters are members of a group of protein-bound clusters designated as bridged assemblies, which in general consist of two discrete fragments that are coupled by one or more covalent bridges. The P-cluster consists of two [Fe_4–S_3] modules linked together via two bridging cysteines and a seventh bridging sulphide. In nitrogenase, the FeMoCo cluster, which is involved in catalysis, is constructed from two [Fe_4–S_3] modules, linked together by sulphides, together with a molybdenum atom which is partially ligated by homocitrate. In the sulphite reductase of *E. coli* a 4Fe–4S cluster is linked via a cysteine to the iron in a sirohaem.

Iron-only hydrogenases catalyse dihydrogen production or oxidation, and contain an unusual [Fe_6–S_6] cluster (the H-cluster) in their active site (Figure 2.16). The H-cluster consists of a novel

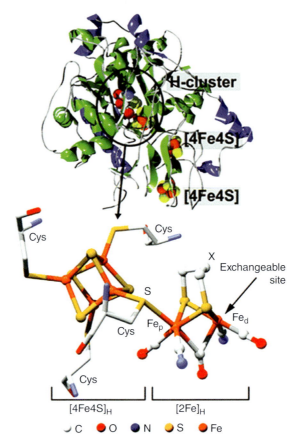

Figure 2.16 *Structure of the [FeFe]-hydrogenase from* D. desulfuricans *(top) and the active site (H-cluster) in the active oxidised state (bottom). The coordinates of the protein structure were taken from the crystal structure published by Nicolet* et al. *(Protein Data Bank entry 1HFE). Coordinates of the H-cluster were combined from structures of the [FeFe]-hydrogenase from* D. desulfuricans *and* C. pasteurianum *(hydrogenase I, Protein Data Bank entry 1C4A)*

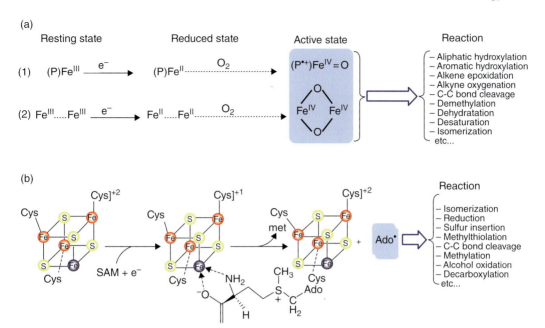

Figure 2.17 *The two strategies for the production of highly oxidant species involved in C–H bond activation. (a) Mechanisms proposed for O_2 activation to yield high-valent-iron-oxo by haem iron enzymes (1) and non-haem iron enzymes (2). P, porphyrin. (b) Mechanism for the reductive cleavage of SAM by [4Fe–4S] cluster of Radical-SAM enzymes to yield 5'-deoxyadenosyl radical Ado·. SAM is ligated through the amino and carboxylate groups to the unique iron (blue) in the [4Fe–4S]$^{+1}$ cluster. e⁻, electron; SAM, S-adenosylmethionine; met, methionine. Reprinted with permission from Atta, M., Arragain, S., Fontecave, M., Mulliez, E., et al. (2012) The methylthiolation reaction mediated by the Radical-SAM enzymes. Biochim. Biophys. Acta, **1824**, 1223–1230; © 2004, American Chemical Society*

dinuclear $[Fe_2–S_2]$ subsite, directly involved in catalysis connected via a Cys-thiol to a classical $[Fe_4–S_4]$ cubane cluster (Silakov *et al.*, 2007). The $[Fe_2–S_2]$ subsite has CO and CN as ligands to the iron atoms, and similar ligands are also involved in the Ni–Fe hydrogenases, where they were first identified using spectroscopy (Pierik *et al.*, 1999).

A prerequisite for C–H bond activation in order to introduce functional groups into organic molecules necessitates the generation of highly oxidant species, and represents one of the greatest challenges in modern bioinorganic chemistry (Atta *et al.*, 2012; Fontecave,*et al.*, 2004). It is achieved essentially by two approaches, both of which require iron as a metal ion catalyst (Figure 2.17). In the first approach, a high-valent iron–oxo complex is generated, either by haem enzymes (as discussed above) or by di-iron enzymes (as discussed below). The second approach involves the reductive activation of S-adenosylmethionine (SAM) by a special $[Fe_4–S_4]^{2+/1+}$ cluster to generate the highly oxidizing 5'-deoxyadenosine radical (Ado$_*$) radical (Fontecave *et al.*, 2001). The reactivity of the Ado$_*$ is transferred to the substrate through abstraction of a hydrogen atom of the C–H target in a wide variety of reactions catalysed by the Radical-SAM superfamily of enzymes (Frey *et al.*, 2008). Members of the Radical-SAM enzyme family are characterised by the presence of a $[Fe_4–S_4]^{1+/2+}$ cluster, whose ligands are three cysteines of a conserved $CysX_5CysXCys$ motif.

2.6   Non-haem, Non-Fe–S Proteins

The third class of proteins consists of a heterogeneous collection which contain iron in a non-haem, non-iron–sulphur form. These proteins can be classified into three categories:

- **Mononuclear non-haem iron enzymes**: These include a large number of enzymes involved in oxygen activation and its incorporation into organic substrates.
- **Dinuclear non-haem iron enzymes**: These include a number of proteins of diverse biological activity, characterised by the presence of iron-oxo-bridged di- or polyiron aggregates at their metallic cores.
- **Proteins of iron storage, transport and metabolism.**

2.6.1   Mononuclear Non-haem Iron Enzymes

Thermodynamically reactions of organic molecules with O_2 are highly favourable and release a significant amount of energy. However, due to the spin mismatch between ground-state oxygen (triplet) and most organic substrates (singlet), the kinetic reactivity of $^3O_2$ is sluggish (Abu-Omar *et al.*, 2005). Nature has found an elegant solution to overcome this kinetic barrier by using transition metal ions, notably iron and copper. There are two classes of iron-containing enzymes involved in dioxygen activation, the first class being the haem enzymes, the prototype of which – cytochrome P450 – was discussed earlier. The second class is the non-haem iron enzymes, which can be further divided into mono- and di-nuclear iron enzymes; the former type will be discussed the following section (for a review, see Bruijnincx *et al.*, 2008).

Dioxygen reduction (oxidase activity) and activation for incorporation into organic substrates are catalysed by a large number of mononuclear non-haem iron enzymes. There are a growing number of crystal structures, and the extraordinary diverse number of reactions catalysed by these enzymes cannot fail to impress (Abu-Omar *et al.*, 2005; Costas *et al.*, 2004; Koehntop *et al.*, 2005). Most importantly, this wealth of structural data has established a superfamily of enzymes involved in the activation of dioxygen, with a new common structural feature motif (Koehntop *et al.*, 2005), which may be one of Nature's recurring motifs, like the haem cofactor and iron–sulphur clusters (Que, 2000). This consists of a mononuclear Fe(II) metal centre coordinated facially to two histidine residues and one carboxylate ligand (either an aspartate or a glutamate) (Figure 2.18a). This structural motif will be referred to as the '2-His-1-carboxylate facial triad' (Que, 2000). Its structural features are also characterised by the triad of three other coordination sites (X,Y and Z in Figure 2.18a) which are either occupied by weakly bound solvent molecules or are vacant – these sites are available for binding by oxygen, substrates and cofactors.

Despite catalysing a very diverse set of reactions, this superfamily of enzymes have a number of common mechanistic features which are shared by all members (Figure 2.18b). First, the typically six-coordinate resting state of the enzyme is rather unreactive towards dioxygen (A). Subsequent binding of substrate or cofactor results in the formation of a coordinatively unsaturated, five-coordinate metal centre, which greatly enhances its dioxygen affinity (B) (Neidig and Solomon, 2004). The coupling of reactivity with substrate binding may protect the enzyme against self-inactivation. In the next step, dioxygen is activated for reaction by direct binding to the metal centre (C). The enzymes employ two different methods of activating dioxygen, and overcome the low one-electron redox potential of dioxygen by acquiring additional reducing equivalents from either a redox-active cofactor or a redox-active substrate (Neidig and Solomon, 2004). The flexibility of the triad allows the binding of dioxygen trans to any of the three endogenous residues, and the different trans-effects have been suggested to modulate the reactivity of the enzyme (Koehntop *et al.*, 2005;

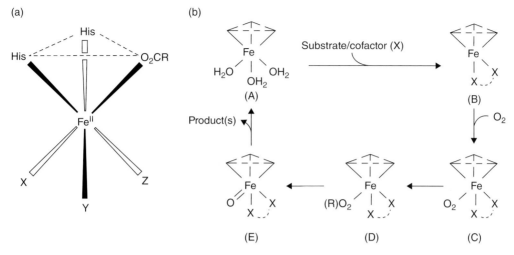

Figure 2.18   *(a) Schematic representation of the 2-His-1-carboxylate facial triad (X, Y and Z denote weakly bound solvent molecules or vacant sites). (b) General mechanistic pathway for reactions catalysed by the 2-His-1-carboxylate facial triad superfamily of non-haem iron(II) enzymes*

Hegg and Que, 1997). Dioxygen is then reduced to the peroxide level (D) and from this point onwards the proposed mechanisms for the different enzymes diverge. In most cases, O–O bond cleavage and the formation of a high-valent iron–oxo species is invoked (E). This iron–oxo species, regardless of whether it is Fe(IV) or Fe(V), is proposed to be the actual oxidizing species.

The enzymes featuring the 2-His-1-carboxylate facial triad can be classified into five different groups based on their structural characteristics, reactivity, and specific requirements for catalysis (Bruijnincx *et al.*, 2008): (i) extradiol-cleaving catechol dioxygenases; (ii) Rieske oxygenases; (iii) α-ketoglutarate-dependent enzymes; (iv) pterin-dependent hydroxylases; and (v) a miscellaneous category.

2.6.1.1   Extradiol-cleaving Catechol Dioxygenases

The catechol dioxygenases are part of Nature's strategy for the degradation of aromatic compounds by bacteria in the environment (Vaillancourt *et al.*, 2006). They catalyse oxidative ring cleavage, involving either extradiol-cleaving enzymes, which use a non-haem Fe(II) active site or intradiol-cleaving catechol dioxygenase counterparts, which represent a minor pathway, with a non-haem iron(III) active site (Figure 2.19). The enzyme–substrate (catechol) complexes of the extradiol enzyme 2,3-dihydroxybiphenyl 1,2-dioxygenase (right, 1KND.pdb) and the intradiol enzyme catechol 1,2-dioxygenase (left, 1DLT.pdb) are also shown in Figure 2.19. The extradiol-cleaving dioxygenases are the more versatile of the two groups, and in addition to catecholic substrates also accept gentisate, salicylate, hydroquinone and 2-aminophenol as substrate. The catechol-cleaving dioxygenases are comprehensively reviewed by Vaillancourt *et al.* (2006).

2.6.1.2   Rieske Oxygenases

A common first step in the biodegradation of aromatic compounds is their conversion into *cis*-dihydroxylated metabolites. The Rieske oxygenases, which require a mononuclear non-haem iron centre and a Rieske-type Fe_2S_2 cluster, are involved in the regio- and stereospecific *cis*-dihydroxylation

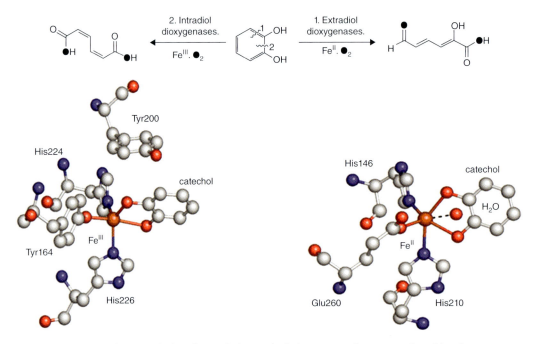

Figure 2.19 *Top: The extradiol and intradiol catechol cleavage pathways catalysed by the respective catechol-cleaving dioxygenases. Bottom: Enzyme–substrate (catechol) complexes of the extradiol enzyme 2,3-dihydroxybiphenyl 1,2-dioxygenase (right, 1KND.pdb) and the intradiol enzyme catechol 1,2-dioxygenase (left, 1DLT.pdb)*

of aromatic hydrocarbons, which are common pollutants of soil and groundwater. The Rieske oxygenases are multicomponent enzymes consisting of a reductase, an oxygenase and, in some cases, a ferredoxin component (Figure 2.20). Substrate oxidation takes place in the oxygenase component, which contains both a Rieske-type [2Fe–2S] cluster and the mononuclear non-haem iron active site. The oxygenase component structures were all shown to be trimers of the α_3 or $\alpha_3\beta_3$ types. Within a single subunit, the Rieske cluster and the non-haem iron centre are too far apart to allow for electron transfer (~45 Å). However, the trimeric quaternary structure allows for electron transfer from a Rieske cluster to a mononuclear iron centre from the neighbouring subunit; these are only ~12 Å apart. It is proposed that electron transfer from the Rieske centre to the mononuclear iron of the neighbouring subunit takes place via a fully conserved aspartic acid residue that bridges the two metal sites, which is involved in gating electron transport. Molecular oxygen has been shown to bind side-on in naphthalene dioxygenase (Figure 2.21).

The general mechanism of dioxygen activation is believed to be the same for all Rieske oxygenases. The binding of dioxygen to the metal is enhanced upon substrate binding through the conversion to a five-coordinate metal centre (Neidig and Solomon, 2004). The reactivity of the ferrous centre is controlled allosterically by the redox state of the Rieske cofactor. Reduction of the cluster leads to conformational changes at the active site, opening up a pathway for the binding of dioxygen (Martins *et al.*, 2005) and electron transfer from the Rieske cluster (Costas *et al.*, 2004; Ferraro *et al.*, 2007). This results in the formation of a side-on iron–(hydro)peroxide complex, consistent with the crystallographically characterised dioxygen adduct (Karlsson *et al.*, 2003). From this point onwards, different mechanisms for the actual oxygen insertion steps have been proposed. A key difference is the fate of the iron(III)–(hydro)peroxide intermediate, which can either act as

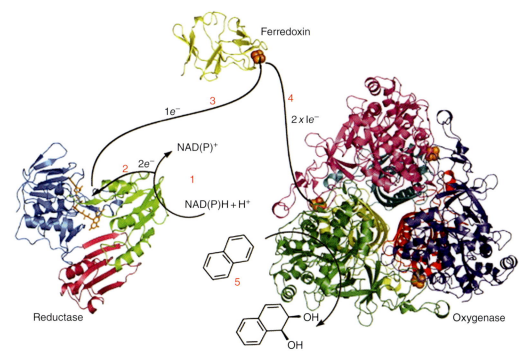

Figure 2.20   *The three components of a Rieske oxygenase system. (1) The reductase (BPDO-R$_{KKS102}$ shown in figure) oxidises NAD(P)H to NADP$^+$ at the NAD(P)H binding site, capturing two electrons. (2) The electrons are stored on the flavin until (3) the reductase completes a one-electron reduction of the ferredoxin component (BPDO-F$_{LB400}$ shown in figure). (4) The ferredoxin shuttles the electron received from the reductase to the oxygenase Rieske cluster (BPDO-O$_{RHA1}$ shown in figure). This step occurs twice for (5) each molecule of product formed at the mononuclear iron site. The flavin is shown as a stick representation, the Rieske cluster and mononuclear iron are shown as spheres. Reproduced with permission from Elsevier from Ferraro, D.J., Gakhar, L. and Ramaswamy, S. (2005) Rieske business: Structure–function of Rieske non-heme oxygenases. Biochem. Biophys. Res. Commun., **334**, 175–190*

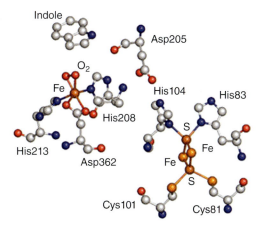

Figure 2.21   *Dioxygen bound side-on to the metal centre in naphthalene dioxygenase (NDO) with bound substrate analogue indole (1O7N.pdb). The [2Fe–2S] Rieske cluster and a conserved aspartate are also shown*

the reactive species itself and directly attack a substrate or, alternatively, first undergo O–O bond cleavage to yield an HO–Fe(V)=O intermediate.

Rieske dioxygenases catalyse a wide variety of reactions, including the oxidation of highly toxic polychlorinated biphenyls, and by evolutionary engineering the substrate scope of these enzymes has been extended to such toxins as dioxin and chlorinated ethenes (Furokawa *et al.*, 2004). Other microbial Rieske dioxygenases are able to degrade several different polycyclic aromatic hydrocarbons, including the well-known carcinogens chrysene, benzopyrene and benzanthracene (Jouanneau *et al.*, 2006; Ferraro *et al.*, 2007). Some Rieske oxygenases show even more versatility, catalysing other oxidations such as monohydroxylation, desaturation, sulfoxidation, O- and N-dealkylation, and amine oxidation.

2.6.1.3 *α-Ketoglutarate-dependent Enzymes*

Ferrous iron and α-ketoglutarate (αKG)-dependent oxygenases were first identified in studies on collagen biosynthesis, where they were found to catalyse the hydroxylation of prolyl and lysyl-residues (Myllyharju and Kivirikko, 2004). Subsequently, the enzymes have been found to be present in most organisms. αKG oxygenases represent the largest subfamily of non-haem iron enzymes with the 2-His-1-carboxylate facial triad (Costas *et al.*, 2004). They catalyse a very wide range of oxidative reactions, probably constituting the most versatile group of oxidizing biological catalysts identified to date. As many of these transformations present an enormous challenge for synthetic organic chemists, the enzymes are of special chemical interest (Clifton *et al.*, 2006; Flashman and Schofield, 2007). In the vast majority of cases they couple the two-electron oxidation of their substrates to the oxidation of αKG to succinate and carbon dioxide. The subfamily catalyses a remarkably diverse set of oxidative transformations including hydroxylation, desaturation, ring closure, ring expansion, epimerisation and many others, which intervene in processes as diverse as the synthesis of antibiotics, DNA repair, oxygen sensing, and the regulation of transcription (Figure 2.22). The most common reaction catalysed is hydroxylation, and there are three classes of hydroxylation reactions which have important medical implications: (i) the repair of alkylated DNA and RNA bases; (ii) histone demethylases; and (iii) proline hydroxylation of hypoxia-inducible factor (HIF). Tumour-derived mutations in the Krebs cycle enzyme isocitrate dehydrogenase reduce α-ketoglutarate levels and cause the accumulation of an α-KG antagonist, 2-hydroxyglutarate, leading to the inhibition of both α-KG-dependent histone lysine demethylases (KDMs) and the TET family of DNA hydroxylases (Yang *et al.*, 2012). These inhibitions alter the epigenetic control of stem and progenitor cell differentiation. As we will see in greater detail in Chapter 9, the hydroxylation of prolyl residues in HIF plays an important role mediating the mammalian response to low oxygen tension (hypoxia) and also contributes an important means of regulating iron homeostasis.

A general, conserved mechanism for the α-KG-dependent oxygenases has been proposed and is presented in Figure 2.23, as exemplified by TauD. The resting enzyme has an octahedral iron(II) metal centre with the facial triad, and three water molecules completing the coordination sphere (Figure 2.23; A). α-Ketoglutarate binds first in a bidentate fashion by displacing two water molecules and the metal centre remains six-coordinate (B), followed by the binding of substrate in the proximity of (but not directly to) the metal ion. On substrate binding the remaining water ligand is lost and the coordination around the ferrous ion changes to five-coordinate square-pyramidal (C). Displacement of the last water molecule is thought to be essential for catalysis, and poises the metal for reaction with dioxygen. The greatly enhanced reactivity of the metal centre towards dioxygen after substrate binding effectively favours the generation of (potentially damaging)

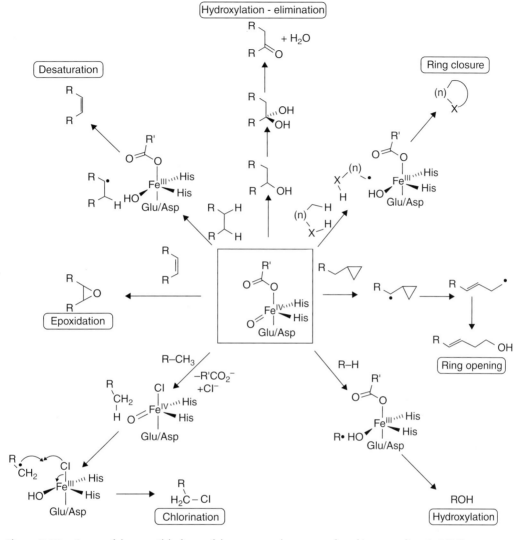

Figure 2.22 *Some of the possible fates of the proposed common ferryl intermediate in 2OG oxygenase catalysis. From Clifton* et al. *(2006)*

reactive intermediates only in the presence of the target substrate, and in this way protects the enzyme from inactivation by self-hydroxylation reactions. Dioxygen now binds, resulting in the formation of an adduct with significant Fe(III)-superoxide radical anion character (D). Nucleophilic attack of the carbonyl carbon atom results in a cyclic ferryl bridged-peroxo species (E). In the next step, decarboxylation and O–O bond cleavage yield succinate, carbon dioxide and a high-valent Fe(IV)=O species (F), which is the intermediate responsible for the substrate oxidation leading to hydroxylation or a related two-electron oxidation. From this point onwards the chemistry of each enzyme diverges, and the different subsequent steps result in the wide variety of oxidative trans-formations that this subgroup catalyses. It has been suggested that the chemistry that follows after

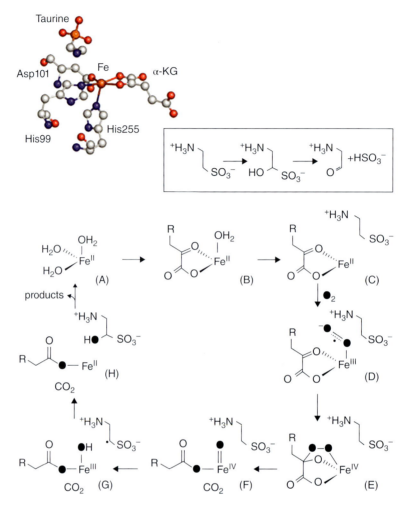

Figure 2.23 *Top: Active site of the ternary TauD–Fe(II)–α-KG–taurine complex (1OS7.pdb). Bottom: Consensus mechanism for α-KG-dependent hydroxylases, exemplified for TauD*

the generation of the pivotal ferryl–oxo species results mainly from the structural characteristics of the specific substrate (reviewed in Bruijnincx *et al.*, 2008).

2.6.1.4 *Pterin-dependent Hydroxylases*

The aromatic amino acid hydroxylases, phenylalanine hydroxylase, tyrosine hydroxylase and tryptophan hydroxylase, represent a very small family of enzymes but they are nonetheless essential for mammalian physiology, with important implications for a number of neurological diseases (as we will see in Chapter 15). They catalyse the regiospecific monohydroxylation of their namesake amino acids, with concomitant oxidation of the pterin cofactor. Tyrosine hydroxylase catalyses the initial step in the biosynthesis of catecholamine neurotransmitters, phenylalanine hydroxylase converts phenylalanine to tyrosine, and tryptophan hydroxylase is involved in the synthesis of the neurotransmitter serotonin. The three enzymes show sequence and structural similarity. Large conformational changes upon pterin and substrate binding are observed, but in contrast to the other subfamilies neither the substrate nor the cofactor binds directly to the metal centre. The monodentate glutamate becomes bidentate, water molecules are lost, and the pterin cofactor is displaced towards the iron (Figure 2.24). The proposed mechanism is shown in Figure 2.24, for phenylalanine hydroxylase. First, a (putative) pterinperoxo–iron(II) species is formed (B), which cleaves heterolytically to yield a reactive iron(IV)–oxo intermediate (C). Electrophilic attack of the substrate then results in a cationic intermediate (D). Kinetic isotope effects have been determined for all three enzymes. In the case of TrpH an inverse isotope effect was found, consistent with the hydroxylation being the rate-limiting step (Moran *et al.*, 2000). For TyrH and PheH, the results obtained for the wild-type enzymes were less straightforward, but in both cases isotope effects could be unmasked by the use of mutant enzymes, which allowed for a partitioning of intermediates via branched pathways (Frantom and Fitzpatrick, 2003). This uncoupling resulted in the observation of the expected isotope effects for both TyrH (Frantom and Fitzpatrick, 2003) and PheH (Pavon and Fitzpatrick, 2005). An NIH-shift and subsequent tautomerisation ultimately resulted in product formation (E, F) (for a review, see Bruijnincx *et al.*, 2008).

2.6.1.5 Miscellaneous Enzymes

The final category is a diverse collection of enzymes that do not fit into the previous four classes, of which only one – isopenicillin N synthase – is discussed. The importance of penicillin- and cephalosporin-related antibiotics in clinical medicine cannot be underestimated, and this has stimulated the study of their biosynthetic pathways. The key steps in the biosynthesis of these antibiotics in some microorganisms are the oxidative ring closure reactions of δ-(L-α-aminoadipoyl)-L-cysteinyl-D-valine (ACV) to form isopenicillin N, the precursor of penicillins and cephalosporins. The enzyme which catalyses this transformation is isopenicillin N synthase (IPNS), which requires Fe(II) and O_2 for activity. IPNS shows a high sequence homology to the α-ketoglutarate-dependent enzymes, but does not require α-ketoglutarate as cofactor and does not incorporate oxygen into the product. The overall reaction utilises the full oxidative potential of O_2, giving two molecules of H_2O for each O_2, and the four electrons required for dioxygen reduction come from the substrate. The active site of the ternary IPNS–Fe(II)–acv–NO complex and the oxidative double ring closure catalysed by IPNS are shown in Figure 2.25.

2.6.2 Dinuclear Non-haem Iron Proteins

A large number of proteins contain non-haem dinuclear iron centres which perform a wide variety of functions. Their common link is that their dimetallic centre is a preferred biological scaffold for binding and activating O_2. Among their functions are iron storage in eukaryotic and bacterial ferritins (see Chapter 8), O_2 transport in haemerythrin, radical generation in ribonucleotide reductases (RNR-R2), peroxide scavenging in rubrerythrin, hydrocarbon desaturation in stearoyl-acyl carrier protein Δ^9 desaturase, and hydrocarbon oxidation in bacterial multicomponent monooxygenases (BMMs) (Kurtz, 1997; Merkx *et al.*, 2001). The latter enzymes include soluble methane monooxygenases (sMMOs), toluene/*o*-xylene monooxygenases, phenol hydroxylases and alkene monooxygenases (reviewed in Sazinsky and Lippard, 2006). More recent additions include the sequential oxidation of aminoarenes to nitroarenes via hydroxylamine and nitroso intermediates (Choi *et al.*, 2008) in the synthesis of the antibiotic aureothin, the ageing-associated protein CLK 1 (Behan and Lippard, 2010), and a cyanobacterial aldehyde decarbonylase (Krebs *et al.*, 2011).

They were originally described as 'di-iron-oxo' proteins, probably due to the common misconception that all members of the family contain an oxo bridge. The original (and for many years the

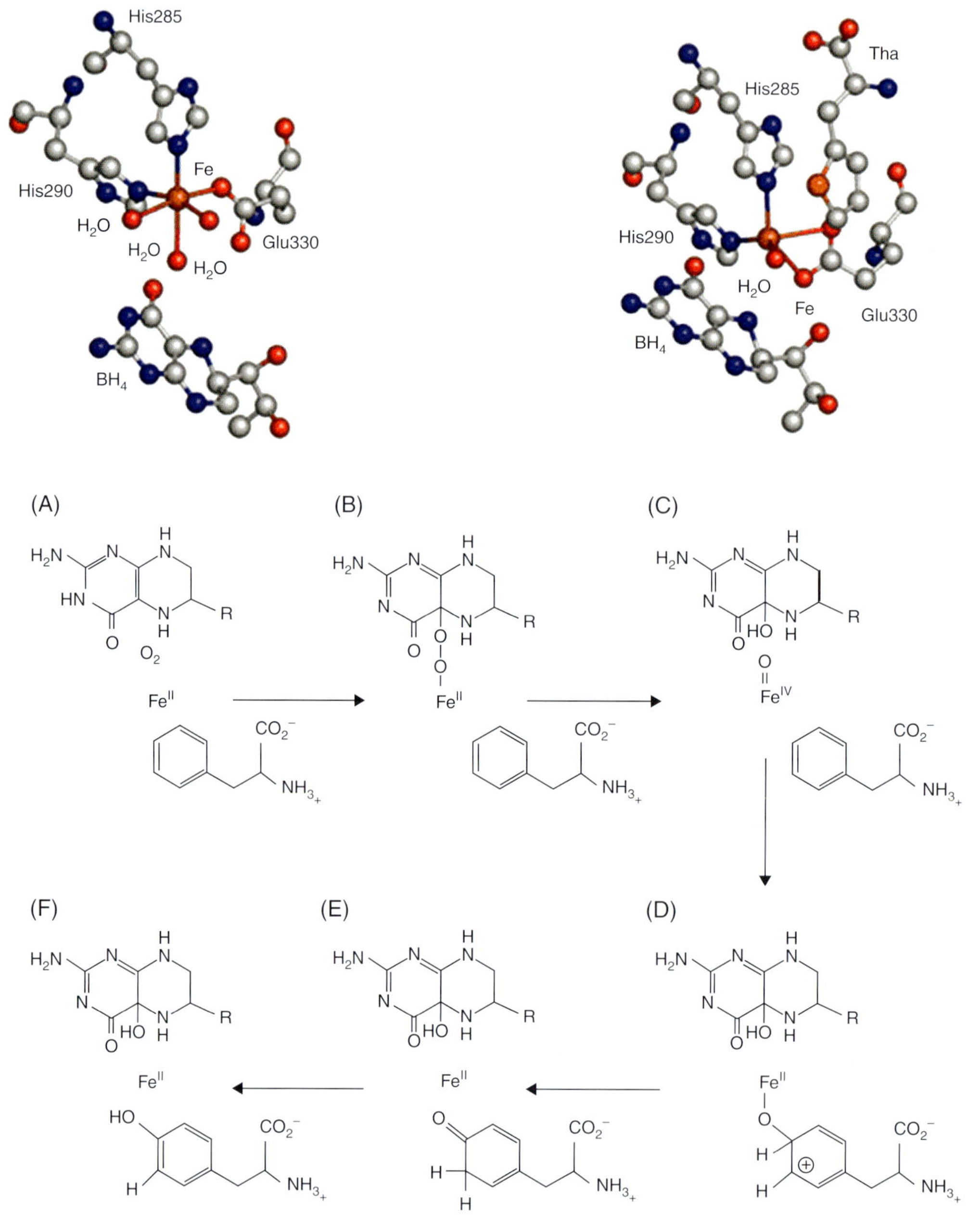

Figure 2.24 *Top: Structural changes upon substrate binding to the active site of phenylalanine hydroxylase: the binary PheH–Fe(II)–BH₄ complex (1J8U.pdb) (left) and the ternary PheH–Fe(II)–BH₄–tha complex (1KW0.pdb) (right). Bottom: Proposed reaction mechanism for the AAAHs, exemplified for PheH. Reproduced with permission from Bruijnincx, P.C., van Koten, G. and Klein Gebbink, R.J. (2008) Mononuclear non-heme iron enzymes with the 2-His-1-carboxylate facial triad: recent developments in enzymology and modeling studies. Chem. Soc. Rev., 37, 2716–2744; © 2008, Royal Society of Chemistry*

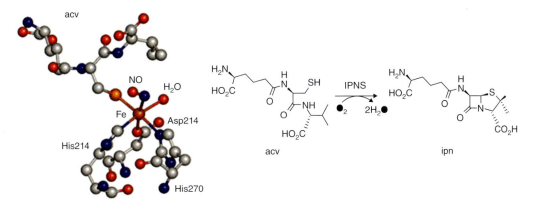

Figure 2.25 *Active site of the ternary IPNS–Fe(II)–acv–NO complex and the oxidative double ring closure catalysed by IPNS*

only) member of this class, haemerythrin, does indeed contain an oxo-bridged di-iron (III) site (Kurtz, 1997), but a more appropriate structural description would be di-iron-carboxylate proteins (Nordlund and Eklund, 1995). The common link in all of these proteins is that their dimetallic centre is a preferred biological scaffold for binding and activating O_2. The carboxylato-bridged di-iron core is contained within a four-helix bundle, with the two iron atoms separated by 0.4 nm or less, and in most cases four of the iron-coordinating ligands are provided by two E(D/H)XXH motifs. The three-dimensional structures of a number of di-iron proteins are shown in Figure 2.26 (Nordlund and Eklund, 1995).

Despite the striking structural similarities, the di-iron proteins represent an enormous functional diversity, and raise the interesting question of how we can correlate the geometry of their di-iron sites with their different reactivities towards O_2 and additional substrates can be correlated. The dioxygen-utilizing di-iron centres of a number of family members in reduced and oxidised states are shown in Figure 2.27. The different functions and activities of these enzymes derive from the surrounding protein environment, which has evolved to control the primary and secondary coordination spheres of the dimetallic centre, introduce active-site pockets, afford substrate access and product egress channels, and create electron-transfer (ET) pathways (Sazinsky and Lippard, 2006). In the following, attention will be focused on the well-characterised di-iron centre of sMMO, before turning briefly to RNR-R2.

Most BMMs, including the sMMO and PH subfamilies, require three proteins for their catalytic activity (Figure 2.28), a large hexameric hydroxylase ($\alpha_2\beta_2\gamma_2$), which contains the carboxylato-bridged di-iron core, a reductase with both [Fe_2–S_2], FAD cofactors which shuttle electrons from NADH to the di-iron centre, and a small regulatory protein which couples electron transport with substrate activation. Among all known BMMs, a universally conserved set of glutamate and histidine ligands are responsible for binding the two iron atoms (Merkx *et al.*, 2001). In the resting di-iron(III) state of MMOH$_{ox}$, one side of the dimetallic unit is formed by two histidine residues, which coordinate to positions distal to the active-site pocket, and a bridging carboxylate ion (Figure 2.27a). This three-amino acid structural motif is conserved in Δ^9 desaturase, RNR-R2, rubrerythrin, haemerythrin, ferritin, and bacterioferritin (Figure 2.27) (Kurtz, 1997). The remaining ligands in the first coordination sphere of MMOH and ToMOH differ significantly from those in the other di-iron proteins. One Fe is coordinated by a monodentate glutamate and a terminal water molecule, while two monodentate carboxylates coordinate to the second Fe. In the resting

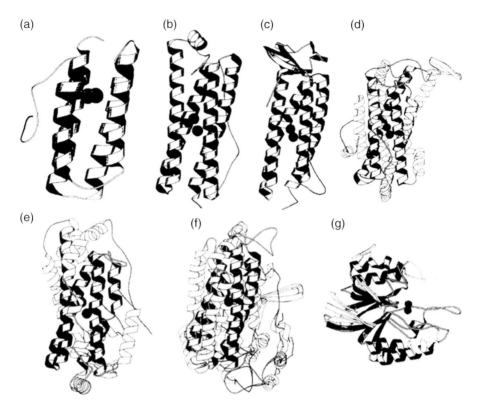

Figure 2.26 *Three-dimensional structures of di-iron proteins. The metals are shown as black balls. (a) Haemerythrin; (b) Bacterioferritin; (c) Rubrerythrin (the iron–sulphur domain is at the top); (d) Ribonucleotide reductase R2; (e) Stearoyl-acyl carrier protein Δ⁹ desaturase; (f) Methane monooxygenase hydrolase a-subunit; (g) Purple acid phosphatase. All helical proteins contain two metal-binding helix pairs (dark shaded in (b–f), the larger proteins have several extra structural elements. Reproduced with permission from Elsevier from Nordlund, P. and Eklund, H. (1995) Diiron-carboxylate proteins.* Curr. Opin. Struct. Biol., **5**, *758–766*

state, hydroxide ions occupy additional bridging positions to complete a pseudooctahedral geometry about the iron atoms, which are separated by 3.0–3.1 Å (Whittington and Lippard, 2001). In different structures of MMOH and ToMOH, product alcohols and monoanions such as formate, acetate and thioglycolate occupy the bridging position facing the hydrophobic active-site pocket, strongly implicating both C−H and O_2 activation at this site (parts A and B of Figure 2.27) (Sazinsky *et al.*, 2004; Whittington and Lippard, 2001; Sazinsky and Lippard, 2005).

For the di-iron sites of Δ⁹ desaturase, RNR-R2, rubrerythrin and bacterioferritin the flanking carboxylate ligands adopt different orientations and coordination modes, suggesting one way in which the chemistry of these enzymes is differentially tuned (Figure 2.27).

Helix E of the MMOH and ToMOH four-helix bundle has a π-helical segment in a region of the protein that contributes a glutamate ligand to the di-iron centre and several residues to the active-site pocket. This 10-amino acid stretch of π helix in the middle of a mostly α-helical segment also occurs in RNR-R2 and rubrerythrin, but is absent in ferritin, bacterioferritin and haemerythrin. The differences in helical structure may be of functional significance, but there is currently no clear understanding of such.

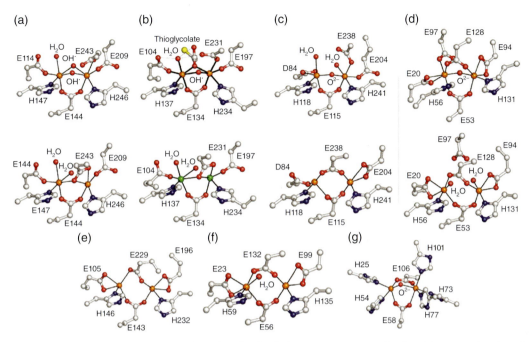

Figure 2.27 *Dioxygen-utilizing carboxylate-bridged di-iron centres. (a) Oxidised (top) and reduced (bottom) MMOH. (b) Oxidised (top) and Mn^{II}-reconstituted ToMOH (bottom). (c) Oxidised (top) and reduced (bottom) RNR-R2. (d) Oxidised (top) and reduced (bottom) rubrerythrin. (e) Reduced stearoyl-ACP Δ^9 desaturase. (f) Reduced bacterioferritin. (g) Methemerythrin. The active site of c. trachomatis RNR-R2 is identical to that of MMOH$_{ox}$, although the bridging species is unknown. Fe1 is on the left, and Fe2 is on the right. All atoms and side chains are depicted in a ball and stick model and are coloured by atom type [carbon (grey), oxygen (red), nitrogen (blue), sulphur (yellow), iron (orange), and manganese (green)]. Reproduced with permission from Elsevier from Sazinsky, M.H. and Lippard, S.J. (2006) Correlating structure with function in bacterial multicomponent monooxygenases and related diiron proteins.* Acc. Chem. Res., **39**, 558–566

Class I ribonucleotide reductases RNRs use a free-radical mechanism, in which a transient cysteine thiyl radical (C$^{\bullet}$) in the active site of the enzyme initiates substrate reduction by abstraction of a hydrogen atom (H$^{\bullet}$) from C3′ of the NDP substrate (Figure 2.1). They consist of two nonidentical homodimeric subunits (R1 and R2, sometimes referred to as α and β) (Figure 2.29), with the di-iron centre and the stable tyrosyl radical ($\gamma Y_{122}^{\bullet}$ in the *E. coli* enzyme), which it generates in close proximity to the di-iron cluster, in the smaller R2 subunit (Ehrenberg and Reichard, 1972; Larsson and Sjöberg, 1986). During catalysis, the radical is continuously shuttled to the cysteine (C439) of the larger R1 subunit, generating the thiyl radical required for activation of the substrate. R1 contains both the catalytic site for ribonucleotide reduction and the allosteric sites for its regulation (Nordlund and Reichard, 2006). The stable tyrosyl radical (Y($\bullet$)) in the R2 subunit of the class Ia RNR is generated by self-assembly from Fe(II)$_2$R2, O$_2$, and reducing equivalents (Ehrenberg and Reichard, 1972; Atkin *et al.*, 1973).

A model of the complex constructed by computer docking, based on X-ray structures of the individual subunits (Uhlin and Eklund, 1994) and subsequently validated by electron–electron double resonance spectroscopic experiments (Bennati *et al.*, 2005; Seyedsayamdost

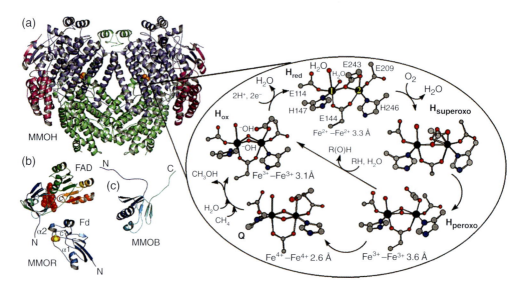

Figure 2.28 *Structures of sMMO components and proposed reaction cycle. (a) MMOH; (b) The MMOR FAD and ferredoxin (Fd) domains; (c) MMOB. The MMOH α, β and γ subunits are coloured blue, green, and purple, respectively. Iron, sulfur and FAD are coloured orange, yellow and red, respectively, and are depicted as spheres. The sMMO reaction cycle is shown on the right with atoms coloured according to type [iron (black), carbon (grey), oxygen (red) and nitrogen (blue)]. Reproduced with permission from Elsevier from Sazinsky, M.H. and Lippard, S.J. (2006) Correlating structure with function in bacterial multicomponent monooxygenases and related diiron proteins.* Acc. Chem. Res., **39**, *558–566*

et al., 2007), indicates (Figure 2.29) a distance of >35 Å between $Y_{122}^{•}$ in the R2 and the $H^{•}$-abstracting C_{439} in R1 (Minnihan *et al.*, 2013). Electron transfer between C_{439} and Y_{122} by a single tunnelling step over such a distance would be far too slow to account for the enzyme's turnover rate ($2–10$ s^{-1}) (Stubbe *et al.*, 2003; Ge *et al.*, 2003). Instead, this long-range intersubunit ET occurs by a multistep 'hopping' mechanism, mediated via the formation of transient amino acid radicals along a chain of strictly conserved aromatic amino acids (Figure 2.30), as originally proposed by Uhlin and Eklund (1994). This long-range, intersubunit radical hopping in class Ia RNR from *E. coli*, is thought to follow a specific pathway comprised of the redox-active aromatic amino acids: $Y_{122}^{•} \leftrightarrow [W_{48}?] \leftrightarrow Y_{356}$ in β2 to $Y_{731} \leftrightarrow Y_{730} \leftrightarrow C_{439}$ in α2 (summarised in Minnihan *et al.*, 2013). Each step necessitates a proton-coupled electron transfer (PCET). The current hypothesis (Figure 2.30) holds that protons move orthogonally to the electron in β2, and colinearly with the electron in α2. The mechanism across the α/β interface is unknown. There is no direct evidence that W_{48} and its putative H^{+} acceptor, D_{237}, participate in long-range PCET during turnover. Recent results strongly suggest that the $(Fe^{III})_{2}$ cluster also actively functions in the catalytic cycle, specifically during translocation of the oxidizing equivalent from its resting position on $Y_{122}^{•}$ in β to the nucleotide reduction site in α. Reduction of $Y_{122}^{•}$ upon forward radical translocation requires transfer of a proton to yield a neutral Y_{122}, which is proposed to be derived from the water molecule bound to the di-iron centre (Wörsdörfer *et al.*, 2013).

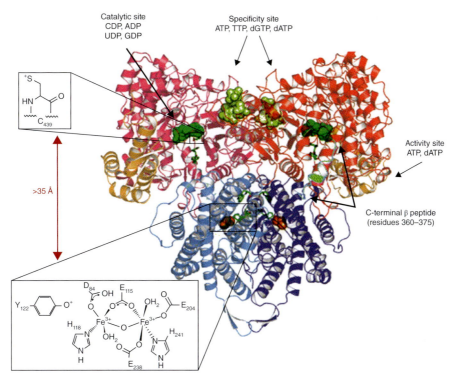

Figure 2.29 *Docking model of the* E. coli *α2β2 complex. α2 (pink and red) contains three nucleotide binding sites. β2 (light and dark blue) contains the diferric-Y• cofactor; residues 340–375 are not resolved in this structure. A peptide corresponding to the C-terminal 20 amino acids of β is bound to each α, a portion of which (residues 360–375) is resolved in the crystal structure (cyan). The 'ATP cone' region of α, which contains the effector site that governs activity, is coloured orange. This model separates Y122• in β2 from C439 in α2 by >35 Å. GDP (green), TTP (yellow), and the Fe₂O core of the diferric cluster (orange) are shown in CPK space-filling models. Residues constituting the RT pathway (green) are shown in sticks. Reprinted with permission from Minnihan, E.C., Nocera, D.G. and Stubbe, J. (2013) Reversible, long-range radical transfer in E. coli class Ia ribonucleotide reductase. Acc. Chem. Res.,* **46**, *2524–2535; © 2013, American Chemical Society*

2.6.3 Proteins of Iron Storage, Transport and Metabolism

These include the iron storage proteins, ferritin and haemosiderin; the iron transport protein, transferrin and its receptor; microbial siderophore receptors, and other receptors involved in iron uptake together with ancillary proteins involved in microbial iron uptake, transport and homeostasis; divalent metal transporters and the iron export protein ferroportin; ferrireductases; iron regulatory proteins and the systemic iron regulatory peptide hepcidin; haem transporters and haem oxygenases, to mention but a few. This final group of proteins will be discussed in greater detail in the chapters related to microbial iron uptake (Chapters 3 and 4), cellular iron uptake and export in mammals (Chapter 6), intracellular iron utilisation (Chapter 8) and cellular and systemic iron homeostasis (Chapter 10).

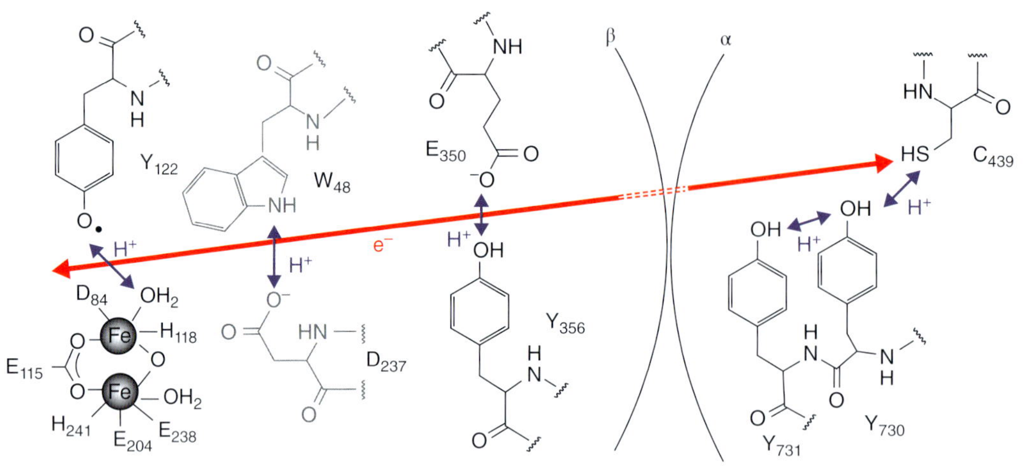

Figure 2.30 *Working mechanism for long-range PCET pathway in* E. coli *class Ia RNR. The current hypothesis holds that protons (blue arrows) move orthogonally to the electron (red arrow) in β2 and colinearly with the electron in α2. The mechanism across the α/β interface is unknown. There is no direct evidence that W_{48} and its putative H^+ acceptor, D_{237}, participate in long-range PCET during turnover, and therefore they are shown in gray. Reprinted with permission from Minnihan, E.C., Young, D.D., Schultz, P.G. and Stubbe, J. (2011) Incorporation of fluorotyrosines into ribonucleotide reductase using an evolved, polyspecific aminoacyl-tRNA synthetase. J. Am. Chem. Soc., **133**, 15942–15945; © 2011, American Chemical Society*

2.7 The Dark Side of Iron: ROS, RNS and NTBI

The appearance of cyanobacteria, capable of using solar energy to split water and evolve molecular dioxygen about 2.7×10^9 years ago, was one of the most momentous events in the evolution of planet Earth. The essentially reducing atmosphere of Earth was progressively transformed into the oxidizing atmosphere that we have today. In a relatively short time on a geological timescale, oxygen became a dominant chemical entity. One of the consequences was that iron, freely available in its reduced Fe(II) form, became much less so, as the product of its oxidation, Fe(III), was hydrolyzed, polymerised and precipitated. Those organisms which developed respiratory chains were able to extract almost 20 times more energy from metabolism than was available using redox-balanced fermentations. However, the downside was that molecular oxygen proved to be toxic, generating oxygen-derived free radicals, reactive oxygen species (ROS) in the presence of iron (and copper). The most potentially dangerous of the ROS is the hydroxyl ion, OH·, a short-lived but highly reactive free radical, which causes enormous damage to biological molecules. In addition to ROS, reactive nitrogen species (RNS) are also generated, notably NO. Under normal conditions, such free radicals will be rapidly detoxified by the body's defence systems described below. However, as we will see, under certain circumstances greater quantities of ROS and RNS are pro-duced, which will ultimately overwhelm the cellular defence mechanisms. This is the so-called oxygen paradox – oxygen is an absolute necessity for an energy-economical anaerobic lifestyle, yet it is a potential toxin. This represents the paradox of aerobic life, the 'Oxygen Paradox' (Davies, 1995), namely that higher eukaryotic aerobic organisms cannot exist without oxygen, yet oxygen is inherently dangerous to their existence. This 'dark side' of oxygen relates directly to the fact that each oxygen atom has one unpaired electron in its outer valence shell, and molecular oxygen has two unpaired electrons. Thus, atomic oxygen is a free radical and molecular oxygen is a (free) bi-radical. Concerted tetravalent reduction of oxygen by the mitochondrial electron-transport chain, to produce water, is considered to be a relatively safe process; however, the univalent reduction of oxygen generates reactive intermediates. The reductive environment of the cellular milieu provides ample opportunities for oxygen to undergo unscheduled univalent reduction. Thus, the superoxide anion radical, hydrogen peroxide and the extremely reactive hydroxyl radical are common products of life in an aerobic environment, and these agents appear to be responsible for oxygen toxicity.

2.7.1   ROS and RNS

ROS and RNS are constantly generated inside cells, and although there are several cellular systems that eliminate ROS, a number of endogenous and exogenous triggers can cause the overproduction of ROS and RNS, leading to a deleterious condition known as 'oxidative stress'. Highly reactive oxidant species such as ozone, hypochlorous acid, peroxynitrite, nitrogen dioxide and the hydroxyl radical are able to oxidise biomolecules irreversibly without preference or specificity (Uchida, 2003). As we will see in later chapters, this represents the 'dark side' of iron, and is thought to be intimately associated with a great number of pathological conditions including many neurode-generative diseases. However, a distinction must be made between the deleterious effects of high levels of ROS and RNS (catalysing pathways which result in essentially irreversible chemical modifications) and their effects at low concentrations which play an important role in cell signalling.

When ROS (particularly hydroxyl radicals) are generated by redox metals in proximity to membrane phospholipids they initiate the peroxidation of polyunsaturated fatty acids in the phospholipids. The lipid hydroperoxides thus generated break down through non-enzymatic Hock cleavage, to form a variety of lipid-derived α,β-unsaturated 4-hydroxyaldehydes (Catala, 2009) of which the most prominent are 4-hydroxynonenal (HNE) and 4-hydroxy-2-hexenal (HHE).

During oxidative stress, numerous post-translational modifications of proteins occur either from the direct oxidation of amino acid residues by highly reactive oxygen species or through the conversion of lipid and carbohydrate derivatives to compounds such as reactive aldehydes, such as HNE and HHE, which react with functional groups on proteins. A consequence is the formation of reactive protein carbonyl derivatives, generically termed 'protein carbonylation,' the level of which is widely used as a marker of oxidative protein damage (Dalle-Donne *et al.*, 2006). Because of their electron-withdrawing functional groups, the double bond of 4-HNE and other α,β-unsaturated aldehydes serves as a site for Michael addition with the sulphur atom of cysteine, the imidazole nitrogen of histidine and, to a lesser extent, the amine nitrogen of lysine. After forming Michael adducts, the aldehyde moiety may in some cases undergo Schiff base formation with amines of adjacent lysines, producing intra- and/or inter-molecular crosslinking.

Of the RNS, nitric oxide itself is only a mildly reactive intermediary, but it can act as a precursor of strong oxidants under pathological conditions associated with oxidative stress. Peroxynitrite, the reaction product of nitric oxide with superoxide radicals, is one of the principal players of nitric oxide-derived toxicity and can modify thiols and oxidise methione residues and nitrate tyrosine residues in proteins.

In contrast, the oxidants which are used at physiological concentrations in signal transduction must not only exhibit substrate specificity but also carry out reversible oxidations. These signalling oxidants include NO, *S*-nitrosothiols (SNOs) and H_2O_2, and act mainly by targeted modifications of cysteine residues in proteins, including S-nitrosylation and S-oxidation. Evidence has accumulated for the existence of an extensive intracellular redox signalling, control and feedback network based on different cysteine-containing proteins and enzymes (Janssen-Heininger *et al.*, 2008; Klomsiri, *et al.*, 2011). Together, these proteins enable the living cell to sense and respond towards external and internal redox changes in a measured, gradual and reversible manner (Chapter 13). The chemical basis of this crucial regulatory 'thiolstat' is the post-translational modification of protein cysteine residues, the complex redox chemistry of the thiol group of which can participate in different redox processes (Miki and Funato, 2012).

2.7.2 NTBI and LPI

Under normal circumstances the vast majority of iron present in plasma is bound to the single chain metal-binding glycoprotein, transferrin. Mean plasma iron and transferrin concentrations are 20 μmol l^{-1} and 30 μmol l^{-1}, respectively, corresponding to a transferrin saturation of approximately 30% (Brissot *et al.*, 2012). However, in the plasma of iron overload patients, another nonphysiological, low-molecular-weight form of iron is found which is not tightly bound to transferrin (Hershko *et al.*, 1978; Graham *et al.*, 1979). Originally designated non-transferrin bound iron (NTBI), since iron levels in the plasma of iron overload patients often supersede the total iron binding capacity (TIBC), it is clear that it represents a pathological source of uncontrolled ingress of iron into cells and the tissue iron loading which subsequently ensues (Hershko *et al.*, 1978; Graham *et al.*, 1979; Pietrangelo, 2007). An important component of NTBI is labile plasma iron (Graham *et al.*, 1979), the plasma counterpart of labile cell iron (LCI), defined as the transitory and exchangeable forms of iron which are important for cellular iron metabolism and homeostasis (Jacobs, 1977; Crichton, 2001; Cabantchik, 2014). LPI constitutes the redox-active and exchangeable forms of iron in plasma which are direct pharmacological targets for chelation (Pootrakul *et al.*, 2004), and also represents a parameter of potential diagnostic and therapeutic value (Cabantchik *et al.*, 2013).

The exact nature of NTBI remains uncertain. Computer simulations have suggested that the main component could be Fe(III) citrate (May and Williams, 1977), while NMR analyses of plasma from haemochromatosis patients indicate that both citrate and acetate could be involved (Grootveld *et al.*, 1989), and more recent studies have indicated dimeric and oligomeric iron citrate complexes (Evans *et al.*, 2008). However, the chemical speciation is likely to vary with the level of iron loading and the natural history of the disease (Silva and Hider, 2009). The determination of LPI and NTBI in the circulation of patients with iron overload poses a number of methodological problems, as is clearly illustrated by the results of an international interlaboratory study (Jacobs *et al.*, 2005). For recent reviews on LPI and NTBI and their clinical evaluation, see Brissot *et al.* (2012) and Cabantchik (2014).

References

Abu-Omar, M.M., Loaiza, A. and Hontzeas, N. (2005) Reaction mechanisms of mononuclear non-heme iron oxygenases. *Chem. Rev.*, **105**, 2227–2252.

Allen, J.W., Jackson, A.P., Rigden, D.J., Willis, A.C., *et al.* (2008) Order within a mosaic distribution of mitochondrial c-type cytochrome biogenesis systems? *FEBS J.*, **275**, 2385–2402.

Armstrong, F.A. (2005) Recent developments in dynamic electrochemical studies of adsorbed enzymes and their active sites. *Curr. Opin. Chem. Biol.*, **9**, 110–117.

Atkin, C.L., Thelander, L., Reichard, P. and Lang, G. (1973) Iron and free radical in ribonucleotide reductase. Exchange of iron and Mössbauer spectroscopy of the protein B2 subunit of the *Escherichia coli* enzyme. *J. Biol. Chem.*, **248**, 7464–7672.

Atta, M., Arragain, S., Fontecave, M., Mulliez, E., *et al.* (2012) The methylthiolation reaction mediated by the Radical-SAM enzymes. *Biochim. Biophys. Acta*, **1824**, 1223–1230.

Banci, L., Bertini, I., Luchinat, C. and Mori, M. (2010) NMR in structural proteomics and beyond. *Prog. Nucl. Magn. Spectrosc.*, **56**, 247–266.

Bashir, K., Nozoye, T., Ishimaru, Y., Nakanishi, H. and Nishizawa, N.K. (2013) Exploiting new tools for iron bio-fortification of rice. *Biotechnol. Adv.*, **31**, 1624–1633.

Behan, R.K. and Lippard, S.J. (2010) The aging-associated enzyme CLK-1 is a member of the carboxylate-bridged diiron family of proteins. *Biochemistry*, **49**, 9679–9681.

Bennati, M., Robblee, J.H., Mugnaini, V., Stubbe, J., *et al.* (2005) EPR distance measurements support a model for long-range radical initiation in *E. coli* ribonucleotide reductase. *J. Am. Chem. Soc.*, **127**, 15014–15015.

Bertini, I., Luchinat, C., Parigi, G. and Pierattelli, R. (2005) NMR spectroscopy of paramagnetic metalloproteins. *ChemBiochem*, **6**, 1536–1549.

Bill, E. (2013) [57]Fe Mössbauer Spectroscopy and Basic Interpretation of Mössbauer Parameters, in *Practical Approaches to Biological Inorganic Chemistry* (eds R.R. Crichton and R.O. Louro), Elsevier, Amsterdam and Oxford, pp. 109–130.

Bohr, C., Hasselbach, K.A. and Krogh, A. (1904) Über Einen in Biologischen Beziehung wichtigen Einfluss, den die Köhlensäurespannung des Blutes auf dessen Sauerstoffbindung übt. *Skand. Arch. Physiol.*, **15**, 401–412.

Bratton, M.R., Pressler, M.A. and Hosler, J.P. (1999) Suicide inactivation of cytochrome *c* oxidase: Catalytic turnover in the absence of subunit III alters the active site. *Biochemistry*, **38**, 16236–16245.

Brissot, P., Ropert, M., Le Lan, C. and Loréal, O. (2012) Non-transferrin bound iron: a key role in iron overload and iron toxicity. *Biochim. Biophys. Acta*, **1820**, 403–410.

Brito, J.A. and Archer, M. (2013) X-ray crystallography, in *Practical Approaches to Biological Inorganic Chemistry* (eds R.R. Crichton and R.O. Louro), Elsevier, Amsterdam and Oxford, pp. 217–255.

Bruijnincx, P.C., van Koten, G. and Klein Gebbink, R.J. (2008) Mononuclear non-heme iron enzymes with the 2-His-1-carboxylate facial triad: recent developments in enzymology and modeling studies. *Chem. Soc. Rev.*, **37**, 2716–2744.

Brzezinski, P. and Johansson, A.L. (2010) Variable proton-pumping stoichiometry in structural variants of cytochrome c oxidase. *Biochim. Biophys. Acta*, **1797**, 710–723.

Cabantchik, Z.I. (2014) Labile iron in cells and body fluids: physiology, pathology and pharmacology. *Front. Pharmacol.*, **13** (5), 45.

Cabantchik, Z.I., Sohn, Y.S., Breuer, W. and Espósito, B.P. (2013) The molecular and cellular basis of iron toxicity in iron overload disorders. Diagnostic and therapeutic approaches. *Thalassemia Reports*, **3**, 7–13.

Carpenter, C. and Payne, S.M. (2014) Regulation of iron transport systems in Enterobacteriaceae in response to oxygen and iron availability. *J. Inorg. Biochem.* **133**, 110–117.

Catala, A. (2009) Lipid peroxidation of membrane phospholipids generates hydroxy-alkenals and oxidized phospholipids active in physiological and/or pathological conditions. *Chem. Phys. Lipids*, **157**, 1–11.

Choi, Y.S., Zhang, H., Brunzelle, J.S., Nair, S.K. and Zhao, H. (2008) In vitro reconstitution and crystal structure of *p*-aminobenzoate N-oxygenase (AurF) involved in aureothin biosynthesis. *Proc. Natl Acad. Sci. USA*, **105**, 6858–6563.

Clifton, I.J., McDonough, M.A., Ehrismann, D., Kershaw, N.J., *et al.* (2006) Structural studies on 2-oxoglutarate oxygenases and related double-stranded beta-helix fold proteins. *J. Inorg. Biochem.*, **100**, 644–669.

Collman, J.P., Boulatov, R., Sunderland, C.J. and Fu, L. (2004) Functional analogues of cytochrome c oxidase, myoglobin, and hemoglobin. *Chem. Rev.*, **104**, 561–588.

Costas, M., Mehn, M.P., Jensen, M.P. and Que, L., Jr (2004) Dioxygen activation at mononuclear nonheme iron active sites: enzymes, models, and intermediates. *Chem. Rev.*, **104**, 939–986.

Cotruvo, J.A. and Stubbe, J. (2011) Class I ribonucleotide reductases: metallocofactor assembly and repair in vitro and in vivo. *Annu. Rev. Biochem.*, **80**, 733–767.

Cotruvo, J.A., Jr and Stubbe, J. (2012) Metallation and mismetallation of iron and manganese proteins in vitro and in vivo: the class I ribonucleotide reductases as a case study. *Metallomics*, **4**, 1020–1036.

Crichton R. (2001) *Inorganic Biochemistry of Iron Metabolism From Molecular Mechanisms to Clinical Consequences*. 2nd edn, Wiley, Chichester, pp. 326.

Crichton, R.R. and Louro, R.O. (eds) (2013) *Practical Approaches to Biological Inorganic Chemistry*. Elsevier, Amsterdam and Oxford, pp. 317.

Dalle-Donne, I., Aldini, G., Carini, M., Colombo, R., *et al.* (2006) Protein carbonylation, cellular dysfunction, and disease progression. *J. Cell. Mol. Med.*, **10**, 389–406.

Daniels, T.R., Bernabeu, E., Rodríguez, J.A., Patel, S., *et al.* (2013) The transferrin receptor and the targeted delivery of therapeutic agents against cancer. *Biochim. Biophys. Acta*, **1820**, 291–317.

Davies, K.J. (1995) Oxidative stress: the paradox of aerobic life. *Biochem. Soc. Symp.*, **61**, 1–31.

Ehrenberg, A. and Reichard, P. (1972) Electron spin resonance of the iron-containing protein B2 from ribonucleotide reductase. *J. Biol. Chem.*, **247**, 3485–3488.

Eisenberg, D. (1994) Max Perutz's achievements: How did he do it? *Protein Sci.*, **3**, 1625–1628.

Evans, R.W., Rafique, R., Zarea, A., Rapisarda C., *et al.* (2008) Nature of non-transferrin-bound iron: studies on iron citrate complexes and thalassemic sera. *J. Biol. Inorg. Chem.*, **13**, 57–74.

Feiters, M.C. and Mayer-Klauke, W. (2013) X-ray absorption spectroscopy in biology (BioXAS), in *Practical Approaches to Biological Inorganic Chemistry* (eds R.R. Crichton and R.O. Louro), Elsevier, Amsterdam and Oxford, pp. 131–160.

Ferraro, D.J., Gakhar, L. and Ramaswamy, S. (2005) Rieske business: Structure-function of Rieske non-heme oxygenases. *Biochem. Biophys. Res. Commun.*, **334**, 175–190.

Ferraro, D.J., Brown, E.N., Yu, C.L., Parales, R.E., *et al.* (2007) Structural investigations of the ferredoxin and terminal oxygenase components of the biphenyl 2,3-dioxygenase from *Sphingobium yanoikuyae* B1. *BMC Struct. Biol.*, **7**, 10.

Flashman, E. and Schofield, C.J. (2007) The most versatile of all reactive intermediates? *Nat. Chem. Biol.*, **3**, 86–87.

Fontecave, M., Mulliez, E. and Ollagnier-de-Choudens, S. (2001) Adenosylmethionine as a source of 5′-deoxyadenosyl radicals. *Curr. Opin. Chem. Biol.*, **5**, 506–511.

Fontecave, M., Atta, M. and Mulliez, E. (2004) S-adenosylmethionine: nothing goes to waste. *Trends Biochem. Sci.*, **29**, 243–249.

Frantom, P.A. and Fitzpatrick, P.F. (2003) Uncoupled forms of tyrosine hydroxylase unmask kinetic isotope effects on chemical steps. *J. Am. Chem. Soc.*, **125**, 16190–16191.

Frey, P.A., Hegeman, A.D. and Ruzicka, F.J. (2008) The radical SAM superfamily. *Crit. Rev. Biochem. Mol. Biol.*, **43**, 63–88.

Furokawa, K., Suenaga, H. and Goto, M. (2004) Biphenyl dioxygenases: functional versatilities and directed evolution. *J. Bacteriol.*, **186**, 5189–5196.

Ge, J., Yu, G., Ator, M.A. and Stubbe, J. (2003) Pre-steady-state and steady-state kinetic analysis of *E. coli* class I ribonucleotide reductase. *Biochemistry*, **42**, 10071–10083.

Graham, G., Bates, G.W., Rachmilewitz, E.A. and Hershko, C. (1979) Nonspecific serum iron in thalassemia: quantitation and chemical reactivity. *Am. J. Hematol.*, **6**, 207–217.

Grootveld, M., Bell, J.D., Halliwell, B., Aruoma, O.I., *et al.* (1989) Non-transferrin-bound iron in plasma or serum from patients with idiopathic hemochromatosis. Characterization by high performance liquid chromatography and nuclear magnetic resonance spectroscopy. *J. Biol. Chem.*, **264**, 4417–4422.

Hagen, W.R. (2006) EPR spectroscopy as a probe of metal centres in biological systems. *Dalton Trans.*, 4415–4434.

Hagen, W.R. (2009) *Biomolecular EPR Spectroscopy*. CRC Press Taylor & Francis Group, Boca Raton, Florida, pp. 249.

Hagen, W.R. (2013) EPR Spectroscopy, in *Practical Approaches to Biological Inorganic Chemistry*. (eds R.R. Crichton and R.O. Louro), Elsevier, Amsterdam and Oxford, pp. 53–75.

Hamilton, F.D. (1974) Ribonucleotide reductase from *Euglena gracilis*. A 5′-deoxyadenosyl-cobalamin-dependent enzyme. *J. Biol. Chem.*, **249**, 4428–4434.

Haurowitz, F. (1938) Des Gleichgewicht zwischen Hähoglobin und Sauerstoff. *Hoppe-Seyler*, **254**, 266–274.

Hegg, E.L. and Que, L., Jr (1997) The 2-His-1-carboxylate facial triad – an emerging structural motif in mononuclear non-heme iron(II) enzymes. *Eur. J. Biochem.*, **250**, 625–629.

Hemp, J. and Gennis, R.B. (2008) Diversity of the heme-copper superfamily in archaea: insights from genomics and structural modeling. *Results Probl. Cell Differ.*, **45**, 1–31.

Hendrickson, W.A. and Love, W.E. (1971) Structure of lamprey haemoglobin. *Nat. New Biol.*, **232**, 197–203.

Hershko, C., Graham, G., Bates, G.W. and Rachmilewitz, E.A. (1978) Non-specific serum iron in thalassaemia: an abnormal serum iron fraction of potential toxicity. *Br. J. Haematol.*, **40**, 255–263.

Högbom, M. (2011) Metal use in ribonucleotide reductase R2, diiron, di-manganese and heterodinuclear – an intricate bioinorganic workaround to use different metals for the same reaction. *Metallomics*, **3**, 110–120.

Huber, C. and Wächtershäuser, G. (2006) alpha-Hydroxy and alpha-amino acids under possible Hadean, volcanic origin-of-life conditions. *Science*, **314** (5799), 630–632.

Huber, R., Epp, O. and Formanek, H. (1969) Elucidation of the molecular structure of insect hemoglobin. *Naturwissenschaften*, **56**, 362–367.

Huber, R., Epp, O., Steigemann, W. and Formanek, H. (1971) The atomic structure of erythrocruorin in the light of the chemical sequence and its comparison with myoglobin. *Eur. J. Biochem.*, **19**, 42–50.

Ishimaru, Y., Kim, S., Tsukamoto, T., Oki, H., *et al.* (2007) Mutational reconstructed ferric chelate reductase confers enhanced tolerance in rice to iron deficiency in calcareous soil. *Proc. Natl Acad. Sci. USA*, **104**, 7373–7378.

Iwata, S., Ostermeier, C., Ludwig, B. and Michel, H. (1995) Structure at 2.8 Å resolution of cytochrome c oxidase from *Paracoccus denitrificans*. *Nature*, **376**, 660–669.

Jacobs, A. (1977) An intracellular transit iron pool. *Blood*, **50**, 4331–4336.

Jacobs, E.M., Hendriks, J.C., van Tits, B.L., Evans, P.J., *et al.* (2005) Results of an international round robin for the quantification of serum non-transferrin-bound iron: need for defining standardization and a clinically relevant isoform. *Anal. Biochem.*, **341**, 241–250.

Janssen-Heidinger, Y.M., Mossman, B.T., Heintz, N.H., Forman, H.J., *et al.* (2008) Redox-based regulation of signal transduction: principles, pitfalls, and promises. *Free Radical Biol. Med.*, **45**, 1–17.

Jordan, A. and Reichard, P. (1998) Ribonucleotide reductases. *Annu. Rev. Biochem.*, **67**, 71–98.

Jouanneau, Y., Meyer, C., Jakoncic, J., Stojanoff, V. and Gaillard, J. (2006) Characterization of a naphthalene dioxygenase endowed with an exceptionally broad substrate specificity toward polycyclic aromatic hydrocarbons. *Biochemistry*, **45**, 12380–12391.

Keilin, D. (1925) On cytochrome, a respiratory pigment, common to animals, yeast and higher plants. *Proc. Roy. Soc. Lond. B*, **98**, 312–339.

Karlsson, A. Parales, J.V., Parales, R.E., Gibson, D.T., *et al.* (2003) Crystal structure of naphthalene dioxygenase: side-on binding of dioxygen to iron. *Science*, **299**, 1039–1042.

Klomsiri, C., Karplus, P.A. and Poole, L.B. (2011) Cysteine-based redox switches in enzymes. *Antioxid. Redox Signal.*, **14**, 1065–1077.

Kirchner, B., Wennmohs, F., Ye, S. and Neese, F. (2007) Theoretical bioinorganic chemistry: the electronic structure makes a difference. *Curr. Opin. Chem. Biol.*, **11**, 134–141.

Kitagawa, T. and Ogura, T. (1998) Time-resolved resonance Raman investigation of oxygen reduction mechanism of bovine cytochrome c oxidase. *J. Bioenerg. Biomembr.*, **30**, 71–79.

Kleinschroth, T., Castellani, M., Trinh, C.H., Morgner, N., *et al.* (2011) X-ray structure of the dimeric cytochrome bc(1) complex from the soil bacterium *Paracoccus denitrificans* at 2.7-Å resolution. *Biochim. Biophys. Acta*, **1807**, 1606–1615.

Koehntop, K.D., Emerson, J.P. and Que, L. Jr (2005) The 2-His-1-carboxylate facial triad: a versatile platform for dioxygen activation by mononuclear non-heme iron(II) enzymes. *J. Biol. Inorg. Chem.*, **10**, 87–93.

Krebs, C., Bollinger, J.M. Jr and Booker, S.J. (2011) Cyanobacterial alkane biosynthesis further expands the catalytic repertoire of the ferritin-like 'diiron-carboxylate' proteins. *Curr. Opin. Chem. Biol.*, **15**, 291–303.

Kurtz, D.M. Jr (1997) Structural similarity and functional diversity in diiron-oxo proteins. *J. Biol. Inorg. Chem.*, **2**, 159–167.

Lamb, D.C. and Waterman, M.R. (2013) Unusual properties of the cytochrome P450 superfamily. *Philos. Trans. R. Soc. Lond. B Biol. Sci.*, **368**, 20120434.

Larsson, A. and Sjöberg, B.M. (1986) Identification of the stable free radical tyrosine residue in ribonucleotide reductase. *EMBO J.*, **5**, 2037–2040.

Léger, C. (2013) An introduction to electrochemical methods for the functional analysis of metalloproteins, in *Practical Approaches to Biological Inorganic Chemistry* (eds R.R. Crichton and R.O. Louro), Elsevier, Amsterdam and Oxford, pp. 179–216.

Lill, R. (2009) Function and biogenesis of iron-sulphur proteins. *Nature*, **460**, 831–838.

Lloyd, S.J., Lauble, H., Prasad, G.S. and Stout, C.D. (1999) The mechanism of aconitase: 1.8 Å resolution crystal structure of the S642a:citrate complex. *Protein Sci.*, **8**, 2655.

Loehr, T.M. and Sanders-Loehr, J. (1993) Techniques for obtaining resonance Raman spectra of metalloproteins. *Methods Enzymol.*, **226**, 431–470.

Louro, R.O. (2013) Introduction to biomolecular NMR and metals, in *Practical Approaches to Biological Inorganic Chemistry* (eds R.R. Crichton and R.O. Louro), Elsevier, Amsterdam and Oxford, pp. 77–107.

Martins, B.M., Svetlitchnaia, T. and Dobbek, H. (2005) 2-Oxoquinoline 8-monooxygenase oxygenase component: active site modulation by Rieske-[2Fe-2S] center oxidation/reduction. *Structure*, **13**, 817–824.

May, P.M. and Williams, D.R. (1977) Computer simulation of chelation therapy. Plasma mobilizing index as a replacement for effective stability constant. *FEBS Lett.*, **78**, 134–138.

McMaster, J. and Oganesyan, V.S. (2010) Magnetic circular dichroism spectroscopy as a probe of the structures of the metal sites in metalloproteins. *Curr. Opin. Struct. Biol.*, **20**, 615–622.

Merkx, M., Kopp, D.A., Sazinsky, M.H., Blazyk, J.L., *et al.* (2001) Dioxygen activation and methane hydroxylation by soluble methane monooxygenase: a tale of two irons and three proteins. *Angew. Chem. Int. Ed. Engl.*, **40**, 2782–2807.

Meyer, J. (2008) Iron–sulfur protein folds, iron-sulfur chemistry, and evolution. *J. Biol. Inorg. Chem.*, **13**, 157–170.

Miki, H. and Funato, Y. (2012) Regulation of intracellular signalling through cysteine oxidation by reactive oxygen species. *J. Biochem.*, **151**, 255–261.

Millo, D., Harnisch, F., Patil, S.A., Ly, H.K., *et al.* (2011) In situ spectroelectrochemical investigation of electrocatalytic microbial biofilms by surface-enhanced resonance Raman spectroscopy. *Angew. Chem. Int. Ed. Engl.*, **50**, 2625–2627.

Minnihan, E.C., Young, D.D., Schultz, P.G. and Stubbe, J. (2011) Incorporation of fluorotyrosines into ribonucleotide reductase using an evolved, polyspecific aminoacyl-tRNA synthetase. *J. Am. Chem. Soc.*, **133**, 15942–15945.

Minnihan, E.C., Nocera, D.G. and Stubbe, J. (2013) Reversible, long-range radical transfer in *E. coli* class Ia ribonucleotide reductase. *Acc. Chem. Res.*, **46**, 2524–2535.

Moran, G.R., Derecskei-Kovacs, A., Hillas, P.J. and Fitzpatrick, P.F. (2000) On the catalytic mechanism of tryptophan hydroxylase. *J. Am. Chem. Soc.*, **122**, 4535.

Mössbauer, R.L (1958a) Kernresonanzabsorption von Gammastrahlung in Ir[191]. *Naturwissenschaften*, **45**, 538–539.

Mössbauer, R.L (1958b) Kernresonanzabsorption von Gammastrahlung in Ir[191]. *Z. Physik.*, **151**, 124–143.

Myllyharju J. and Kivirikko, K.I. (2004) Collagens, modifying enzymes and their mutations in humans, flies and worms. *Trends Genet.*, **20**, 33–43.

Neese, F. (2003) Quantum chemical calculations of spectroscopic properties of metalloproteins and model compounds: EPR and Mössbauer properties. *Curr. Opin. Chem. Biol.*, **7**, 125–135.

Neidig, M.L. and Solomon, E.I. (2004) Structure-function correlations in oxygen activating non-heme iron enzymes. *Chem. Commun. (Camb)*., **21**, 5843–5863.

Nordlund, P. and Eklund, H. (1995) Diiron-carboxylate proteins. *Curr. Opin. Struct. Biol.*, **5**, 758–766.

Nordlund, P. and Reichard, P. (2006) Ribonucleotide reductases. *Annu. Rev. Biochem.*, **75**, 681–706.

Ogura, T. and Kitagawa, T. (2004) Resonance Raman characterization of the P intermediate in the reaction of bovine cytochrome c oxidase. *Biochim. Biophys. Acta*, **1655**, 290–297.

Ortiz de Montellano, P.R. (2005) *Cytochrome P450, structure, mechanism and biochemistry*. 3rd edn, Kluwer Academic/Plenum Publishers, New York.

Ostermeier, C., Harrenga, A., Ermler, U. and Michel, H. (1997) Structure at 2.7 Å resolution of the *Paracoccus denitrificans* two-subunit cytochrome c oxidase complexed with an antibody FV fragment. *Proc. Natl Acad. Sci. USA*, **94**, 10547–10553.

Pavon, J.A. and Fitzpatrick, P.F. (2005) Insights into the catalytic mechanisms of phenylalanine and tryptophan hydroxylase from kinetic isotope effects on aromatic hydroxylation. *Biochemistry*, **45**, 11030–11037.

Pereira, M.M., Santana, M. and Teixeira, M. (2001) A novel scenario for the evolution of haem-copper oxygen reductases. *Biochim. Biophys. Acta*, **1505**, 185–208.

Perutz, M.F. (1970) Stereochemistry of cooperative effects in haemoglobin. *Nature*, **228**, 726–739.

Perutz, M.F. (1979) Regulation of oxygen affinity of hemoglobin: influence of structure of the globin on the heme iron. *Annu. Rev. Biochem.*, **48**, 327–386.

Perutz, M.F. (1980) The origins of molecular biology. *New Scientist*, **85**, 326–329.

Perutz, M.F., Wilkinson, A.J., Paoli, M. and Dodson, G.G. (1998) The stereochemical mechanism of the cooperative effects in hemoglobin revisited. *Annu. Rev. Biophys. Biomol. Struct.*, **27**, 1–34.

Pietrangelo, A. (2007) Iron chelation beyond transfusion iron overload. *Am. J. Hematol.*, **82**, 1142–1146.

Pierik, A.J., Roseboom, W., Happe, R.P., Bagley, K.A. and Albracht, S.P. (1999) Carbon monoxide and cyanide as intrinsic ligands to iron in the active site of [NiFe]-hydrogenases. NiFe(CN)$_2$CO, Biology's way to activate H2. *J. Biol. Chem.*, **274**, 3331–3337.

Polyakov, K.M., Boyko, K.M., Tikhonova, T.V., Slutsky, A., *et al.* (2009) High-resolution structural analysis of a novel octaheme cytochrome c nitrite reductase from the haloalkaliphilic bacterium *Thioalkalivibrio nitratireducens*. *J. Mol. Biol.*, **389**, 846–862.

Pootrakul, P., Breuer, W., Sametband, M., Sirankapracha, P., *et al.* (2004). Labile plasma iron (LPI) as an indicator of chelatable plasma redox activity in iron overloaded beta-thalassaemia/HbE patients treated with an oral chelator. *Blood*, **104**, 1504–1510.

Poulos, T.L., Finze, B.C. and Howard, A.J. (1986) Crystal structure of substrate-free *Pseudomonas putida* cytochrome P-450. *Biochemistry*, **25**, 5314–5322.

Proshlyakov, D.A., Pressler, M.A. and Babcock, G.T. (1998) Dioxygen activation and bond cleavage by mixed-valence cytochrome c oxidase. *Proc. Natl Acad. Sci. USA*, **95**, 8020–8025.

Qin, L., Hiser, C., Mulichak, A., Garavito, R.M. and Ferguson-Miller, S. (2006) Identification of conserved lipid/detergent-binding sites in a high-resolution structure of the membrane protein cytochrome c oxidase. *Proc. Natl Acad. Sci. USA*, **103**, 16117–16122.

Que, L., Jr (2000) One motif – many different reactions. *Nat. Struct. Biol.*, **7**, 182–184.

Robson, R.L. (2013) Genetic and molecular biology approaches for the study of metals in biology, in *Practical Approaches to Biological Inorganic Chemistry* (eds R.R. Crichton and R.O. Louro), Elsevier, Amsterdam and Oxford, pp. 257–304.

Sazinsky, M.H. and Lippard, S.J. (2005) Product bound structures of the soluble methane monooxygenase hydroxylase from *Methylococcus capsulatus* (Bath): protein motion in the alpha-subunit. *J. Am. Chem. Soc.*, **127**, 5814–5825.

Sazinsky, M.H. and Lippard, S.J. (2006) Correlating structure with function in bacterial multicomponent monooxygenases and related diiron proteins. *Acc. Chem. Res.*, **39**, 558–566.

Sazinsky, M.H., Bard, J., Di Donato, A. and Lippard, S.J. (2004) Crystal structure of the toluene/*o*-xylene monooxygenase hydroxylase from *Pseudomonas stutzeri* OX1. Insight into the substrate specificity, substrate channeling, and active site tuning of multicomponent monooxygenases. *J. Biol. Chem.*, **279**, 30600–30610.

Sevrioukova, I.F. and Poulos, T.L. (1999) Structural biology of redox partner interactions in P450cam monooxygenase: a fresh look at an old system. *Arch. Biochem. Biophys.*, **507**, 66–74.

Sevrioukova, I.F. and Poulos, T.L. (2013) Understanding the mechanism of cytochrome P450 3A4: recent advances and remaining problems. *Dalton Trans.*, **42**, 3116–3126.

Seyedsayamdost, M.R., Xie, J., Chan, C.T., Schultz, P.G. and Stubbe, J. (2007) Site-specific insertion of 3-aminotyrosine into subunit alpha2 of *E. coli* ribonucleotide reductase: direct evidence for involvement of Y730 and Y731 in radical propagation. *J. Am. Chem. Soc.*, **129**, 15060–15071.

Sharma, S., Cavallaro, G. and Rosato, A. (2010) A systematic investigation of multiheme *c*-type cytochromes in prokaryotes. *J. Biol. Inorg. Chem.*, **15**, 559–571.

Silakov, A., Reijerse, E.J., Albracht, S.P., Hatchikian, E.C. and Lubitz, W. (2007) The electronic structure of the H-cluster in the [FeFe]-hydrogenase from *Desulfovibrio desulfuricans*: a Q-band ^{57}Fe-ENDOR and HYSCORE study. *J. Am. Chem. Soc.*, **129**, 11447–11458.

Silva, A.M. and Hider, R.C. (2009). Influence of non-enzymatic post-translation modifications on the ability of human serum albumin to bind iron. Implications for non-transferrin-bound iron speciation. *Biochim. Biophys. Acta*, **1794**, 1449–1458.

Simon, J., Kern, M., Hermann, B., Einsle, O. and Butt, J.N. (2011) Physiological function and catalytic versatility of bacterial multihaem cytochromes c involved in nitrogen and sulfur cycling. *Biochem. Soc. Trans.*, **39**, 1864–1870.

Smith, D.W. and Williams, R.J.P. (1970) The spectra of ferric haems and haemoproteins. *Struct. Bonding*, **7**, 1–45.

Sousa, F.L., Alves, R.J., Ribeiro, M.A., Pereira-Leal, J.B., *et al.* (2012) The superfamily of heme-copper oxygen reductases: types and evolutionary considerations. *Biochim. Biophys. Acta*, **1817**, 629–637.

Strange, R.W. and Feiters, M.C. (2008) Biological X-ray absorption spectroscopy (BioXAS): a valuable tool for the study of trace elements in the life sciences. *Curr. Opin. Biol.*, **18**, 609–616.

Stubbe, J. and Riggs-Gelasco, P. (1998) Harnessing free radicals: formation and function of the tyrosyl radical in ribonucleotide reductase. *Trends Biochem. Sci.*, **23**, 438–443.

Stubbe, J., Ge, J. and Yee, C.S. (2001) The evolution of ribonucleotide reduction revisited. *Trends Biochem. Sci.*, **26**, 93–99.

Stubbe, J., Nocera, D.G., Yee, C.S. and Chang, M.C. (2003) Radical initiation in the class I ribonucleotide reductase: long-range proton-coupled electron transfer? *Chem. Rev.*, **103**, 2167–2201.

Svensson-Ek, M., Abramson, J., Larsson, G., Törnroth, S., *et al.* (2002) The X-ray crystal structures of wild-type and EQ(I-286) mutant cytochrome c oxidases from *Rhodobacter sphaeroides*. *J. Mol. Biol.*, **321**, 329–339.

Tsukihara, T., Aoyama, H., Yamashita, E., Tomizaki, T., *et al.* (1996) The whole structure of the 13-subunit oxidized cytochrome c oxidase at 2.8 Å. *Science*, **272**, 1136–1144.

Tsukihara, T., Shimokata, K., Katayama, Y., Shimada, H., *et al.* (2003) The low-spin heme of cytochrome c oxidase as the driving element of the proton-pumping process. *Proc. Natl Acad. Sci. USA*, **100**, 15304–15309.

Uchida, K. (2003) 4-Hydroxy-2-nonenal: a product and mediator of oxidative stress. *Prog. Lipid Res.*, **42**, 318–343.

Uhlin, U. and Eklund, H. (1994) Structure of ribonucleotide reductase protein R1. *Nature*, **370**, 533–539.

Vaillancourt, F.H., Barbosa, C.J., Spiro, T.G., Bolin, J.T., *et al.* (2006) Definitive evidence for monoanionic binding of 2,3-dihydroxybiphenyl to 2,3-dihydroxybiphenyl 1,2-dioxygenase from UV resonance Raman spectroscopy, UV/Vis absorption spectroscopy, and crystallography. *J. Am. Chem. Soc.*, **124**, 2485–2496.

Venkateswara Rao, P. and Holm, R.H. (2004) Synthetic analogues of the active sites of iron-sulfur proteins. *Chem. Rev.*, **104**, 1135–1158.

Weng, L.C. and Baker, G.M. (1991) Reaction of hydrogen peroxide with the rapid form of resting cytochrome oxidase. *Biochemistry*, **30**, 5727–5733.

Whittington, D.A. and Lippard, S.J. (2001) Crystal structures of the soluble methane monooxygenase hydroxylase from *Methylococcus capsulatus* (Bath), demonstrating geometrical variability at the dinuclear iron active site. *J. Am. Chem. Soc.*, **123**, 827–838.

Wikström, M. (1981) Energy-dependent reversal of the cytochrome oxidase reaction. *Proc. Natl Acad. Sci. USA*, **78**, 4051–4054.

Wikström, M. (2004) Cytochrome c oxidase: 25 years of the elusive proton pump. *Biochim. Biophys. Acta*, **1655**, 241–247.

Wikström, M. (2012) Active site intermediates in the reduction of O(2) by cytochrome oxidase, and their derivatives. *Biochim. Biophys. Acta*, **1817**, 468–475.

Williams, R.J.P. (1961) Nature and properties of metal ions of biological interest and their coordination compounds. *Fed. Proc.*, **20** (Suppl. 3), 10–15.

World Health Organization (2002) World Health Report 2002. http://wwwwhoint/whr/2002/.

Wörsdörfer, B., Conner, D.A., Yokoyama, K., Livada, J., *et al.* (2013) Function of the diiron cluster of *Escherichia coli* class Ia ribonucleotide reductase in proton-coupled electron transfer. *J. Am. Chem. Soc.*, **135**, 8585–8593.

Yang, H., Ye, D., Guan, K.L. and Xiong, Y. (2012) IDH1 and IDH2 mutations in tumorigenesis: mechanistic insights and clinical perspectives. *Clin. Cancer Res.*, **18**, 5562–5571.

Yoshikawa, S., Shinzawa-Itoh, K. and Tsukihara, T. (1998) Crystal structure of bovine heart cytochrome c oxidase at 2.8 Å resolution. *J. Bioenerg. Biomembr.*, **30**, 7–14.

3

Microbial Iron Uptake

3.1 Introduction

Bacteria are surrounded by rigid cell walls which give them their characteristic shapes – spherical for cocci, rod-shaped for bacilli and coiled for spirilla – but which also enables them to live in hypotonic environments without swelling and lysing their plasma membranes. The thick peptidoglycan layer (about 25 nm) in the cell wall that encases the cell membrane of *Gram-positive bacteria* takes up and retains the crystal violet stain used in the Gram staining method of bacterial differentiation (Gram, 1884), making positive identification possible. In contrast, *Gram-negative bacteria*, in which the peptidoglycan layer is much thinner (about 3 nm) and sandwiched between an inner cell membrane and a bacterial outer membrane, cannot retain the violet stain (Figure 3.1). This defines four compartments in Gram-negative bacteria: the outer membrane; the periplasm; the plasma membrane; and the cytosol. As we will see later in the chapter, this poses a challenge for iron uptake and its regulation.

Since the solubility of ferric iron is far below the concentration required for bacterial growth, bacteria have developed an incredible number and variety of iron uptake systems, which probably reflect the type of iron sources present in their particular environment at a given time. The standard laboratory strain used for the elucidation of *Escherichia coli* physiology, genetics, and molecular biology, *E. coli* K-12,[1] has many chromosomal-encoded and plasmid-encoded iron transport systems, although it only synthesises one siderophore itself, namely enterobactin. This strain has maintained all of these iron transport systems during years of cultivation in the laboratory since its

---

[1] Discovered in 1885 by the German paediatrician Theodor Escherich, the K12 strain was subsequently used by Edward Tatum in his classic experiments on tryptophan biosynthesis (Tatum and Lederberg, 1947).

Iron Metabolism – From Molecular Mechanisms to Clinical Consequences, Fourth Edition. Robert Crichton.
© 2016 John Wiley & Sons, Ltd. Published 2016 by John Wiley & Sons, Ltd.

(a)
Gram-positive bacteria

(b)
Gram-negative bacteria

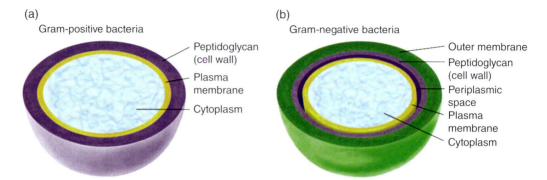

Figure 3.1 *Schematic diagram comparing the cell envelopes of (a) Gram-positive bacteria and (b) Gram-negative bacteria. (Figure 11.35 Voet and Voet.) Reproduced with permission from John Wiley & Sons, Ltd from Voet, D. and Voet, J.G. (2004)* Biochemistry, *3rd edn, John Wiley & Sons, Inc., Hoboken, NJ, pp. 1591*

original isolation from the stool of a convalescent diphtheria patient in 1922 (Bachman, 1972). K-12 is a debilitated strain which does not normally colonise the human intestine, survives poorly in the environment, and has a history of safe commercial use.

Most of the nutrients required for Gram-negative bacteria diffuse passively across the outer membrane into the periplasm through general or specific porins. Porins are β-barrel proteins composed of adjacent antiparallel β sheets connected by extracellular loops and periplasmic turns, which form hydrophilic channels, open on both sides of the outer membrane through which molecules can diffuse. However, scarce metals such as iron and cobalt (in the form vitamin B_{12}), need to be actively transported across each layer of the cell envelope. In the case of iron, this is frequently achieved by synthesizing and secreting strong and highly specific Fe^{3+}-complexing compounds, termed *siderophores*, which are taken up by specific transport systems. Many microorganisms also use ambient iron sources, such as Fe^{3+}-loaded siderophores (which they do not themselves synthesise and are therefore termed xenosiderophores) from other bacteria and fungi, and in the case of organisms which can grow anaerobically, they also have uptake systems for Fe^{2+}. As we will see in Chapter 4, a motley and often deadly collection of pathogenic bacteria can also acquire the iron of haem, bound to haemoglobin, haemoglobin-haptoglobin, myoglobin or hemopexin from their mammalian hosts, or can even use iron-bound host iron-binding proteins, transferrin or lactoferrin.

Dedicated outer membrane receptors are involved in the uptake of ferric siderophores and vitamin B_{12} (cyanocobalamin). The energy they require for their passage though the outer membrane receptors are supplied by the TonB–ExbB–ExbD complex (designated as the TonB system), which is anchored in the cytoplasmic membrane. These outer membrane receptors belong to a large family known collectively as the TonB-dependent transporters (TBDTs). Once in the periplasm, nutrients which are either actively or passively transported are sequestered by specific periplasmic binding proteins (PBPs) and brought across the periplasm to the cytosolic membrane where their cargo is delivered to their respective cytosolic membrane (CM) ABC transporter for translocation of the substrate into the cytoplasm (Figure 3.2). Transport systems in Gram-positive bacteria look the same (Figure 3.3) except that, in the absence of an outer membrane, the TBDTs and the TonB system are lacking and the PBP is a lipoprotein which, in most cases, is attached to the outer leaflet

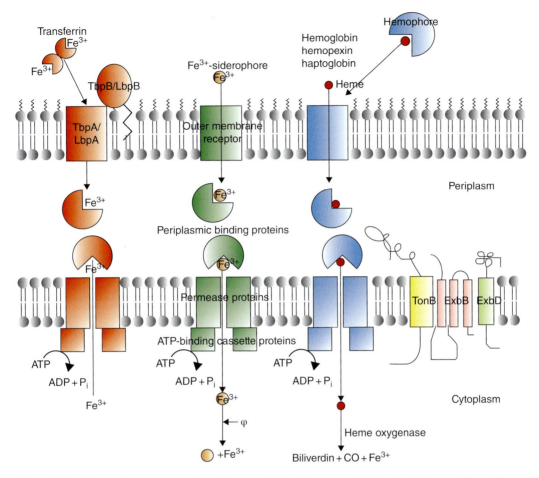

Figure 3.2 *Schematic representation of iron uptake in Gram-negative bacteria. Iron uptake pathways from transferrin, siderophores, or haem require an outer membrane receptor, a PBP, and an inner-membrane ABC transporter. Transport through the outer membrane receptor requires the action of the TonB system (TonB, ExbB, ExbD). Reproduced with permission from Elsevier from Krewulak, K.D. and Vogel, H.J. (2008) Structural biology of bacterial iron uptake.* Biochim. Biophys. Acta, **1778**, *1781–1804*

of the CM. After capturing the substrate, the PBP delivers it to the CM ABC transporter for transport into the cytoplasm. Under anoxic and/or reducing conditions, Fe^{2+} diffuses freely through the porins of the outer membrane and is transported by the Feo system, which differs from the Fe^{3+} transport systems.

In this chapter, emphasis is placed on the common principles of bacterial iron transport, without attempting to cover the multiple facets of the solutions that bacteria have evolved to solve their iron supply problems. Those systems that have been most extensively studied genetically and biochemically will be discussed. With the rapidly increasing body of information deriving from the sequencing of bacterial genomes, the great temptation is to assume that sequence similarities indicate similar functions. While genomics/proteomics approaches, with their *in-silico* extrapolations,

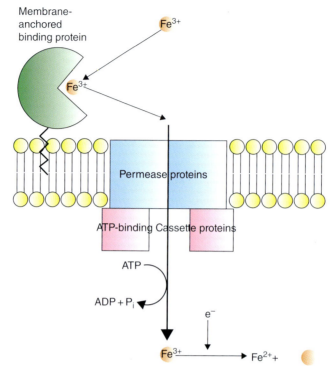

Figure 3.3 *Schematic representation of iron uptake in Gram-positive bacteria which, unlike Gram-negative bacteria, lack an outer membrane. Therefore, the uptake of iron from haem, siderophore or transferrin involves a membrane-anchored binding protein and a membrane-associated ABC transporter. Reproduced with permission from Elsevier from Krewulak, K.D. and Vogel, H.J. (2008) Structural biology of bacterial iron uptake.* Biochim. Biophys. Acta, **1778**, *1781–1804*

may be the 'flavour of the month,' biochemical and physiological data will still ultimately be needed to establish exactly what is going on in a particular bacterial species. Recent reviews on microbial iron uptake have been produced by Braun and Hantke (2011, 2013), Miethke (2013), Chakrabarty (2013), and Carpenter and Payne (2014).

3.2 Iron Uptake from Siderophores

3.2.1 Siderophores

Siderophores are low-molecular-weight (typically 500–1500 Da) iron-complexing molecules, which are synthesised by bacteria, fungi and grasses, and secreted into their environment to enable them to acquire iron. In addition to a high affinity for Fe(III), siderophores have almost exclusive specificity for Fe(III) – the only other biologically important trivalent metal ion is the kinetically inert Co(III). All natural siderophores are designed to selectively chelate Fe(III) which, under aerobic conditions, is the predominant and potentially bioaccessible form of iron in the environment (see Chapter 1). This means that they usually contain 'hard' oxygen donor atoms as ligands, and form thermodynamically extremely stable complexes with Fe(III)[2] More than 500 different sidero-phores have now been identified, and a compilation of structures known since 2009 lists more than 279 siderophores (Hider and Kong, 2010). They utilise a range of bidentate ligands to solubilise insoluble ferric iron, including the three major functional groups – hydroxamates, catecholates and carboxylates – which can be incorporated into hexadentate structures, like the three hydroxamates in ferrioxamine (Figure 3.4). As we will see in Chapter 10, the iron-free desferrioxamine is used therapeutically to chelate excess iron in patients with iron overload. The structures of a number of other siderophores are shown in Figure 3.4.

Enterobactin (pFe = 35.5) (Figure 3.4b) is the prototype of the catecholate siderophores, pro-duced by many enteric bacteria such as *E. coli*, and is a cyclic trimer of 2,3-dihydroxybenzoylser-ine. Its synthesis, encoded by the *entA, B, C, D, E* and *F* genes, involves six enzymes, starting from the common precursor of quinones and aromatic amino acids, chorismate. In the first step, choris-mate is converted by isochorismate synthase, Ent C, to isochorismate, a reaction on the path to menaquinone, catalysed by Men F (Kwon *et al.*, 1996). However, while catalysing the same reaction, the Ent C product is channelled to enterobactin synthesis, whereas the isochorismate produced by Men F is used exclusively for menaquinone synthesis. Until recently, it was thought that enterochelin was essential for the growth of *E. coli*. However, lipocalin-2, a protein of the innate immune system, produced by epithelial cells during inflammation and found in granules of neutrophils, binds enterobactin, effectively sequestering the siderophore from the bacteria (Kjeldsen *et al.*, 1993; Flo *et al.*, 2004) and contributing to the antibacterial iron-depletion defence system. Klaus Hantke and his colleagues have shown that enterobactin can be glucosylated in *Salmonella* species, in *Shigella dysenteriae*, and by some *E. coli*, such as uropathogenic *E. coli*, producing modified catechols termed salmochelins (Figure 3.4) (reviewed in Müller *et al.*, 2009). The enzymes responsible and their transport proteins are the products of the *iroBCDEN* genes (Hantke *et al.*, 2003). IroB glucosylates enterobactin and the resulting salmochelin is secreted by IroC (Müller *et al.*, 2009). Since lipocalin-2 cannot bind the glucosylated enterobactin, this gives salmochelin-producing pathogens an advantage over their mammalian host (Fischbach *et al.*, 2006). This has led to these modified bacterial siderophores (which also include the petrobactins of *B. anthracis* and *B. cereus*) being described as 'stealth siderophores' (Abergel *et al.*, 2008).

Many members of the Gram-positive *Bacillus* species, including *B. anthracis* and *B. cereus*, synthesise two hexadentate siderophores, bacillibactin and petrobactin. Bacillibactin is a 2,3-dihydroxybenoyl-Gly-Thr trilactone siderophore, and like its Gram-positive equivalent enterobactin, it exhibits a phenomenally high and selective affinity for iron with a pFe of 33.1 (Dertz *et al.*, 2006). Petrobactin (Figure 3.4; Wilson *et al.*, 2006), which was originally identified as a sidero-phore produced by the oil-degrading marine bacterium *Marinobacter hydrocarbonoclasticus* (Barbeau *et al.*, 2002), is an unusual citrate- and 3,4-catecholate-based ligand (Bergeron *et al.*, 2003), and is the only natural hexadentate 3,4-catecholate siderophore observed in a pathogenic bacterium. In marked contrast to bacillibactin, petrobactin and its photoproduct have pFe-values of −23.0 and 24.4, respectively, which is surprisingly low for catecholate compounds (Abergel *et al.*, 2008).

Ferrichrome (pFe = 25.2) is a hydroxamate siderophore common to numerous fungal species. The fungi do not synthesise ferrichrome; rather, it is transported across the outer membrane of

---

[2] The stability of Fe(III)–siderophore complexes can be most conveniently addressed in an empirical approach which does not require knowledge of the K_a of the ligand groups, nor the denticity of the complex (Raymond *et al.*, 1984). The pM value, in this case, the pFe, is defined from an equilibrium reaction (Telford and Raymond, 1996) as the negative logarithm of the free or uncomplexed Fe^{3+}_{aq} concentration (pFe = $-\log[Fe^{3+}_{aq}]$, calculated from the formation constant for a fixed set of experimental conditions: pH 7.4, a total ligand concentration of 10 µM and $[Fe^{3+}_{aq}]_{tot}$ of 1 µM. The larger the pM value for a particular ligand, the more stable is the metal complex under these standard conditions.

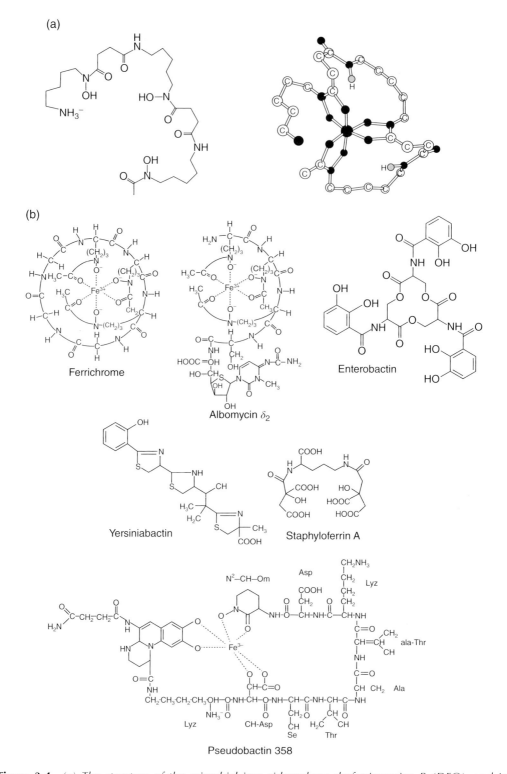

Figure 3.4 (a) The structure of the microbial iron siderophore desferrioxamine B (DFO), and its complex with Fe(III) (ferrioxamine). (b) The structures of selected siderophores to illustrate the major structural classes. The hydroxamate siderophore ferrichrome is shown in its complex with iron, together with the corresponding structure of the antibiotic, albomycin. The others – enterobactin (catecholate), staphyloferrin (carboxylate) and yersiniabactin and pseudobactin (heterocyclic) – are shown in their iron-free forms. (c) The structure of salmochelin and (d) three citrate-based siderophores, aerobactin, petrobactin achromobactin. Reprinted with permission from Elsevier from Wilson, M.K., Abergel, R.J., Raymond, K.N., Arceneaux, J.E. and Byers, B.R. (2006) Siderophores of Bacillus anthracis, Bacillus cereus, and Bacillus thuringiensis. Biochem. Biophys. Res. Commun., **348**, 320–325

(c)

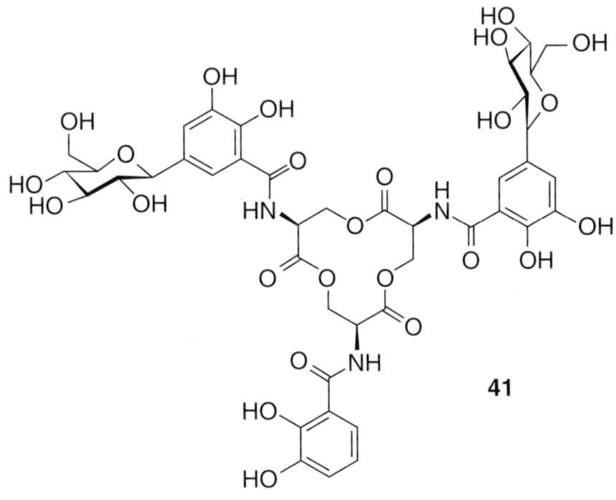

41

(d)

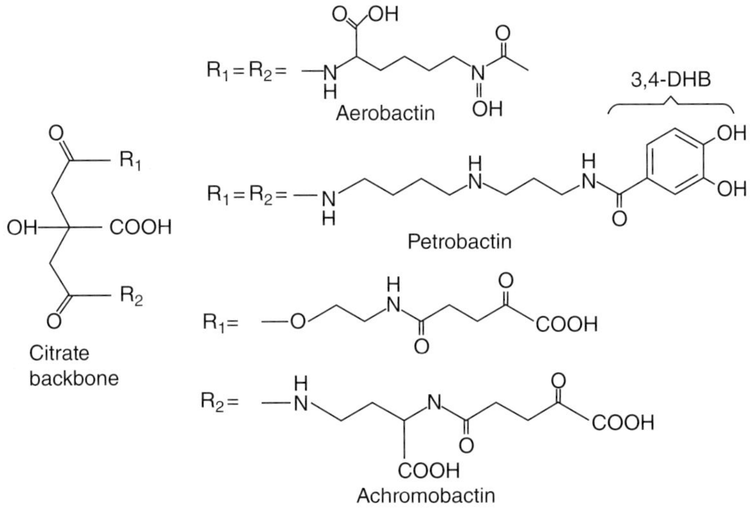

Figure 3.4 *(Continued)*

many bacteria by the multifunctional transporter FhuA. FhuA also transports the structurally similar antibiotic albomycin, the structurally diverse rifamycin analogue CGP4832, the peptide antibiotic microcin J25 and colicin M, and serves as a receptor for the bacteriophages T1, T5, and φ80.

Staphyloferrin A (Figure 3.4b) belongs to the family of carboxylate siderophores and is a highly hydrophilic molecule composed of two molecules of citrate bridged by a molecule of D-ornithine (Konetschny-Rapp *et al.*, 1990; Beasley and Heinrichs, 2010). It is produced by many clinically relevant pathogenic species of the Gram-positive staphylococcal family, including *S. aureus* and *S. epidermidis*.

Aerobactin (Figure 3.4d), a mixed citrate–hydroxamate siderophore, was first discovered as a virulence factor in invasive strains of *E. coli* encoded by the ColV plasmid (Williams, 1979). Despite having a much lower affinity for Fe(III) than enterobactin (as we will see in Chapter 4), it confers on the strains that produce it an enhanced capacity to infect their mammalian host.

Pyoverdines (Abdallah, 1991; Boukhalfa *et al.*, 2006) are the characteristic fluorescent sidero-phores produced by the Gram-negative *Pseudomonas aeruginosa* and its relatives. They form a large class of mixed catecholate–hydroxamate siderophores characterised by a conserved dihy-droxyquinoline-derived chromophore to which a peptide chain of variable length and composition is attached (Meyer *et al.*, 2002). Pyoverdines are high-affinity siderophores which are essential for causing acute infections by *Pseudomonas* strains; the latter also produce pyochelin, which has a much lower affinity for iron than pyoverdine (as discussed in Chapter 4).

Although it can hardly be considered to be a siderophore, a TBDT system exists in many bacte-ria for ferric citrate uptake, which is also used extensively by plants (see chapter 5). In *E. coli*, transcription of the ferric citrate transport operon encoding the genes *fecABCDE* is controlled by a signal transduction mechanism that starts at the cell surface. (Fe^{3+} citrate)$_2$ binds to the outer mem-brane protein FecA, and without further transport into the cell induces transcription of the *fec* transport genes (Härle *et al.*, 1995; Kim *et al.*, 1997) (see below). This type of signal receptor/transducer is present in a variety of Gram-negative bacteria (Koebnik, 2005); indeed, the first ferric citrate pathway to be found in a pathogenic Gram-positive bacterium, namely *B. cereus*, will be described in Chapter 4.

3.2.2 Iron Transport across the Outer Membrane in Gram-negative Bacteria

The transport of many nutrients across the outer membrane of Gram-negative bacteria involves passive transport through channels formed by porins, with low specificity and high rates of trans-port. In contrast, the transport of iron is an active process, and regardless of whether iron is deliv-ered to the outer membrane as siderophores, haem, transferrin or lactoferrin, the iron ligands are tightly bound to surface-exposed regions of their transporters with high affinities ($K_m \sim 1$ nM). The uptake of metal chelates, whether in the form of siderophores, haem, transferrin, lactoferrin or vitamin B$_{12}$, by Gram-negative bacteria require a TonB-dependent outer membrane receptor, a periplasmic binding protein (PBP), a cytoplasmic membrane ATP-binding cassette (ABC) trans-porter, and TonB/ExbB/ExbD. A schematic representation of the TonB-dependent uptake of cya-nocobalamin (vitamin B$_{12}$) is shown in Figure 3.5.

At this point, we review siderophore iron transport across the outer membrane in Gram-negative bacteria, notably *E. coli*. The crystal structure of the first outer membrane siderophore transporter to be determined was FhuA, the ferrichrome receptor (Ferguson *et al.*, 1998; Locher *et al.*, 1998). Since then, the crystallographic structures of a growing number of other outer membrane metal chelate transporters have been determined and the basic structural design of FhuA has been found in all of them (Braun and Hantke, 2013). They include FepA, the ferric enterobactin receptor (Buchanan *et al.*, 1999), FecA, the receptor for ferric citrate (Ferguson *et al.*, 2002; Yue *et al.*, 2003), BtuB, the vitamin B$_{12}$ receptor (Chimento *et al.*, 2003), and FptA and FpvA, respectively receptors for the *Pseudomonas aeruginosa* siderophores, pyochelin and pyoverdine (Cobessi *et al.*, 2004, 2005a, b; Wirth *et al.*, 2007). However, this protein superfamily is much larger, as there are many transmembrane transporters which, like the siderophore receptors, have a TonB box, and are classed as TonB-dependent transporters (TBDTs). They are involved in the uptake of not only iron sources, including siderophores, haem, transferrin lactoferrin and vitamin B$_{12}$, and also nickel, carbohydrates, bacteriophages and colicines (Killmann *et al.*, 1995; Neugebauer *et al.*, 2005; Blanvillain *et al.*, 2007; Cascales *et al.*, 2007; Schauer *et al.*, 2007, 2008).

All of these proteins have a unique fold composed of two domains, a C-terminal β-barrel and an N-1 domain, called the plug or cork, which fits tightly into the channel formed by the β-barrel from the periplasmic side, completely closing it (Krewulak and Vogel, 2007; Noinaj *et al.*, 2010).

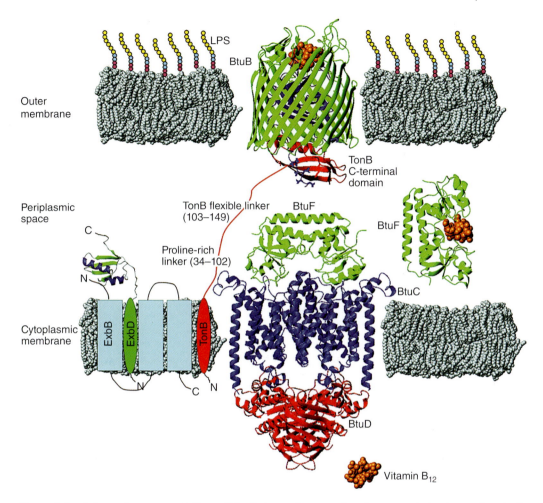

Figure 3.5 *Schematic representation of TonB-dependent uptake of cyanocobalamin or vitamin B_{12} (orange in the Web version and in space-filling format) by Gram-negative bacteria. The structures of the outer membrane receptor BtuB bound to TonB (PDB accession code 2GSK) (Shultis et al., 2006), the PBP BtuF bound to vitamin B_{12} (PDB accession code 1N4A) (Karpowich et al., 2003), BtuCD bound to BtuF (PDB accession code 2QI9) (Lewinson et al., 2010), and the C-terminal domain of ExbD (PDB accession code 2PFU) (Garcia-Herrera et al., 2007) are shown above. The lipid bilayer is created from a PDB file from Tieleman and Berendsen (1998). The displayed periplasmic space and proteins are not to scale. This figure was created using MolMol (Koradi et al., 1996). Reproduced with permission from NRC Research Press from Krewulak, K.D. and Vogel, H.J. (2011) TonB or not TonB: is that the question? Biochem. Cell. Biol., **89**, 87–97*

Bacteria, mitochondria and chloroplasts all have outer membranes which contain β-barrel proteins. In the case of the TBDT siderophore receptors, the elliptical-shaped β-barrel is composed of 22 anti-parallel β-strands embedded in the outer membrane, some 5.5–7.0 nm in height with an elliptical cross-section of between 3.5 and 4.5 nm (see Figure 3.6). This figure shows a comparison of the crystal structures of ribbon representations of outer membrane siderophore receptors from *E. coli* and *P. aeruginosa* of (a) vitamin B_{12} (BtuB), (b) *E. coli* ferric-citrate (FecA),

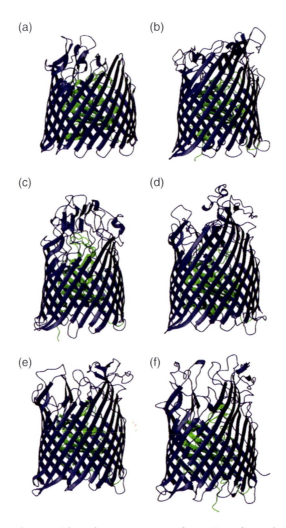

Figure 3.6 *Outer membrane siderophore receptors from* E. coli *and* P. aeruginosa. *Ribbon representations of the (a) vitamin B$_{12}$ (BtuB), (b)* E. coli *ferric-citrate (FecA), (c) ferric-enterobactin (FepA), (d) ferric-hydroxamate (FhuA), (e)* P. aeruginosa *pyochelin (FptA), and (f)* P. aeruginosa *pyoverdin (FpvA) receptors. Reproduced with permission from Elsevier from Krewulak, K.D. and Vogel, H.J. (2008) Structural biology of bacterial iron uptake.* Biochim. Biophys. Acta, **1778**, *1781–1804*

(c) ferric-enterobactin (FepA), (d) ferric-hydroxamate (FhuA), (e) *P. aeruginosa* pyochelin (FptA), and (f) *P. aeruginosa* pyoverdin (FpvA) receptors. The mixed α–β globular (cork) domain is coloured green, while the 22-strand β-barrel is coloured blue. All of the siderophore TBDTs consist of 11 extracellular loops and 10 periplasmic β-turns, with a large part of the β-barrel (including the metal chelate binding site) protruding above the outer membrane lipid bilayer. The 22-strand β-barrels are structurally similar when the Cα backbones of the β-barrels are overlayed, as is the angle of the β-strands relative to the axis of the β-barrel (45°), although the height of the β-barrel varies considerably, with the extracellular loops extending 0.3–0.4 nm above the outer membrane, forming a pocket which binds the iron ligand from the exterior medium. As for all known outer membrane proteins, two bands of aromatic residues line the membrane-embedded surface of the transporters and mark the boundary of an apolar cylindrical zone on the barrel surface, which extends into the lipid bilayer and delineates the border between the lipid hydrocarbon chains of the outer membrane, and their polar head groups. Direct crystallographic studies of FhuA bound to a single ordered lipopolysaccharide molecule have clearly defined the membrane-embedded and solvent-accessible surfaces of this transporter, and also showed electrostatic interactions between the phosphorylated glucosamine moieties and van der Waals contacts with the acyl side chains of the lipopolysaccharide and the protein (Ferguson *et al.*, 2000). The strands of the β-barrel that extend above the lipid bilayer are stabilised by inter-strand hydrogen bonds, together with salt bridges connecting strands 1 and 22. There is also a highly conserved C-terminal Phe (or Trp), which is important for folding and insertion into the outer membrane (Struyve *et al.*, 1991).

The N-terminal domain, which effectively closes the channel through the β-barrel, consists of a central mixed four-strand β-sheet surrounded by loops and helices. Above the cork, and accessible to solvent, is a cone-shaped extracellular pocket which contains the binding site, with loops of the cork pointing upwards and into the extracellular pocket, contributing to the metal chelate binding site. The electrostatic lining of this pocket differs for each transporter, and is complementary to the charge of the metal chelate. Below the mixed β-sheet of the cork is a second pocket, which opens to the periplasm, and contains a highly conserved sequence of seven amino acid residues, known as the TonB box. This has a consensus sequence: acidic-Thr-hydrophobic-hydrophobic-Val-polar-Ala (Krewulak and Vogel, 2011), which distinguishes this family of outer membrane proteins as TonB-gated transporters (Lundrigan and Kadner, 1986; Schramm *et al.*, 1987; Postle, 2002). Biochemical and biophysical studies have shown that the TonB boxes of this family of transporters interact directly with the cytoplasmic membrane protein TonB (Larsen *et al.*, 1997; Ogierman and Braun, 2003; Shirley and Lamont, 2009). In addition to the binding domain for ligands and the TonB box, in FecA and FpvA the plug domain contains an N-terminal extension, which regulates transcription.

The crystal structures of FhuA, FecA, FpvA, FptA and BtuB have been determined in both the free and the metal chelate bound forms. What is particularly noteworthy is that while they all undergo major structural changes upon ligand binding, this does not result in channel opening. Figure 3.7 (Schalk *et al.*, 2004) shows the structural differences between the FecA$_{apo}$, FecA$_{Cit}$ and FecA$_{FeCit}$. Upon binding of the metal chelate, it appears (as illustrated for FecA in Figure 3.7) that the apices of the extracellular channel and other regions of the plug move towards the metal chelate, while several extracellular loops (notably 7 and 8) change their relative arrangement and conformation. This results in the top of the β-barrel closing, sequestering the metal chelate from the external medium, and closing the gated channel. In addition, in FecA$_{FeCit}$, the TonB-box becomes disordered, though this may form part of the signalling mechanism for any subsequent interaction with TonB; transfer of the metal chelate into the periplasmic space can occur in the next energy-dependent step.

For this to occur, the plug must move and the conformation of the binding site must change so that the ferric siderophore, haem or Fe^{3+} can be released into the periplasmic space. The K_d of the metal chelates bound to their transporters is in the nanomolar range (Newton *et al.*, 1999), and clearly the release from the binding site and transport across the outer membrane requires energy; however, this energy cannot be derived from the outer membrane, which lacks an energy source. Gram-negative bacteria have overcome this problem by supplying the energy required for the outer membrane via the proton motive force of the cytoplasmic membrane, using the TonB system which couples the two membranes. This comprises the protein complex formed by TonB, ExbB and ExbD, which is located in the cytoplasmic membrane, the location and transmembrane topology

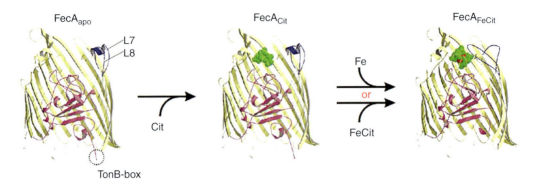

Figure 3.7 *Structural differences between the FecA$_{apo}$, FecA$_{Cit}$ and FecA$_{FeCit}$ crystal structures. Comparison between FecA$_{apo}$ and FecA$_{Cit}$ suggests that FecA binds iron-free citrate (Cit) in the first step. Comparison between FecA$_{Cit}$ and FecA$_{FeCit}$ suggests that the bound iron-free dicitrate in FecA$_{Cit}$ may extract iron (Fe) from another iron source (note the Fe^{3+} would be chelated to another molecule in this case) or be displaced by diferric dicitrate (FeCit). Compared to FecA$_{apo}$ and FecA$_{Cit}$, large conformational changes are observed in the extracellular loops L7 and L8 (blue) of FecA$_{FeCit}$. In addition, the TonB-box (circled) becomes disordered in FecA$_{FeCit}$, which may be part of the signalling mechanism for subsequent interaction with TonB. Reprinted from Schalk, I.J., Yue, W.W. and Buchanan, S.K. (2004) Recognition of iron-free siderophores by TonB-dependent iron transporters.* Mol. Microbiol., **54**, *14–22*

of which are shown in Figure 3.5. Most of the TonB protein, which interacts with both the cytoplasmic membrane and the outer membrane, is located in the periplasm, with its N terminus in the cytoplasmic membrane, as is ExbD, while ExbB is anchored in the cytoplasmic membrane (Figure 3.5).

TonB, ExbB and ExbD are found in a ratio of 1:7:2 in the cell over a wide range of growth conditions (Higgs *et al.*, 2002), although an ExbB :ExbD complex with a stoichiometry of ExbB$_4$–ExbD$_2$ has been recently purified (Sverzinsky *et al.*, 2014). While it is assumed that ExbB$_6$ forms the platform on which the final complex is assembled (Pramanik *et al.*, 2010), the actual *in-vivo* stoichiometry of the complex is not fully established. ExbB is a 26 kDa protein with three helical transmembrane domains anchored in the cytoplasmic membrane, and the majority of its soluble domain in the cytoplasm (Kampfenkel and Braun, 1993; Karlsson *et al.* 1993): its detailed molecular structure has yet to be determined. ExbD (17 kDa) has one helical N-terminal transmembrane domain in the cytoplasmic membrane, and its soluble C-terminal domain is located in the periplasm (Hannavy *et al.*, 1990; Roof *et al.*, 1991; Kampfenkel and Braun, 1992). The NMR solution structure of the periplasmic domain (residues 44–141) presents three clearly distinct regions: (i) an N-terminal flexible tail (residues 44–63); (ii) a well-defined folded region (residues 64–133); and (iii) a small C-terminal flexible region (residues 134–141). The folded region is formed by two alpha-helices, located on one side of a single beta-sheet composed of five beta-strands, with a mixed parallel and antiparallel arrangement, which closely resembles that found in the C-terminal lobe of the siderophore-binding proteins FhuD and CeuE (Garcia-Herrero *et al.*, 2007) (Figure 3.8). TonB is a 26 kDa protein composed of three functional domains. Like ExbD, it has a single helical transmembrane domain (residues 1–32), modelled as an α-helix, which contains a hydrophobic signal sequence that facilitates the translocation of TonB into the cytoplasmic membrane. The second functional domain is a proline-rich spacer (residues 66–102, composed of a series of proline and glutamic acid residues followed by several Pro-Lys repeats), which is located in the periplasm. Beyond the proline-rich region is another extended region spanning residues 103 to 149.

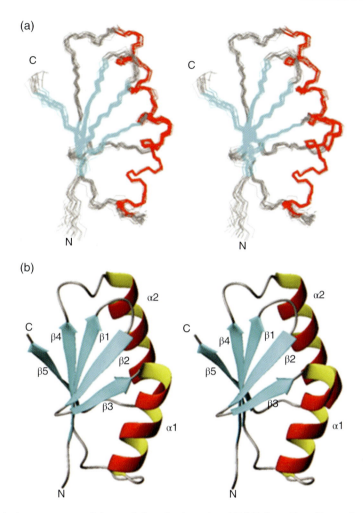

Figure 3.8 *Solution structure of the periplasmic domain of ExbD from* E. coli. *(a) Stereo-view of the bundle of 20 conformers obtained in the last cycle of the CYANA structure calculation; the backbone heavy atoms of residues 64–133 were superimposed for minimal RMSD. The residues are coloured according to their secondary structure (red for α-helical, blue for β-stranded, dark grey for undefined secondary structure). The region 135–141 and the His6-tag have no regular structure and are not shown in this diagram. (b) Ribbon diagram of the core domain (residues 64–133) of the conformer with the lowest CYANA target function. The positions of the N-terminal and C-terminal ends are indicated in the diagram. Reproduced with permission from John Wiley & Sons, Ltd from Garcia-Herrera, A., Peacock, R.S., Howard, S.P. and Vogel, H.J. (2007) The solution structure of the periplasmic domain of the TonB system ExbD protein reveals an unexpected structural homology with siderophore-binding proteins.* Mol. Microbiol., **66**, *872–889*

This entire region is thought to confer flexibility to TonB, allowing it to stretch across the periplasmic space and span the outer membrane for TonB-dependent receptors. Long-range distance measurements by spin-label pulsed electron paramagnetic resonance (EPR) and circular dichroism (CD) spectroscopy show that the proline-rich segment of TonB exists in a polyproline helix H

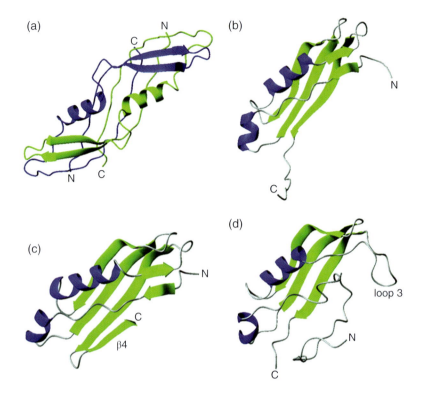

Figure 3.9 *The structures of the C-terminal domain of TonB. (a) The first X-ray crystallographic structure of E. coli TonB (residues 165–239) reveals an intertwined dimer, which is likely a result of domain swapping (PDB accession code 1IHR) (Chang et al., 2001). The monomers in the dimer are coloured differently in the Web version. (b) Both the X-ray crystallographic structure of a longer fraction of the C-terminal domain of E. coli TonB (residues 150–239) (PDB accession code 1U07) (Ködding et al., 2005). (c) The NMR structure of a similar length fraction (residues 151–239) (Peacock et al., 2005) (PDB accession code 1XX3) have an overall structure of a four-stranded antiparallel β-sheet in front of two α-helices. (d) Overall topology of the V. anguillarum TonB2 structure (residues 121–206) (PDB accession code 2K9K) (López et al., 2009) is similar to that of the C-terminal domain of E. coli TonB. The β4 strand found at the C terminus of TonB is absent in V. anguillarum TonB2. Additionally, loop 3 is extended by 9 Å. Reproduced with permission from NRC Research Press from Krewulak, K.D. and Vogel, H.J. (2011) TonB or not TonB: is that the question?* Biochem. Cell. Biol., **89**, 87–97

conformation which spans the periplasm of Gram-negative bacteria (Köhler *et al.*, 2010). The third functional domain is the C-terminal domain (residues 150–239), which is essential for interacting with the TonB box of the outer membrane transporters (see below).

The structures of the isolated C-terminal domains from *E. coli* and *Vibrio anguilarum* have been determined (Figure 3.9). The structures of the longer (residues 150–239) *E. coli* domain determined by crystallography and nuclear magnetic resonance (NMR) have the overall structure of a four-stranded antiparallel β-sheet in front of two α-helices (Ködding *et al.*, 2005; Peacock *et al.*, 2005), whereas the crystallographic structure (Chang *et al.*, 2001) of the shorter (165–239) *E. coli* domain is an intertwined dimer, which may represent the result of domain swapping. The overall topology of the *V. anguilarum* structure (residues 121–2006) (López *et al.*, 2009) is similar to that of the longer *E. coli* domain, although the β4 strand of TonB is absent in *V. anguilarum* TonB. It is suggested that an absence of this helix prevents dimer formation in *V. anguilarum* TonB. Bioinformatic analysis of TonB proteins in sequenced bacterial genomes suggests that this β4 strand is not present in most TonB proteins (Chu *et al.*, 2007), indicating that dimer formation may not be functionally important. Recent studies have indicated that monomeric TonB and the Ton box are required for the formation of a high-affinity transporter–TonB complex (Freed *et al.*, 2013).

ExbB and ExbD are thought to couple the proton motive force to conformational changes in TonB. Since TonB binds to a specific region – the TonB box – of the outer membrane transporter, which is exposed to the periplasm, it is hypothesised that this forms the basis of energy transduction between the outer and cytoplasmic membranes. TonB mutants are defective in all energy-requiring processes at the outer membrane, whether it be high-affinity transport of metal chelates, infection by bacteriophages, or infection by colicins (Cao and Klebba, 2002). While the role of ExbB is not well understood, contact between the periplasmic domains of TonB and ExbD is required, with the conformational response of TonB to the presence or absence of proton motive force being modulated through ExbD. Protonation/deprotonation may change the conformation of the complex, and clearly negatively charged amino acid residues would be reasonable candidates for such a protonation/deprotonation cycle in response to the proton motive force across the cytoplasmic membrane, as observed for membrane-bound H^+-ATPases. Asp25 in the transmembrane region of ExbD is a good candidate to be on such a proton translocation pathway (Ollis and Postle, 2012). The energised form of TonB could then allosterically change the conformation of the outer membrane transporter, resulting in the de-energisation of TonB, which would then be re-energised by the proton motive force to complete the cycle (Braun and Hantke, 2013). Three stages in the energisation of TonB have been identified based on the effects of ExbD mutations L132Q in the periplasmic domain and D25N in the transmembrane domain and H20A in TonB (Ollis and Postle, 2012).

Four models have been proposed to explain the interaction of TonB with the outer membrane transporters (Krewulak and Vogel, 2011), as briefly outlined below:

- The *propellor* model, based on homology between ExbB/ExbD and the flagellar motor proteins MotA and MotB (Cascales *et al.*, 2001), was supported by the strand-exchanged dimer structure construct found in the shorter C-terminal domain of TonB (Chang *et al.*, 2001). Recent fluorescence microscopy studies suggest a rotational movement of TonB (Jordan *et al.*, 2013). The model depends on the assumption that TonB is a dimer but, as was pointed out above, this may be the consequence of undesired domain swapping (Liu and Eisenberg, 2002; Rousseau *et al.*, 2003, 2012), and current evidence suggests that dimer formation is not important for TonB function.
- The *shuttle* model, was based on cellular fractionation studies in which TonB was found to be associated with both the outer membrane and the cytoplasmic membrane (Letain and Postle, 1997), together with *in-vivo* labelling experiments which showed that the N terminus of TonB is exposed to the periplasm (Larsen *et al.*, 2003). Whereas in other models, TonB remains attached to the cytoplasmic membrane during energy transduction, in the shuttle model the TonB N terminus leaves the cytoplasmic membrane to deliver conformationally stored potential energy to outer membrane transporters. More recent studies from the authors of the hypothesis (Gresock *et al.*, 2011) have led to a reinterpretation of the earlier results, and they now conclude that TonB does not shuttle, but rather suggest the existence of a signal transduction pathway from outer membrane to cytoplasm.
- The *pulling* model is based on studies which demonstrate that the mechanical stability and unfolding pathway of a protein strongly depend on the linkage through which the mechanical

force is applied (Brockwell *et al.*, 2001; Carrion-Vazquez *et al.*, 2003). Since both the plug domain of the outer membrane receptor and the TonB–TonB-box complex are four-stranded β-sheet structures (similar to the proteins used in these unfolding studies), the proposal is made that the TonB system exerts a vectorial force on the complexed β-sheet and plug domain to unfold the β-sheet (a perpendicular orientation requires negligible force, whereas a parallel force requires much greater force). Although steered molecular dynamics simulations *in silico* demonstrate how pulling by TonB on BtuB may occur (Gumbart *et al.*, 2007), at present there is no *in-vivo* experimental data to support this mechanism.

- The *Periplasmic-Binding Protein (PBP)-assisted* model is based on the observation that TonB not only forms a complex with FhuA (Carter *et al.*, 2006a) but also forms a 1:1 complex with the periplasmic siderophore binding protein (PDP) FhuD of the metal hydroxamate (Carter *et al.*, 2006b). The addition of FhuD to a preformed TonB–FhuA complex resulted in the formation of a ternary complex (Carter *et al.*, 2006b). TonB is then thought to act as a scaffold which presents FhuD to its outer membrane receptor FhuA, facilitating transfer of the siderophore. At the same time, TonB binds to the TonB box, resulting in a conformational change of the plug domain, followed by translocation of the siderophore. A similar interaction has been reported for the B_{12} periplasmic binding protein BtuF and TonB (James *et al.*, 2009). While this model could explain the actions of all of the proteins involved in translocation of the substrate, it does not account for the energy requirement (Krewulak and Vogel, 2011).

As has been pointed out in the article, delightfully entitled 'TonB or not TonB: is that the question?' (Krewulak and Vogel, 2011), while all of these models tick some of the boxes, none of them tick all of the boxes. So, it is still not clear how TonB and the TonB complex react to the proton motive force, and how they interact with the outer membrane transporters to induce conformational changes resulting in pore opening and substrate release (Krewulak and Vogel, 2011; Braun and Hantke, 2013).

3.2.3 Transport across the Periplasm and Cytoplasmic Membrane in Gram-negative Bacteria

Once in the periplasm, nutrients which have been transported across the outer membrane of Gram-negative bacteria bind to PBPs and are then delivered to their respective cytoplasmic membrane (CM) ABC transporter. The genes encoding the outer membrane and cytoplasmic membrane ABC transporter and the PBP of a given transport system are usually located on a single operon. Formation of the PBP–CM ABC transporter complex allows the subsequent transport of substrates across the cytoplasmic membrane. This involves charge–charge interactions between surface-exposed acidic residues on the PBP and basic residues on the periplasmic face of the cytoplasmic membrane ABC transporter (Hollenstein *et al.*, 2007; Hvorup *et al.*, 2007).

Periplasmic binding proteins[3] are members of a widely distributed protein superfamily which mediate chemotaxis and solute uptake in bacteria. They bind a wide variety of ligands, including carbohydrates, amino acids, anions, metal ions, organic metal ion complexes, di- and oligo-peptides. Quiocho and Ledvina (1996) identified two groups (I and II), which, despite huge disparities of size and low amino acid sequence identity, were characterised by three major structural characteristics, namely two distinct globular domains of mixed α/β structure, a binding cleft (either deep or

---

[3] Many of PBPs are so-called 'Venus fly trap' proteins. The Venus fly trap is a white-flowered swamp flower of the sundew family, native to the Carolinas, having leaves with two hinged blades which snap shut to trap insects.

shallow) in which the substrate was bound, and hinge-bending motions between the two domains, which gave the substrate access to the binding pocket (Quiocho and Ledvina, 1996; Chu and Vogel, 2011). The two domains, which can be further divided into subdomains (a consequence of the domains not being folded from one contiguous polypeptide segment) are connected by two or three β-strands, which allow bending motions between the two domains upon binding and release of their ligands. Type I and II PBPs, including FbpA, a type II PBP which binds an Fe^{3+}-ion scavenged from human transferrin and lactotransferrin by *Neisseria meningitides* (Perkins-Balding *et al.*, 2004), show large 'Venus flytrap' opening and closing domain movements on ligand binding (30–40°) (Quiocho and Ledvina, 1996).

Elucidation of the structures of two PBPs, FhuD (Clarke *et al.*, 2000) and TroA (Lee *et al.*, 1999), responsible respectively for the transport of hydroxamate siderophores and of zinc, led to the recognition of a third class of PBPs (class III), characterised by a similar bilobal fold in which the two independently folded N- and C-terminal domains, each composed of a central β-sheet flanked by α-helices, are connected by a long (some 20 amino acid residues) α-helical linker (Krewulak *et al.*, 2004). Type III PBPs are thought to be more restricted in their domain movements, on account of the structural rigidity imposed by the long α-helix which links the N- and C-terminal domains. For FhuD and TroA, only 2–4° hinge bending and/or rotation on ligand binding is observed (Krewulak *et al.*, 2009), although BtuF undergoes some 10° hinge closing motion upon vitamin B_{12} binding (Karpowich *et al.*, 2003), and an even greater degree of intradomain movements has been found in other siderophore- and haem-binding PBPs, notably from Gram-positive organisms (reviewed in Chu and Vogel, 2011).

One important difference between outer membrane transporters, which typically import only a single metal chelate (though they may transport other ligands, like bacteriophages and colicins), and the PBPs, is that the latter can transport metal chelates from a number of different groups of transporters. Thus, FhuD transports all of the hydroxamate siderophores imported by the TonB-gated transporters – FhuA (ferrichrome), FhuE (coprogen, rhodotorulic acid and ferrioxamine) and IutA (aerobactin) to the ABC transporter, FhuBC, while FepB transports all of the catecholate siderophores imported by FepA (enterobactin) and Cir and Fiu (a number of other catecholates, including dihydroxybenzoylserine) to the cytoplasmic membrane complex FepCDEG (Figure 3.10).

Structural studies have given greater insight into how class III PBPs bind their corresponding ligands (reviewed in Chu and Vogel, 2011). The structure of FhuD, which transports hydroxamate siderophores across the periplasm, has been determined in both the apo form and with the ferrichrome homologue gallichrome bound (Clarke *et al.*, 2000, 2002). The crystal structure of *E. coli* BtuF, the PBP for the vitamin B_{12} transporter BtuCD has also been determined in the apo state and with vitamin B_{12} bound (Karpowich *et al.*, 2003), revealing a functionally important reduction in mobility upon ligand binding, as illustrated in Figure 3.11 for BtuF in its apo- and vitamin B_{12}-bound forms. The structure of BtuF is similar to that of the FhuD and TroA PBPs (*vide infra*), and is composed of two α/β domains linked by a rigid α-helix. Vitamin B_{12} is bound in the 'base-on' or vitamin conformation in a wide acidic cleft located between these domains. While no structure for the *E. coli* enterobactin PBP, FepB, has been reported, structural studies for the related catecholate-binding PBPs – CeuE from the Gram-negative *Campylobacter jejuni* (Müller *et al.*, 2006) and FeuA (Peuckert *et al.*, 2009) and YclQ (Zawadza *et al.*, 2009), both from the Gram-positive *B. subtilis* – have shown that the net −3 charge of the ferric enterobactin complex is compensated by a triad of basic residues, all three of them Arg in CeuA and YclQ, whereas Feu uses two Lys residues and one Arg residue. Tro is the general transition metal uptake PBP in *Treponema pallidum* (Lee *et al.*, 1999, 2002), and structural alignment of apo and holo (Zn^{2+})-TroA (Lee *et al.*, 2002), and many high-resolution structures of TroA-like proteins from both Gram-positive and Gram-negative

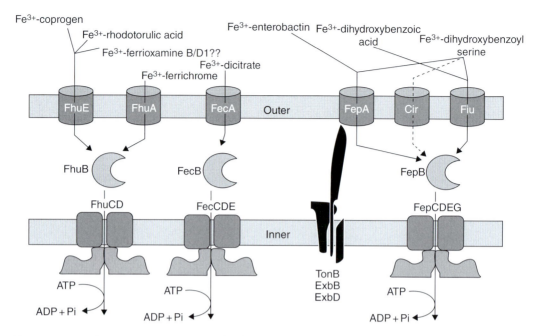

Figure 3.10 *Schematic representation of siderophore-mediated iron uptake systems in* E. coli *K-12. Note that the TonB–ExbB–ExbD complex energises and interacts with all the outer membrane receptors (not just FepA). Reprinted with permission from Elsevier from Andrews, S.C., Robinson, A.K. and Rodriguez-Quinones, F. (2003) Bacterial iron homeostasis.* FEMS Microbiol. Rev., ***27***, *215–237*

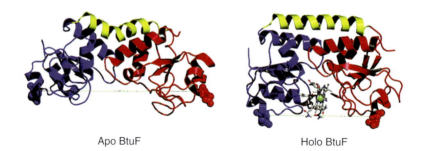

Figure 3.11 *Structures of the vitamin B$_{12}$-binding PDP BtuF in its apo- and holoforms. The dynamics of BtuF has been analyzed using multicopy molecular dynamics simulations of these two forms of the protein. BtuF was found to be more flexible than previously assumed, displaying clear opening and closing motions which are more pronounced in the apo form. The protein behaviour is compatible with a PBP functional model which postulates a closed conformation for the ligand-bound state, whereas the empty form fluctuates between open and closed conformations. Reprinted from Kandt, C., Xu, Z. and Tieleman, D.P. (2006) Opening and closing motions in the periplasmic vitamin B12 binding protein BtuF.* Biochemistry, ***45***, *13284–13292*

bacteria have been determined recently. In general they are able to bind Zn^{2+} or Mn^{2+} with four or five coordinating ligands provided by histidines or acidic residues (Ma *et al.*, 2009).

FhuD can bind to various hydroxamate siderophores including ferrichrome, coprogen, ferrioxamine B and rhodoturulic acid. The structures of *E. coli* FhuD bound to gallium-bound ferrichrome (gallichrome) and to a number of other hydroxymate-type siderophores have been determined (Clarke *et al.*, 2000, 2002). The three-dimensional structures of FhuD bound to ferrichrome, albomycin, ferrioxamine B and ferric coprogen show that the binding pockets are very similar, with only subtle rearrangements of the side chains (for a more detailed discussion, see Krewulak and Vogel, 2007).

ATP-binding cassette (ABC) transporters constitute a large superfamily of integral membrane proteins with diverse functions. They convert the energy gained from ATP hydrolysis into a transbilayer movement of substrates either into the cytoplasm (import) or out of the cytoplasm (export). A pair of highly conserved cytoplasmic ABCs (also termed nucleotide-binding domains, NBDs) provide the nucleotide-dependent engine which drives the transport. In contrast, translocation of the substrate is facilitated by a pair of transmembrane domains (TMDs) which are much more variable. ABC transporters can be classified into exporters and two subtypes of importers (type I and type II), based on their transmembrane architectures and topologies (Hollenstein *et al.*, 2007; Locher, 2009). Whereas exporters are expressed in all cells, ABC importers are only found in prokaryotes (Davidson and Chen, 2004). Bacterial ABC importers are generally assembled from separate subunits, whereas both bacterial and eukaryotic ABC exporters consist of ABC and MSD domains fused into one single polypeptide chain. Type II importers have a TMD architecture distinct from those of type I, with 10 helices in each TMD for a total of 20 transmembrane segments in the assembled transporter. The architecture was revealed in the crystal structure of the *E. coli* vitamin B_{12} transporter BtuCD (Locher *et al.*, 2002; Locher, 2004). Two copies of the membrane-spanning BtuC subunit and two ABC domains (BtuD subunits) assemble to form the functional heterotetramer ($BtuC_2D_2$). Crystal structures have been determined for the homologous HIF protein (HI1470/1) from *Haemophilus influenzae* (Pinkett *et al.*, 2007), and the BtuCD protein in complex with BtuF (Hvorup *et al.*, 2007). The structures demonstrate that a subset of TM helices (3–5a) can adopt one of two conformations (Figure 3.12b). In BtuCD, both the TMDs adopt conformation 1, resulting in an outward-facing translocation pathway. In HIF, they adopt conformation 2, resulting in an inward-facing translocation pathway. In BtuCD-F, one TMD adopts conformation 1, whereas the other adopts conformation 2, resulting in an occluded translocation pathway. The structures of BtuCD and HiF show how these gates can adopt open or closed conformations, thereby producing inward-facing or outward-facing conformations of the translocation pathway (Figure 3.12a). The type II PBPs BtuCD-F and Hi1470/1 are similar to each other in terms of sequence conservation, yet are relatively distant from the type I ABC transporters for maltose, molybdate, histidine and methionine, which also share a core fold of their membrane-spanning domain (Locher, 2009; Rees *et al.*, 2009), that is distinct from the fold shared by BtuCD-BtuF and Hi1470/1. Another dimension has been added to this picture by a study of the dynamics of complex formation, which highlight substantial mechanistic differences between BtuCD–BtuF, and probably also Hi1470/1, and the better characterised maltose and related type I ABC transport systems (Lewinson *et al.*, 2010). The structure of the transporter-binding protein complex BtuCD–BtuF (BtuCD-F) trapped in a β-γ-imidoadenosine 5′-phosphate (AMP-PNP)-bound intermediate state reveals that, although the ABC domains form the expected closed sandwich dimer, the membrane-spanning BtuC subunits adopt a new conformation, with the central translocation pathway sealed by a previously unrecognised cytoplasmic gate. A fully enclosed cavity is formed approximately halfway across the membrane and contains bound B_{12} (Khorkov *et al.*, 2012). Together with engineered disulfide crosslinking and functional assays, this suggests an unexpected peristaltic transport mechanism (Locher, 2004) that is distinct from those observed in other ABC transporters. This is illustrated in Figure 3.13, which presents a ribbon diagram of ADP-bound BtuCD and B_{12}-bound BtuF. The latter has been manually orientated to place the bound B_{12} over the entrance to the

(a)

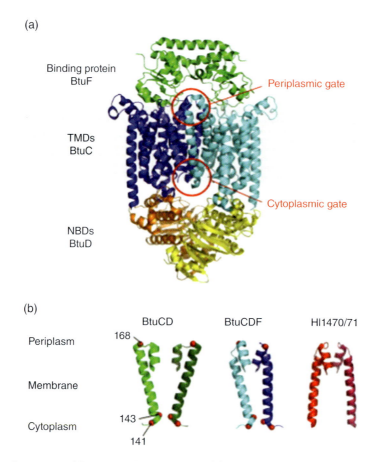

Binding protein
BtuF

Periplasmic gate

TMDs
BtuC

Cytoplasmic gate

NBDs
BtuD

(b)

BtuCD   BtuCDF   HI1470/71

Periplasm

168

Membrane

Cytoplasm

143

141

Figure 3.12 *Structures of Type II ABC importers and location of gates and mutations in BtuCD. (a) Ribbon diagram of the BtuCD–F complex (pdb ID 2QI9), with the two gates indicated. (b) The three conformations of the central TM helices lining the translocation pathway, as observed in the crystal structures of BtuCD and the homologous HiF protein. BtuCD–F is a hybrid conformation of the inward-facing HiF and the outward-facing BtuCD. The BtuC side chains mutated to cysteines were residues 141 and 143 at the cytoplasmic gate, and residue 168 at the periplasmic gate. The C_α atoms of these residues are depicted as red spheres, with numbers indicated. Reprinted with permission from Elsevier from Goetz, B.A., Perozo, E. and Locher, K.P. (2009) Distinct gate conformations of the ABC transporter BtuCD revealed by electron spin resonance spectroscopy and chemical cross-linking. FEBS Lett.,* **583**, *266–270*

translocation pathway (at the interface of the two membrane-spanning BtuC subunits). In the nucleotide-free and ADP-bound states of the transporter, this pathway is open to the periplasm but closed to the cytoplasm by a gate region. In order for transport to occur, B_{12} is released from its binding site, travels through the transport pathway, passes the gate, and exits at the large intersubunit gap evident at the centre of BtuCD. Support for this suggestion is derived from EPR and modelling studies (Goetz *et al.*, 2009; Joseph *et al.*, 2011, 2014; Kandt and Tieleman, 2010).

The reaction mechanism of BtuCD-F-catalysed vitamin B_{12} transport into *E. coli* has been recently clarified by the determination of the structure of the last missing state in the form of

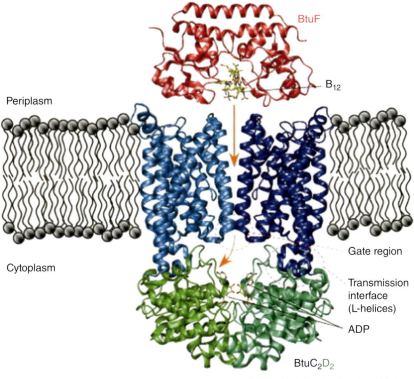

Figure 3.13 *Ribbon diagram of ADP-bound BtuCD and B_{12}-bound BtuF. The latter has been manually orientated to place the bound B_{12} over the entrance to the translocation pathway (at the interface of the two membrane-spanning BtuC subunits). In the nucleotide free and ADP bound states of the transporter, this pathway is open to the periplasm but closed to the cytoplasm by a gate region. For transport to occur, B_{12} is released from its binding site, travels through the transport pathway, passes the gate, and exits at the large intersubunit gap evident at the centre of BtuCD (orange arrow). Reprinted with permission from Elsevier from Locher, K.P. (2004) Structure and mechanism of ABC transporters. Curr. Opin. Struct. Biol., **14**, 426–431*

AMP–PNP-bound BtuCD, trapped by a disulfide crosslink (Korkhov *et al.*, 2014). The structural and biochemical data allow a consistent mechanism to be formulated, which is presented in Figure 3.14. A productive cycle of B_{12} transport starts with ATP-bound BtuCD (state 1), which is based on the AMP–PNP-bound BtuCD structure (Korkhov *et al.*, 2014). ATP binding triggers closure of the BtuD dimer, thus resulting in the opening of cytoplasmic gate I and simultaneous closing of cytoplasmic gate II. Subsequent docking of B_{12}-bound BtuF to BtuCD leads to state 2 (PDB 4FI3) (Korkhov *et al.*, 2012), an occluded conformation in which B_{12} can be trapped in a central, low-affinity ('Teflon') cavity. Docking of B_{12}-bound BtuF to BtuCD invariably triggers the release of B_{12} because there is insufficient space in the distorted binding pocket of BtuCD-bound BtuF. In a nonproductive cycle, B_{12} is lost on the external side. The transition from state 2 to state 3 is triggered by hydrolysis of ATP and the release of inorganic phosphate and ADP, which in turn disrupt the closed sandwich dimer conformation of the BtuD subunits. The coupling helices and

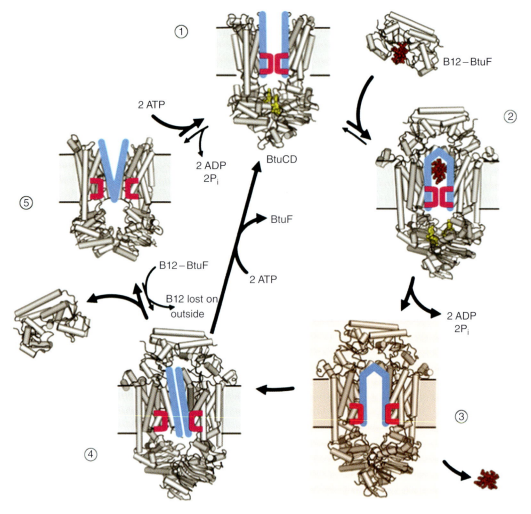

Figure 3.14 *Grey cylinder cartoons illustrate the structures of BtuCD, BtuF or BtuCD–F. Numbers indicate states as discussed in text. Yellow ball-and-stick models represent nucleotides; red ball-and-stick models depict vitamin B$_{12}$. Thick blue lines depict transmembrane helices 5 in each BtuC subunit, which form the periplasmic gate and the cytoplasmic gate I. Magenta brackets depict cytoplasmic gate II in each BtuC subunit. P$_i$, inorganic phosphate. Reprinted with permission from Nature Publishing Group from Korkhov, V.M., Mireku, S.A., Veprintsev, D.B. and Locher, K.P. (2014) Structure of AMP-PNP-bound BtuCD and mechanism of ATP-powered vitamin B$_{12}$ transport by BtuCD-F. Nat. Struct. Mol. Biol., **21**, 1097–1099*

cytoplasmic gate II are pulled open, thus leading to the formation of a transient, inward-facing conformation allowing B$_{12}$ release into the cytoplasm.

3.2.4 Iron Uptake by Gram-positive Bacteria

Whereas in Gram-negative bacteria the bilayer which constitutes the outer membrane is where solute transporters reside and interact with the external environment, Gram-positive bacteria have no outer membrane. Rather, in its place is a thick matrix of peptidoglycan embedded with covalently bound proteins that confronts the outside world. The cell wall of Gram-positive bacteria not only functions as a cytoskeleton but also promotes interactions between bacteria and their environment and, as the environment changes, microbes respond with alterations in envelope structure and function. Cell wall peptidoglycan is covalently and noncovalently decorated with teichoic acids, polysaccharides, and proteins. The sum of these molecular decorations provide bacterial envelopes with species- and strain-specific properties which, as we will see in Chapter 4, are ultimately responsible for bacterial virulence, interactions with host immune systems, and the development of disease symptoms or successful outcomes of infections (Marraffini *et al.*, 2006).

The cytoplasmic membrane in Gram-positive bacteria provides the main barrier to entry into the cytoplasm for small molecules such as Fe(III)–siderophore complexes. As such, Fe(III)–siderophores are brought into the cytoplasm through an active process involving ABC transporters that use the hydrolysis of ATP to provide the energy required for transport across the membrane. ABC transporter systems are comprised of a substrate-binding protein, a transmembrane permease, and an ATPase. The ATPase interacts with the permease and couples active transport to ATP hydrolysis (for a review, see Davidson *et al.*, 2008). Fe(III)–siderophore-binding proteins in Gram-positive bacteria are lipoproteins tethered to the lipid bilayer of the cytoplasmic membrane via acylation to a conserved cysteine residue which resides at the end of the cleavable signal peptide, within the so-called 'lipobox' domain (consensus: LXXC) (Hutchings *et al.*, 2009; Beasley and Heinrichs, 2010). They form part of the type III periplasmic binding protein (PBP) family (based, as we saw earlier, on their location in the periplasm of Gram-negative bacteria), and although they can be described by the more general term 'substrate-binding proteins' (Berntsson *et al.*, 2010) they will be referred to here as PBPs, as they are structurally and functionally homologous to the PBPs of Gram-positive bacteria (Chu and Vogel, 2011). In the case of Feu A, a 19-residue flexible linker links the folded part of the PBP with the membrane-bound acyl groups.

3.3 Fe^{2+} Transport Systems

The solubility of Fe^{3+} at pH 7 (0.1 M) is much greater than that of Fe^{3+} (10^{-18} M), and in anaerobic/microaerophilic conditions and/or at low, pH iron is mostly in the Fe^{2+} form. *E. coli* can grow in the gut, where such conditions prevail. In 1987, Klaus Hantke discovered a Fe^{2+} transport system in *E. coli* K-12 consisting of three genes, *feoA*, *feoB* and *feoC* (Hantke, 1987, 2003; Kammler *et al.*, 1993), arranged in this order. Since then, the Feo system has been found to be widely distributed in bacterial genomes (Cartron *et al.*, 2006). Residing upstream of *feoA*, *feoB* and *feoC* are the *fnr* and *fur* regulatory elements (Kammler *et al.*, 1993; Cartron *et al.*, 2006). As we will see later in this chapter, Fnr is an anaerobically induced transcriptional activator, whereas Fur is an iron-dependent transcriptional repressor. Fur and Fnr each play a crucial role in maintaining cellular iron homeostasis and preventing the formation of damaging free radicals.

It is assumed that Fe diffuses into the periplasm via undefined porins, and is then transported across the cytoplasmic membrane into the cytoplasm by FeoB in an ATP/GTP-driven active transport process (Figure 3.15). Only the 84 kDa G protein-coupled transmembrane protein FeoB is essential for Fe^{2+} transport. *E. coli* FeoB consists of a hydrophilic N-terminal domain (residues 1–270) exposed to the cytosol, and a C-terminal integral-membrane domain (residues 271–773) which is predicted to consist of eight transmembrane α-helices containing two 'Gate' motifs, which may function as the Fe^{2+} permease. Prediction of the topology of FeoB suggests that the two Gate motifs have opposite orientations, reminiscent of the iron permease of yeast FRp1 (see

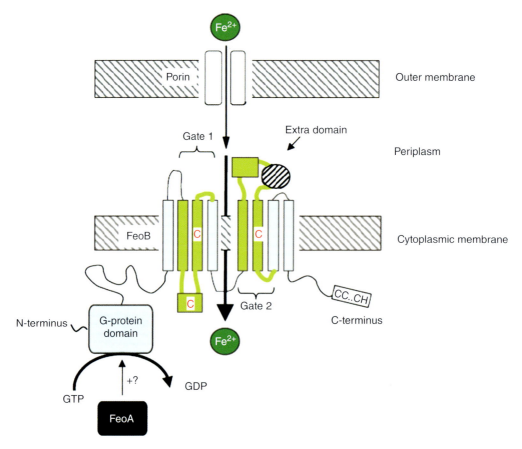

Figure 3.15 *Schematic representation of ferrous iron uptake by the Feo of* E. coli. *Extracellular iron diffuses through undefined porins and is transported into the cytoplasm by FeB, which has a G protein domain at its N terminus and two 'Gate' motifs (light green). Highly conserved Cys residues (red) and a Cys/His-rich region (red hatched) are shown. FeoA is thought to be required for maximal FeoA activity. Reproduced with permission from Springer from Cartron, M.L., Maddocks, S., Gillingham, P. et al. (2006) Feo-transport of ferrous iron into bacteria.* Biometals, **19**, *143–157*

Chapter 5), which also possesses a duplicated motif (the metal-binding 'RExLE' motif; Severance *et al.*, 2004) with opposite orientations within the membrane. The N-terminal domain contains a G protein region with a GTP-binding site (residues 1–160) (Marlovits *et al.*, 2002), linked by a poorly conserved spacer (residues 160–270), which may function as a GDP dissociation inhibitor (Eng *et al.*, 2008). The intracellular domain of FeoB has been crystallised from *E. coli* (Guilfoyle *et al.*, 2009), from the thermophiles *Methanococcus jannaschii* (Köster *et al.*, 2009), *Thermatoga maritima* (Hattori *et al.*, 2009), *Pyrococcus furiosus* (Hung *et al.*, 2010) and *Streptococcus thermophilus* (*St*NFeoB) (Ash *et al.*, 2010), as well as from the pathogens *Klebsiella pneumoniae* (Hung *et al.*, 2010) and *Legionella pneumophila* (Petermann *et al.*, 2010). The structures show that the GTPase domain and the GDP dissociation inhibitor domain form a large interface with hydrophobic and polar interactions, and that GDP binding to the GTPase is stabilised by interaction of the GTPase with the GDP dissociation inhibitor. This may represent the 'off state' of the FeoB transporter, with the GTP bound state being the 'on state'.

G proteins (GTPases) play an important role in prokaryotic and eukaryotic signal transmission. The G protein cycle, which involves binding of GTP, activation of downstream effector molecules and hydrolysis of GTP to GDP, is brought to a halt after GTP hydrolysis, and requires the release of GDP before a new cycle can be initiated. In eukaryotic G proteins, the nucleotide release mechanism has been shown to be facilitated at least in part by a structural change in the G5 loop, one of the five guanine nucleotide binding motifs (G1–G5) which characterise G proteins. Prokaryotic FeoBs GTPases contain these five characteristic sequence motifs responsible for nucleotide recognition, coordination and catalysis (Figure 3.16a), including the G4-motif NXXD responsible for guanine nucleotide specificity. A large conformational change in the G5 motif of *St*NFeoB is also observed when the structures of nucleotide-free (apo) and nucleotide-bound protein are compared (Ash *et al.*, 2010; Guilfoyle *et al.*, 2014) (Figure 3.16b).

In contrast to typical G proteins, GTP hydrolysis by *E. coli* FeoB occurs far too slowly to serve as an energy source to drive iron uptake, whereas the association and dissociation of GDP is much too fast to regulate the open/closed state (Marlovits *et al.*, 2002). This suggests that additional proteins are involved in the regulation of FeoB activity, possibly (as discussed below) FeoA and FeoC (Cartron *et al.*, 2006). Sequence alignment of the G5 loop (Figure 3.16c) shows that *E. coli* FeoB is the only G protein in which the second residue is Ser rather than Ala. Previous studies of HRas and Gα proteins with the corresponding mutation (Feig and Cooper, 1988; Iiri *et al.*, 1994; Posner *et al.*, 1998), and mutation of Ala to Ser in *St*NFeoB (Guilfoyle *et al.*, 2014) are also associated with lower affinity for GDP and accelerated GDP release rates.

FeoA and FeoC are required components of the *Vibrio cholera* ferrous iron uptake system, and FeoC has been shown to interact with the cytoplasmic domain of FeoB (Weaver *et al.*, 2013). *E. coli* FeoC is a small 78-residue protein with a winged-helix fold (Cartron *et al.*, 2006; Hung *et al.*, 2012a), characteristic of a family of DNA-binding, proteins, of which Fur is an example. It has been reported to contain a [4Fe–4S] cluster (Hsueh *et al.*, 2013), and it is proposed that it may be an [Fe–S] cluster-dependent transcriptional regulator of the *feo* operon. The crystal structure of a tight complex between the intracellular domain of FeoB and FeoC from *Klebsiella pneumoniae* (Hung *et al.*, 2012b), in which KpFeoC binds between the GTPase domain and the GDP dissociation inhibitor domain of KpFeoB, has been determined. It was also shown that the binding of KpFeoC disrupts pore formation by interfering with KpFeoB trimerisation.

The structure of the 75-residue *E. coli* FeoA protein has been determined (Su *et al.*, 2010; Lau *et al.*, 2013). The structure reveals a Src-homology 3 (SH3)-like fold, composed of a β-barrel with two α-helices where one helix is positioned over the barrel. FeoB has a potassium-activated GTPase which is essential for regulating iron import (Ash *et al.*, 2011), and enzymatic assays with FeoB suggest that FeoA may not act as a GTPase-activating protein, as previously proposed (Cartron *et al.*, 2006; Su *et al.*, 2010). Together with bioinformatics and structural analyses, it is suggested that FeoA may have a different role, possibly interacting with the cytoplasmic domain of the highly conserved core portion of the FeoB transmembrane region (Lau *et al.*, 2013). To date, no structural or functional studies have been reported on the transmembrane domain, which comprises most of the FeoB protein.

A new type of ferrous iron transport has been described in *E. coli* encoded by the *efe*UOB operon (Grosse *et al.*, 2006; Cao *et al.*, 2007). EfeUOB is a tripartite, acid-induced and CpxAR-regulated low pH Fe^{2+} transporter which is cryptic in *E. coli* K-12 but functional in *E. coli* O157:H7 (Cao *et al.*, 2007), which has similarities to the oxidase-dependent Fe^{2+} transporter of *Saccharomyces cerevisiae* (Askwith and Kaplan, 1997) (described in detail in Chapter 5). EfeU is homologous to the high-affinity iron permease Ftr1p of *Saccharomyces cerevisiae*, EfeO and EfeB are periplasmic: the former has a cupredoxin N-terminal domain while the latter is haem peroxide-like

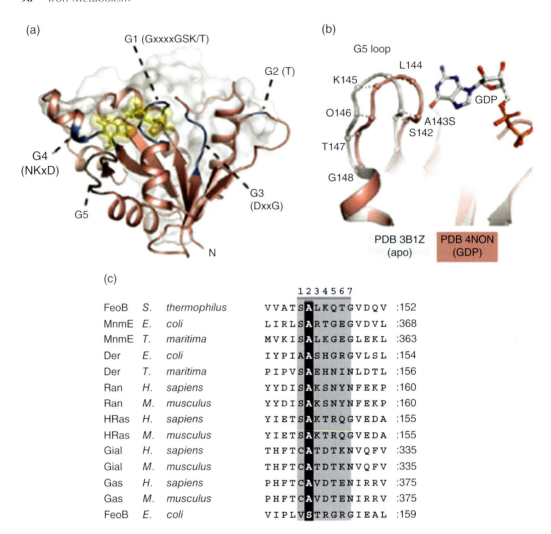

(a)

G1 (GxxxxGSK/T)

G2 (T)

G4
(NKxD)

G5

G3
(DxxG)

N

(b)

G5 loop

L144

K145

O146

T147

A143S
S142

GDP

G148

PDB 3B1Z
(apo)

PDB 4NON
(GDP)

(c)

```
                                1 2 3 4 5 6 7
FeoB    S.   thermophilus      V V A T S A L K Q T G V D Q V  :152
MnmE    E.   coli              L I R L S A R T G E G V D V L  :368
MnmE    T.   maritima          M V K I S A L K G E G L E K L  :363
Der     E.   coli              I Y P I A A S H G R G V L S L  :154
Der     T.   maritima          P I P V S A E H N I N L D T L  :156
Ran     H.   sapiens           Y Y D I S A K S N Y N F E K P  :160
Ran     M.   musculus          Y Y D I S A K S N Y N F E K P  :160
HRas    H.   sapiens           Y I E T S A K T R Q G V E D A  :155
HRas    M.   musculus          Y I E T S A K T R Q G V E D A  :155
Gial    H.   sapiens           T H F T C A T D T K N V Q F V  :335
Gial    M.   musculus          T H F T C A T D T K N V Q F V  :335
Gas     H.   sapiens           P H F T C A V D T E N I R R V  :375
Gas     M.   musculus          P H F T C A V D T E N I R R V  :375
FeoB    E.   coli              V I P L V S T R G R G I E A L  :159
```

Figure 3.16 *Overall structure and G protein nucleotide sequence motifs. (a) The overall structure of S. thermophilus NFeoB. The core G protein domain is shown in pink cartoon representation, whereas the helical domain of NFeoB is shown in surface rendering for clarity. The GDP molecule is shown as a yellow ball-and-stick representation, and the nucleotide binding motifs are highlighted in blue with the amino acid sequence of the respective motifs indicated. (b) Superposition of the G5 loop of apo- (gray) and GDP- bound (pink) StNFeoB. The positions of the residues in the G5 loop are indicated by spheres, and the GDP molecule is shown as a ball-and-stick representation. (c) Sequence alignment of the G5 motif from representative eukaryotic and prokaryotic G proteins. The residues, here defined as the G5 loop, are numbered and shaded in gray, whereas the residue investigated in the present study is highlighted in black. Reprinted from Guilfoyle, A., Deshpande, C.N., Vincent, K., et al. (2014) Structural and functional analysis of a FeoB A143S G5 loop mutant explains the accelerated GDP release rate. FEBS J., **281**, 2254–2265*

(Cao *et al.*, 2007). In the soil bacterium *Bacillus subtilis*, EfeUOB employs an unprecedented dual-mode mechanism for the acquisition of ferrous and ferric iron (Miethke *et al.*, 2013). The binding protein EfeO and the permease EfeU form a minimal complex for ferric iron uptake, whilst the third haemoprotein component EfeB oxidises ferrous iron to ferric iron for uptake by EfeUO, thereby promoting growth under microaerobic conditions where ferrous iron is more abundant.

As we will see in Chapter 4, Fe^{2+} transport systems are often associated with virulence in bacterial pathogens. Some obvious examples are pathogenic strains of *E. coli* which, in common with many other pathogenic Gram-negative bacteria, express a second Fe^{2+} transport system encoded by the *sitABCD* genes (Fisher *et al.*, 2009).

3.4 Iron Release from Siderophores in the Cytoplasm

In view of the coordination chemistry of ferric siderophores, with a predominance of hard oxygen ligands, it might reasonably be assumed that the reduction of Fe^{3+} to Fe^{2+} would decrease the binding constant substantially, and would therefore represent a logical mechanism for iron release in the cytosol. The reduction of complexed Fe^{3+} results in a weak Fe^{2+}–chelate complex from which the Fe^{2+} can dissociate relatively easily. We can distinguish two types of ferric reductase, namely assimilatory and dissimilatory. The former are essential components of the iron assimilatory pathway which generates soluble ferrous iron, for incorporation into cellular proteins, whereas the dissimilatory ferric reductases are essential terminal reductases of the iron respiratory pathway in iron-reducing bacteria (Schröder *et al.*, 2003). The ferric reductases which act in the reduction of ferrisiderophores are either NADPH-dependent flavoproteins or iron–sulphur proteins (for reviews, see Schröder *et al.*, 2003; Miethke, 2013).

In the flavoprotein reductases, reduction is generally independent of the structural nature of the ferric siderophore, and may only be limited by its redox potential and possible steric hindrances during electron transfer. These ferric siderophore reductases are perhaps better described as *flavin reductases* in which reduced flavin is used to reduce ferric iron (Fontecave *et al.*, 1994). It seems that most of these enzymes generate reduced flavins from electrons supplied by NAD(P)H, presumably because the redox potential of the $NAD(P)^+$/NAD(P)H couple is not able to reduce the ferric chelates directly. They include the NAD(P)H flavin oxidoreductase Fre (Coves and Fontecave, 1993; Ingelman *et al.*, 1999) and the sulphite reductase SiR (Coves and Fontecave, 1993) of *E. coli*, the *P. aeruginosa* ferripyoverdine reductase (Halle and Meyer, 1992a,b), and the flavin reductases FerA and FeR in *Paracoccus denitrificans* and *Magnetospirillum gryphiswaldense*, respectively (Mazoch *et al.*, 2004; Xia *et al.*, 2007). The reduced flavins can transfer electrons either in their hydroquinone or their semiquinone forms, and their different redox potentials may lead to the reduction of diverse ferric siderophore species.

Flavin reductases use flavins as substrates, and unlike flavoenzymes the flavin cofactor is not tightly bound. The reduced flavin can serve to reduce ferric complexes and iron proteins. In *E. coli*, reactivation of the di-iron centre of ribonucleotide reductase is achieved by reduced flavins produced by flavin reductase. The crystal structure of *E. coli* flavin reductase (Ingelman *et al.*, 1999) reveals that the enzyme structure is similar to the structures of the ferredoxin reductase family of flavoproteins, despite very low sequence similarities. The crystal structure of the ferric reductase (FeR) from *Archaeoglobus fulgidus* has also been determined (Chiu *et al.*, 2001).

The best characterised example of the second category of ferrisiderophore reductase is the *E. coli* ferric hydroxamate reductase FhuF, which has a [2Fe–2S] cluster (Müller *et al.*, 1998). The cluster has a midpoint redox potential of approximately −0.31 V, which is within or near the effective range for electron transfer to complexes such as ferrichrome, coprogen or ferrioxamine B, all of which belong to the set of substrates reduced by FhuF (Matzanke *et al.*, 2004). Since ferric enterobactin has a low potential it does not belong to the substrate spectrum of FhuF. The ferric reductase from the schizokinen-producing Gram-positive alkaliphile *Bacillus halodurans* was found to cluster with a ferric citrate–hydroxamate uptake system and to catalyse iron release efficiently from Fe[III]-dicitrate, Fe[III]-schizokinen, Fe[III]-aerobactin, and ferrichrome (Miethke *et al.*, 2011a). It also contains a [2Fe–2S] cluster with a midpoint potential of about −0.35 V, and its close relationship with FhuF suggests a similar mode of action.

Flavin reductases use flavins as substrates and are distinct from flavoenzymes, which have tightly bound flavins. The reduced flavin can serve to reduce ferric complexes and iron proteins. In *E. coli*, the reactivation of ribonucleotide reductase is achieved by reduced flavins produced by flavin reductase. The crystal structure of *E. coli* flavin reductase reveals that the enzyme structure is similar to the structures of the ferredoxin reductase family of flavoproteins, despite very low sequence similarities. The crystal structure of the ferric reductase (FeR) from *Archaeoglobus fulgidus* has been determined (Chiu *et al.*, 2001), and it catalyses the flavin-mediated reduction of ferric iron complexes, using NAD(P)H as the electron donor.

Early studies in *E. coli* showed that Fe^{3+}–enterobactin requires the esterase Fes, encoded within the enterobactin operon, for iron release (Earhart, 1996). Fes hydrolyzes the ester bonds of ferric enterobactin to produce ferric dihydrobenzoyl serine (Brickman and McIntosh, 1992), and similar observations have been reported for Fe^{3+}–salmochelin by the Fes analogue IroD (Zhu *et al.*, 2005; Lin *et al.*, 2005). Iron acquisition mediated by the Gram-positive trilactone-based catecholate siderophore bacillibactin also necessitates enzymatic hydrolysis of the scaffold for successful intracellular iron delivery, and this is catalysed by the esterase BesA (Wen *et al.*, 2011). However, BesA can hydrolyze the trilactones of both siderophores, while only the tri-l-serine trilactone is a substrate of Fes (Miethke *et al.*, 2006; Abergel *et al.*, 2008). The trilactone hydrolases usually have a conserved GxSxG motif characteristic of serine esterases, which is part of the classic catalytic S-H-E/D triad. Crystal structures of *Shigella flexneri* and *Salmonella typhimurium* Fes (PDB entries 3C87 and 3MGA), and *Bacillus cereus* BesA (PDB entry 2QM0) have been determined.

The subsequent step in iron release from the hydrolyzed ferric triscatecholate scaffold requires a ferrireductase, which in *E. coli* is YqjH (Miethke *et al.*, 2011a,b). YqjH has high sequence similarity with a number of known siderophore-interacting proteins and its structure was solved (Bamford *et al.*, 2008) by molecular replacement using the siderophore-interacting protein ViuB from *Shewanella putrefaciens* (PDB 2GPJ). Like ViuB, it is a member of the NAD(P)H:flavin oxidoreductase family. YdjH catalyses iron release from a variety of siderophores, most effectively from ferri-(2,3-dihydroxybenzoylserine), the product of esterase hydrolysis of ferri-enterobactin. It can also release iron from ferric dicitrate, and has been shown to be a Fur-regulated protein (Wang *et al.*, 2011).

3.5 Intracellular Iron Metabolism

Once iron has been assimilated within the bacterial cell, it is made available for intracellular functions. While iron from siderophore uptake and from lactoferrin and transferrin is directly available, haem iron must be released by the action of haem oxygenase (discussed in Chapter 8). Once iron is available within the bacteria, it can be made available for intracellular functions. However, in many bacteria it can constitute an intracellular reserve, by its incorporation into a number of iron storage proteins (Andrews *et al.*, 2003), which can make iron available for growth when extracellular sources of iron are limiting. Three types of iron storage protein are found in bacteria, characterised by a similar molecular architecture, composed of a roughly spherical protein shell surrounding a central cavity within which a mineral core of iron is deposited. These three proteins, which can all exist in the same bacterium, are: (i) ferritins, which are also found in eukaryotes; (ii) haem-containing bacterioferritins, found in eubacteria; and (iii) the smaller Dps proteins, present only in prokaryotes (Andrews *et al.*, 2003). As discussed in greater detail in Chapter 9, they are composed of either 24 (ferritins and bacterioferritins) or 12 (Dps proteins) similar – if not identical – subunits folded in a central bundle of four parallel and antiparallel α-helices. Although they form evolutionarily distinct families, they have many structural and functional similarities (this will be discussed in greater detail in Chapter 9). The subunits assemble to form a roughly spherical protein shell that surrounds a central cavity within which iron is stored (up to 4500 iron atoms per 24mer in ferritins and bacterioferritins, and around 500 iron atoms in the smaller Dps protein 12mer).

Iron in these proteins is stored in the ferric form, but is taken up as Fe^{2+}, and subsequently oxidised by ferroxidase sites. In ferritins and bacterioferritins these ferroxidase centres, which are composed of a number of highly conserved residues, are located in the central region of each subunit (Chapter 9). Two Fe^{2+} bind to the ferroxidase centre, where they are oxidised to an oxo bridged diferric intermediate, characteristic of the (μ-carboxylato)di-iron protein family, of which ferritins are members (see Chapter 2). The Fe^{3+} then migrates to the interior cavity of the protein to form either a ferrihydrite core or, if phosphate is present, an amorphous ferric phosphate core.

The ferritins in bacteria such as *E. coli*, *Campylobacter jejuni* and *Helicobacter pylori* appear to fulfil the classical role of iron storage proteins – that is, they accumulate iron when it is in excess for future use under conditions of iron penury (Andrews *et al.*, 2003). This is reflected in the expression pattern of the ferritin A gene, *ftnA* in *E. coli*, which is induced by iron (as described later in this chapter). It may also play a role in iron detoxification.

The bacterioferritins (Bfrs) are more common in bacteria than ferritins, but their physiological role is less clear (Andrews *et al.*, 2003). They all contain haem, normally as protoporphyrin IX, although bacterioferritin from *Desulfovibrio desulfuricans* Bfr has coproporphyrin III (Romao *et al.* 2000), with the iron coaxially ligated by two methionine residues, a haem coordination unique to bacterioferritin. The haem iron is low-spin, the redox potential of the Bfr of *Azotobacter vinelandii* (Watt *et al.*, 1986) is relatively low (–225 mV), and recent studies have argued that the haem bound to *E. coli* BFR accelerates iron core formation by an electron transfer-based mechanism (Wong *et al.*, 2012). The association of a ferredoxin with Bfr in many bacteria (Quail *et al.*, 1996), or in *Desulfovibrio desulfuricans* of a rubredoxin (Da Costa *et al.*, 2001), has led to the suggestion that these iron–sulphur proteins may act as iron-starvation-induced bacterioferritin reductases, which ensure the release of iron from Bfr under conditions of iron restriction. A possible direct role for the haem cofactor in iron mobilisation has also been proposed (Yasmin *et al.*, 2011).

The Dps protein was isolated from three day-old cultures of *E. coli* in 1992 (Almiron *et al.*, 1992), designated *D*NA-binding *p*rotein from *s*tarved cells, and during the stationary phase of *E. coli* growth Dps was the most abundant protein in the bacterial cytoplasm (Wolf *et al.*, 1999; Frenkiel-Krispin *et al.*, 2001). It is widely distributed in bacteria, with a highly conserved tertiary and quaternary structure composed of a central four-helix bundle (A–D) as the core, with a small BC helix linking the B and C helices (Figure 3.17a).

The highly conserved ferroxidase centre is the most distinctive structural signature of Dps proteins (Chiancone and Ceci, 2010), located at the interface of twofold symmetry of related subunits (Figure 3.17b) instead of within the four-helix bundle of a single subunit, as in all known

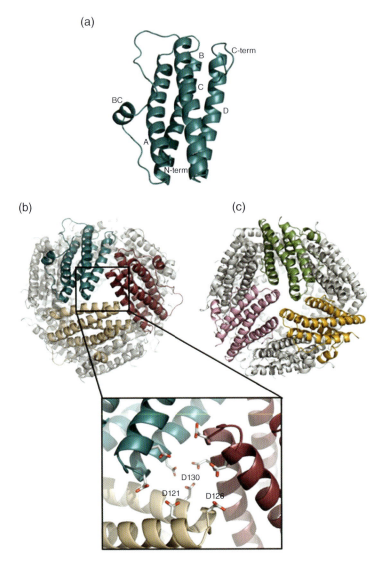

Figure 3.17 *Structural organisation of Dps proteins. Dps fold (a), 12-mer assembly: view along the ferritin-like (b) and Dps-type (c) pores formed respectively by the N- and C-terminal regions of the subunits. In (b) the blow-up shows the aspartate residues lining of the ferritin-like pore in* L. innocua *Dps. Reprinted with permission of Elsevier from Chiancone, E. and Ceci, P. (2010) The multifaceted capacity of Dps proteins to combat bacterial stress conditions: Detoxification of iron and hydrogen peroxide and DNA binding.* Biochim. Biophys. Acta., ***1800**, 798–805*

ferroxidases (Ilari *et al.*, 2000). The residues involved in iron binding are well conserved in Dps proteins from different bacterial species (see Chapter 8). However, whereas typically, most ferritins use O_2 as an oxidant for the ferroxidase centre, Dps proteins use H_2O_2 (Zhao *et al.*, 2002). This suggests that the primary role of Dps in *E. coli*, rather than its iron storage function, is to protect DNA against the toxicity of the hydroxyl radical produced by the Fenton reaction, via the concomitant removal of Fe^{2+} and H_2O_2 (Chiancone and Ceci, 2010). It therefore seems likely that the role of this family of proteins is to: (i) act as an anti-redox agent against Fenton chemistry; and (ii) physically protect DNA (Chiancone *et al.*, 2004; Chiancone and Ceci, 2010). Based on the X-ray structure, the DNA-interacting element of *E. coli* Dps is the highly mobile N-terminal region of the protein, which reaches out from the surface of the protein with three Lys residues which can interact with the phosphate groups in DNA. Mutant Dps lacking all three Lys residues cannot bind to or condense DNA (Ceci *et al.*, 2004). Mobility is also essential, since *A. tumefaciens* Dps, which has all three Lys residues, is unable to interact with DNA since the N-terminal regions are immobilised on the surface of the dodecamer by the formation of hydrogen bonds and salt bridges with symmetry-related subunits (Ceci *et al.*, 2003). Some 20 members of the Dps family have N-terminal sequences similar to that of *E. coli*, as underlined by studies on studies on *M. smegmatis* Dps2 and on *D. radiodurans* Dps1 (Roy *et al.*, 2008; Grove and Wilkinson, 2005; Bhattacharyya and Grove, 2007). Two other DNA-binding signatures have been identified. *M. smegmatis* Dps2 has a truncated N terminus and a flexible 26 residue-long C terminus containing five positively and four negatively charged amino acids. Deletion of the last 16 residues eliminates DNA binding (Gupta and Chatterji, 2003; Roy *et al.*, 2007). *H. pylori* Dps, unlike other Dps proteins, has a positively charged protein surface that is used to bind DNA (Ceci *et al.*, 2007), and a similar mechanism may be operative in the Dps protein from *Trichodesmium erythraeum*, a marine N_2-fixing cyanobacterium (Castruita *et al.*, 2006).

3.6 Control of Gene Expression by Iron

Iron transport systems in bacteria needs to be tightly regulated in response to iron availability, and in the Enterobacteriaceae this is carried out by Fur, the principal transcriptional regulator of iron transport genes (Hantke, 1981, 1984; Bagg and Neilands, 1987). The transcriptional regulation of gene expression in prokaryotes involves regulatory proteins which either bind to DNA to repress or activate expression of specific genes or groups of genes, or else bind to somewhat degenerate sequences or structural motifs, thus spreading DNA interactions along extended nucleotide sequences. This feature is shared by the Fur protein of *E. coli*, which displays both those properties found in specific transcriptional factors and those found in more global regulators. The striking phenotype of the first *fur* mutants isolated was not only the overexpression of the outer membrane receptors for siderophore iron transport, but also the excretion of siderophores under iron-rich growth conditions, indicating that not only the uptake of siderophores but also their biosynthesis was regulated by Fur (Figure 3.18). However, the Fur protein controls the iron-dependent expression not only of genes involved in iron acquisition – siderophore biosynthesis, ferric-siderophore and ferrous iron uptake (at least 35) – but also of many others; in *E. coli* strains, more than 90 genes are under its control (Escolar *et al.*, 1999; Hantke, 2001). These include genes with 'non-iron' functions, such as respiration, motility, intermediary metabolism, including glycolysis, the tricarboxylic acid cycle, methionine biosynthesis, DNA synthesis, purine metabolism, phage DNA packaging, resistance to redox stress and, as will be seen later, a small noncoding RNA, RyhB (Stojiljkovic *et al.*, 1994; Park and Gunsalus, 1995; Vassinova and Kozyrev, 2000; Touati, 1988; Wassarman *et al.*, 2001).

The Fur protein from *E. coli* can be isolated in one step due to its high affinity for metal chelate columns loaded with zinc (Wee *et al.*, 1988). The essential role of Fur proteins is to act as a transcriptional repressor, binding as a dimer to specific palindromic A/T-rich sequences upstream of the transcription start site of iron-regulated promoters, using iron or another metal as corepressor

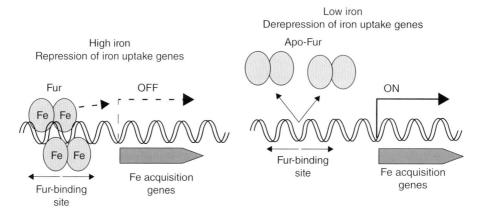

Figure 3.18 *Schematic representation of Fur-mediated gene repression. Reprinted with permission from Elsevier from Andrews, S.C., Robinson, A.K. and Rodriguez-Quinones, F. (2003) Bacterial iron homeostasis.* FEMS Microbiol. Rev., **27***, 215–237*

(Bagg and Neilands, 1987; Escolar *et al.*, 1999). *E. coli* Fur is a dimer made up of two identical 17 kDa subunits, acting as a positive transcriptional repressor when it interacts with its corepressor Fe^{2+}, and causing derepression in the absence of Fe^{2+}. The Fur protein was shown to bind the DNA between −35 and −10 bases from the initiation site in the promoter region of Fur-repressed genes. This 19 base pair palindromic[4] consensus sequence, called the Fur box (Escolar *et al.*, 1999), is GATAATGATAATCATTATC (although this exact sequence is not found anywhere in the *E. coli* genome, and most Fur binding sites only match, at best, 11 of the 19 base pairs). *In vitro* binding is dependent on a divalent cation, with Fe^{2+} clearly the physiologically relevant one.

Fur from *E. coli* was the first member described of the by now large Fur and Fur-like family of metal-uptake regulators that control the homeostasis not only of iron (Fur) but also of zinc (Zur) (Patzer and Hantke, 1998), nickel (Nur) (An *et al.*, 2009) and manganese (Mur) (Díaz-Mireles *et al.*, 2004; An *et al.*, 2009). Two other members of the Fur family are the peroxide-sensing protein PerR of *B. subtilis* (Faulkner *et al.*, 2012), which plays a major role in the response to oxidative stress and a special haem-dependent protein, Irr, which regulates haem iron homeostasis in *Bradyrhizobium* (Small *et al.*, 2009). Although these proteins show a wide diversity of metal selectivity and biological functions, they share a common fold with an average length of between 130 and 160 amino acids comprising two domains: an N-terminal winged-helix DNA-binding domain (ca. 80 residues; DBD); and a C-terminal domain (ca. 70 residues) responsible for the dimerisation and binding of divalent metal ions, connected by a short interdomain loop. This is illustrated for *Pseudomonas aeruginosa* PaFur (Pohl *et al.*, 2003) in Figure 3.19. Members of this superfamily are recognised by a His-rich motif $HHHXHX_2CX_2C$ located at the beginning of the dimerisation domain after the loop that links the N- and C-terminal domains. A second CXXC motif close to the C terminus is found in some Fur proteins and all Zur and PerR proteins reported to date. The Fur family is ubiquitous in prokaryotes with close to 10 000 sequences distributed between 4091 different bacteria and archae in the Pfam database (http://pfam.sanger.ac.uk/family/PF01475) (Fillat, 2014).

---

[4] Palindromes are words, phrases or sentences which read the same backwards as forwards, e.g. 'Able was I ere I saw Elba'.

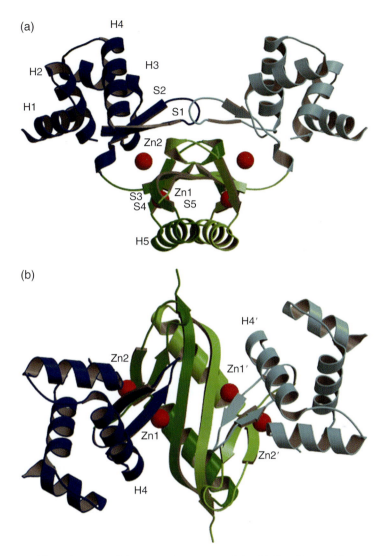

Figure 3.19 *(a) Ribbon diagram of the crystal structure of the PA-Fur dimer with secondary structural elements annotated. The view shown is approximately perpendicular to the crystallographic twofold axis. The DNA-binding domains are depicted in blue, and the dimerisation domain in green. The symmetry-related second monomer is shown in light blue and green. (b) View along the crystallographic twofold axis. Reprinted from Pohl, E., Haller, J.C., Mijovilovich, A. et al. (2003) Architecture of a protein central to iron homeostasis: crystal structure and spectroscopic analysis of the ferric uptake regulator.* Mol. Microbiol., **47**, *903–915*

Structural information is available for three full-length Fur proteins, the *Pseudomonas aeruginosa* PaFur (Pohl *et al.*, 2003) the *Vibrio cholerae*, VcFur (Sheikh and Taylor, 2009) and *Helicobacter pylori* HpFur (Dian *et al.*, 2011) and for the DBD of *E. coli*, EcFur (Pecqueur *et al.*, 2006). Crystal structures of the *Mycobacterium tuberculosis* zinc uptake regulator MtZur (Lucarelli *et al.*, 2007), the *B. subtilis* peroxide-regulon repressor BsPerR (Traoré *et al.*, 2006; Jacquamet *et al.*, 2009) and

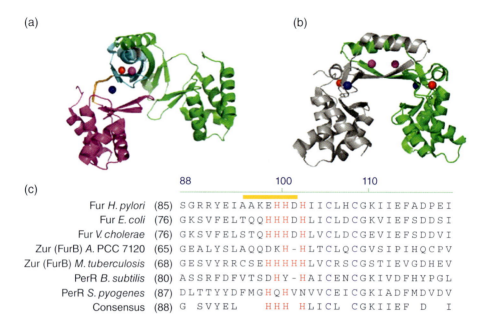

(a)

(b)

(c)

		88	100	110
Fur *H. pylori*	(85)	SGRRYEIAAKE	HHD	HIICLHCGKIIEFADPEI
Fur *E. coli*	(76)	GKSVFELTQQ	HHHDH	LICLDCGKVIEFSDDSI
Fur *V. cholerae*	(76)	GKSVFELSTQ	HHHDH	LVCLDCGEVIEFSDDVI
Zur (FurB) *A.* PCC 7120	(65)	GEALYSLAQQDK	H-H	LTCLQCGVSIPIHQCPV
Zur (FurB) *M. tuberculosis*	(68)	GESVYRRCSE	HHHHH	LVCRSCGSTIEVGDHEV
PerR *B. subtilis*	(80)	ASSRFDFVTSD	HY-H	AICENCGKIVDFHYPGL
PerR *S. pyogenes*	(87)	DLTTYYDFMG	HQH	VNVVCEICGKIADFMDVDV
Consensus	(88)	G SVYEL	HHH	HLICL CGKIIEF D I

Figure 3.20 *Ribbon representation of the Fur dimer from* H. pylori *(PDB ID 1MZB) showing the three metal ions generated with PyMol. Structural zinc (site 1) is shown as a red sphere. The zinc coordinated in the regulatory site (site 2) is represented in dark blue, and the metal ion in site 3 is coloured magenta. (a) Dimer showing the DNA-binding domain of the A chain in magenta, the inter-domain loop is represented in orange, and the dimerisation domain in cyan. The B chain is coloured in green. (b) Different orientation of the Fur dimer showing the A chain in gray and the B chain in green. (c) Sequence alignment of the histidine-rich motifs from different FUR paralogues. The yellow bar on the top indicates the position of the amino acids involved in the inter-domain loop in the primary sequence. Reprinted with permission from Elsevier from Fillat, M.F. (2014) The FUR (ferric uptake regulator) superfamily: diversity and versatility of key transcriptional regulators. Arch. Biochem. Biophys.,* **546**, *41–52*

the *Streptomyces coelicolor* nickel uptake regulator ScNur (An *et al.*, 2009) confirm the structural homology between the members of this family.

Fur and Fur-like proteins contain two and sometimes three metal-binding sites. While there has been much debate about which of the metal-binding sites is the iron-binding site (Dian *et al.*, 2011; Fleischhacker and Kiley, 2011), it seems that metal-binding site S2, in the hinge region between the DNA-binding domain and the dimerisation domain, corresponds to the high-affinity metal-sensing site and engages amino acids from both domains of the regulator (Dian *et al.*, 2011). As illustrated for HpFur in Figure 3.20, the other two sites (S1 and S3) are embedded in the dimerisation domain. The two Zn^{2+}-binding sites S2 and S3 correspond to the PaFur Zn^{2+}-binding sites, 2 and 1, respectively (Pohl *et al.*, 2003). The coordination geometry of the Zn^{2+} ion in S2 seems to be conserved in all Fur and Fur-like proteins with some flexibility in the coordination sphere, using between four and six ligands to coordinate the metal ion, when the structures of PaFur, BsPerR and HpFur are compared (Pohl *et al.*, 2003; Jacquamet *et al.*, 2009; Dian *et al.*, 2011). In the Fur and PerR proteins, the metal-responsive S2 site is penta-coordinated by three histidine residues and two acidic residues. The variability in the coordination sphere may reflect the nature of the metal occupying the site. Thus, HpFur is active in DNA-binding with Fe^{2+}, but also with Mn^{2+}, Zn^{2+}, Ni^{2+}

and Co^{2+}, while a Cys ligand present in MtZur may reflect its specificity for Zn^{2+} and the presence of four His in ScNur may explain its preference for Ni^{2+} (Lucarelli *et al.*, 2007; An *et al.*, 2009). The site S1, previously identified as the structural Zn^{2+} site (Vitale *et al.*, 2009), is close to the C terminus, with the Zn^{2+} ion tetra-coordinated by two CX_2C motifs stabilizing the β3–β4–β5 sheet. The zinc located at site 3 seems to play a role in stabilizing the dimeric form of the regulator, and is located in the core of the dimerisation domain (Lucarelli *et al.*, 2007; Dian *et al.*, 2011; Ma *et al.*, 2011; Shin *et al.*, 2011; Butcher *et al.*, 2012).

While Fur is the major regulator of iron metabolism, in certain bacterial groups other regulators are involved in this important function. They include the RirA protein in the Rhizobiales and the Rhodobacterales (Johnston *et al.*, 2007), a member of the Rrf2 proteins which include an Fe–S cluster, although in *Caulobacter* there is evidence for Fur as the general iron regulator (da Silva Neto *et al.*, 2009). Low-GC, Gram-positive bacteria, such as *Baccillus* and *Staphylococcus* species, use Fur as their major iron regulator whereas in the high-GC, Gram-positive bacteria, *Corynebacterium*, *Mycobacterium* and *Streptomyces*, DtxR (*d*iphtheria *t*oxin *r*egulator) regulates iron metabolism (Wennerhold and Bott, 2006; Günther-Seeboth and Schupp, 1995). Despite the lack of sequence homology to Fur, the α-helical DNA-binding domain of DtxR is similar to that of Fur (Gonzalez de Peredo *et al.*, 2001: Pohl *et al.*, 2003); however, the position of both domains with respect to each other in the functional dimer is completely different.

The DNA-binding site of Fur is in the N-terminal domain in an unusual helix-turn-helix motif (Holm *et al.*, 1994; Stojiljkovic and Hantke, 1995; Pohl *et al.*, 2003), composed of four helices followed by a two-stranded antiparallel β-sheet (Figure 3.20), and contains the typical winged helix (WH) motif found in other prokaryotic transcription regulators (Huffmann and Brennan, 2002), in which the three-helix bundle H2, H3 and H4 contains the putative DNA-binding helix H4 (Gly 50–Ala 64). The dimerisation domain of each monomer consists of an α/β-domain with three antiparallel strands (S3, S4, S5) covering one long α-helix (H5). Ultraviolet crosslinking and mass spectroscopy studies have indicated that Tyr55 of *E. coli*, as well as the thymines at positions 18 and 19 of the consensus Fur box, are involved in binding (Tiss *et al.*, 2005).

Another important conclusion is that, like DtxR, two dimers of Fur may bind to the operator (Lavrrar and McIntosh, 2003). The crystal structure of the cobalt-activated DtxR bound to a 21-bp DNA duplex has been determined, in which two DxtR dimers surround the DNA duplex, which is distorted compared to classical B-DNA (Pohl *et al.*, 1999). Fur has never been shown to protect less than 27–30 bp in DNase 1 protection assays (Ochsner and Vasil, 1996), which would be consistent with the binding of two Fur dimers. This might explain why there are so many Fur molecules per cell (5000–10 000), yet only a three- to fourfold decrease in the level of Fur causes derepression of iron starvation-inducible genes and increased susceptibility to oxidative stress (Ochsner *et al.*, 1999; Zheng *et al.*, 1999).

Although the majority of iron-regulated genes are repressed, Fe^{2+}-Fur regulates a number of genes positively: in *E. coli* these include the genes for the TCA cycle enzymes aconitase, fumarase and succinate dehydrogenase, both ferritins FtnA and Bfr, and the Fe-superoxide dismutase, sodB, all of which encode for proteins that contain iron or have iron–sulphur clusters (Escolar *et al.*, 1999; Hantke, 2001). The explanation comes from the discovery of small noncoding RNAs (Wassarman *et al.*, 2001) in all organisms, mostly as regulators of translation and message stability. In *E. coli* there are more than 50, which corresponds to 1–2% of the number of protein-coding genes in this organism (Gottesman, 2004). One of these, RyhB, was found to repress genes encoding proteins that require iron (Figure 3.21), and it was shown that Fur represses the *ryhB* gene (Massé and Gottesman, 2002). Logically, therefore, when Fur is active, the transcription of RyhB RNA is repressed and, in its absence, the mRNAs for the proteins found to be upregulated are no

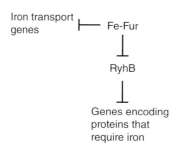

Figure 3.21 *Schematic representation of Fur-mediated gene repression. Reprinted with permission from Elsevier from Carpenter, C. and Payne, S.M. (2014) Regulation of iron transport systems in Enterobacteriaceae in response to oxygen and iron availability. J. Inorg. Biochem.,* **133**, *110–117*

longer degraded and are expressed (for reviews on small RNAs that modulate intracellular iron utilisation in different organisms, see Massé *et al.*, 2005; Oglesby-Sherrouse and Murphy, 2013).

Iron transport genes are regulated primarily by the availability of iron in the environment, but the amount of oxygen also modulates their expression via the transcription factors ArcA and Fnr. ArcA is part of a two-component regulatory system of aerobic and microaerobic metabolism (Iuchi and Weinar, 1996; Alexeeva *et al.*, 2003). ArcB, a membrane-anchored sensor kinase, autophosphorylates under anoxic or reducing conditions and subsequently transfers the phosphoryl group to ArcA, thereby stimulating its DNA-binding activity, resulting in the repression or activation of genes involved in a variety of catabolic pathways. Under oxic conditions, ubiquinones oxidise the cysteine residues of ArcB, resulting in intermolecular disulfide bond formation and the inactivation of ArcB kinase activity. In contrast, when a shift from oxic to microoxic or anoxic conditions occurs the ubiquinone pool is replaced by menaquinones, which reduce the cysteine residues of ArcB; this results in the cleavage of intermolecular disulfide bonds and the activation of ArcB kinase activity (Georgellis *et al.*, 2001; Bekker *et al.*, 2010; Alvarez *et al.*, 2013).

Fnr is a cytoplasmic sensor–regulator which contains an oxygen-responsive [4Fe–4S] cluster, and is the major regulator of anaerobic metabolism, regulating many genes with widely different functions (Unden and Bongaerts, 1997). Fnr binds specifically to DNA as a dimer under anoxic conditions, and exposure to oxygen causes oxidation of the [4Fe–4S] iron–sulphur cluster to a [2Fe–2S] cluster; this results in dissociation to the monomer, which is unable to bind DNA (Melville and Gunsalus, 1996; Lazazzera *et al.*, 1996; Green *et al.*, 1996). ArcA and Fnr regulate the expression of iron transport systems, and as we will see in Chapter 4, they play an important role in many pathogens.

Whereas Fur and DtxR act negatively, repressing gene transcription when cellular iron requirements are satisfied, additional regulatory devices are known which act positively, inducing the transcription of transport genes only when the ferric siderophores themselves are present (Braun, 1997; Venturi *et al.*, 1995). The best studied system is the *Fec* operon, which is involved in the uptake of iron from ferric citrate (Braun, 1997).

Analysis of the ferric citrate transport genes in *E. coli* K-12 revealed a novel type of transcriptional regulation, in which the inducer – ferric citrate – binds to an outer membrane protein and does not need to be transported into the cells to initiate transcription of the ferric citrate transport system, consisting of the *fec ABCDE* genes. Instead, a signalling cascade from the cell surface across the outer membrane, the periplasm, and the cytoplasmic membrane into the cytoplasm transmits information on the presence of the inducer in the culture medium into the cytoplasm,

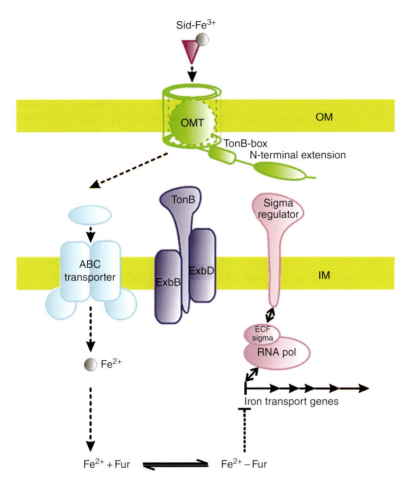

Figure 3.22 *Siderophore transport and transcription induction by OMT_Ns. Ferric siderophore (Sid–Fe^{3+}) from the extracellular medium is recognised by an OMT_N, which serves two functions. First, the OMT_N transports Sid–Fe^{3+} into the periplasm, and from there into the cytoplasm via an ABC transporter. Second, the OMT_N regulates the transcription induction of iron uptake genes. This latter process is initiated by the binding of Sid–Fe^{3+} to the OMT_N, and involves the N-terminal extension of the OMT_N, which interacts with an inner membrane regulator protein. This results in the activation of a cytoplasmic ECF sigma factor, which initiates transcription of iron transport genes for the Sid–Fe^{3+} by RNA polymerase (RNA pol). Both functions require energy transduction by the TonB/ExbB/ExbD system. Reproduced with permission from John Wiley & Sons Ltd*

where gene transcription occurs (Figure 3.22). Under iron-limiting growth conditions, the transcription of ferric citrate transport is induced in the presence of ferric citrate.

FecA, the outer membrane transporter (OMT) for ferric citrate – unlike the other ferric siderophore OMTs described above – has an N-terminal extension of about 70 residues (Pressler *et al.*, 1988), the removal of which results in a complete disruption of the induction of the transport genes, while retaining full transport activity (Kim *et al.*, 1997). Thus, FecA protein exerts two distinct activities, functioning not only as an OMT for dinuclear ferric citrate [$(Fe^{3+}$ citrate$)_2$] across the outer membrane, but also as the sensor and signal transmitter for the initiation of transcription of the ferric transport genes. The signal for transcription is transmitted from the cell surface to the cytoplasm by a mechanism which requires three components: the OMT itself with its ferric ligand bound; a cytosolic sigma factor, FecI, belonging to the extracytoplasmic function (ECF) family (Braun, 1997); and its cognate signalling protein, FecR (Braun and Mahren, 2005). TonB-dependent binding of Fe^{3+}-dicitrate to FecA results in a structural change in FecR, anchored in the cytoplasmic membrane by a single transmembrane helix, which leads to the proteolytic degradation of FecR by the site-2 protease RseP. The resulting cytoplasmic FecR fragment binds to FecI, which activates it to recruit RNA polymerase to the promoter of the *fec* operon. Transcription of the *fecI* and *fecR* regulatory genes is repressed by Fe^{2+} bound to the Fur repressor protein. Under iron-limiting conditions, Fur is not loaded with Fe^{2+}, the *fecI* and *fecR* genes are transcribed, and the FecI and FecR proteins are synthesised and respond to the presence of ferric citrate in the medium when ferric citrate binds to the FecA protein (Braun, 1997; Braun, V. *et al.*, 2003, 2006; Braun and Mahren, 2005).

Regulation of the *fec* genes represents the paradigm of a growing number of gene regulation systems involving transmembrane signalling across two or three cellular compartments (reviewed in Braun and Endriss, 2007; Brooks and Buchanan, 2008), involving a subset of sigma factors which respond to a changing environment by recruiting RNA polymerase to appropriate response genes. As these sigma factors are involved in regulating the expression of proteins residing in the outer membrane or periplasmic space, they are called extracytoplasmic function (ECF) sigma factors (Lonetto *et al.*, 1994).

The examination of TonB-dependent outer membrane iron transporters in a large number of pathogenic bacteria has shown that there is a subfamily (designated OMT$_N$) which, like FecA, has the additional N-terminal domain (Schalk *et al.*, 2004), and these are discussed in greater detail in Chapter 4.

References

Abdallah, M. (1991) Pyoverdins and pseudobactins, in *Handbook of Microbial Iron Chelates* (ed. G. Winkelmann), CRC Press, pp. 139–153.

Abergel, R.J., Zawadzka, A.M. and Raymond, K.N. (2008) Petrobactin-mediated iron transport in pathogenic bacteria: coordination chemistry of an unusual 3,4-catecholate/citrate siderophore. *J. Am. Chem. Soc.*, **130**, 2124–2125.

Alexeeva, S., Hellingwerf, K.J. and Teixeira de Mattos, M.J. (2003) Requirement of ArcA for redox regulation in *Escherichia coli* under microaerobic but not anaerobic or aerobic conditions. *J. Bacteriol.*, **185**, 204–209.

Almiron, M., Link, A.J. and Furlong, D. (1992) A novel DNA-binding protein with regulatory and protective roles in starved *Escherichia coli*. *Genes Dev.*, **6**, 2646–2654.

Alvarez, A.F., Rodriguez, C. and Georgellis, D. (2013) Ubiquinone and menaquinone electron carriers represent the yin and yang in the redox regulation of the ArcB sensor kinase. *J. Bacteriol.*, **195**, 3054–3061.

An, Y.J., Ahn, B.E. Roe, J.H. and Cha, S.S. (2009) Crystallization and preliminary X-ray crystallographic analyses of Nur, a nickel-responsive transcription regulator from *Streptomyces coelicolor*. *Acta Crystallogr. Sect. F Struct. Biol. Cryst. Commun.*, **64**, 130–132.

Andrews, S.C., Robinson, A.K. and Rodriguez-Quinones, F. (2003) Bacterial iron homeostasis. *FEMS Microbiol Rev.*, **27**, 215–237.

Ash, M. R., Guilfoyle, A., Clarke, R.J., *et al.* (2010) Potassium-activated GTPase reaction in the G protein-coupled ferrous iron transporter B. *J. Biol. Chem.*, **285**, 14594–14602.

Askwith, C. and Kaplan, J. (1997) An oxidase-permease-based iron transport system in *Schizosaccharomyces pombe* and its expression in *Saccharomyces cerevisiae*. *J. Biol. Chem.*, **272**, 401–405.

Bachman, B.J. (1972) Pedigrees of some mutant strains of *Escherichia coli* K-12. *Bacteriol. Rev.*, **36**, 525–557.

Bagg, A. and Neilands, J.B. (1987) Ferric uptake regulation protein acts as a repressor, employing iron (II) as a cofactor to bind the operator of an iron transport operon in *Escherichia coli*. *Biochemistry*, **26**, 5471–5477.

Bamford, V.A., Armour, M., Mitchell, S.A., *et al.* (2008) Preliminary X-ray diffraction analysis of YqjH from *Escherichia coli*: a putative cytoplasmic ferri-siderophore reductase. *Acta Crystallogr. Sect. F Struct. Biol. Cryst. Commun.*, **64**, 792–796.

Barbeau, K., Zhang, G.P., Live, D.H. and Butler, A. (2002) Petrobactin, a photoreactive siderophore produced by the oil-degrading marine bacterium *Marinobacter hydrocarbonoclasticus*. *J. Am. Chem. Soc.*, **124**, 378–379.

Beasley, F.C. and Heinrichs, D.H. (2010) Siderophore-mediated iron acquisition in the staphylococci. *J. Inorg. Biochem.*, **104**, 282–288.

Bekker, M., Alexeeva, S., Laan, W., *et al.* (2010) The ArcBA two-component system of *Escherichia coli* is regulated by the redox state of both the ubiquinone and the menaquinone pool. *J. Bacteriol.*, **192**, 746–754.

Bergeron, R., Bergeron, R.J., Huang, G.F., *et al.* (2003) Total synthesis and structure revision of petrobactin. *Tetrahedron*, **59**, 2007–2014.

Berntsson, R.P., Smits, S.H., Schmitt, L., Slotboom, D.J. and Poolman B. (2010) A structural classification of substrate-binding proteins. *FEBS Lett.*, **584**, 2606–2617.

Bhattacharyya, G. and Grove, A. (2007) The N-terminal extensions of *Deinococcus radiodurans* Dps-1 mediate DNA major groove interactions as well as assembly of the dodecamer. *J. Biol. Chem.*, **282**, 11921–11930.

Blanvillain, S., Meyer, D., Boulanger A, *et al.* (2007) Plant carbohydrate scavenging through tonB-dependent receptors: a feature shared by phytopathogenic and aquatic bacteria. *PLoS One*, **2**, e224.

Braun, V. (1997) Surface signaling: novel transcription initiation mechanism starting from the cell surface. *Arch. Microbiol.*, **167**, 325–331.

Braun, V. and Mahren, S. (2005) Transmembrane transcriptional control (surface signalling) of the *Escherichia coli* type. *FEMS Microbiol. Rev.*, **29**, 673–684.

Braun, V. and Endriss, F. (2007) Energy-coupled outer membrane transport proteins and regulatory proteins. *Biometals*, **20**, 219–231.

Braun, V. and Hantke, K. (2011) Recent insights into iron import by bacteria. *Curr. Opin. Chem. Biol.*, **15**, 328–334.

Braun, V. and Hantke, K. (2013) The Tricky Ways Bacteria Cope with Iron limitation, in *Iron Uptake in Bacteria with Emphasis on E. coli and Pseudomonas* (eds R. Chakrabarty, K. Hantke, V. Braun and P. Cornelis), Springer, Dordrecht, pp. 31–66.

Braun, V., Mahren, S. and Ogierman, M. (2003) Regulation of the FecI-type ECF sigma factor by transmembrane signalling. *Curr. Opin. Microbiol.*, **6**, 173–180.

Braun, V., Mahren, S. and Sauter, A. (2006) Gene regulation by transmembrane signaling. *Biometals*, **19**, 103–113.

Brickman, T.J. and McIntosh, M.A. (1992) Overexpression and purification of ferric enterobactin esterase from *Escherichia coli*. Demonstration of enzymatic hydrolysis of enterobactin and its iron complex. *J. Biol. Chem.*, **267**, 12350–12355.

Brockwell, D.J., Paci, E., Zinober, R.C., *et al.* (2003) Pulling geometry defines the mechanical resistance of a beta-sheet protein. *Nat. Struct. Biol.*, **10**, 731–737.

Brooks, B.E. and Buchanan, S.K. (2008) Signaling mechanisms for activation of extracytoplasmic function (ECF) sigma factors. *Biochim. Biophys. Acta*, **1778**, 1930–1945.

Buchanan, S.K., Smith, B.S., Venkatramani, L., *et al.* (1999) Crystal structure of the outer membrane active transporter FepA from *Escherichia coli*. *Nat. Struct. Biol.*, **6**, 56–63.

Butcher, J., Sarvan, S., Brunzelle, J.S., Couture, J.F. and Stintzi, A. (2012) Structure and regulon of *Campylobacter jejuni* ferric uptake regulator Fur define apo-Fur regulation. *Proc. Natl Acad. Sci. USA*, **109**, 10047–10052.

Cao, Z. and Klebba, P.E. (2002) Mechanisms of colicin binding and transport through outer membrane porins. *Biochimie*, **84**, 399–412.

Cao, J., Woodhall, M.R., Alvarez, J., Cartron, M.L. and Andrews, S.C. (2007) EfeUOB (YcdNOB) is a tripartite, acid-induced and CpxAR-regulated, low-pH Fe^{2+} transporter that is cryptic in *Escherichia coli* K-12 but functional in *E. coli* O157:H7. *Mol. Microbiol.*, **65**, 857–875.

Carpenter, C. and Payne, S.M. (2014) Regulation of iron transport systems in Enterobacteriaceae in response to oxygen and iron availability. *J. Inorg. Biochem.*, **133**, 110–117.

Carrion-Vazquez, M., Li, H., Lu, H., *et al.* (2003) The mechanical stability of ubiquitin is linkage-dependent. *Nat. Struct. Biol.*, **10**, 738–743.

Carter, D.M., Gagnon, J.N., Damlaj, M., *et al.* (2006a) Phage display reveals multiple contact sites between FhuA, an outer membrane receptor of *Escherichia coli*, and TonB. *J. Mol. Biol.*, **357**, 236–251.

Carter, D.M., Miousse, I.R., Gagnon, J.N., *et al.* (2006b) Interactions between TonB from *Escherichia coli* and the periplasmic protein FhuD. *J. Biol. Chem.*, **281**, 35413–35424.

Cartron, M.L., Maddocks, S., Gillingham, P., *et al.* (2006) Feo-transport of ferrous iron into bacteria. *Biometals*, **19**, 143–157.

Cascales, E., Lioubes, R. and Sturgis, J.N. (2001) The TolQ-TolR proteins energize TolA and share homologies with the flagellar motor proteins MotA-MotB. *Mol. Microbiol.*, **42**, 795–807.

Cascales, E., Buchanan, S.K., Duché, D., *et al.* (2007) Colicin biology. *Microbiol. Mol. Biol. Rev.*, **71**, 158–229.

Castruita, M., Saito, M., Schottel, P.C., *et al.* (2006) Overexpression and characterization of an iron storage and DNA-binding Dps protein from *Trichodesmium erythraeum*. *Appl. Environ. Microbiol.*, **72**, 2918–2924.

Ceci, P., Ilari, A., Falvo, E. and Chiancone, E. (2003) The Dps protein of *Agrobacterium tumefaciens* does not bind to DNA but protects it toward oxidative cleavage: X-ray crystal structure, iron binding, and hydroxyl-radical scavenging properties. *J. Biol. Chem.*, **278**, 20319–20326.

Ceci, P., Cellai, S., Falvo, E., *et al.* (2004) DNA condensation and self-aggregation of *Escherichia coli* Dps are coupled phenomena related to the properties of the N-terminus. *Nucleic Acids Res.*, **32**, 5935–5944.

Ceci, P., Mangiarotti, L., Rivetti, C. and Chiancone, E. (2007) The neutrophil-activating Dps protein of *Helicobacter pylori*, HP-NAP, adopts a mechanism different from *Escherichia coli* Dps to bind and condense DNA. *Nucleic Acids Res.*, **35**, 2247–2256.

Chakrabarty, R. (2013) Ferric Siderophore transport via outer membrane receptors of *Escherichia coli*: Structural advancement and a tribute to Dr. Dick van der Helm – an 'Ironman' of siderophore biology, in Iron Uptake in Bacteria, with Emphasis on E. coli and Pseudomonas (eds R. Chakrabarty, K. Hantke, V. Braun and P. Cornelis), Springer, Dordrecht, pp. 1–29.

Chang, C., Mooser, A., Pluckthun, A. and Wlodawer, A. (2001) Crystal structure of the dimeric C-terminal domain of TonB reveals a novel fold. *J. Biol. Chem.*, **276**, 27535–27540.

Chiancone, E. and Ceci, P. (2010) The multifaceted capacity of Dps proteins to combat bacterial stress conditions: Detoxification of iron and hydrogen peroxide and DNA binding. *Biochim. Biophys. Acta*, **1800**, 798–805.

Chiancone, E., Ceci, P., Ilari, A. *et al.* (2004) Iron and proteins for iron storage and detoxification. *Biometals*, **17**, 197–202.

Chimento, D.P., Mohanty, A.K., Kadner, R.J. and Wiener, M.C. (2003) Substrate-induced transmembrane signaling in the cobalamin transporter BtuB. *Nat. Struct. Biol.*, **10**, 394–401.

Chiu, H.J., Johnson, E., Schröder, I. and Rees, D.C. (2001) Crystal structures of a novel ferric reductase from the hyperthermophilic archaeon *Archaeoglobus fulgidus* and its complex with NADP$^+$. *Structure*, **9**, 311–319.

Chu, B.C. and Vogel, H.J. (2011) A structural and functional analysis of type III periplasmic and substrate binding proteins: their role in bacterial siderophore and heme transport. *Biol. Chem.*, **392**, 39–52.

Chu, B.C., Peacock, R.S. and Vogel, H.J. (2007) Bioinformatic analysis of the TonB protein family. *Biometals*, **20**, 467–483.

Clarke, T.E., Ku, S.Y., Dougan, D.R., *et al.* (2000) The structure of the ferric siderophore binding protein FhuD complexed with gallichrome. *Nat. Struct. Biol.*, **7**, 287–291.

Clarke, T.E., Braun, V., Winkelmann, G., *et al.* (2002) X-ray crystallographic structures of the *Escherichia coli* periplasmic protein FhuD bound to hydroxamate-type siderophores and the antibiotic albomycin. *J. Biol. Chem.*, **277**, 13966–13972.

Cobessi, D., Celia, H. and Pattus, F. (2004) Crystallization and X-ray diffraction analyses of the outer membrane pyochelin receptor FptA from *Pseudomonas aeruginosa*. *Acta Crystallogr. D*, **60**, 1919–1921.

Cobessi, D., Celia, H. and Pattus, F. (2005a) Crystal structure at high resolution of ferric-pyochelin and its membrane receptor FptA from *Pseudomonas aeruginosa*. *J. Mol. Biol.*, **352**, 893–904.

Cobessi, D., Celia, H., Folschweiler, N., *et al.* (2005b) The crystal structure of the pyoverdine outer membrane receptor FpvA from *Pseudomonas aeruginosa* at 3.6 angstroms resolution. *J. Mol. Biol.*, **347**, 121–134.

Coves, J. and Fontecave, M. (1993) Reduction and mobilization of iron by a NAD(P)H:flavin oxidoreductase from *Escherichia coli*. *Eur. J. Biochem.*, **211**, 635–641.

Da Costa, P.N., Romao, C., Le Gall, J., *et al.* (2001) The genetic organization of *Desulfovibrio desulphuricans* ATCC 27 774 bacterioferritin and rubredoxin-2 genes: involvement of rubredoxin in iron metabolism, *Mol. Microbiol.*, **41**, 217–227.

Da Silva Neto, J.F., Braz, V.S., Italiani, V.C. and Marques, M.V. (2009) Fur controls iron homeostasis and oxidative stress defense in the oligotrophic alpha-proteobacterium *Caulobacter crescentus*. *Nucleic Acids Res.*, **37**, 4812–4825.

Davidson, A.L. and Chen, J. (2004) ATP-binding cassette transporters in bacteria. *Annu. Rev. Biochem.*, **73**, 241–268.

Davidson, A.L., Dassa, E., Orelle, C. and Chen. J. (2008) Structure, function, and evolution of bacterial ATP-binding cassette systems. *Microbiol. Mol. Biol. Rev.*, **72**, 317–364.

Dertz, E.A., Xu, J., Stintzi, A. and Raymond, K.N. (2006) Siderophores of *Bacillus anthracis, Bacillus cereus*, and *Bacillus thuringiensis*. *J. Am. Chem. Soc.*, **128**, 22–23.

Díaz-Mireles, E., Wexler, M., Sawers, G., *et al.* (2004) The Fur-like protein Mur of *Rhizobium leguminosarum* is a Mn(2+)-responsive transcriptional regulator. *Microbiology*, **150**, 1447–1456.

Dian, C., Vitale, S., Leonard, G.A., *et al.* (2011) The structure of the *Helicobacter pylori* ferric uptake regulator Fur reveals three functional metal binding sites. *Mol. Microbiol.*, **79**, 1260–1275.

Earhart, C.F. (1996) in Escherichia coli *and* Salmonella*: Cellular and molecular biology* (ed. F.C. Neidhard), ASM Press, pp. 1075–1090.

Eng, E.T., Jalilian, A.R., Spasov, K.A. and Unger, V.M. (2008) Characterization of a novel prokaryotic GDP dissociation inhibitor domain from the G protein coupled membrane protein FeoB. *J. Mol. Biol.*, **375**, 1086–1097.

Escolar, L., Perez-Martin, J. and de Lorenzo, V. (1999) Opening the iron box: transcriptional metalloregulation by the Fur protein. *J. Bacteriol.*, **181**, 6223–6229.

Faulkner, M.J., Ma, Z., Fuangthong, M. and Helmann, J.D. (2012) Derepression of the *Bacillus subtilis* PerR peroxide stress response leads to iron deficiency. *J. Bacteriol.*, **194**, 1226–1235.

Feig, L.A. and Cooper, G.M. (1988) Relationship among guanine nucleotide exchange, GTP hydrolysis, and transforming potential of mutated ras proteins. *Mol. Cell Biol.*, **8**, 2472–2478.

Ferguson, A., Hofmann, D.E., Coulton, J.W., *et al.* (1998) Siderophore-mediated iron transport: crystal structure of FhuA with bound lipopolysaccharide. *Science*, **282**, 2215–2220.

Ferguson, A.D., Welte, S., Hofmann, E., *et al.* (2000) A conserved structural motif for lipopolysaccharide recognition by procaryotic and eucaryotic proteins. *Structure*, **8**, 585–592.

Ferguson, A.D., Chakraborty, R., Smith, B.S., *et al.* (2002) Structural basis of gating by the outer membrane transporter FecA. *Science*, **295**, 1715–1719.

Fillat, M.F. (2014) The FUR (ferric uptake regulator) superfamily: diversity and versatility of key transcriptional regulators. *Arch. Biochem. Biophys.*, **546**, 41–52.

Fischbach, M.A., Lin, H., Liu, D.R. and Walsh C.T. (2006) How pathogenic bacteria evade mammalian sabotage in the battle for iron. *Nat. Chem. Biol.*, **2**, 132–138.

Fisher, C.R., Davies, N.M., Wyckoff, E.E., *et al.* (2009) Genetics and virulence association of the *Shigella flexneri* sit iron transport system. *Infect. Immun.*, **77**, 1992–1999.

Fleischhacker, A.S. and Kiley, P.J. (2011) Iron-containing transcription factors and their roles as sensors. *Curr. Opin. Chem. Biol.*, **15**, 335–341.

Flo, T.H., Smith, K.D., Sato, S., Rodriguez, D.J., *et al.* (2004) Lipocalin 2 mediates an innate immune response to bacterial infection by sequestrating iron. *Nature*, **432**, 917–921.

Fontecave, M., Coves, J. and Pierre, J.-L. (1994) Ferric reductases or flavin reductases? *BioMetals*, **7**, 3–8.

Frenkiel-Krispin, D., Ben-Avraham, I., Englander, J., *et al.* (2001) Nucleoid restructuring in stationary-state bacteria. *Mol. Microbiol.*, **51**, 395–405.

Freed, D.M., Lukasik, S.M., Sikora, A., Mokdad, A. and Cafiso, D.S. (2013) Monomeric TonB and the Ton box are required for the formation of a high-affinity transporter-TonB complex. *Biochemistry*, **52**, 2638–2648.

Garcia-Herrera, A., Peacock, R.S., Howard, S.P. and Vogel, H.J. (2007) The solution structure of the periplasmic domain of the TonB system ExbD protein reveals an unexpected structural homology with siderophore-binding proteins. *Mol. Microbiol.*, **66**, 872–889.

Georgellis, D., Kwon, O. and Lin, E.C. (2001) Quinones as the redox signal for the arc two-component system of bacteria. *Science*, **292**, 2314–2316.

Goetz, B.A., Perozo, E. and Locher, K.P. (2009) Distinct gate conformations of the ABC transporter BtuCD revealed by electron spin resonance spectroscopy and chemical cross-linking. *FEBS Lett.*, **583**, 266–270.

Gonzalez de Peredo, A., Saint-Pierre, C., Latour, J.M., Michaud-Soret, I. and Forest, E. (2001) Conformational changes of the ferric uptake regulation protein upon metal activation and DNA binding; first evidence of structural homologies with the diphtheria toxin repressor. *J. Mol. Biol.*, **310**, 83–91.

Gottesman, S. (2004) The small RNA regulators of *Escherichia coli*: roles and mechanisms. *Annu. Rev. Microbiol.*, **58**, 303–328.

Gram, H.C.J. (1884) Über die isolierte Färbung der Schizomyceten in Schnitt- und Trockenpräparaten. *Fortschritte der Medizin*, **2**, 185–189.

Green, J., Bennett, B., Jordan, P., *et al.* (1996) Reconstitution of the [4Fe-4S] cluster in FNR and demonstration of the aerobic-anaerobic transcription switch in vitro. *Biochem. J.*, **316** , 887–892.

Gresock, M.G., Savenkova, M.I., Larsen, R.A., Ollis, A.A. and Postle K. (2011) Death of the TonB Shuttle Hypothesis. *Front. Microbiol.*, **2**, 206.

Grosse, C., Scherer, J., Koch, D., *et al.* (2006) A new ferrous iron-uptake transporter, EfeU (YcdN), from *Escherichia coli. Mol. Microbiol.*, **62**, 120–131.

Grove, A. and Wilkinson, S.P. (2005) Differential DNA binding and protection by dimeric and dodecameric forms of the ferritin homolog Dps from *Deinococcus radiodurans. J. Mol. Biol.*, **347**, 495–508.

Guilfoyle, A., Maher, M.J., Rapp, M., *et al.* (2009) Structural basis of GDP release and gating in G protein-coupled Fe^{2+} transport. *EMBO J.*, **28**, 2677–2685.

Guilfoyle, A., Deshpande, C.N., Vincent, K., *et al.* (2014) Structural and functional analysis of a FeoB A143S G5 loop mutant explains the accelerated GDP release rate. *FEBS J.*, **281**, 2254–2265.

Gumbart, J., Wiener, M.C. and Tajkhorshid, E. (2007) Mechanics of force propagation in TonB-dependent outer membrane transport. *Biophys. J.*, **93**, 496–504.

Günter-Seeboth, K. and Schupp, T. (1995) Cloning and sequence analysis of the *Corynebacterium diphtheriae* dtxR homologue from *Streptomyces lividans* and *S. pilosus* encoding a putative iron repressor protein. *Gene*, **166**, 117–119.

Gupta, S. and Chatterji, G. (2003) Bimodal protection of DNA by *Mycobacterium smegmatis* DNA-binding protein from stationary phase cells. *J. Biol. Chem.*, **278**, 5235–5241.

Hallé, F. and Meyer, J.M. (1992a) Ferrisiderophore reductases of *Pseudomonas*. Purification, properties and cellular location of the *Pseudomonas aeruginosa* ferripyoverdine reductase. *Eur. J. Biochem.*, **209**, 613–620.

Hallé, F. and Meyer, J.M. (1992b) Iron release from ferrisiderophores. A multi-step mechanism involving a NADH/FMN oxidoreductase and a chemical reduction by $FMNH_2$. *Eur. J. Biochem.*, **209**, 621–627.

Hannavy, K., Barr, G.C., Dorman, C.J., *et al.* (1990) TonB protein of *Salmonella typhimurium*. A model for signal transduction between membranes. *J. Mol. Biol.*, **216**, 897–910.

Hantke, K. (1981) Regulation of ferric iron transport in *Escherichia coli* K12: isolation of a constitutive mutant. *Mol. Gen. Genet.*, **182**, 288–292.

Hantke, K. (1984) Cloning of the repressor protein gene of iron-regulated systems in *Escherichia coli* K12. *Mol. Gen. Genet.*, **197**, 337–341.

Hantke, K. (1987) Ferrous iron transport mutants in *Escherichia coli* K-12. *FEMS Microbiol. Lett.*, **44**, 53–57.

Hantke, K. (2001) Iron and metal regulation in bacteria. *Curr. Opin. Microbiol.*, **4**, 172–177.

Hantke, K. (2003) Is the bacterial ferrous iron transporter FeoB a living fossil? *Trends Microbiol.*, **11**, 192–195.

Hantke, K., Nicholson, G., Rabsch, W. and Winkelmann, G. (2003) Salmochelins, siderophores of *Salmonella enterica* and uropathogenic *Escherichia coli* strains, are recognized by the outer membrane receptor IroN. *Proc. Natl Acad. Sci. USA*, **100**, 3677–3682.

Härle, C., Kim, J., Angerer, A. and Braun, V. (1995) Signal transfer through three compartments: transcription initiation of the *Escherichia coli* ferric citrate transport system from the cell surface. *EMBO J.*, **14**, 1430–1438.

Hattori, M, Jin, Y., Nishimasu, H., *et al.* (2009) Structural basis of novel interactions between the small-GTPase and GDI-like domains in prokaryotic FeoB iron transporter. *Structure*, **17**, 1345–1355.

Hider, R.C and Kong, X. (2010) Chemistry and biology of siderophores. *Nat. Prod. Rep.*, **27**, 637–657.

Higgs, P.I., Larsen, R.A. and Postle, K. (2002) Quantification of known components of the *Escherichia coli* TonB energy transduction system: TonB, ExbB, ExbD and FepA. *Mol. Microbiol.*, **44**, 271–281.

Hollenstein, K., Frei, D.C. and Locher, K.P. (2007) Structure of an ABC transporter in complex with its binding protein. *Nature*, **446**, 213–216.

Holm, L., Sander, C., Rüterjans, H., *et al.* (1994) LexA repressor and iron uptake from *Escherichia coli*: new members of the CAP-like DNA binding domain superfamily. *Protein Eng.*, **7**, 1449–1453.

Hsueh, K.L., Yu, L.K., Chen, Y.H., *et al.* (2013) FeoC from *Klebsiella pneumoniae* contains a [4Fe–4S] cluster. *J. Bacteriol.*, **195**, 4726–4734.

Huffman, J.L. and Brennan, R.G. (2002) Prokaryotic transcription regulators: more than just the helix-turn-helix motif. *Curr. Opin. Struct. Biol.*, **12**, 98–106.

Hung, K.W., Chang, Y.W., Eng, E.T., *et al.* (2010) Structural fold, conservation and Fe(II) binding of the intracellular domain of prokaryote FeoB. *J. Struct. Biol.*, **170**, 501–512.

Hung, K.W., Juan, T.H., Hsu, Y.L. and Huang, T.H. (2012a) NMR structure note: the ferrous iron transport protein C (FeoC) from *Klebsiella pneumoniae*. *J. Biomol. NMR*, **53**, 161–165.

Hung, K.W., Tsai, J.Y., Juan, T.H., *et al.* (2012b) Crystal structure of the *Klebsiella pneumoniae* NFeoB/FeoC complex and roles of FeoC in regulation of Fe²⁺ transport by the bacterial Feo system. *J. Bacteriol.*, **194**, 6518–6526.

Hutchings, M.I., Palmer, T., Harrington, D.J. and Sutcliffe, I.C. (2009) Lipoprotein biogenesis in Gram-positive bacteria: knowing when to hold 'em, knowing when to fold 'em. *Trends Microbiol.*, **17**, 13–21.

Hvorup, R.N., Goetz, B.A. and Niederer, M. (2007) Asymmetry in the structure of the ABC transporter-binding protein complex BtuCD-BtuF. *Science*, **317**, 1387–1390.

Iiri, T., Herzmark, P., Nakamoto, J.M., van Dop, C. and Bourne, H.R. (1994) Rapid GDP release from Gs alpha in patients with gain and loss of endocrine function. *Nature*, **371**, 164–168.

Ilari, A., Stefanini, S., Chiancone, E. and Tsernoglou, D. (2000) The dodecameric ferritin from *Listeria innocua* contains a novel intersubunit iron-binding site. *Nat. Struct. Biol.*, **7**, 38–43.

Ingelman, M., Ramaswamy, S., Nivière, V., Fontecave, M. and Eklund, H. (1999) Crystal structure of NAD(P) H:flavin oxidoreductase from *Escherichia coli*. *Biochemistry*, **38**, 7040–7049.

Iuchi, S. and Weinar, L. (1996) Cellular and molecular physiology of *Escherichia coli* in the adaptation to aerobic environments. *J. Biochem.*, **120**, 1055–1063.

Jacquamet, L., Traoré, D.A., Ferrer, J.L., *et al.* (2009) Structural characterization of the active form of PerR: insights into the metal-induced activation of PerR and Fur proteins for DNA binding. *Mol. Microbiol.*, **73**, 20–31.

James, K.J., Hancock, M.A., Gagnon, J.N. and Coulton, J.W. (2009) TonB interacts with BtuF, the *Escherichia coli* periplasmic binding protein for cyanocobalamin. *Biochemistry*, **48**, 9212–9220.

Johnston, A.W., Todd, J.D., Curson, A.R., *et al.* (2007) Living without Fur: the subtlety and complexity of iron-responsive gene regulation in the symbiotic bacterium *Rhizobium* and other alpha-proteobacteria. *Biometals*, **20**, 501–511.

Jordan, L.D., Zhou, Y., Smallwood, C.R., *et al.* (2013) Energy-dependent motion of TonB in the Gram-negative bacterial inner membrane. *Proc. Natl Acad. Sci. USA* , **110**, 11553–11558.

Joseph, B., Jeschke, G., Goetz, B.A., Locher, K.P. and Bordignon, E. (2011) Transmembrane gate movements in the type II ATP-binding cassette (ABC) importer BtuCD-F during nucleotide cycle. *J. Biol. Chem.*, **286**, 41008–41017.

Joseph, B., Korkhov, V.M., Yulikov, M., Jeschke, G. and Bordignon, E. (2014) Conformational cycle of the vitamin B_{12} ABC importer in liposomes detected by double electron-electron resonance (DEER). *J. Biol. Chem.*, **289**, 3176–3185.

Kammler, M., Schön, C., and Hantke, K. (1993) Characterization of the ferrous iron uptake system of *Escherichia coli*. *J. Bacteriol.*, **175**, 6212–6219.

Kampfenkel, K. and Braun, V. (1992) Membrane topology of the *Escherichia coli* ExbD protein. *J. Bacteriol.*, **174**, 5485–5487.

Kampfenkel, K. and Braun, V. (1993) Topology of the ExbB protein in the cytoplasmic membrane of *Escherichia coli*. *J. Biol. Chem.*, **268**, 6050–6057.

Kandt, C. and Tieleman, D.P. (2010) Holo-BtuF stabilizes the open conformation of the vitamin B_{12} ABC transporter BtuCD. *Proteins*, **78**, 738–753.

Karlson, M., Hannavy, K. and Higgins, C.F. (1993) ExbB acts as a chaperone-like protein to stabilize TonB in the cytoplasm. *Mol. Microbiol.*, **8**, 389–396.

Karpowich, N.K., Huang, H.H., Smith, P.C. and Hunt, J.F. (2003) Crystal structures of the BtuF periplasmic-binding protein for vitamin B_{12} suggest a functionally important reduction in protein mobility upon ligand binding. *J. Biol. Chem.*, **278**, 8429–8434.

Killmann, H., Videnov, G., Jung, G., Schwarz, H. and Braun, V. (1995) Identification of receptor binding sites by competitive peptide mapping: phages T1, T5, and phi 80 and colicin M bind to the gating loop of FhuA. *J. Bacteriol.*, **177**, 694–698.

Kim, I., Stiefel, A., Plantör, S., Angerer, A. and Braun, V. (1997) Transcription induction of the ferric citrate transport genes via the N-terminus of the FecA outer membrane protein, the Ton system and the electrochemical potential of the cytoplasmic membrane. *Mol. Microbiol.*, **23**, 333–344.

Kjeldsen, S.E., Petrin, J., Weder, A.B. and Julius, S. (1993) Contrasting effects of epinephrine on forearm hemodynamics and arterial plasma norepinephrine. *J. Biol. Chem.*, **268**, 10425–10432.

Koebnik, R. (2005) TonB-dependent trans-envelope signalling: the exception or the rule? *Trends Microbiol.*, **13**, 343–347.

Ködding, J., Killig, F., Polzer, P. *et al.* (2005) Crystal structure of a 92-residue carboxy-terminal fragment of TonB from *Escherichia coli* reveals significant conformational changes compared to structures of smaller TonB fragments. *J. Biol. Chem.*, **280**, 3022–3028.

Köhler, S.D., Weber, A., Howard, S.P., Welte, W. and Drescher, M. (2010) The proline-rich domain of TonB possesses an extended polyproline II-like conformation of sufficient length to span the periplasm of Gram-negative bacteria. *Protein Sci.*, **19**, 625–630.

Konetschny-Rapp, S., Jung, G., Meives, J. and Zähner, H. (1990) Staphyloferrin A: a structurally new siderophore from staphylococci. *Eur. J. Biochem.*, **191**, 65–74.

Koradi, R., Billeter, M. and Wüthrich, K. (1996) MOLMOL: a program for display and analysis of macromolecular structures. *J. Mol. Graph.*, **14**, 51–55.

Korkhov, V.M., Mireku, S.A. and Locher, K.P. (2012) Structure of AMP-PNP-bound vitamin B_{12} transporter BtuCD-F. *Nature*, **490**, 367–372.

Korkhov, V.M., Mireku, S.A., Veprintsev, D.B. and Locher, K.P. (2014) Structure of AMP-PNP-bound BtuCD and mechanism of ATP-powered vitamin B_{12} transport by BtuCD-F. *Nat. Struct. Mol. Biol.*, **21**, 1097–1099.

Köster, S., Wehner, M., Herrmann, C., Kühlbrandt, W. and Yildiz, O. (2009) Structure and function of the FeoB G-domain from *Methanococcus jannaschii*. *J. Mol. Biol.*, **392**, 405–419.

Krewulak, K.D. and Vogel, H.J. (2007) Structural biology of bacterial iron uptake. *Biochim. Biophys. Acta*, **1778**, 1781–1804.

Krewulak, K.D. and Vogel, H.J. (2011) TonB or not TonB: is that the question? *Biochem. Cell Biol.*, **89**, 87–97.

Krewulak, K.D., Peacock, R.S. and Vogel, H.J. (2004) Periplasmic binding proteins involved in bacterial iron uptake, in *Iron Transport in Bacteria* (eds J.H. Crosa, A.R. Mey and S.M. Payne), ASM Press, Washington DC, pp. 375–386.

Krewulak, K.D., Koster, W. and Vogel, H.J. (2009) Siderophore-binding protein FhuD and related periplasmic proteins involved in bacterial iron uptake, in *Handbook of Metalloproteins* (ed. A. Messerschmidt), Wiley New York.

Kwon, O., Hudspeth, M.E. and Meganathan, R. (1996) Anaerobic biosynthesis of enterobactin *Escherichia coli*: regulation of entC gene expression and evidence against its involvement in menaquinone (vitamin K2) biosynthesis. *J. Bacteriol.*, **178**, 3252–3259.

Larsen, R.A., Foster-Hartnett, D., McIntosh, M.A. and Postle K. (1997) Regions of *Escherichia coli* TonB and FepA proteins essential for in vivo physical interactions. *J. Bacteriol.*, **179**, 3213–3221.

Larsen, R.A., Letain, T.E. and Postle, K. (2003) *In vivo* evidence of TonB shuttling between the cytoplasmic and outer membrane in *Escherichia coli*. *Mol. Microbiol.*, **49**, 211–218.

Lau, C.K., Ishida, H., Liu, Z. and Vogel, H.J. (2013) Solution structure of *Escherichia coli* FeoA and its potential role in bacterial ferrous iron transport. *J. Bacteriol.*, **195**, 46–55.

Lavrrar, J.L. and McIntosh, M.A. (2003) Architecture of a fur binding site: a comparative analysis. *J. Bacteriol.*, **185**, 2194–2202.

Lazazzera, B.A., Beinert, H., Khoroshilova, N., Kennedy, M.C. and Kiley, P.J. (1996) DNA binding and dimerization of the Fe-S-containing FNR protein from *Escherichia coli* are regulated by oxygen. *J. Biol. Chem.*, **271**, 2762–2768.

Lee, Y.-H., Deka, R.K., Norgard, M.V., *et al.* (1999) *Treponema pallidum* TroA is a periplasmic zinc-binding protein with a helical backbone. *Nat. Struct. Biol.*, **6**, 628–633.

Lee, Y.-H., Dorwart, M.R., Hazlett, K.R.O., *et al.* (2002) The crystal structure of Zn(II)-free *Treponema pallidum* TroA, a periplasmic metal-binding protein, reveals a closed conformation. *J. Bacteriol.*, **184**, 2300–2304.

Letain, T.E. and Postle, K. (1997) TonB protein appears to transduce energy by shuttling between the cytoplasmic membrane and the outer membrane in Gram-negative bacteria. *Mol. Microbiol.*, **24**, 271–283.

Lewinson, O., Lee, A.T., Locher, K.P. and Rees, D.C. (2010) A distinct mechanism for the ABC transporter BtuCD-BtuF revealed by the dynamics of complex formation. *Nat. Struct. Mol. Biol.*, **17**, 332–338.

Lin, H., Fischbach, M.A., Liu, D.R. and Walsh, C.T. (2005) In vitro characterization of salmochelin and enterobactin trilactone hydrolases IroD, IroE, and Fes. *J. Am. Chem. Soc.*, **127**, 11075–11084.

Liu, Y. and Eisenberg, D. (2002) 3D domain swapping: as domains continue to swap. *Protein Sci.*, **11**, 1285–1299.

Locher, K.P. (2004) Structure and mechanism of ABC transporters. *Curr. Opin. Struct. Biol.*, **14**, 426–431.

Locher, K.P. (2009) Review. Structure and mechanism of ATP-binding cassette transporters. *Philos. Trans. R. Soc. Lond. B Biol. Sci.*, **364**, 239–245.

Locher, K.P., Rees, B., Koebnik, R., *et al.* (1998) Transmembrane signaling across the ligand-gated FhuA receptor: crystal structures of free and ferrichrome-bound states reveal allosteric changes. *Cell*, **95**, 771–778.

Locher, K.P., Lee, A.T. and Rees, D.C. (2002) The *E. coli* BtuCD structure: a framework for ABC transporter architecture and mechanism. *Science*, **296**, 1091–1098.

Lonetto, M.A., Brown, K.L., Rudd, K.E. and Buttner, M.J. (1994) Analysis of the *Streptomyces coelicolor* sigE gene reveals the existence of a subfamily of eubacterial RNA polymerase sigma factors involved in the regulation of extracytoplasmic functions. *Proc. Natl Acad. Sci. USA*, **91**, 7573–7577.

López, C.S., Peacock, R.S., Crosa, J.H. and Vogel, H.J. (2009) Molecular characterization of the TonB2 protein from the fish pathogen *Vibrio anguillarum*. *Biochem. J.*, **418**, 49–59.

Lucarelli, D., Russo, S, Garman, E., *et al.* (2007) Crystal structure and function of the zinc uptake regulator FurB from *Mycobacterium tuberculosis*. *J. Biol. Chem.*, **282**, 9914–9922.

Lundrigan, M.D. and Kadner, R.J. (1986) Nucleotide sequence of the gene for the ferrienterochelin receptor FepA in *Escherichia coli*. Homology among outer membrane receptors that interact with TonB. *J. Biol. Chem.*, **261**, 10797–10801.

Ma, L., Kaserer, W., Annamalai, R., Scott, D.C., *et al.* (2007) Evidence of ball-and-chain transport of ferric enterobactin through FepA. *J. Biol. Chem.*, **282**, 397–406.

Ma, Z., Jacobsen, F.E. and Giedroc, D.P. (2009) Coordination chemistry of bacterial metal transport and sensing. *Chem. Rev.*, **109**, 4644–4681.

Ma, Z., Gabriel, S.E. and Helmann, J.D. (2011) Sequential binding and sensing of Zn(II) by *Bacillus subtilis* Zur. *Nucleic Acids Res.*, **39**, 9130–9138.

Marlovits, T.C., Haase, W., Herrmann, C., Aller, S.G. and Unger, V.M. (2002) The membrane protein FeoB contains an intramolecular G protein essential for Fe(II) uptake in bacteria. *Proc. Natl Acad. Sci. USA*, **99**, 16243–16248.

Marraffini, L.A., Dedent, A.C. and Schneewind, O. (2006) Sortases and the art of anchoring proteins to the envelopes of gram-positive bacteria. *Microbiol. Mol. Biol. Rev.*, **70**, 192–221.

Massé, E. and Gottesman, S. (2002) A small RNA regulates the expression of genes involved in iron metabolism in *Escherichia coli*. *Proc. Natl Acad. Sci. USA*, **99**, 4620–4625.

Massé, E., Salvail, H., Desnoyers, G. and Arguin, M. (2005) Small RNAs controlling iron metabolism. *Curr. Opin. Microbiol.*, **10**, 140–145.

Matzanke, B.F., Annemuller, S., Schünemann, V., Trautwein, A.X. and Hantke, K. (2004) FhuF, part of a siderophore-reductase system. *Biochemistry*, **43**, 1386–1392.

Mazoch, J., Tesarík, R., Sedlácek, V., Kucera, I. and Turánek, J. (2004) Isolation and biochemical characterization of two soluble iron(III) reductases from *Paracoccus denitrificans*. *Eur. J. Biochem.*, **271**, 553–562.

Melville, S.B. and Gunsalus, R.P. (1996) Isolation of an oxygen-sensitive FNR protein of *Escherichia coli*: interaction at activator and repressor sites of FNR-controlled genes. *Proc. Natl Acad. Sci. USA*, **93**, 1226–12231.

Meyer, J.M., Geoffroy, V.A., Baysse, C., *et al.* (2002) Siderophore-mediated iron uptake in fluorescent *Pseudomonas*: characterization of the pyoverdine-receptor binding site of three cross-reacting pyoverdines. *Arch. Biochem. Biophys.*, **397**, 179–183.

Miethke, M. (2013) Molecular strategies of microbial iron assimilation: from high-affinity complexes to cofactor assembly systems. Molecular strategies of microbial iron assimilation: from high-affinity complexes to cofactor assembly systems. *Metallomics*, **5**, 15–28.

Miethke, M., Klotz, O., Linne, U., *et al.* (2006) Ferri-bacillibactin uptake and hydrolysis in *Bacillus subtilis*. *Mol. Microbiol.*, **61**, 1413–1427.

Miethke, M., Hou, J. and Marahiel, M.A. (2011a) The siderophore-interacting protein YqjH acts as a ferric reductase in different iron assimilation pathways of *Escherichia coli*. *Biochemistry*, **50**, 10951–10964.

Miethke, M., Pierik, A.J., Peuckert, F., Seubert, A. and Marahiel, M.A. (2011b) Identification and characterization of a novel-type ferric siderophore reductase from a gram-positive extremophile. *J. Biol. Chem.*, **286**, 2245–2260.

Miethke, M., Monteferrante, C.G., Marahiel, M.A. and van Dijl, J.M. (2013) The *Bacillus subtilis* EfeUOB transporter is essential for high-affinity acquisition of ferrous and ferric iron. *Biochim. Biophys. Acta*, **1833**, 2267–2278.

Müller, A., Wilkinson, A.J., Wilson, K.S. and Duhme-Klair, A.K. (2006) An [{Fe(mecam)}$_2$]$_6$- bridge in the crystal structure of a ferric enterobactin binding protein. *Angew. Chem. Int. Ed. Engl.*, **45**, 5132–5136.

Müller, K., Matzanke, B.F., Schünemann, V., Trautwein, A.X. and Hantke, K. (1998) FhuF, an iron-regulated protein of *Escherichia coli* with a new type of [2Fe–2S] center. *Eur. J. Biochem.*, **258**, 1001–1008.

Müller, S.I., Valdebenito, M. and Hantke, K. (2009) Salmochelin, the long-overlooked catecholate sidero-phore of *Salmonella*. *Biometals*, **22**, 691–695.

Neugebauer, H., Herrmann, C., Kammer, W., *et al.* (2005) ExbBD-dependent transport of maltodextrins through the novel MalA protein across the outer membrane of *Caulobacter crescentus*. *J. Bacteriol.*, **187**, 8300–8311.

Newton, S.M., Igo, J.D., Scott, D.C. and Klebba, P.E. (1999) Effect of loop deletions on the binding and transport of ferric enterobactin by FepA. *Mol. Microbiol.*, **32**, 1153–1165.

Noinaj, N., Gullier, M.N., Barnard, T.J. and Buchanan, S.K. (2010) TonB-dependent transporters: regulation, structure, and function. *Annu. Rev. Microbiol.*, **64**, 43–60.

Ochsner, U.A. and Vasil, M.L. (1996) Gene repression by the ferric uptake regulator in *Pseudomonas aeruginosa*: cycle selection of iron-regulated genes. *Proc. Natl Acad. Sci. USA*, **93**, 4409–4414.

Ochsner, U.A., Vasil, A.I., Johnson, Z. and Vasil, M.L. (1999) *Pseudomonas aeruginosa* fur overlaps with a gene encoding a novel outer membrane lipoprotein, OmlA. *J. Bacteriol.*, **181**, 1099–1109.

Ogierman, M. and Braun, V. (2003) Interactions between the outer membrane ferric citrate transporter FecA and TonB: studies of the FecA TonB box. *J. Bacteriol.*, **185**, 1870–1885.

Oglesby-Sherrouse, A.G. and Murphy, E.R. (2013) Iron-responsive bacterial small RNAs: variations on a theme. *Metallomics*, **5**, 276–286.

Ollis, A.A. and Postle, K. (2012) Identification of functionally important TonB-ExbB periplasmic domain interactions in vivo. *J. Bacteriol.*, **194**, 3078–3087.

Park, S.-J. and Gunsalus, R.P. (1995) Oxygen, iron, carbon, and superoxide control of the fumarase fumA and fumC genes of *Escherichia coli*: role of the arcA, fnr, and soxR gene products. *J. Bacteriol.*, **177**, 6255–6262.

Patzer, S. and Hantke, K. (2001) Dual repression by Fe(2+)-Fur and Mn(2+)-MntR of the mntH gene, encoding an NRAMP-like Mn(2+) transporter in *Escherichia coli*. *J. Bacteriol.*, **183**, 4806–4813.

Peacock, R.S., Weljie, A.M., Howard, S.P., *et al.* (2005) The solution structure of the C-terminal domain of TonB and interaction studies with TonB box peptides. *J. Mol. Biol.*, **345**, 1185–1197.

Pecqueur, L., d'Autréaux, B., Dupuy, J., *et al.* (2006) Structural changes of *Escherichia coli* ferric uptake regulator during metal-dependent dimerization and activation explored by NMR and X-ray crystallography. *J. Biol. Chem.*, **281**, 21286–21295.

Perkins-Balding, D., Ratliff-Griffin, M. and Stojiljkovic, I. (2004) Iron transport systems in *Neisseria meningitidis*. *Microbiol. Mol. Biol. Rev.*, **68**, 154–171.

Petermann, N., Hansen, G., Schmidt, C.L. and Hilgenfeld, R. (2010) Structure of the GTPase and GDI domains of FeoB, the ferrous iron transporter of *Legionella pneumophila*. *FEBS Lett.*, **584**, 733–738.

Peukert, F., Miethke, M., Albrecht, A.G., Essen, L.O. and Marahiel, M.A. (2009) Structural basis and stereochemistry of triscatecholate siderophore binding by FeuA. *Angew. Chem. Int. Ed. Engl.*, **48**, 7924–7927.

Pinkett, H.W., Lee, A.T., Lum, P., Locher, K.P. and Rees, D.C. (2007) An inward-facing conformation of a putative metal-chelate-type ABC transporter. *Science*, **315**, 373–377.

Pohl, E., Holmes, R.K. and Hol, W.G. (1999) Crystal structure of a cobalt-activated diphtheria toxin repressor-DNA complex reveals a metal-binding SH3-like domain. *J. Mol. Biol.*, **292**, 653–667.

Pohl, E., Haller, J.C., Mijovilovich, A., *et al.* (2003) Architecture of a protein central to iron homeostasis: crystal structure and spectroscopic analysis of the ferric uptake regulator. *Mol. Microbiol.*, **47**, 903–915.

Posner, B.A., Mixon, M.B., Wall, M.A., Sprang, S.R. and Gilman, A.G. (1998) The A326S mutant of Gialpha1 as an approximation of the receptor-bound state. *J. Biol. Chem.*, **273**, 21752–21758.

Postle, K. (2002) Close before opening *Science*, **295**, 1658–1659.

Pramanik, A., Zhang, F., Schwarz, H., Schreiber, F. and Braun V. (2010) ExbB protein in the cytoplasmic membrane of *Escherichia coli* forms a stable oligomer. *Biochemistry*, **49**, 8721–8728.

Pressler, U., Staudenmaier, H., Zimmermann, L. and Braun, V. (1988) Genetics of the iron dicitrate transport system of *Escherichia coli*. *J. Bacteriol.*, **170**, 2716–2724.

Quail, M.A., Jordan, P., Grogan, J.M., *et al.* (1996) Spectroscopic and voltammetric characterisation of the bacterioferritin-associated ferredoxin of *Escherichia coli. Biochem. Biophys. Res. Commun.*, **229**, 635–642.

Quiocho, F.A. and Ledvina, P.S. (1996) Atomic structure and specificity of bacterial periplasmic receptors for active transport and chemotaxis: variation of common themes. *Mol. Microbiol.*, **20**, 17–25.

Raymond, K.N., Müller, G. and Matzanke, B.F. (1984) in *Topics in Current Chemistry* (ed. F.L. Boschke), Springer-Verlag, Berlin, pp. 49–102.

Rees, D.C., Johnson, E. and Lewinson, O. (2009) ABC transporters: the power to change. *Nat. Rev. Mol. Cell Biol.*, **10**, 218–227.

Romao, C.V., Louro, R., Timkovich, R., *et al.* (2000) Iron-coproporphyrin III is a natural cofactor in bacterioferritin from the anaerobic bacterium *Desulfovibrio desulfuricans. FEBS Lett.*, **480**, 213–216.

Roof, S.K., Allard, J.D., Bertrand, K.P. and Postle, K. (1991) Analysis of *Escherichia coli* TonB membrane topology by use of PhoA fusions. *J. Bacteriol.*, **173**, 5554–5557.

Rousseau, F., Schymkowitz, J.W. and Itzhaki, L.S. (2003) The unfolding story of three-dimensional domain swapping. *Structure*, **11**, 243–251.

Rousseau, F., Schymkowitz, J.W. and Itzhaki, L.S. (2012) Implications of 3D domain swapping for protein folding, misfolding and function. *Adv. Exp. Med. Biol.*, **747**, 137–152.

Roy, S., Saraswathi, R., Gupta, S., *et al.* (2007) Role of N- and C-terminal tails in DNA binding and assembly in Dps: structural studies of *Mycobacterium smegmatis* Dps deletion mutants. *J. Mol. Biol.*, **370**, 752–767.

Roy, S., Saraswathi, R., Chatterji, D. and Vijayan, M. (2008) Structural studies on the second *Mycobacterium smegmatis* Dps: invariant and variable features of structure, assembly and function. *J. Mol. Biol.*, **375**, 948–959.

Schalk, I.J., Yue, W.W. and Buchanan, S.K. (2004) Recognition of iron-free siderophores by TonB-dependent iron transporters. *Mol. Microbiol.*, **54**, 14–22.

Schauer, K., Gouget, B., Carriere, M., Labigne, A. and de Reuse, H. (2007) Novel nickel transport mechanism across the bacterial outer membrane energized by the TonB/ExbB/ExbD machinery. *Mol. Microbiol.*, **63**, 1054–1068.

Schauer, K., Rodionov, D.A. and de Reuse, H. (2008) New substrates for TonB-dependent transport: do we only see the 'tip of the iceberg'? *Trends Biochem. Sci.*, **33**, 330–338.

Schramm, E., Mende, J., Braun, V. and Kamp, R.M. (1987) Nucleotide sequence of the colicin B activity gene cba: consensus pentapeptide among TonB-dependent colicins and receptors. *J. Bacteriol.*, **169**, 3350–3357.

Schröder, I., Johnson, E. and de Vries, S. (2003) Microbial ferric iron reductases. *FEMS Microbiol. Rev.*, **27**, 427–447.

Severance, S., Chakraborty, S. and Kosman, D.J. (2004) The Ftr1p iron permease in the yeast plasma membrane: orientation, topology and structure-function relationships. *Biochem. J.*, **380**, 487–496.

Sheikh, M.A. and Taylor, G.L. (2009) Crystal structure of the *Vibrio cholerae* ferric uptake regulator (Fur) reveals insights into metal co-ordination. *Mol. Microbiol.*, **72**, 1208–1220.

Shin, J.H., Jung, H.J., An, Y., *et al.* (2011) Graded expression of zinc-responsive genes through two regulatory zinc-binding sites in Zur. *Proc. Natl Acad. Sci. USA*, **108**, 5045–5050.

Shirley, M. and Lamont, I.L. (2009) Role of TonB1 in pyoverdine-mediated signaling in *Pseudomonas aeruginosa. J. Bacteriol.*, **191**, 5634–5640.

Shultis, D.D., Purdy, M.D., Banchs, C.N. and Wiener, M.C. (2006) Outer membrane active transport: structure of the BtuB:TonB complex. *Science*, **312**, 1396–1399.

Small, S.K., Puri, S. and O'Brian, M.R. (2009) Heme-dependent metalloregulation by the iron response regulator (Irr) protein in *Rhizobium* and other Alpha-proteobacteria. *Biometals*, **22**, 89–97.

Stojiljkovic, I. and Hantke, K. (1995) Functional domains of the *Escherichia coli* ferric uptake regulator protein (Fur). *Mol. Gen. Genet.*, **247**, 199–205.

Stojiljkovic, I., Baumler, A.J. and Hantke, K. (1994) Fur regulon in gram-negative bacteria. Identification and characterization of new iron-regulated *Escherichia coli* genes by a fur titration assay. *J. Mol. Biol.*, **236**, 531–546.

Struyve, M., Moons, M. and Tommassen, J. (1991) Carboxy-terminal phenylalanine is essential for the correct assembly of a bacterial outer membrane protein. *J. Mol. Biol.*, **218**, 141–148.

Su, Y.C., Chin, K.H., Hung, H.C., *et al.* (2010) Structure of *Stenotrophomonas maltophilia* FeoA complexed with zinc: a unique prokaryotic SH3-domain protein that possibly acts as a bacterial ferrous iron-transport activating factor. *Acta Crystallogr. F*, **66**, 636–642.

Sverzinsky, A., Fabre, L., Cottreau, A.L., *et al.* (2014) Coordinated rearrangements between cytoplasmic and periplasmic domains of the membrane protein complex ExbB–ExbD of *Escherichia coli*. *Structure*, **22**, 797–797.

Tatum E.L. and Lederberg, J. (1947) Gene recombination in the bacterium *Escherichia coli*. *J. Bacteriol.*, **53**, 673–684.

Telford, J.R. and Raymond, K.N. (1996) in Comprehensive Supramolecular Chemistry, Vol. **1** (eds J.M. Lehn and G.W. Gokel), Pergamon Press, London, pp. 245–266.

Tieleman, D.P. and Berendsen, H.J. (1998) A molecular dynamics study of the pores formed by *Escherichia coli* OmpF porin in a fully hydrated palmitoyloleoylphosphatidylcholine bilayer. *Biophys. J.*, **74**, 2786–2801.

Tiss, A., Barre, O., Michaud-Soret, I. and Forest, E. (2005) Characterization of the DNA-binding site in the ferric uptake regulator protein from *Escherichia coli* by UV crosslinking and mass spectrometry. *FEBS Lett.*, **579**, 5454–5460.

Touati, D. (1988) Transcriptional and posttranscriptional regulation of manganese superoxide dismutase biosynthesis in *Escherichia coli*, studied with operon and protein fusions. *J. Bacteriol.*, **170**, 2511–2520.

Traoré, D.A., El Ghazouani, A., Ilango, S., *et al.* (2006) Crystal structure of the apo-PerR-Zn protein from *Bacillus subtilis*. *Mol. Microbiol.*, **61**, 1211–1219.

Unden, G. and Bongaerts, J. (1997) Alternative respiratory pathways of *Escherichia coli*: energetics and transcriptional regulation in response to electron acceptors. *Biochim. Biophys. Acta*, **1320**, 217–234.

Vassinova, N. and Kozyrev, D. (2000) A method for direct cloning of fur-regulated genes: identification of seven new fur-regulated loci in *Escherichia coli*. *Microbiology*, **146**, 3171–3182.

Venturi, V., Weisbeek, P. and Koster, M. (1995) Gene regulation of siderophore-mediated iron acquisition in *Pseudomonas*: not only the Fur repressor. *Mol. Microbiol.*, **17**, 603–610.

Vitale, S., Fauquant, C., Lascoux, D., *et al.* (2009) A ZnS(4) structural zinc site in the *Helicobacter pylori* ferric uptake regulator. *Biochemistry*, **48**, 5582–5591.

Voet, D. and Voet, J.G. (2004) *Biochemistry*, 3rd edition, John Wiley & Sons, Inc., Hoboken, NJ, pp. 1591.

Wang, S., Wu, Y. and Outten, F.W. (2011) Fur and the novel regulator YqjI control transcription of the ferric reductase gene yqjH in *Escherichia coli*. *J. Bacteriol.*, **193**, 563–574.

Wassarman, K.M., Repoila, F., Rosenow, C., *et al.* (2001) Identification of novel small RNAs using comparative genomics and microarrays. *Genes Dev.*, **15**, 1637–1651.

Watt, G.D., Frankel, R.B., Papaefthymiou, G.C., *et al.* (1986) Redox properties and Mossbauer spectroscopy of *Azotobacter vinelandii* bacterioferritin. *Biochemistry*, **25**, 4330–4336.

Weaver, E.A., Wyckoff, E.E., Mey, A.R., Morrison, R. and Payne, S.M. (2013) FeoA and FeoC are essential components of the *Vibrio cholerae* ferrous iron uptake system, and FeoC interacts with FeoB. *J. Bacteriol.*, **195**, 4826–4835.

Wee, S., Neilands, J.B., Bittner, M.L., *et al.* (1988) Expression, isolation and properties of Fur (ferric uptake regulation) protein of *Escherichia coli* K 12. *Biol. Met.*, **1**, 62–68.

Wen, Y., Wu, X., Teng, Y., *et al.* (2011) Identification and analysis of the gene cluster involved in biosynthesis of paenibactin, a catecholate siderophore produced by *Paenibacillus elgii* B69. *Environ. Microbiol.*, **13**, 2726–2737.

Wennerhold, J. and Bott, M. (2006) The DtxR regulon of *Corynebacterium glutamicum*. *J. Bacteriol.*, **188**, 2907–2918.

Williams, P.H. (1979) Novel iron uptake system specified by ColV plasmids: an important component in the virulence of invasive strains of *Escherichia coli*. *Infect. Immun.*, **26**, 925–932.

Wilson, M.K., Abergel, R.J., Raymond, K.N., Arceneaux, J.E. and Byers, B.R. (2006) Siderophores of *Bacillus anthracis*, *Bacillus cereus*, and *Bacillus thuringiensis*. *Biochem. Biophys. Res. Commun.*, **348**, 320–325.

Wirth, C., Meyer-Klaucke, W., Pattus, F. and Cobessi, D. (2007) From the periplasmic signaling domain to the extracellular face of an outer membrane signal transducer of *Pseudomonas aeruginosa*: crystal structure of the ferric pyoverdine outer membrane receptor. *J. Mol. Biol.*, **368**, 398–406.

Wolf, S.G., Frenkiel, D., Arad, T., *et al.* (1999) DNA protection by stress-induced biocrystallization. *Nature*, **400**, 83–85.

Wong, S.G., Abdulqadir, R., Le Brun, N.E., Moore, G.R. and Mauk, A.G. (2012) Fe-haem bound to *Escherichia coli* bacterioferritin accelerates iron core formation by an electron transfer mechanism. *Biochem. J.*, **444**, 553–560.

Xia, M., Wei, J., Lei, Y. and Ying, L. (2007) A novel ferric reductase purified from *Magnetospirillum gryphiswaldense* MSR-1. *Curr. Microbiol.*, **55**, 71–75.

Yasmin, S., Andrews, S.C., Moore, G.R. and Le Brun, N.E. (2011) A new role for heme, facilitating release of iron from the bacterioferritin iron biomineral. *J. Biol. Chem.*, **286**, 3473–3483.

Yue, W.W., Grizot, S. and Buchanan, S.K. (2003) Structural evidence for iron-free citrate and ferric citrate binding to the TonB-dependent outer membrane transporter FecA. *J. Mol. Biol.*, **332**, 353–368.

Zawadza, A.M., Kim, Y., Maltseva N., *et al.* (2009) Characterization of a *Bacillus subtilis* transporter for petrobactin, an anthrax stealth siderophore. *Proc. Natl Acad. Sci. USA*, **106**, 21854–21859.

Zhao, G.H., Ceci, P., Ilari, A. *et al.* (2002) Iron and hydrogen peroxide detoxification properties of DNA-binding protein from starved cells. A ferritin-like DNA-binding protein of *Escherichia coli. J. Biol. Chem.*, **277**, 27689–27696.

Zheng, M., Doan, B., Schneider, T.D. and Storz, G. (1999) OxyR and SoxRS regulation of fur. *J. Bacteriol.*, **181**, 4639–4643.

Zhu, M., Valdebenito, M., Winkelmann, G. and Hantke, K. (2005) Functions of the siderophore esterases IroD and IroE in iron-salmochelin utilization. *Microbiology*, **151**, 2363–2372.

4

Iron Acquisition by Pathogens

4.1 Introduction

Improved treatments for malignant diseases, advances in intensive care interventions and organ transplantations have contributed greatly to prolonged life expectancy. However, this has resulted in an increase in various opportunistic microbial infections, notably fungal infections (Yapar, 2014). The number of elderly, critically ill and immunocompromised patients at risk for fungal infections caused by *Candida* species has increased dramatically (Brown *et al.*, 2012). In a survey of healthcare-associated infections reported to the National Healthcare Safety Network during 2009–2010 in the USA (Sievert *et al.*, 2013), the top four pathogen groups were *Staphylococcus aureus*, *Enterococcus* spp., *Escherichia coli* and coagulase-negative staphylococci; *Candida* species occupied the fifth place. Yet, on account of difficulties in the diagnosis of invasive fungal infections and the limited efficacy of existing drugs, both mortality and morbidity caused by *Candida* and other human pathogenic yeasts are unacceptably high (Luo *et al.*, 2013).

In surveys carried out between 2001 and 2004, some 30% of the USA population were found to have innocuous nasal colonisation by *S. aureus* (Kuehnert *et al.*, 2006). Yet, if this initial site of colonisation is breached, *S. aureus* can infect nearly every tissue of the human body, causing disorders ranging in severity from superficial wound infections to septicaemia, toxic shock and endocarditis (David and Daum, 2010). *S. aureus* is the most frequent cause of nosocomial infections in the USA, and the percentage of infections caused by methicillin-resistant *S. aureus* (MRSA) is growing precipitously (Todd, 2006). Indeed, it has increased dramatically during the past two decades in populations who have not had identifiable exposure to healthcare institutions (David and Daum, 2010).

These two examples illustrate the urgent need to identify and develop new targets for antimicrobial therapy to treat this threat of infections (Haley and Skaar, 2012). A promising strategy would be to prevent the pathogens procuring from their host the nutrients that they require for their growth and proliferation (nutritional immunity). Iron is a cofactor in many important biological systems, and is essential for almost all living organisms; with the exception of non-pathogenic lactobacilli (Archibald, 1983) and pathogenic *Borrelia burgdorferi* (Posey and Gherardini, 2000), all groups of protozoa, fungi and bacteria require iron for survival and replication (Weinberg, 2009). Since iron is the only nutrient known to be generally growth-limiting and to play an important role in microbial virulence, the iron uptake systems of pathogens are a particularly interesting target. Pathogenic bacteria and fungi have developed sophisticated strategies to acquire iron from their hosts. While these include siderophore synthesis and transport, an interesting collection of often deadly pathogens can also acquire from haem, whether bound to haemoglobin, haemoglobin–haptoglobin, myoglobin or haemopexin (Wandersman and Delepelaire, 2004, 2012), from the host iron-binding proteins, transferrin or lactoferrin or by reduction of ferric to ferrous iron.[1] This information is presented in this chapter, starting with bacteria and then turning to fungi.

4.2 Host Defence Mechanisms, Nutritional Immunity

The relationship between iron supply and the growth of bacteria in animal models was recognised in early studies (Weinberg 1978, 1990; Bullpen and Griffith, 1987; Wooldridge and Williams, 1993). Indeed, low environmental levels of available iron often act as a signal for the induction of virulence genes in pathogenic bacteria. The importance of iron acquisition to ensure the proliferation and growth of bacteria makes iron *withholding* by mammalian hosts a logical defensive strategy which is widely applied to limit the growth of invading parasitic organisms. A number of iron-binding proteins, notably transferrin, lactoferrin, ferritin, haemoglobin, haptoglobin, haemopexin and lipocalin (NGAL, siderocalin) serve to withdraw iron and prevent bacterial growth. For bacteria which are unable to mobilise the iron deposited in these proteins, iron withdrawal is a very effective strategy (Bullen *et al.*, 2005; Weinberg, 2009). The first reaction of the body to bacterial infection and its associated inflammation is to withdraw iron from the circulation (hypoferraemia). This is achieved by the release of inflammatory cytokines – notably interleukin (IL) 6 – which elicit increased biosynthesis and secretion of the key systemic homeostatic regulator, hepcidin (reviewed in Chapter 10) into the serum. Iron uptake from the gut and its release from iron stores in the liver and the macrophages into the circulation is blocked, and the resulting iron deprivation reduces bacterial multiplication to the level which enables the innate and acquired immune system to eradicate the infection (Ganz, 2006). Lactoferrin, a major component of the innate immune system of mammals, is promptly released from storage granules in circulating neutrophils to sites of microbial invasion, where it effectively scavenges iron at pH values as low as 3.5, and exerts direct antimicrobial activities against a large panel of microorganisms, together with anti-inflammatory activities (Weinberg, 2007). Lactoferrin also prevents biofilm development by the opportunistic pathogen *Pseudomonas aeruginosa*, which is of considerable importance, since the transition from a free-living, independent existence to a biofilm lifestyle can be devastating, particularly for pathogens, because biofilms notoriously resist killing by host defence mechanisms and antibiotics (Singh *et al.*, 2002).

---

[1] Among the members of this collection of killers, which employ host iron sources and do not use siderophores, can be counted, in addition to the charmers mentioned in the text, *Yersinia pestis, Yersinia entercolitica, Neisseria gonorrhoeae, E. coli* O157, and *Vibrio cholera*.

Siderocalin (Scn) is also secreted by host cells at sites of inflammation (reviewed in Correnti and Strong, 2012). Scn, the only mammalian siderophore-binding protein currently known, is an antibacterial protein which acts by sequestering ferric siderophore complexes away from their bacterial siderophore receptors (Clifton *et al.*, 2009), often binding siderophores with subnanomolar affinities (Correnti and Strong, 2012). The possibility that endogenous mammalian siderophores may participate in siderocalin-mediated iron transport independently of the well-characterised transferrin pathway is discussed in Chapter 6.

All members of this functional group of proteins belong to the lipocalin family of binding proteins and so are known as 'siderocalins' for 'siderophore-binding lipocalins', sequestering iron away from the infecting bacteria as ferric siderophore complexes. The lipocalin family of binding proteins displays a conserved eight-stranded β-barrel fold, which encompasses a highly sculpted binding site known as a calyx, often lined with positively charged lysine and arginine side chains to interact, through cation-π and coulombic interactions, with negatively charged siderophores with aromatic catecholate groups. Pathogenic bacteria have evolved responses to these defences by using multiple siderophores, including siderophores that do not bind to Scn, or by modifying siderophores (e.g. by glucosylation, as we saw for the diglucosylated enterochelin, salmochelin) to block Scn binding, allowing iron to be acquired even in the presence of Scn. For instance, as we will see later, Scn does not bind aerobactin. Although siderocalin can bind many catechol siderophores with high efficiency, it was reported that it could not bind vibriobactin of *Vibrio cholerae*, which includes an oxazoline adjacent to a catechol (Li *et al.*, 2012), implying that vibriobactin is a 'stealth siderophore'. It has now been shown (Allred *et al.*, 2013) that this chelating unit binds iron either in a catecholate or a phenolate–oxazoline coordination mode (Figure 4.1). Although the phenolate–oxazoline coordination mode is present at physiological pH and is not bound by Scn, nonetheless, Scn binding shifts the coordination to the catecholate mode and thereby inactivates vibriobactin. Hence, vibriobactin is not a stealth siderophore.

Despite these host withdrawal mechanisms, the battle for iron to enable bacterial proliferation is a constant struggle. As we will see, commensal and pathogenic bacteria have developed systems which enable them to synthesise specific virulence-associated siderophores together with their corresponding iron transport systems, to mobilise iron from its tightly bound form in transferrin and lactoferrin ($K_D = 10^{-23}$ M^{-1}), or to obtain the iron they so desperately need from haemoglobin, haemopexin and the haemoglobin–haptoglobin complex.

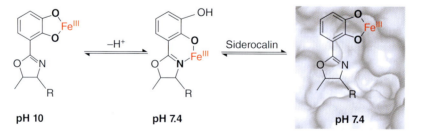

Figure 4.1 *Although the phenolate–oxazoline coordination mode of vibriobactin is present at physiological pH and is not bound by siderocalin (Scn), nonetheless, Scn binding shifts the coordination to the catecholate mode and thereby inactivates the siderophore. Reprinted from Allred, B.E., Correnti, C., Clifton, M.C., Strong, R.K. and Raymond, K.N. (2013) Siderocalin outwits the coordination chemistry of vibriobactin, a siderophore of* Vibrio cholerae. *ACS Chem. Biol.,* **8**, *1882–1887; © 2013, American Chemical Society*

4.3 Pathogenicity and PAIs

Bacterial genomes evolve through mutations, rearrangements or horizontal gene transfer (HGT). As whole-genome sequences of more and more bacterial species (particularly pathogens) are determined, it has become clear that, in addition to the core sequences encoding essential metabolic housekeeping functions, with a fairly homogeneous G + C content and codon usage, there are sequences which differ in both their G + C content and codon usage. These have been acquired via HGT and they harbour a number of accessory genes that can be beneficial under specific environmental conditions. HGT is defined as the transfer of genetic material between bacterial cells which is not coupled with cell division (Lawrence, 2005). Genetic exchange by HGT is a major force in microbial evolution, as illustrated by the demonstration that comparison of pathogenic and non-pathogenic strains of *E. coli* share only 40% of their genome (Welch *et al.*, 2002), indicating that the rest has been acquired horizontally during evolution. These regions of the bacterial genome have been designated as *genomic islands* (Juhas *et al.*, 2009; Juhas, 2015), and the horizontal transfer of genes which frequently encode for accessory functions has a tremendous impact on the genome plasticity, adaptation and, in particular, the evolution of pathogenic bacteria. Horizontally transferred mobile genetic elements are involved in the dissemination of antibiotic resistance and virulence genes, thus contributing to the emergence of novel 'superbugs'. The mechanisms of HGT have been reviewed recently (Juhas, 2015), with special focus on the novel multiresistant and hypervirulent 'superbugs' *Clostridium difficile*, *E. coli* and MRSA, which have caused serious outbreaks of infection and currently represent a major threat to public health.

The term pathogenicity island (PAI) was introduced by Hacker *et al.* (1990) to describe regions in the genomes of certain pathogens that are absent in the non-pathogenic strains of the same or closely related species, and which contain large continuous blocks of virulence genes. PAIs represent a distinctive subset of genomic islands comprising specific gene clusters, which code for several bacterial virulence factors, such as adhesins, iron-scavenging siderophores, capsules, endo- and exotoxins, type III and type IV secretion systems (Dobrindt *et al.*, 2004).

PAIs are found in both animal and plant pathogens, can be transmitted between bacteria of different species or even different genera, and are often inserted into tRNA genes (reviewed in Hacker and Kaper, 2000). PAIs can be detected *in silico* within a given DNA sequence by their GC-content, deviations in codon usage, insertion sequences and/or tRNA flanking regions, together with transpososon coding genes (Hacker and Kaper, 2000; Guy, 2006). More recently, a novel software suite has been designed for the prediction of PAIs, which utilises multiple features for PAI detection in an integrative manner (Soares *et al.*, 2012).

The genetic repertoire contained within PAIs can be divided into several functional groups (Gal-Mor and Finlay, 2006). These include: (i) adherence factors, which enable bacteria to attach to host surfaces, facilitating the infection process; (ii) siderophores such as yersiniabactin and aerobactin, which escape detection by siderocalins; (iii) exotoxins such as haemolysins, which destroy or affect the function of host cells; (iv) invasion genes, which mediate bacterial entry into host cells; and (v) type III and IV secretion systems, which deliver bacterial effector proteins capable of modulating host functions. Type III secretion systems (T3SS) are found in PAIs of a number of pathogens including *Salmonella*, *Shigella*, *Yersinia* and pathogenic strains of *E. coli*, while PAIs harbouring type IV secretion systems (T4SS) include *Legionella pneumophila*, *Helicobacter pylori*, *Bordetella pertussis* and *Brucella* spp. Certain PAIs are rather promiscuous, like the high-pathogenicity island (HPI) of *Yersinia*, a genomic island essential for the virulence phenotype in *Yersinia* and indispensable for the pathogenicity of *Yersinia* and certain pathotypes of *E. coli*. In contrast to most genomic islands, the HPI is widely disseminated among members of the family of

Enterobacteriaceae. It contains the genes responsible for an integrase which, together with an excisionase and recombination sites, make up the genetic mobility module of the island, while the siderophore yersiniabactin biosynthesis and uptake system comprises its functional part with respect to fitness and pathogenicity (Schubert *et al.*, 2004). One species of bacteria may have more than one PAI (e.g. *Salmonella* has at least five). The genetic organisation of three representative PAIs (Gal-Mor and Finlay, 2006), in *E. coli*, *H. pylori* and *S. aureus* are illustrated in Figure 4.2.

The locus of enterocyte enhancement (LEE) for PAI in *E. coli* (Figure 4.2a) contains 41 open reading frames (ORFs) organised in five polycistronic operons, and consists of: (i) a T3SS, which is used as a molecular syringe to translocate effector proteins into host cells; (ii) three secreted translocator proteins, required for translocating effectors into host cells; (iii) an adhesin (intimin), which mediates attachment of the effector protein Tir to the host cell cytosol membrane; and (iv) another series of six effector proteins, including Tir, and the intimin receptor, together with a chaperone. Translocation of these molecules into the host cell by T3SS results in changes of the cytoskeleton and the formation of actin-rich pedestals with the Tir effector located at their tip. This structure allows a direct interaction of Tir with the bacterial outer membrane protein intimin, as well as the host cytoskeleton (Zaharik *et al.*, 2002).

The human gastric pathogen *H. pylori* colonises over half of the world's population, and the *cag* PAI is a well-defined virulence factor, associated with severe gastric diseases, such as peptic ulcers (Censini *et al.*, 1996). The *cag* PAI (Figure 4.2b) encodes some 27 ORFs, the majority of which are required for the formation of a functional T4SS which is used to translocate the bacterial

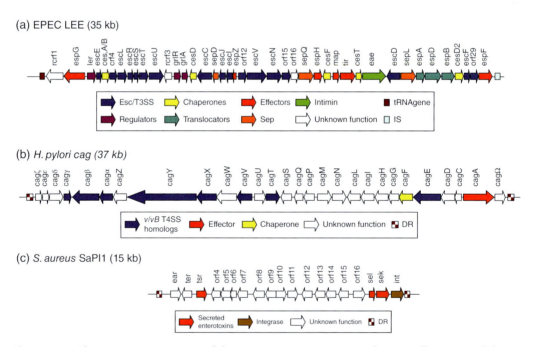

Figure 4.2 *The genetic organisation of three representative PAIs. A schematic illustration of the LEE PAI from EPEC (a), the cag PAI of H.pylori (b), and the SaPI1 of S.aureus (c) is shown. The genetic nomenclature of the EPEC LEE is based on the suggested terminology by Pallen* et al. *(2005). The organisation of the cag PAI is according to Fischer* et al. *(2001), and the organisation of the SaPI1 is based on Novick (2003). Reproduced with permission from John Wiley & Sons, Ltd*

effector protein, CagA into host cells where it interacts with a number of host proteins, and to induce the synthesis and secretion of chemokines, notably IL-8.

Although PAIs in Gram-positive pathogens are apparently less abundant than in Gram-negative bacteria, they play a similar role (Gill *et al.*, 2005). Pathogenic strains of *S. aureus* are responsible for a range of acute and pyogenic infections caused by a variety of toxins, including haemolysins, exotoxins and superantigens (SAgs). Staphylococcal SAgs are potent stimulatory agents for CD4+ T lymphocytes, leading to nonspecific activation of a large proportion of T cells with the release of inflammatory cytokines. The SaPIs are 15- to 17-kb mobile pathogenicity islands in staphylococci, and the SaP11 of *S. aureus* is shown in Figure 4.2c. They usually carry two or more superantigens and are responsible for most superantigen-related human diseases, especially staphylococcal toxic shock syndrome. SaPIs are extremely common in *S. aureus*, with all but one of the sequenced genomes containing one or more (Novick and Subedi, 2007).

4.4 Pathogen-specific Iron Uptake Systems

4.4.1 Siderophores Associated with Virulence

The ability to secrete siderophores and to internalise ferric-siderophore complexes is critical for the virulence of many bacterial pathogens (reviewed recently in Saha *et al.*, 2012). The earliest iron-acquisition mechanism to be identified as specific to bacterial pathogens was the synthesis of virulence-specific siderophores, together with their corresponding ferric-siderophore-dependent iron-transport proteins. One of the first such systems was the aerobactin transport system, which allows invasive *E. coli* of human and animal origin to grow in serum (Williams, 1979; Crosa, 1984). The genes for this system constitute an operon including those for the synthesis of this hydroxamate siderophore and the IutA outer membrane receptor, and are carried on the pColV-K30 plasmid (Williams and Warner, 1980; Warner *et al.*, 1981). Whereas in pathogenic *E. coli* strains the aerobactin operon is plasmid-associated, in *Shigella boydii* DNA sequence analysis revealed a PAI containing a conserved aerobactin operon associated with a P4 prophage-like integrase gene and numerous insertion sequences (Purdy and Payne, 2001). Although it binds iron with a lower affinity than the primary siderophore of many enteric bacteria enterobactin, aerobactin is associated with virulence since it is able to evade siderocalin (Scn)2 sequestration.

The fish pathogen *Vibrio anguillarum* is the causative agent of a fatal hemorrhagic septicaemia in salmon, and many strains harbour a 65 kbp plasmid encoding an iron-sequestering system essential for virulence. The genes involved in the biosynthesis of the siderophore anguibactin are encoded by both the plasmid and the chromosome, while those involved in the transport of the ferric-siderophore complex, including the outer membrane receptor, are plasmid-encoded (Lopez and Crosa, 2007). However, as was pointed out earlier, vibriobactin does not evade sequestration by siderocalin (Allred *et al.*, 2013).

Yersinia enterocolitica can only kill mice when it synthesises yersiniabactin and a related iron-repressible outer membrane transport protein (Heesemann *et al.*, 1993). This iron-scavenging system is present in one of the most widely distributed PAIs, the Yersinia High-Pathogenicity Island (HPI), first described in the plague agent *Yersinia pestis* (Buchreisser *et al.*, 1998). It confers a highly pathogenic phenotype to a number of human pathogenic *Yersiniae*, and is the only known PAI which crosses species borders, having been detected in other members of the Enterobacteriaceae family including *Escherichia*, *Klebsiella*, *Enterobacter*, *Citrobacter*, *Salmonella* and *Serratia* (Olsson *et al.*, 2003; Oelschläger *et al.*, 2003; Schubert *et al.*, 2000; Bach *et al.*, 2000). Moreover, it displays a highly conserved genetic organisation in these genera with 98–100% nucleotide identity between *Yersinia* and *E. coli* (Rakin *et al.*, 1995). Whereas it had been assumed that yersiniabactin (Ybt) is the solely functional endogenous siderophore iron uptake system in highly virulent *Yersinia*, it has been recently suggested that two other siderophores – pseudochelin (Pch) and yersiniachelin – may operate in highly virulent *Yersinia* (Rakin *et al.*, 2012), efficiently substituting and/or supplementing yersiniabactin.

Pyoverdines are the characteristic composite siderophores of fluorescent *Pseudomonas* species (Meyer, 2000; Ravel and Cornelis, 2003; Visca *et al.*, 2007), and are composed of a peptide chain, which is highly variable even within a species (Meyer *et al.*, 2008), and a chromophore, which provides the catecholate function responsible for Fe^{3+} binding with very high affinity. They can displace iron from transferrin, and their production is absolutely required to cause infection in mouse models; pyoverdine is also a signal molecule which triggers the production of extracellular virulence factors and is involved in the establishment of mature biofilms (reviewed in Cornelis and Dingemans, 2013). Pyochelin, the second siderophore of *P. aeruginosa*, is produced by all *P. aeruginosa* isolates, and has a much lower affinity for iron than pyoverdine (Brandel *et al.*, 2012). It is produced at higher iron concentrations, and pyoverdine synthesis is only initiated when iron concentrations are extremely low (Dumas *et al.*, 2013). Pyochelin iron can redox cycle, and in the presence of pycocyanin it can generate hydroxyl radicals, causing oxidative damage and inflammation (Britigan *et al.*, 1997; Coffman *et al.*, 1990). *P. aeruginosa* has more than 30 genes encoding for TonB-dependent transporters (TBDTs) (Cornelis and Bodilis, 2009). In addition to the pyoverdine and pyochelin receptors, *P. aeruginosa* is therefore able to utilise a vast range of different siderophores produced by other microorganisms (reviewed in Cornelis and Dingemans, 2013). This siderophore piracy may be advantageous *P. aeruginosa* in polymicrobial infections (Traxler *et al.*, 2012), depriving competitors of iron since they would be unable to recognise the complex pyoverdine siderophore.

B. cereus is the first Gram-positive bacterium in which a ferric citrate periplasmic binding protein (PBP), FctC, has been described (Fukushima *et al.*, 2012). Earlier genome studies in *B. subtilis* had shown the presence of a Fur-regulated ferric citrate uptake system (Olinger *et al.*, 2006) encoded by the *yfmCDEF* operon. FctC shows the tightest binding of any *B. cereus* siderophore-binding protein (K_d = 2.6 nM), and FctC binds both Fe_3Cit_3 and Fe_2Cit_2. However, it selectively binds Fe_3Cit_3 even though this species is naturally present only at very low concentration.

Some Gram-negative TBDTs and Gram-positive lipoprotein PBPs involved in iron transport have been found to bind not only Fe-siderophores but also apo-siderophores (Schalk *et al.*, 1999; Hoegy *et al.*, 2005; Zawadka *et al.*, 2009a,b; Fukushima *et al.*, 2012). What function this might serve is puzzling, since an apo-siderophore is structurally and electronically different from a Fe-siderophore, and receptor proteins usually precisely recognise a specific substrate. For Gram-negative bacteria a 'siderophore-shuttle' model was demonstrated to explain this (Stintzi *et al.*, 2000). This involves a ligand exchange mechanism at the cell surface involving the exchange of iron from a ferric siderophore to an iron-free siderophore already bound to the receptor. Recently, a similar siderophore-shuttle system has been reported in the Gram-positive *B. cereus* (Fukushima *et al.*, 2013) with the siderophore-binding protein YxeB facilitating iron-exchange from Fe-siderophore to apo-siderophore bound to the receptor.

4.4.2 Transferrin/lactoferrin Iron Uptake

The Neisseriaceae (e.g. *Neisseria gonorrheae* and *Neisseria meningitidis*) and Pasteurellaceae (e.g. *Haemophilius influenzae*) families include a variety of bacterial pathogens that are important in both human and veterinary medicine. They do not synthesise siderophores, but they can use xenosiderophores such as aerobactin, enterobactin and salmochelin that are produced by neighbouring organisms. To do so, they express outer membrane TBDTs. However, the major source of iron for this collection of pathogens involves a siderophore-independent Fe^{3+} transport system (Meitzner *et al.*, 1998), which directly targets host iron-binding proteins (transferrin and lactoferrin). These transport systems are highly specific; only human, but not bovine or porcine transferrins, support growth of the human pathogens *Neisseria meningitidis* and *Haemophilus influenzae*, and only primate transferrins bind to the human pathogens (Gray-Owen and Schryvers, 1996). Unlike the siderophore uptake systems, this involves a two-component transporter system composed of a TBDT, which mediates iron transport, as well as a coreceptor, which is attached by a lipid anchor to the outer leaflet of the outer membrane and participates in capturing the iron-containing substrates. In both systems, energy for transport is supplied by the TonB system, and substrates are then shuttled across the periplasm by periplasmic carrier proteins to an ATP-binding cassette (ABC) transporter for transport across the inner membrane (IM) into the cytoplasm. Highly species-specific transferrin or lactoferrin receptors (TfR and LfR) are expressed at their outer membrane which bind the host iron-binding proteins with micromolar affinities, extracting the iron directly from both host proteins (Gray-Owen and Schryvers, 1996).

The best characterised is the TbpA/TpbB transport system for transferrin iron uptake in *Neisseria meningitides*. TbpA, the outer membrane TBDT, binds both iron-loaded and apotransferrin with the same affinity, whereas TbpB, the lipoprotein coreceptor, binds only diferric transferrin. TbpA alone suffices to transport iron, but in the presence of TdpB iron uptake is more efficient. The crystal structures of both neisserial Tf-binding proteins have been recently reported in complex with human Tf (Calmettes *et al.*, 2012; Noinaj *et al.*, 2012a), providing molecular insight into how *Neisseria* are able to steal iron from Tf and import it across the outer membrane for survival and virulence. TbpB, anchored to the surface of the cell by its N-terminal lipid anchor, consists of two structurally similar domains, each containing an eight-stranded β-barrel with an adjacent four-stranded β-rich handle domain (Calmettes *et al.*, 2012). The TbpB–transferrin complex indicates structural features consistent with its specificity for human transferrin and for binding holotransferrin rather than apotransferrin. The TbpA structure (Noinaj *et al.*, 2012a) shows, as predicted (Boulton *et al.*, 2000; Oakhill *et al.*, 2005), that TbpA is indeed a TBDT, with a large N-terminal plug domain and a 22-stranded β-barrel transmembrane domain (Figure 4.3), albeit with a number of unique features. Whereas in other TBDTs the plug is buried in the β-barrel (see Chapter 3), in the complex of TbpA with human apotransferrin (Noinaj *et al.*, 2012a) there are a number of very long extracellular loops which interact with the C-lobe of transferrin. In particular, there is an unusually long plug loop implicated in iron uptake (Jost-Daijev and Cornelissen, 2004; Noto and Cornelissen, 2008) which protrudes some 2.5 nm above the cell surface and interacts directly with the CI subdomain and a helix finger at the apex of extracellular loop 3, which is inserted directly into the cleft between the CI and C2 subdomains of the transferrin C-lobe and appears to be involved in catalysing iron release. These interactions induce a partial opening of the iron-binding cleft in the transferrin C-lobe, distorting the iron coordination and thereby facilitating iron release and its transfer to TbpA. The α-helix in TbpA extracellular loop 3 contains residues found only in human transferrin, which may explain the specificity of *Neisseria* TbpA for human transferrin. The X-ray and small-angle X-ray scattering (SAXS) structures of TbpB and the TbpB–Fe_2–transferrin complex show that TbpB also binds to the C-lobe of transferrin, but at sites that differ from TbpA. According to current models for transferrin iron import, after binding of transferrin to TbpB, the latter escorts transferrin to TbpA for iron release and import, which involves the formation of a quaternary iron import complex (TbpA–TbpB–transferrin). Based on the X-ray structure of TbpA–apoTf and the SAXS solution structure of Tbp–Fe_2–Tf, an *in-silico* model of the TbpA–TbpB–Fe_2–Tf

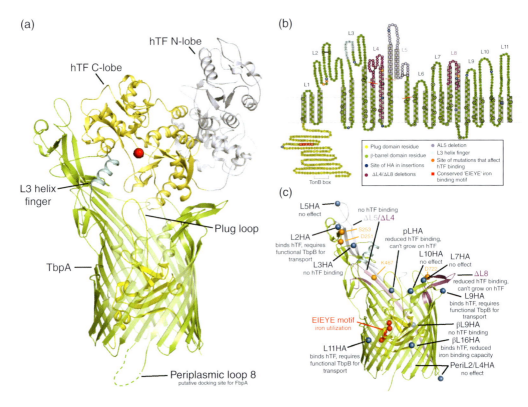

Figure 4.3 *Molecular details of the interactions between neisserial TbpA and human transferrin. (a) The complex crystal structure of neisserial TbpA and human transferrin (apo form) (PDB code 3V8X) is shown in ribbon representation with the beta-domain of TbpA in green, the plug domain in red, the helix finger of loop 3 (L3) in purple, and transferrin in gold (C-lobe) and light blue (N-lobe). The location of iron (red sphere) was modelled based on the diferric transferrin crystal structure (PDB code 3V83) and the putative docking site for FbpA along disordered periplasmic loop 8 (dashed green line) is indicated. (b) 2D-topology diagram of TbpA highlighting selected mutations, regions of sequence conservation and sequence diversity (adapted from Boulton et al., 2000). Plug domain residues are highlighted in yellow, beta-domain residues are in green, L3 helix finger residues are in cyan, residues that affect hTF binding when mutated are in orange, sites of HA tag insertions are in blue, and the iron-binding motif EIEYE is shown as red squares. Deleted loops are shown in dark purple (loop 4 and loop 8) and in light blue (loop 5). The solid red bars indicate the start and end-points for the loop 4+5 construct which retained hTF binding when individually expressed and purified, while the dashed red bar indicates the start point for the loop 5 only construct. Boldface circled residues are aromatics and boldface squared residues are those that are conserved among all TbpA proteins (even in other species). (c) The structure of TbpA (green ribbon) depicting the locations of HA-insertions (blue spheres), and deletions (purple and light blue) and the resulting effect on transferrin binding and iron import. The locations of mutations that affected transferrin binding are indicated by orange spheres and the putative iron binding motif EIEYE is shown by red spheres. Reproduced with permission from John Wiley & Sons, Ltd*

complex was formed which is shown in Figure 4.4. The model was tested by single particle electron microscopy using the triple complex assembled from its components. The X-ray, SAXS and electron microscopy (EM) structures support a consistent arrangement of the triple complex, one

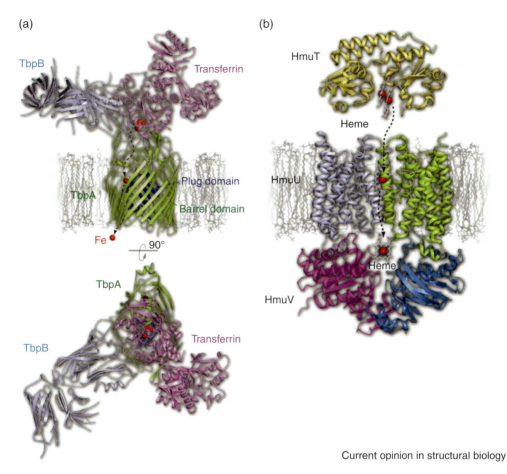

(a)

TbpB

Transferrin

TbpA

Plug domain

Barrel domain

TbpB

Fe

90°

TbpA

Transferrin

TbpB

(b)

HmuT

Heme

HmuU

HmuV

Heme

Current opinion in structural biology

Figure 4.4 *Structural insights into iron transport by TbpA/B and HmuUV in pathogenic bacteria. (a) Iron (red sphere) is extracted from transferrin (magenta) by a concerted effort from TbpA (green), a TonB-dependent transporter, and its lipoprotein coreceptor TbpB (cyan), both found in the outer membrane. On the basis of the crystal structures of transferrin with TbpA and TbpB separately, a model is shown here of the TbpA–TbpB–transferrin triple complex. The proposed pathway for iron import is indicated by dashed arrows. A view in the membrane is shown at the top, while a view from the surface is shown at the bottom. (b) Haem transfer into the cytosol is mediated by the inner membrane protein HmuUV, composed of two membrane-integrated HmuU subunits (cyan and green) and two periplasmic nucleotide exchange subunits called HmuV (magenta and blue). The periplasmic haem carrier protein, HmuT (gold), delivers haem to HmuUV for import, which follows the proposed pathway indicated by the dashed arrows. Haem is shown in stick and iron as a red sphere. Reprinted with permission from Elsevier from Noinaj, N. and Buchanan, S.K. (2014) Structural insight into the transport of small molecules across membranes. Curr. Opin. Struct. Biol., **27C**, 8–15*

consequence of which is the formation of an enclosed chamber with a volume of around 1000 Å, which is located directly above the plug domain of TbpA (Figure 4.5). This chamber may serve two important roles for iron absorption: (i) it may prevent the diffusion of iron released from transferrin; and (ii) it may guide the iron towards the β-barrel domain of TbpA for subsequent transport.

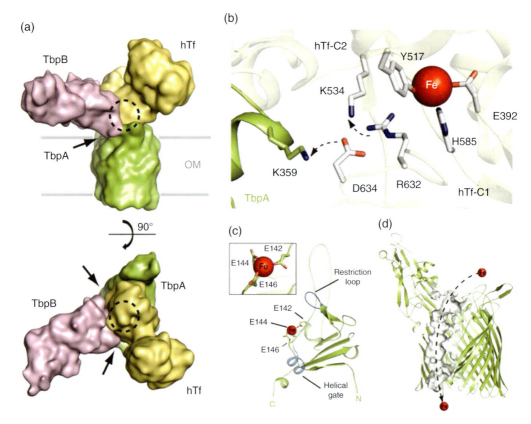

Figure 4.5 *The role of TbpA in iron extraction from transferrin and import across the outer membrane. (a) Model for the neisserial TbpA–TbpB–transferrin triple complex in the outer membrane (OM). TbpA is shown in green surface representation, TbpB in purple, and human transferrin in gold. Dashed circles indicate the approximate location of the enclosed chamber (~1000Å³) formed by the union of the triple complex, and black arrows indicate regions of putative interactions between TbpA and TbpB. (b) Proposed mechanism for TbpA-mediated iron release from transferrin, where K359 of TbpA neutralises the negative charge of D634 of transferrin, producing a charge–charge repulsion of K534 and R632 and leading to a conformational change in transferrin and iron release. (c) A model for the role of the TbpA plug domain (green) in serving as a transient docking site during iron transport. The inset shows a top-down view of the iron coordination. (d) Molecular dynamics simulations designed to mimic the role of the Ton system demonstrated a systematic unfolding of the plug domain and formation of a pore (grey surface) that could facilitate iron passage. Reproduced with permission from John Wiley & Sons, Ltd*

A stepwise model for iron import in *Neisseria* species involving both TbpA and TbpB has been proposed (Nionaj *et al.*, 2012b), which is presented in Figure 4.6. Initially, at the cell surface TbpB would preferentially bind iron-loaded transferrin, locking it in a closed state to ensure the iron is not prematurely released. Then, TbpB would transfer transferrin to TbpA where a transient triple complex would be formed. TbpA then catalyses a conformational change in transferrin in an energy-dependent mechanism mediated by the TonB system (Cornelissen and Sparling, 1994), which results in Fe^{3+} release from transferrin, and the subsequent dissociation of apotransferrin, facilitated by TbpB. The interaction of TonB with TbpA

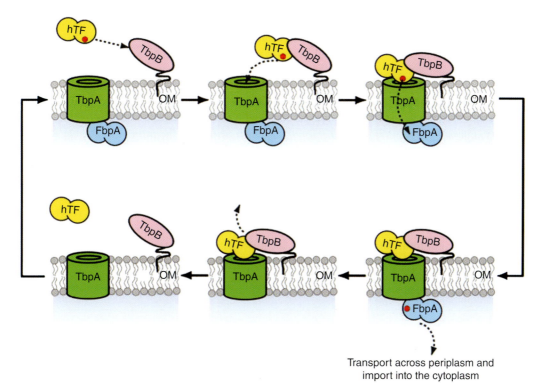

Figure 4.6 *Stepwise mechanism for the acquisition of iron from lactoferrin by* Neisseria. *Based on similarities to the hTF acquisition system, a stepwise mechanism can be postulated. Once within the host, the neisserial coreceptor LbpB would bind soluble hLF and shuttle it to the iron transporter LbpA. Upon the LbpA–hLF complex docking onto LbpA and combined with the Ton system, a conformational change within the plug domain of LbpA would catalyse iron release and import through the β-domain, where it would immediately bind to FbpA and be further shuttled across the periplasm and into the cytoplasm by FbpB/C. Reproduced with permission from John Wiley and Sons, Ltd*

is expected to lead to systematic TonB-dependent conformational changes within the entire plug domain, which would then allow the formation of a transient docking site for iron. Further unravelling of the plug domain would eventually allow the transport of iron through the beta-domain to the periplasm (Figure 4.4), from where it would be transferred to the ferric ion-binding protein (FbpA), docked on the periplasmic face of TbpA. FbpA then transfers the iron across the periplasm where it would be transported into the cytoplasm. Based on similarities to the hTF acquisition system, a similar mechanism has been postulated for human lactoferrin (Noinaj *et al.*, 2013).

The most likely mechanism for iron release involves a conserved lysine residue, K359, within the helix finger of loop 3 of TbpA, which may serve to catalyse the release of iron by hijacking the pH-sensing triad of the C-lobe of transferrin (described in greater detail in Chapter 6). K359 of TbpA could sequester the negative charge of D634 of transferrin (Figure 4.5), leading to charge repulsion between K534 and R632 which mediates a conformation change and eventual iron release. D634 typically serves the role of neutralizing this positive charge, and when this transferrin residue is mutated to alanine, iron release increases approximately 100-fold (Steere *et al.*, 2012).

However, it has been shown that the mutation of Lys534 or Arg632 to an alanine severely retards iron release from that lobe, essentially locking iron in the C-lobe (Halbrooks *et al.*, 2003).

Fe³⁺ is transported from the periplasm to the cytosol by the FbpABC transporter consisting of the PBP FbpA, a permease, and an ATP-binding protein. The structures of a number of Fbps have been determined, and they all belong to the class II PBPs (as described in Chapter 3) (Quiocho and Ledvina, 1996). Overall, PBPs are built of two α/β domains, with a central β-sheet of five β-strands flanked by α-helices. The two domains are connected by a hinge-region, with the ligand-binding site buried in between the two domains. In the absence of ligand, the protein is flexible with the two domains rotating around the hinge, and it exists largely in the open conformation with both domains separated. Upon substrate binding, the closed conformation is stabilised, and the ligand is trapped at the interface between the domains in the so-called 'Venus Fly-trap' mechanism. Comparison of the structures of iron-free and iron-loaded *H. influenzae* FbpA (apo and holo-FbpA) reveals a 20° rotation of the two structural domains about the central β-strands (Figure 4.7). The Fe³⁺ ion binds in a cleft between the two domains, coordinated by two oxygens from Tyr195 and Tyr196, an imidazole nitrogen from His9, a carboxylate oxygen from Glu57, an oxygen atom from an exogenous phosphate, and an oxygen atom from a water molecule. As we will see in Chapter 6, the mammalian iron transport protein transferrin has not only a similar three-dimensional fold as Fbp but also a rather similar Fe³⁺ coordination geometry.

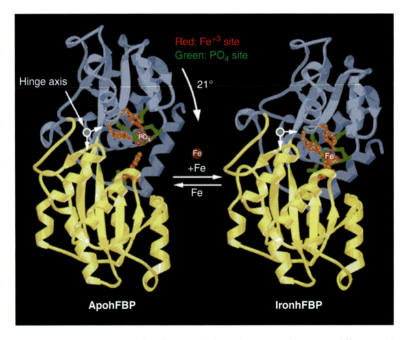

Figure 4.7 *Hinge motion upon iron binding in hFbp. The most dramatic difference between apo-hFbp and iron-hFbp is a large relative rotation of the two structural domains. The C-terminal iron half-site (top) retains the same structure in both the apo and iron forms, including the presence of a phosphate ion (pre-existing complementarity), while the N-terminal half-site reorganises upon iron binding (induced fit). Reprinted with permission from Bruns, C.M., Nowalk, A.J., Arvai, A.S. et al. (1997) Structure of* Haemophilus influenza *Fe(+3)-binding protein reveals convergent evolution within a superfamily.* Nat. Struct. Biol., **4**, *919–924; © 2014, American Chemical Society*

4.4.3 Haem Iron Uptake

Roughly two-thirds of the total body iron in humans is in haemoglobin, within the circulating erythrocytes, and it is therefore not surprising that pathogenic bacteria have evolved numerous strategies to acquire this most abundant source of iron from their host. Tetrameric haemoglobin in the serum dissociates to methaemoglobin (MetHb), an α/β dimer with the iron in the ferric form, which is irreversibly bound to haptoglobin (Hp), thus preventing both haem dissociation from MetHb and oxidative damage (Wandersman, 2010). Both, MetHb and the MetHb–Hp complex represent the predominant host sources of iron for bacteria, while any free haem is bound to haemopexin (Wandersman and Delepelaire, 2004). While most pathogens assimilate only haem iron, some bacteria (e.g. *H. influenzae*) that cannot synthesise the tetrapyrrole ring require haem not only as a source of iron but also of protoporphyrin. Some well-known pathogens are able to secrete haemolysins, which lyse the erythrocyte membrane, releasing intracellular haemoglobin.

There are two mechanisms for bacterial iron acquisition from haem. The first mechanism uses secreted haem-scavenging proteins, known as haemophores, while the second involves direct uptake via membrane-bound or cell wall-embedded haemoprotein receptors (Stojiljkovic and Perkins-Balding, 2002; Wandersman and Delepelaire, 2004, 2012; Contreras *et al.*, 2014). Haem uptake by haemophores is considered first.

A number of Gram-negative bacteria synthesise specialised extracellular proteins called haemophores (by analogy with siderophores), which acquire haem from various sources and bring it to a specific outer membrane receptor. In *Serratia marcescens*[2] the system has been particularly well characterised (Ghigo *et al.*, 1997; Wandersman and Delepelaire, 2004, 2012). All of the proteins involved, including the haemophore itself, HasA, the outer membrane receptor, HasR, and the TonB paralogue, HasB, are encoded (as in most other species including *Pseudomonas* and *Yersinia*) by an operon which is repressed by Fe^{2+}–Fur.

HasA binds haem tightly (K_d = 18 pM); it can also bind haem from haemoglobin, haemopexin and myoglobin without forming stable complexes with these proteins (Wandersman, 2010; Wandersman and Stojiljkovic, 2000). The mechanism of haem scavenging has been studied in detail using $HasA_{sm}$. The structures of holo-HasA and of apo-HasA from *S. marcescens* (Arnoux *et al.*, 1999, 2000; Wolff *et al.*, 2008) are shown in Figure 4.8. Holo-HasA (Figure 4.8A) is a globular monomer of 19 kDa with two opposite faces; one face is composed of four α-helices, and the other of seven β-strands. Haemin is bound by two axial iron ligands, His32 and Tyr75, located on two loops which separate the two faces (Arnoux *et al.*, 1999) (Figure 4.8A). Tyr75 is stabilised in the tyrosinate state (which makes it a better iron ligand) by His83, to which it is hydrogen-bonded. It follows that His83 influences haem binding (Caillet-Saguy *et al.*, 2008). Upon haem binding, the general secondary structure elements are conserved and there is a drastic change in the conformation of the loop 32 that contains His32, one of the iron axial ligands (3 nm movement). *Pseudomonas aeruginosa* holo-HasA (HasAp) shows a similar fold with the same axial haem iron ligands (Alontaga *et al.*, 2009). HasA from *Yersinia pestis* retains its ability to bind haem despite the replacement of His32 by a non-coordinating Gln (Kumar *et al.*, 2013), and $HasA_{sm}$ retains its ability to bind haem despite the loss of either of the axial ligands, coordination probably compensated by water (Wandersman, 2010). It has been recently reported that replacing the axial ligand Tyr75 or its hydrogen-bonded partner His83, only minimally affects haemin acquisition by HasAp from *P. aeruginosa* (Kumar *et al.*, 2014).

---

[2]While not mentioned earlier among pathogens, *S. marcescens* is not the most convivial of visitors, being associated with nosocomial (hospital-acquired) infections, such as urinary and respiratory tract infections, endocarditis, osteomyelitis, septicaemia, wound infections, eye infections and meningitis.

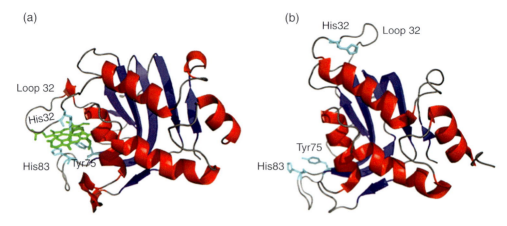

Figure 4.8 *Crystal structure of holo-HasA (a) and a representative model of nuclear magnetic resonance structure of apo-HasA (b) from S. marcescens. Helices are in red, strands in blue, coils in grey, and haem in green. Upon haem binding, the general secondary structure elements are conserved and there is a drastic change in the conformation of loop 32 that contains His-32, one of the iron axial ligands (30Å movement). The two haem iron axial ligands are His32 and Tyr75, with the latter residue stabilised in its tyrosinate form by nearby His83 (all in cyan) (PDB 1B2V and 1YBJ). Reproduced with permission from John Wiley & Sons, Ltd*

Once haem has been bound to HasA-type haemophores, it is then delivered to the outer membrane receptor HasR, which actively transports haem through this membrane (Ghigo *et al.*, 1997), despite having a much lower affinity for haem than HasA. Upon binding of HasA to HasR, both of the axial ligands to haem are broken (Krieg *et al.*, 2009), allowing haem to bind to the low-affinity site of HasR. Only haem is internalised, while the apohaemophore remains outside. HasR receptors belong to the family of TonB-dependent receptors, and HasR$_{sm}$ structure determination (in the HasA–HasR complex) has shown that it has a similar fold, with a plug and barrel organisation (Figure 4.9) (Krieg *et al.*, 2009). In the HasA$_{sm}$–HasR$_{sm}$ haem complex, haem is bound to HasR$_{sm}$ by two conserved histidines, His189 and His603; the former is located on the extracellular face of the N-terminal plug, whereas His603 is located on an extracellular loop of the β-barrel (Figure 4.9). The two His residues are close enough to simultaneously ligate haem iron. Haem uptake by HasA only occurs under strongly iron-limiting conditions, and involves transcription of the *hasA* and *hasB* genes, with haem-loaded HasA serving as inducer: HasB is also required for induction (Benvides-Matos and Biville, 2010). The transfer of haem to the cytosol involves a specific haem-binding periplasmic protein and an ABC transporter in the cytosolic membrane. The structure of the ABC transporter of *Y. pestis* HmuUV has been recently determined (Woo *et al.*, 2012), and shown to consist of two copies each of the transmembrane domain HmuU and the nucleotide-binding domain HmuV. Each HmuU subunit contains 10 transmembrane helices, with HmuV interacting noncovalently via a conserved cytoplasmic coupling helix. Unlike type I ABC transporters, an outward-facing conformation was observed in the absence of nucleotide (Oldham *et al.*, 2007; Dawson and Locher, 2006). A cavity, which is open in the periplasm but closed to the cytoplasm, was found at the interface between the two HmuU subunits, revealing the site where HmuT, the periplasmic haem export protein, interacts with HmuUV for haem exchange and subsequent translocation (Mattle *et al.*, 2010).

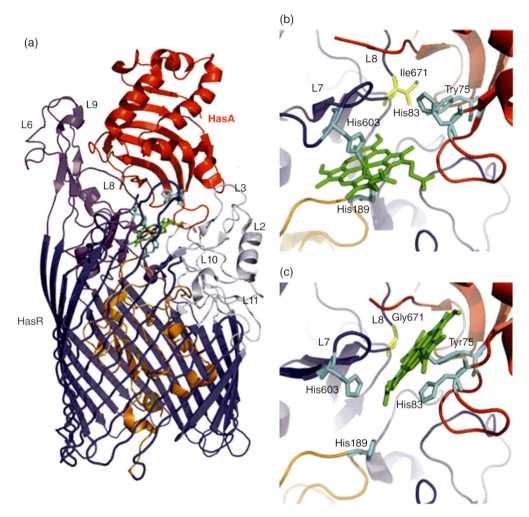

Figure 4.9 *Crystal structure of the complex resulting from the association of holo-HasA with apo-HasR. (a) The HasA–haem–HasR complex. (b) Close-up of the haem-binding region of the wild-type complex. (c) Close-up of a mutant complex unable to transfer haem from HasA to HasR. (A) HasA is in red, while HasR has the classical plug-barrel organisation of the TonB-dependent transporters receptors; barrel is in blue, plug in orange (strands 1–8 are shown as thin ribbon). The interaction surface on HasR is defined by long extracellular loops L6, L8 and L9 (purple) on the one hand, and L2, L3, L10 and L11 (gray-blue) on the other hand. HasA has conserved most of its structure with the exception of the loop that contains His32 (cf. Figure 4.8), which is not seen in the electron density map; haem is on its binding site on HasR defined (B) by the two His residues 189 from the plug and 603 from the loop 7 (L7) of the barrel, that are the haem iron axial ligands; His83 from HasA has pivoted away from its initial position (see Figure 4.8); Ile671 from the HasR loop 8 (L8) (in yellow) is in the HasA haem-binding pocket. In the mutant complex (C) resulting from the association of holo-HasA with HasR mutant Ile671Gly (in yellow), haem stays on HasA, still liganded by HasA Tyr75, but not by His32 (PDB 3CSL and 3DDR). Reproduced with permission from John Wiley & Sons, Ltd*

Haemophilus influenza can scavenge haem from the host haem–haemopexin complex via the Hxu system (Cope *et al.*, 1998), encoded by an operon of three genes: *hxuC*, *hxuB* and *hxuA* (Morton *et al.*, 2007). The *hxuC* gene encodes the HxuC protein, an outer membrane TonB-dependent receptor with the signatures of a haem transporter, whereas the *hxuB* and *hxuA* genes encode a two-component secretion system (Tps), with the haemophore HxuA exported across the cell envelope by HxuB. Following interaction between haem–haemopexin and HxuA, haem is no longer bound to its initial high-affinity site and becomes accessible to its cognate haem receptor, HxuC (Fournier *et al.*, 2011).

Whereas Gram-negative bacteria have an outer membrane to which TonB-dependent receptors are bound, Gram-positive bacteria lack an outer membrane and therefore do not require a TonB energy-coupled transport system; as we will see later, they also have ABC transporters for haem transport in their cytosol membrane. Instead, they are enveloped in a thick matrix of peptidoglycan, in which covalently bound proteins are embedded. In Gram-positive bacteria, proteins are displayed on the cell surface using sortases; these are cysteine transpeptidases which join proteins bearing an appropriate sorting signal to strategically positioned amino groups on the cell surface (Spirig *et al.*, 2011). Based on extensive studies with *S. aureus*, we now have a detailed understanding of the intricate vectorial cascade of haem transfer across the thick cell wall (Mazmanian *et al.*, 2003; Grigg *et al.*, 2010; Contreras *et al.*, 2014). This involves a cascade of Isd proteins (*iron-regulated surface determinant*) which are tethered to unique positions within the cell wall such that haem moves from one protein to the next until it reaches the cytosolic membrane (Figure 4.10). There are nine Isd proteins, the transcription of which is controlled by the Fur repressor. All cell wall-anchored Isd proteins (IsdA, IsdB, IsdC and IsdH) contain structurally conserved NEAT domains, which bind haem. These domains were first identified 'in silico' as a poorly conserved ORF repeated from one to five times in the neighbourhood of genes encoding siderophore transporters (Andrade *et al.*, 2002), and therefore designated NEAT (near transporter) domains. They have been found in putative ABC transporters in Gram-positive bacteria including *Streptococcus*, *Bacillus*, *Listeria* and *Clostridium* species (Andrade *et al.*, 2002). IsdA and IsdC have one NEAT domain, IsdB has two, and IsdH has three (Andrade *et al.*, 2002; Mazmanian *et al.*, 2003). They are secreted by the Sec pathway: IsdA, IsdB and IsdH have an LPXGT motif and are anchored to the peptidoglycan by sortase A, whereas IsdC, which has an NPQTN motif, is attached by sortase B (Mazmanian *et al.*, 2002). NEAT domains have similar immunoglobulin-like β-sandwich folds (Grigg *et al.*, 2010), as illustrated for IsdA with haem bound in Figure 4.11a. The haem-binding sites of IsdA, IsdC and IsdH are also shown in the other panels of Figure 4.11.

Two of the Isd proteins, IsdB and IsdH, are haemophores and although in Figure 4.10 IsdB and IsdH are shown interacting with only one protein ligand, IsdB also binds Hp–Hb and IsdH also binds metHb. IsdE and IsdF are the binding protein and permease components of an ABC transporter, respectively, IsdD is a membrane protein of unknown function, and IsdG and IsdI are cytoplasmic haem-degrading enzymes. From IsdB and IsdH, haem is transferred either directly to IsdE, located in the cytoplasmic membrane, or through IsdA and IsdC. From IsdE, haem is then transferred to Isd F, which is thought to form the permease, a homodimeric integral membrane protein (Mazmanian *et al.*, 2003). The final component required to drive haem uptake across the cytosol membrane is an ATP hydrolase. However, the *S. aureus* Isd system lacks an obvious ATPase encoded in the *isd* locus; in fact, several iron-compound ABC transporters from *S. aureus* lack a corresponding ATPase, including the siderophore transporters HtsABC and SirABC (Dale *et al.*, 2004; Speciali *et al.*, 2006). In the Hts and Sir systems, FhuC provides the ATPase function, and evidence suggests that FhuC also serves as the ATPase for the Isd system (Speciali *et al.*, 2006; Beasley *et al.*, 2009). Figure 4.12 presents the X-ray structure of IsdE (PDB ID: 2q8q) docked against a model of IsdF and FhuC. The vectorial transport of haem along the chain of proteins is

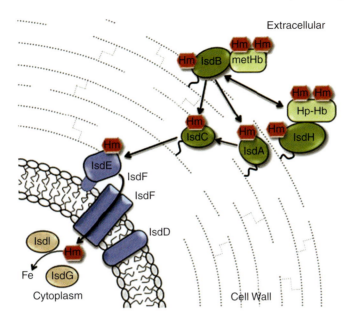

Figure 4.10 *Schematic representation of the Isd system haem transport components. Haem transport and iron liberation is accomplished by the coordinated effort of nine Isd proteins. IsdA, IsdB, IsdC, and IsdH (green) are covalently anchored to the cell wall. IsdE and IsdF (blue) are the binding protein and permease components of an ABC transporter, respectively. IsdE is shown in the haem-bound state prior to complexation with IsdF for transport. IsdD (blue) is a membrane protein of unknown function. IsdG and IsdI are cytoplasmic haem-degrading enzymes. The ligand preferences for each member are illustrated as Hm (haem), metHb (methaemoglobin) and Hp (haptoglobin–haemoglobin). For simplicity, IsdB and IsdH are shown interacting with only one protein ligand, but in fact, IsdB also binds Hp–Hb and IsdH also binds metHb. The predominant haem transfer path in the Isd system is represented by arrows. Reprinted with permission from Elsevier from Grigg, J.C., Ukpabi, G., Gaudin, C.F. and Murphy, M.E. (2010) Structural biology of heme binding in the* Staphylococcus aureus *Isd system.* J. Inorg. Biochem., **104**, *341–348*

unidirectional and rapid, and once in the cytosol iron is released from haem by two haem oxygenases, IsdG and IsdI. This sequence of events, as first proposed by Mazmanian *et al.* (2003), has been corroborated by more recent studies (Muryoi *et al.*, 2008; Tiedemann *et al.*, 2012), essentially confirming that haem transport from the cell wall-anchored IsdH/IsdB proteins proceeds directly to IsdE in the cytoplasmic membrane, with IsdC acting as the central cog-wheel that facilitates haem transfer from IsdA to IsdE.

As we will see in Chapter 8, conventional haem oxygenases (see Chapter 8) catalyse the oxidation of haem to biliverdin, carbon monoxide and ferrous iron in a seven-electron process which requires three molecules of dioxygen, together with an impressive amount of reducing power supplied by NADPH. Bacterial haem oxygenases (for a review, see Wilks and Ikedo-Saito, 2014) from a number of pathogenic bacteria, including *Corynebacterium diphtheriae*, *N. meningitis* and *P. aeruginosa*, were found to be structurally and mechanistically similar (Zhu *et al.*, 2000; Ratliff *et al.*, 2001). However, as illustrated in Figure 4.13, the *S. aureus* IsdG and *M. tuberculosis* MhuD haem oxygenases give rise to different degradation products. The *S. aureus* IsdG converts haem to the novel chromophore staphylobilin, where the β- or δ-*meso*-carbon is released as formaldehyde (Reniere *et al.*, 2010; Matsui *et al.*, 2013). The structurally related MhuD cleaves haem to mycobilin, where the *meso*-carbon is retained as an aldehyde (Nambu *et al.*, 2013).

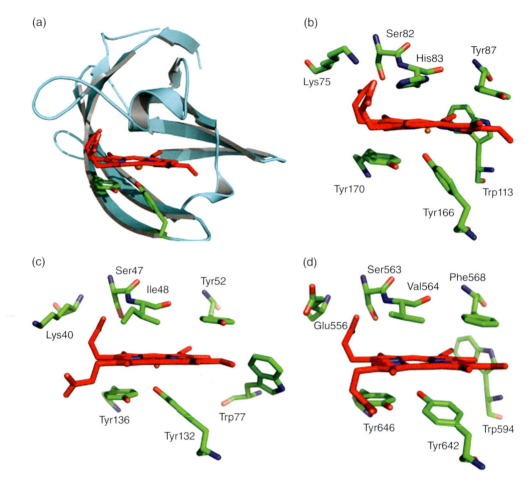

Figure 4.11 *Haem binding by IsdA, IsdC and IsdH. (a) The X-ray crystal structure of IsdA-N1 (PDB ID:2itf) is shown in cyan cartoon, looking into the binding pocket for orientation reference. (b) The IsdA-N1 (PDB ID:2itf) binding pocket residues and haem are shown as sticks. Oxygen (red), nitrogen (blue), iron (orange), haem carbon (red) and side-chain carbon (green) atoms are coloured accordingly. Residues are numbered based on the full-length protein sequence in the NCBI database (NCBI ID: YP_001332075). (c) The IsdC-N1 (PDB ID: 2o6p) binding pocket, oriented as in (a). Residues are numbered according to NCBI ID: YP_001332076. (d) The IsdH-N3 (PDB ID: 2z6f) binding pocket, oriented as in (a). Residues are numbered according to NCBI ID: YP_001332658. Reprinted with permission from Elsevier from Grigg, J.C., Ukpabi, G., Gaudin, C.F. and Murphy, M.E. (2010) Structural biology of heme binding in the* Staphylococcus aureus *Isd system. J. Inorg. Biochem., **104**, 341–348*

4.4.4 Ferrous Iron Uptake

Fe^{2+} transport systems are often associated with the colonisation or virulence of enteric pathogens. However, whereas non-pathogenic *E. coli* strains use the Feo system, some pathogenic strains of *E. coli*, like many other pathogenic Gram-negative bacteria (e.g. *Salmonella*, *Shigella* and *Yersinia*) express a second Fe^{2+} transport system, Sit (Janakiraman and Slauch, 2000; Runyen-Janecky *et al.*, 2003; Fetherston *et al.*, 2012). The Sit iron transport system is encoded by the *sitABCD* genes (Fisher *et al.*, 2009), and is present within PAIs in all *Shigella* spp. and some

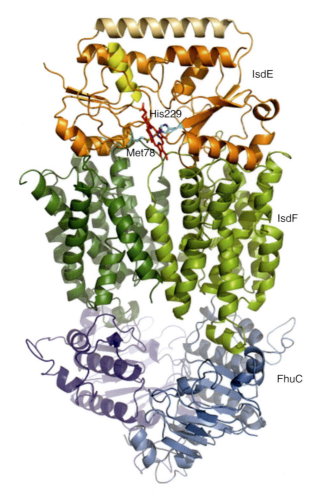

Figure 4.12 *Model of the haem ABC transporter of the Isd system composed of IsdEF and FhuC. The X-ray crystal structure of IsdE (orange, PDB ID: 2q8q) is shown docked against a model of the IsdF (green) and FhuC (blue). The model complex was generated by superposition over the BtuCD-F crystal structure (PDB ID: 2qi9). The backbones are shown as cartoons, with each homodimer chain shown in a different shade of the same colour. In the IsdE structure, the domain-spanning α-helix (light orange), the propionate-stabilizing α-helix (yellow) and the haem–iron-coordinating side chains (cyan) are shown. Reprinted with permission from Elsevier from Grigg, J.C., Ukpabi, G., Gaudin, C.F. and Murphy, M.E. (2010) Structural biology of heme binding in the* Staphylococcus aureus *Isd system.* J. Inorg. Biochem., **104**, 341–348*

pathogenic *E. coli* strains. Characterisation of the *sitABCD* genes in *S. flexneri* indicates that they encode a ferrous iron transport system, although the genes are induced aerobically. *Shigella* spp. are intracellular pathogens, invading and replicating within human colonic epithelial cells, and the *sit* genes provide a competitive advantage to *S. flexneri* growing within epithelial cells (Carpenter and Payne, 2014).

In *Y. pestis*, the Yfe (Sit) and Feo ferrous iron transport systems are both required for efficient growth under static, low-oxygen conditions, and for disease in a bubonic plaque model. The effects

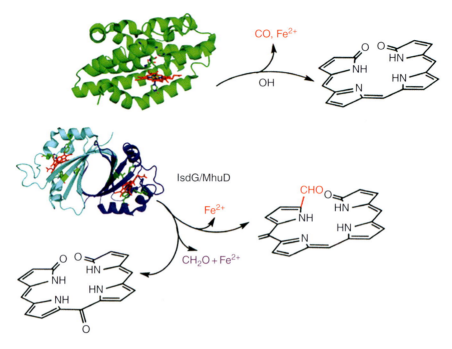

Figure 4.13 *Whereas canonical pathogen haem oxygenases (top), like their eukaryotic counterparts, cleave haem to biliverdin, releasing iron and CO, the noncanonical haem oxygenases IsdG of* S. aureus *and MhuD of* Mycobacterium tuberculosis *(bottom) convert haem to staphylobilin and formaldehyde and to mycobilin, respectively. Reprinted with permission from Wilks, A. and Ikeda-Saito M. (2014)* Heme utilization by pathogenic bacteria: not all pathways lead to biliverdin. Acc. Chem. Res., *May 29, Abstract Figure; © 2014, American Chemical Society*

of mutations in these systems were additive, and the double mutant had a more severe phenotype in an experimental infection than either of the single mutants (Fetherston *et al.*, 2012). Taken together, the results of studies on the role of ferrous iron transporters in virulence of enteric pathogens suggest that ferrous iron transport is important in certain stages of infection and that, although the Feo and Sit/Yfe systems both transport ferrous iron, they are not fully redundant (Carpenter and Payne, 2014).

The Gram-negative *P. aeruginosa* is one of the most frequent causes of opportunistic infections, including colonisation of the lungs of cystic fibrosis patients. The cystic fibrosis lung mucus, where *P. aeruginosa* forms biofilms (Worlitzsch *et al.*, 2002) presents a microaerobic or anaerobic environment that is particularly favourable to the uptake of Fe^{2+}. Phenazine-1-carboxylic acid (PCA) is the precursor of pyocyanin, a blue-green compound typical of *P. aeruginosa*, and both phenazine compounds can redox-cycle (Wang and Newman, 2008). PCA, and to a lesser extent pyocyanin, is able to reduce Fe^{3+} bound to host proteins to Fe^{2+}, allowing the uptake of iron in biofilms via the Feo system (Wang *et al.*, 2011). Reduced PCA is excreted from the cell where it reduces Fe^{3+} to Fe^{2+}; the oxidised phenazine is then recycled inside the cell where it is reduced by NADH (Wang *et al.*, 2011). It was recently shown that both phenazines and Fe^{2+} accumulate in the lungs of cystic fibrosis patients when their condition deteriorates (Hunter *et al.*, 2012, 2013).

4.4.5   Ferric Citrate Uptake by *Bacillus cereus*

Although neither a particularly powerful nor distinctive chelator, ferric citrate can serve as an iron-delivery agent for many bacteria and plants to fulfil their nutritional requirement for iron. As we saw in Chapter 3, the *E. coli* ferric citrate outer membrane transport protein FecA has been characterised, together with the associated ferric citrate transporters. Although the ferric citrate-uptake machinery FecABCDE is conserved in other Gram-negative bacteria such as *Pseudomonas* and *Shigella*, less is known about Gram-positive ferric citrate transport systems. The Gram-positive bacterium, *B. subtilis*, possesses ferric citrate-uptake machinery in the form of YfmC (ferric citrate-binding protein), YfmD and YfmE (membrane transporters), and YfmF (ATPase) (Ollinger *et al.*, 2006)).

Recently, a unique siderophore-binding protein FctC from the Gram-positive pathogen *B. cereus* has been described (Fukushima *et al.*, 2012), which binds multinuclear ferric citrate complexes with a dissociation constant (K_d) of 2.6 nM. Whereas FctC binds diferric dicitrate and triferric tricitrate, it does not bind ferric dicitrate, ferric monocitrate, or citrate alone. Significantly, the protein selectively binds triferric tricitrate even though this species is naturally present at very low equilibrium concentrations.

4.5   Role of Fur and Fur Homologues in Virulence

As we saw in Chapter 3, Fur and Fur homologues are involved in controlling the uptake of iron and other metals (Zur, Mur and Nur), but also control defence against oxidative stress (PerR). This is equally true for pathogenic bacteria, but in addition Fur family members are important for virulence in numerous animal and plant models of infection (reviewed in Troxell and Hassan, 2013; Fillat, 2014). Fur plays a crucial role in pathogenesis, controlling the expression of virulence factors in host–microbe interactions, as well as in the regulation of toxin production in free-living and environmental bacteria such as *Vibrio* spp., *P. aeruginosa*, *Legionella pneumophila* and the toxigenic cyanobacterium *Microcystis aeruginosa*. During recent years intense studies have been dedicated to understanding the relationship between Fur and virulence (Carpenter *et al.*, 2009; Troxell and Hassan, 2013; Fillat, 2014). The requirement of a functional *fur* gene for pathogenesis, the colonisation of host cells and virulence has been well established in *H. pylori*, *S. aureus*, *Listeria monocytogenes* and *V. cholerae* and *Campylobacter jejuni* (reviewed in Fillat, 2014). Fur-controlled genes are also involved in the control of pathogenesis of *N. meningitidis* and *N. gonorrhoeae* (Yu and Genco, 2012). Fur also plays a crucial role in the defence against oxidative and nitrosative insults imposed by the host. Beyond the control of iron homeostasis and the closely related response to oxidative stress, Fur is involved in the regulation of processes that appear to be independent of the status of iron, including the acid tolerance response in *Salmonella typhimurium* and *H. pylori* (Gancz *et al.*, 2006; Hall and Foster, 1996) and the tolerance to nitrite and osmotic stresses in *Desulfovibrio vulgaris* (Bender *et al.*, 2007). In *Pseudomonas* spp., Fur has been related to the formation of mature biofilms (Banin *et al.*, 2005) and the regulation of quorum sensing (Oglesby *et al.*, 2008). The central role of Fur in the metabolism of prokaryotes through the modulation of a plethora of genes involved in different functional categories in response to different stimuli is illustrated schematically in Figure 4.14.

4.6   Role of Pathogen ECF Sigma Factors

We saw in Chapter 3 that, unlike other ferric siderophore outer membrane transporters (OMTs), Fec A has an N-terminal extension of about 70 residues (Pressler *et al.*, 1988) which is implicated in inducing the transcription of the transport genes when ferric citrate is bound. The signal for

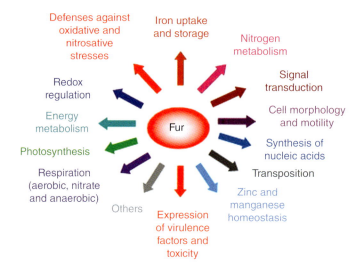

Figure 4.14 *Overview of the cellular processes which are modulated by Fur. Reproduced with permission from Elsevier from Fillat, M.F. (2014) The FUR (ferric uptake regulator) superfamily: diversity and versatility of key transcriptional regulators.* Arch. Biochem. Biophys., **546**, 41–52

transcription is transmitted from the cell surface to the cytoplasm by a mechanism which requires three components: the OMT itself with its ferric ligand bound; a cytoplasmic membrane regulator protein; and a cytosolic sigma factor, belonging to the extracytoplasmic function (ECF) family (Braun, 1997).

Sequence alignments have identified a subfamily of OMTs, designated OMT_Ns, which have similar N-terminal extensions to FecA of 70–80 residues (Figure 4.15), and are involved in the regulation of iron uptake from ferric siderophores or from haem. These include the ferric-pyoverdine (Pvd) transporter FpvA (Figure 4.16) and the ferrioxamine transporter FiuA of *P. aeruginosa* (Poole *et al.*, 1993; Visca *et al.*, 2002), the pseudobactin BN7 and BN8 transporters PupA and PupB of *P. putida* (Koster *et al.*, 1993, 1994), the haemophore transporter HasR of *Serratia marcescens* (Biville *et al.*, 2004), and BfrZ, a putative siderophore transporter from *Bordetella bronchiseptica* (Pradel and Locht, 2001). A conserved motif is found in the N-terminal domain of OMT_Ns at residues 50–59 (numbering for FecA), which may play a role in interactions between the transporter and regulator proteins (Figure 4.15). The presence of an N-terminal elongation of the OMT protein by 70–80 residues associated with the presence of the FecI/FecR pair reveals itself to be a good indication of ECF sigma factor regulation, which is found in many Gram-negative bacteria.

As we saw earlier in Chapter 3, proteolytic digestion of the cytoplasmic membrane regulator protein is the trigger for the activation of the ECF sigma factor, and in the FecA system, the site-2 protease RseP plays a key role. Detailed studies have shown that in the pyoverdine, ferrichrome and desferrioxamine siderophore uptake systems of *P. aeruginosa*, RseP is once again required for the induction of signal transduction (Draper *et al.*, 2011). Once again, the siderophore receptor interacts with the sigma regulator protein which extends from the periplasm into the cytoplasm to control the activity of the cognate sigma factor. When pyoverdine is present, the sigma regulator FpvR undergoes proteolysis resulting in the activation of two sigma factors PvdS and FpvI, and expression of the genes for pyoverdine synthesis and uptake. When pyoverdine is absent, subfragments of FpvR inhibit PvdS and FpvI. Similarly, subfragments of the sigma regulators FoxR and FiuR are formed in the absence of desferrioxamine and ferrichrome, but are much less abundant

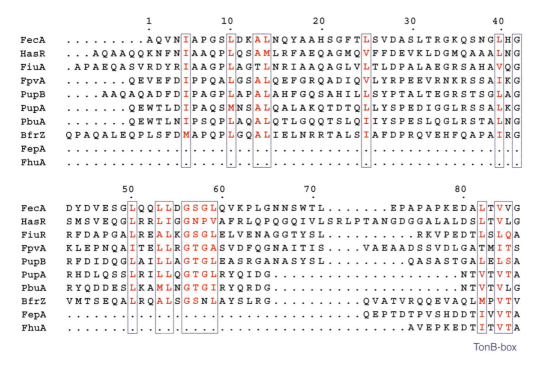

Figure 4.15 *The OMT$_N$ N-terminal extension. Sequence alignment of the N-terminal extension in E. coli FecA, S. marcescens HasR, P. aeruginosa FiuA, P. aeruginosa FpvA, P. putida PupB, P. putida PupA, P. fluorescence M114 PbuA, and B. bronchiseptica BfrZ transporters. The N-terminal sequences of E. coli FepA and FhuA, which do not contain the extension region, are included for comparison. The predicted TonB-box motifs for the transporters are indicated. Regions of high sequence similarity are boxed in blue. Identical or similar residues are coloured in red. Numbering refers to the FecA amino acid sequence. Sequences shown correspond to the mature proteins (without signal sequences). Sequences were aligned using ClustalW and the figure was prepared with ESPript (Gouet et al., 1999). Reproduced with permission from John Wiley & Sons, Ltd from Schalk, I.J., Yue, W.W. and Buchanan, S.K. (2004) Recognition of iron-free siderophores by TonB-dependent iron transporters. Mol. Microbiol., **54**, 14–22*

when the siderophores are present, and downstream gene expression takes place. In all three systems, RseP (MucP/YaeL) is required for complete proteolysis of the sigma regulator and sigma factor activity. These findings underline the important role of regulated proteolysis as a general mechanism for signal transduction in cell-surface signalling.

A feature of characterised OMT$_N$ family members is their ability to bind the corresponding iron-free and iron-loaded (ferric-) ligands with similar affinities. This has been observed for a ferric-citrate transporter (Yue *et al.*, 2003), a ferric-Pvd transporter (Schalk *et al.*, 1999) and a haemophore transporter (Rossi *et al.*, 2003), although the biological function of binding an iron-free ligand is unknown.

4.7 Fungal Pathogens

The three best-studied opportunistic fungal pathogens are the saprotroph mould *Aspergillus fumigatus*, responsible for invasive pulmonary aspergillosis, the polymorphic fungus *Candida albicans*, the cause of skin or mucosal infections and invasive candidiasis, and the yeast *Cryptococcus*

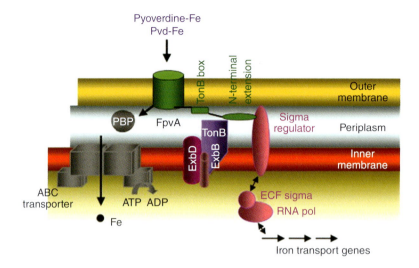

Figure 4.16 *Proteins involved in the PvdI uptake pathway in* P. aeruginosa. *Ferric pyoverdine I (PvdI–Fe³⁺) from the extracellular medium is recognised by the specific outer membrane transporter FpvAI, which serves two functions. First, FpvAI transports PvdI–Fe³⁺ into the periplasm. Second, FpvAI is involved in a signalling cascade regulating the transcription of genes encoding proteins involved in iron uptake by the PvdI pathway and of genes encoding virulence factors. This signalling cascade is initiated by the binding of PvdI–Fe³⁺ to FpvAI, and involves several components: the N-terminal extension of FpvAI, the inner membrane sigma-regulator protein FpvR, and the cytoplasmic ECF sigma factor, FpvI. Both transport and induction functions require energy transduction from the TonB–ExbB–ExbD complex in the inner membrane. PvdI–Fe dissociation occurs in the periplasm, via a mechanism involving iron reduction and the transfer of Fe²⁺ from PvdI to a periplasmic binding protein. Iron is then probably transported by an ABC transporter specific for Fe²⁺. This inner membrane transporter has not yet been identified. Reproduced with permission from Elsevier from Schalk, I.J. (2008) Metal trafficking via siderophores in Gram-negative bacteria: specificities and characteristics of the pyoverdine pathway.* J. Inorg. Biochem., *102, 1159–1169*

neoformans, responsible for cryptococcosis, a life-threatening meningoencephalitis (Caza and Kronstad, 2013). A brief discussion is provided here of the current understanding of the strategies used by fungal pathogens to acquire iron. A more detailed account of fungal iron uptake will be presented in Chapter 5.

Fungi produce a large number of structurally very different siderophores (Winkelmann, 2007) and indeed, historically the first siderophore to be isolated was ferrichrome from culture filtrates of the smut fungus *Ustilago sphaerogena* (Neilands, 1952). Siderophore-mediated iron acquisition has been shown to be essential for virulence, and has been particularly well studied in *Aspergillus* species (Haas, 2012; Moore, 2013). *A. fumigatus* produces four hydroxamate siderophores (Figure 4.17) all based on N5-hydroxy-N5-acyl-L-ornithine. Ferricrocin and hydroxyferricrocin are intracellular siderophores found respectively in hyphae during filamentous growth, and within the conidial spores that are the infectious particles, (Schrettl *et al.*, 2007; Wallner *et al.*, 2009). They are believed to function in iron storage (Schrettl *et al.*, 2007). In contrast, fusarinine C (FSC) and its N-acetylated derivative, *N′*, *N″*, *N‴*-triacetylfusarinine C (TAFC) are secreted (Haas, 2012) in response to iron deprivation. They function in extracellular binding and, like most fungi, they use transporters of the major facilitator superfamily rather than ABC transporters for siderophore inter-nalisation (Haas *et al.*, 2003, 2008), and the uptake of ferri-TAFC is mediated by MirB, whereas the

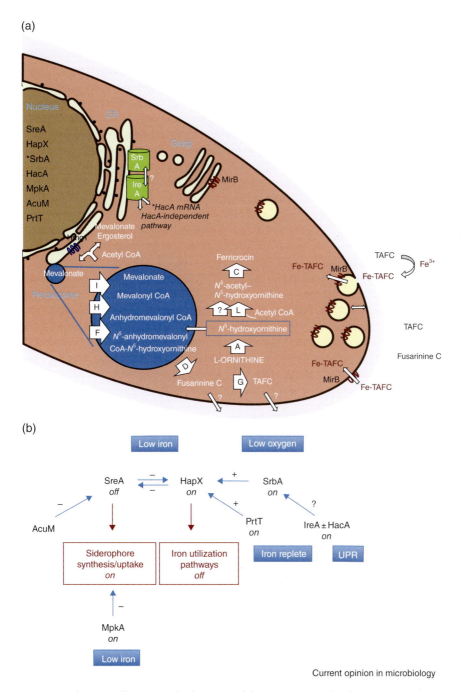

Figure 4.17 *(a) Schematic illustrating the location of the proteins involved in siderophore biosynthesis and uptake in hyphae of* A. fumigatus. *Siderophore biosynthetic enzymes are denoted by letters inside block white arrows. Transcription factors implicated in siderophore regulation are listed in the nucleus. *indicates the active form of the molecule and '?' indicates interactions that have not been experimentally confirmed. (b) Transcription factors shown to be involved in regulating siderophore-mediated iron acquisition in* A. fumigatus. *'+' and '−' indicate activation and repression, respectively. Effects on ergosterol biosynthesis not indicated in this figure but are described in the text. Reproduced with permission from Elsevier from Moore, M.M. (2013) The crucial role of iron uptake in* Aspergillus fumigatus *virulence. Curr. Opin. Microbiol.,* **16**, *692–699*

specific membrane transporter of ferri-FSC is not known. After internalisation, the intracellular release of iron from ferri-TAFC is facilitated by hydrolysis of the trilactone ring of TAFC by EstB (Kragl *et al.*, 2007). The enzymes involved in siderophore biosynthesis and uptake are compartmentalised in peroxisomes and endosome-like vesicles, respectively. Gene and protein expression studies have revealed a coordinated regulation of siderophore and sterol metabolism linked to the common precursor mevalonate. Iron starvation causes extensive transcriptional remodelling involving two central transcription factors in *A. fumigatus*, which are interconnected in a negative transcriptional feedback loop. During iron sufficiency SreA represses iron uptake, including reductive iron assimilation and siderophore-mediated iron uptake, whereas in iron starvation HapX represses iron-consuming pathways, including haem biosynthesis and respiration, and activates the synthesis of siderophores, the latter partly by ensuring supply of the precursor, ornithine (Haas, 2012).

The pathogenic yeasts *C. albicans* and *C. neoformans* do not produce siderophores, but can scavenge xenosiderophores from other microbes, using specific siderophore receptors in their outer membranes (Heymann *et al.*, 2002; Tongen *et al.*, 2007).

The strategy of secreting haemolysins to lyse red blood cells in order to access sources of host haem, which is employed by a number of pathogenic bacteria, is also used by fungi. Both, *A. fumigatus* and *C. albicans* have haemolytic activity, although *C. neoformans* reportedly does not (Yokoto *et al.*, 1977; Manns *et al.*, 1994). *C. albicans* has several specific receptors for haem/haemoglobin, two of which – Rbt5 and Rtb51 – are extracellular, glycosylphosphatidylinositol-anchored proteins which have a CFEM domain composed of eight Cys residues of conserved spacing which are found in a number of fungal membrane proteins (Kulkarni *et al.*, 2003) and may be involved in haem binding (Weissman and Kornitzer, 2004). Haem degradation appears to involve the haem oxygenase CaHmx1 (Pendrak *et al.*, 2004; Weissman *et al.*, 2008), since CaHmx1 is required for full virulence in a mouse model of disseminated candidiasis (Navarathna and Roberts, 2010). *C. neoformans* can also grow on haemoglobin and haem as sole iron source (Jung and Kronstad, 2008), and a first candidate fungal haemophore, the mannoprotein Cig1, has been recently identified in *C. neoformans* (Cadieux *et al.*, 2013).

Transferrin and lactoferrin were found to have an inhibitory effect on the growth of all three of the pathogenic fungi discussed here (Caza and Kronstad, 2013). However, it seems that both *C. albicans* and *C. neoformans* can take up transferrin iron using a high-affinity uptake system which includes an iron permease and a reductase (Ramanan and Wang, 2000; Jung *et al.*, 2008). Recent studies have shown that *C. neoformans* overcomes iron limitation by multiple mechanisms targeting transferrin and haem, and mediated by an interconnected set of transcription factors which integrate iron homeostasis with a myriad of other functions including pH-sensing, nutrient and stress signalling pathways, virulence factor elaboration, and cell wall biogenesis (Kronstad *et al.*, 2013).

As we discuss in greater detail in Chapter 5 for the yeast *S. cerevisiae*, fungi have high-affinity systems for iron uptake that consist of reductases, a multicopper oxidase and a ferric iron permease. All three fungi discussed above have this system, in which the reduction of ferric iron by the reductase supplies ferrous iron to the oxidase/permease complex (reviewed in Caza and Kronstad, 2013).

References

Allred, B.E., Correnti, C., Clifton, M.C., Strong, R.K. and Raymond, K.N. (2013) Siderocalin outwits the coordination chemistry of vibriobactin, a siderophore of *Vibrio cholerae*. *ACS Chem. Biol.*, **8**, 1882–1887.

Alontaga, A.Y., Rodriguez, J.C., Schönbrunn, E., *et al.* (2009) Structural characterization of the hemophore HasAp from *Pseudomonas aeruginosa*: NMR spectroscopy reveals protein–protein interactions between Holo-HasAp and hemoglobin. *Biochemistry*, **48**, 96–109.

Andrade, M.A., Ciccarelli, F.D., Perez-Iratxeta, C. and Bork, P. (2002) NEAT: a domain duplicated in genes near the components of a putative Fe^{3+} siderophore transporter from Gram-positive pathogenic bacteria. *Genome Biol.* **3**, research0047;1- research0047;5.

Archibald, F. (1983) *Lactobacillus plantarum*, an organism not requiring iron. *FEMS Microbiol. Lett.*, **19**, 29–32.

Arnoux, P., Haser, R., Izadi, N., *et al.* (1999) The crystal structure of HasA, a hemophore secreted by *Serratia marcescens*. *Nat. Struct. Biol.*, **6**, 516–520.

Arnoux, P., Haser, R., Izadi-Pruneyre, N., *et al.* (2000) Functional aspects of the heme-bound hemophore HasA by structural analysis of various crystal forms. *Proteins*, **41**, 202–210.

Bach, S., de Almeida, A. and Carniel, E. (2000) The Yersinia high-pathogenicity island is present in different members of the family Enterobacteriaceae. *FEMS Microbiol. Lett.*, **183**, 289–294.

Banin, E., Vasil, M.L. and Greenberg, E.P. (2005) Iron and *Pseudomonas aeruginosa* biofilm formation. *Proc. Natl Acad. Sci. USA*, **102**, 11076–11081.

Beasley, F.C., Vinés, E.D., Grigg, J.C., *et al.* (2009) Characterization of staphyloferrin A biosynthetic and transport mutants in *Staphylococcus aureus*. *Mol. Microbiol.*, **72**, 947–963.

Bender, K.S., Yen, H.C., Hemme, C.L., *et al.* (2007) Analysis of a ferric uptake regulator (Fur) mutant of *Desulfovibrio vulgaris* Hildenborough. *Appl. Environ. Microbiol.*, **73**, 5389–5400.

Benevides-Matos, N. and Biville, F. (2010) The Hem and Has haem uptake systems in *Serratia marcescens*. *Microbiology*, **156**, 1749–1757.

Biville, F., Cwerman, H., Létoffé, S., *et al.* (2004) Haemophore-mediated signalling in *Serratia marcescens*: a new mode of regulation for an extra cytoplasmic function (ECF) sigma factor involved in haem acquisition. *Mol. Microbiol.*, **53**, 1267–1277.

Boulton, I.C., Yost, M.K., Anderson, J.E. and Cornelissen, C.N. (2000) Identification of discrete domains within gonococcal transferrin-binding protein A that are necessary for ligand binding and iron uptake functions. *Infect. Immun.*, **68**, 6988–6996.

Brandel, J., Humbert, N., Elhabiri, M., *et al.* (2012) Pyochelin, a siderophore of *Pseudomonas aeruginosa*: physicochemical characterization of the iron(III), copper(II) and zinc(II) complexes. *Dalton Trans.*, **41**, 2820–2834.

Braun, V. (1997) Surface signaling: novel transcription initiation mechanism starting from the cell surface. *Arch. Microbiol.*, **167**, 325–331.

Britigan, B.E., Rasmussen, G.T. and Cox, C.D. (1997) Augmentation of oxidant injury to human pulmonary epithelial cells by the *Pseudomonas aeruginosa* siderophore pyochelin. *Infect. Immun.*, **65**, 1071–1076.

Brown, G.D., Denning, D.W., Gow, N.A., *et al.* (2012) Hidden killers: human fungal infections. *Sci. Transl. Med.*, **4**, 165rv13.

Bruns, C.M., Nowalk, A.J., Arvai, A.S., *et al.* (1997) Structure of *Haemophilus influenza* Fe(+3)-binding protein reveals convergent evolution within a superfamily. *Nat. Struct. Biol.*, **4**, 919–924.

Buchreisser, C., Prentice, M. and Carniel, E. (1998) The 102-kilobase unstable region of *Yersinia pestis* comprises a high-pathogenicity island linked to a pigmentation segment which undergoes internal rearrangement. *J. Bacteriol.*, **180**, 2321–2329.

Bullen, J.J. and Griffith, E. (eds) (1987) *Iron and Infection. Molecular, Physiological and Clinical Aspects.* John Wiley & Sons, Inc., New York, pp. 325.

Bullen, J.J., Rogers, H.J., Spalding, P.B. and Ward, C.G. (2005) Iron and infection: the heart of the matter. *FEMS Immunol. Med. Microbiol.*, **43**, 325–330.

Cadieux, B., Lian, T., Hu, G., *et al.* (2013) The Mannoprotein Cig1 supports iron acquisition from heme and virulence in the pathogenic fungus *Cryptococcus neoformans*. *J. Infect. Dis.*, **207**, 1339–1347.

Caillet-Saguy, C., Turano, P., Piccioli, M., *et al.* (2008) Deciphering the structural role of histidine 83 for heme binding in hemophore HasA. *J. Biol. Chem.*, **287**, 26932–26943.

Calmettes, C., Alcantara, J., Yu, R.H., Schryvers, A.B. and Moraes, T.F. (2012) The structural basis of transferrin sequestration by transferrin-binding protein B. *Nat. Struct. Mol. Biol.*, **19**, 358–360.

Carniel, E., Guilvout, I. and Prentice, M. (1996) Characterization of a large chromosomal 'high-pathogenicity island' in biotype 1B *Yersinia enterocolitica*. *J. Bacteriol.*, **178**, 6743–6751.

Carpenter, B.M., Whitmire, J.M. and Merrell, D.S. (2009) This is not your mother's repressor: the complex role of fur in pathogenesis. *Infect. Immun.*, **77**, 2590–2601.

Carpenter, C. and Payne, S.M. (2014) Regulation of iron transport systems in Enterobacteriaceae in response to oxygen and iron availability. *J. Inorg. Biochem.*, **133**, 110–117.

Caza, M. and Kronstad, J.W. (2013) Shared and distinct mechanisms of iron acquisition by bacterial and fungal pathogens of humans. *Front. Cell. Infect. Microbiol.*, **3**, 80.

Censini, S., Lange, C., Xiang, Z., *et al.* (1996) cag, a pathogenicity island of *Helicobacter pylori*, encodes type I-specific and disease-associated virulence factors. *Proc. Natl Acad. Sci. USA*, **93**, 14648–14653.

Clifton, M.C., Correnti, C. and Strong, R.K. (2009) Siderocalins: siderophore-binding proteins of the innate immune system. *Biometals*, **22**, 557–564.

Coffman, T.J., Cox, C.D., Edeker, B.L. and Britigan, B.E. (1990). Possible role of bacterial siderophores in inflammation. Iron bound to the *Pseudomonas* siderophore pyochelin can function as a hydroxyl radical catalyst. *J. Clin. Invest.*, **86**, 1030–1037.

Contreras, H., Chim, N., Credali, A. and Goulding, C.W. (2014) Heme uptake in bacterial pathogens. *Curr. Opin. Chem. Biol.*, **19C**, 34–41.

Cope, L.D., Thomas, S.E., Hrkal, Z. and Hansen, E.J. (1998) Binding of heme-hemopexin complexes by soluble HxuA protein allows utilization of this complexed heme by *Haemophilus influenzae*. *Infect. Immun.*, **66**, 4511–4516.

Cornelis, P. and Bodilis, J. (2009). A survey of TonB-dependent receptors in fluorescent pseudomonads. *Environ. Microbiol. Reports*, **1**, 256–262.

Cornelis, P. and Dingemans, J. (2013) *Pseudomonas aeruginosa* adapts its iron uptake strategies in function of the type of infections. *Front. Cell. Infect. Microbiol.*, **3**, 75.

Cornelissen, C.N. and Sparling, P.F. (1994) Iron piracy: acquisition of transferrin-bound iron by bacterial pathogens. *Mol. Microbiol.*, **14**, 843–850.

Correnti, C. and Strong, R.K. (2012) Mammalian siderophores, siderophore-binding lipocalins, and the labile iron pool. *J. Biol. Chem.*, **287**, 13524–13531.

Crosa, J.H. (1984) The relationship of plasmid-mediated iron transport and bacterial virulence. *Annu. Rev. Microbiol.*, **38**, 69–89.

Dale, S.E., Sebulsky, M.T. and Heinrichs, D.E. (2004) Involvement of SirABC in iron siderophore import in *Staphylococcus aureus*. *J. Bacteriol.*, **186**, 8356–8362.

David, M.Z. and Daum, R.S. (2010) Community-associated methicillin-resistant *Staphylococcus aureus*: epidemiology and clinical consequences of an emerging epidemic. *Clin. Microbiol. Rev.*, **23**, 616–687.

Dawson, R.J. and Locher, K.P. (2006) Structure of a bacterial multidrug ABC transporter. *Nature*, **443**, 180–185.

Dobrindt, U., Hochhut, B., Hentschel, U. and Hacker, J. (2004) Genomic islands in pathogenic and environmental microorganisms. *Nat. Rev. Microbiol.*, **2**, 414–424.

Draper, R.C., Martin, L.W., Beare, P.A. and Lamont, I.L. (2011) Differential proteolysis of sigma regulators controls cell-surface signalling in *Pseudomonas aeruginosa*. *Mol. Microbiol.*, **82**, 1444–1453.

Dumas, Z., Ross-Gillespie, A. and Kümmerli R. (2013). Switching between apparently redundant iron-uptake mechanisms benefits bacteria in changeable environments. *Proc. R. Soc. B*, **280**, 20131055.

Fetherston, J.D., Mier, I. Jr, Truszczynska, H. and Perry, R.D. (2012) The Yfe and Feo transporters are involved in microaerobic growth and virulence of *Yersinia pestis* in bubonic plague. *Infect. Immun.*, **80**, 3880–3891.

Fillat, M.F. (2014) The FUR (ferric uptake regulator) superfamily: diversity and versatility of key transcriptional regulators. *Arch. Biochem. Biophys.*, **546**, 41–52.

Fischer, W., Puls, J., Buhrdorf, R., *et al.* (2001) Systematic mutagenesis of the *Helicobacter pylori* cag pathogenicity island: essential genes for CagA translocation in host cells and induction of interleukin-8. *Mol. Microbiol.*, **42**, 1337–1348.

Fisher, C.R., Davies, N.M., Wyckoff, E.E., *et al.* (2009) Genetics and virulence association of the *Shigella flexneri* sit iron transport system. *Infect. Immun.*, **77**, 1992–1999.

Fournier, C., Smith, A. and Delepelaire, P. (2011) Haem release from haemopexin by HxuA allows *Haemophilus influenzae* to escape host nutritional immunity. *Mol. Microbiol.*, **80**, 133–148.

Fukushima, T., Sia, A.K., Allred, B.E., *et al.* (2012) *Bacillus cereus* iron uptake protein fishes out an unstable ferric citrate trimer. *Proc. Natl Acad. Sci. USA*, **109**, 16829–16834.

Fukushima, T., Allred, B.E., Sia, A.K., *et al.* (2013) Gram-positive siderophore-shuttle with iron-exchange from Fe-siderophore to apo-siderophore by *Bacillus cereus* YxeB. *Proc. Natl Acad. Sci. USA*, **110**, 13821–13826.

Gal-Mor, O. and Finlay, B.B. (2006) Pathogenicity islands: a molecular toolbox for bacterial virulence. *Cell. Microbiol.*, **8**, 1707–1719.

Gancz, H., Censini, S. and Merrell, D.S. (2006) Iron and pH homeostasis intersect at the level of Fur regulation in the gastric pathogen *Helicobacter pylori*. *Infect. Immun.*, **74**, 602–614.

Ganz, T. (2006) Hepcidin – a peptide hormone at the interface of innate immunity and iron metabolism. *Curr. Top. Microbiol. Immunol.*, **306**, 183–198.

Ghigo, J.M., Létoffé, S. and Wandersman, C. (1997) A new type of hemophore-dependent heme acquisition system of *Serratia marcescens* reconstituted in *Escherichia coli*. *J. Bacteriol.*, **179**, 3572–3579.

Gill, S.R., Fouts, D.E., Archer, G.L., *et al.* (2005) Insights on evolution of virulence and resistance from the complete genome analysis of an early methicillin-resistant *Staphylococcus aureus* strain and a biofilm-producing methicillin-resistant *Staphylococcus epidermidis* strain. *J. Bacteriol.*, **187**, 2426–2438.

Gray-Owen, S.D. and Schryvers, A.B. (1996) Bacterial transferrin and lactoferrin receptors. *Trends Microbiol.*, **4**, 185–191.

Grigg, J.C., Ukpabi, G., Gaudin, C.F. and Murphy, M.E. (2010) Structural biology of heme binding in the *Staphylococcus aureus* Isd system. *J. Inorg. Biochem.*, **104**, 341–348.

Guy, L. (2006) Identification and characterization of pathogenicity and other genomic islands using base composition analyses. *Future Microbiol.*, **1**, 309–316.

Haas, H. (2012) Iron – A key nexus in the virulence of *Aspergillus fumigatus*. *Front. Microbiol.*, **3**, 28.

Haas, H., Schoeser, M., Lesuisse, E., *et al.* (2003) Characterization of the *Aspergillus nidulans* transporters for the siderophores enterobactin and triacetylfusarinine C. *Biochem. J.*, **371**, 505–513.

Haas, H., Eisendle, M. and Turgeon, B.G. (2008) Siderophores in fungal physiology and virulence. *Annu. Rev. Phytopathol.*, **46**, 149–187.

Hacker, J. and Kaper, J.B. (1999) in *Pathogenicity Islands and Other Mobile Virulence Elements* (eds J.B. Kaper and J. Hacker), American Society of Microbiology, Washington, DC, pp. 1–11.

Hacker, J. and Kaper, J.B. (2000) Pathogenicity islands and the evolution of microbes. *Annu. Rev. Microbiol.*, **54**, 641–679.

Hacker, J., Bender, L., Ott, M., *et al.* (1990) Deletions of chromosomal regions coding for fimbriae and hemolysins occur *in vitro* and *in vivo* in various extraintestinal *Escherichia coli* isolates. *Microb. Pathog.*, **8**, 213–225.

Halbrooks, P.J., He, Q.Y., Briggs, S.K., *et al.* (2003) Investigation of the mechanism of iron release from the C-lobe of human serum transferrin: mutational analysis of the role of a pH sensitive triad. *Biochemistry*, **42**, 3701–3707.

Haley, K.P. and Skaar, E.P. (2012) A battle for iron: host sequestration and *Staphylococcus aureus* acquisition. *Microbes Infect.*, **14**, 217–227.

Hall, H.K. and Foster, J.W. (1996) The role of fur in the acid tolerance response of *Salmonella typhimurium* is physiologically and genetically separable from its role in iron acquisition. *J. Bacteriol.*, **178**, 5683–5691.

Heesemann, J., Hantke, K., Vocke, T., *et al.* (1993) Virulence of *Yersinia enterocolitica* is closely associated with siderophore production, expression of an iron-repressible outer membrane polypeptide of 65,000 Da and pesticin sensitivity. *Mol. Microbiol.*, **8**, 397–408.

Heymann, P., Gerads, M., Schaller, M., *et al.* (2002) The siderophore iron transporter of *Candida albicans* (Sit1p/Arn1p) mediates uptake of ferrichrome-type siderophores and is required for epithelial invasion. *Infect. Immun.*, **70**, 5246–5255.

Hoegy, F., Celia, H., Mislin, G.L., *et al.* (2005) Binding of iron-free siderophore, a common feature of siderophore outer membrane transporters of *Escherichia coli* and *Pseudomonas aeruginosa*. *J. Biol. Chem.*, **280**, 20222–20230.

Hunter, R.C,, Klepac-Ceraj, V., Lorenzi, M.M., *et al.* (2012) Phenazine content in the cystic fibrosis respiratory tract negatively correlates with lung function and microbial complexity. *Am. J. Respir. Cell. Mol. Biol.*, **47**, 738–745.

Hunter, R.C., Asfour, F., Dingemans, J., *et al.* (2013) Ferrous iron is a significant component of bioavailable iron in cystic fibrosis airways. *MBio.*, **4**, pii: e00557-13.

Janakiraman, A. and Slauch, J.M. (2000) The putative iron transport system SitABCD encoded on SPI1 is required for full virulence of *Salmonella typhimurium*. *Mol. Microbiol.*, **35**, 1146–1155.

Jost-Daijev, M.K. and Cornelissen, C.N. (2004) Determination of surface-exposed, functional domains of gonococcal transferrin-binding protein A. *Infect. Immun.*, **72**, 1775–1785.

Juhas, M. (2015) Horizontal gene transfer in human pathogens. *Crit. Rev. Microbiol.*, **41**, 101–108.

Juhas, M., van der Meer, J.R., Gaillard, M., *et al.* (2009) Genomic islands: tools of bacterial horizontal gene transfer and evolution. *FEMS Microbiol. Rev.*, **33**, 376–393.

Jung, W.H. and Kronstad, J.W. (2008) Iron and fungal pathogenesis: a case study with *Cryptococcus neoformans*. *Cell Microbiol.*, **10**, 277–284.

Jung, W.H., Sham, A., Lian, T., *et al.* (2008) Iron source preference and regulation of iron uptake in *Cryptococcus neoformans*. *PLoS Pathog.*, **4**, e45.

Koster, M., van de Vossenberg, J., Leong, J. and Weisbeek, P.J. (1993) Identification and characterization of the pupB gene encoding an inducible ferric-pseudobactin receptor of *Pseudomonas putida* WCS358. *Mol. Microbiol.*, **8**, 591–601.

Koster, M., van Klompenburg, W., Bitter, W., Leong, J. and Weisbeek, P. (1994) Role for the outer membrane ferric siderophore receptor PupB in signal transduction across the bacterial cell envelope. *EMBO J.*, **13**, 2805–2813.

Kragl, C., Schrettl, M., Abt, B., *et al.* (2007) EstB-mediated hydrolysis of the siderophore triacetylfusarinine C optimizes iron uptake of *Aspergillus fumigatus*. *Eukaryot. Cell*, **6**, 1278–1285.

Krieg, S., Huché, F., Diederichs, K., *et al.* (2009) Heme uptake across the outer membrane as revealed by crystal structures of the receptor–hemophore complex. *Proc. Natl Acad. Sci. USA*, **106,** 1045–1050.

Kronstad, J.W., Hu, G. and Jung, W.H. (2013) An encapsulation of iron homeostasis and virulence in *Cryptococcus neoformans*. *Trends Microbiol.*, **21**, 457–465.

Kuehnert, M.J., Kruszon-Moran, D., Hill, H.A., *et al.* (2006) Prevalence of *Staphylococcus aureus* nasal colonization in the United States, 2001–2002. *J. Infect. Dis.*, **193**, 172–179.

Kulkarni, R.D., Kelkar, H.S. and Dean, R.A. (2003) An eight-cysteine-containing CFEM domain unique to a group of fungal membrane proteins. *Trends Biochem. Sci.*, **28**, 118–121.

Kumar, R., Lovell, S., Matsumura, H., *et al.* (2013) The hemophore HasA from *Yersinia pestis* (HasAyp) coordinates hemin with a single residue, Tyr75, and with minimal conformational change. *Biochemistry*, **52**, 2705–2707.

Kumar, R., Matsumura, H., Lovell, S., *et al.* (2014) Replacing the axial ligand tyrosine 75 or its hydrogen bond partner histidine 83 minimally affects hemin acquisition by the Hemophore HasAp from *Pseudomonas aeruginosa*. *Biochemistry*, **53**, 2112–2125.

Lawrence, J.G. (2005) Horizontal and vertical gene transfer: the life history of pathogens. *Contrib. Microbiol.*, **12**, 255–271.

Li, N., Zhang, C., Li B, *et al.* (2012) Unique iron coordination in iron-chelating molecule vibriobactin helps *Vibrio cholerae* evade mammalian siderocalin-mediated immune response. *J. Biol. Chem.*, **287**, 8912–8919.

Lopez, C.S. and Crosa, J.H. (2007) Characterization of ferric-anguibactin transport in *Vibrio anguillarum*. *Biometals*, **20**, 393–403.

Luo, S., Skerka, C., Kurzai, O. and Zipfel, P.F. (2013) Complement and innate immune evasion strategies of the human pathogenic fungus *Candida albicans*. *Mol. Immunol.*, **56**, 161–169.

Manns, J.M., Mosser, D.M. and Buckley, H.R. (1994) Production of a hemolytic factor by *Candida albicans*. *Infect. Immun.*, **62**, 5154–5156.

Matsui, T., Nambu, S., Ono, Y., *et al.* (2013) Heme degradation by *Staphylococcus aureus* IsdG and IsdI liberates formaldehyde rather than carbon monoxide. *Biochemistry*, **52**, 3025–3027.

Mattle, D., Zeltina, A., Woo, J.S., Goetz, B.A. and Locher, K.P. (2010) Two stacked heme molecules in the binding pocket of the periplasmic heme-binding protein HmuT from *Yersinia pestis*. *J. Mol. Biol.*, **404**, 220–231.

Mazmanian, S.K., Ton-That, H., Su, K. and Schneewind, O. (2002) An iron-regulated sortase anchors a class of surface protein during *Staphylococcus aureus* pathogenesis. *Proc. Natl Acad. Sci. USA*, **99**, 2293–2298.

Mazmanian, S.K., Skaar, E.P., Gaspar, A.H., *et al.* (2003) Passage of heme-iron across the envelope of *Staphylococcus aureus*. *Science*, **299**, 906–909.

Meyer, J.M. (2000) Pyoverdines: pigments, siderophores and potential taxonomic markers of fluorescent *Pseudomonas* species. *Arch. Microbiol.*, **174**, 135–142.

Meyer, J.M., Gruffaz, C., Raharinosy, V., *et al.* (2008) Siderotyping of fluorescent *Pseudomonas*: molecular mass determination by mass spectrometry as a powerful pyoverdine siderotyping method. *Biometals*, **21**, 259–271.

Mietzner, T.A., Tencza, S.B., Adhikari, P. *et al.* (1998) Fe(III) periplasm-to-cytosol transporters of gram-negative pathogens. *Curr. Topics Microbiol. Immunol.*, **228**, 113–135.

Moore, M.M. (2013) The crucial role of iron uptake in *Aspergillus fumigatus* virulence. *Curr. Opin. Microbiol.*, **16**, 692–699.

Morton, D.J., Seale, T.W., Madore, L.L., *et al.* (2007) The haem-haemopexin utilization gene cluster (hxuCBA) as a virulence factor of *Haemophilus influenzae*. *Microbiology*, **153**, 215–224.

Muryoi, N., Tiedemann, M.T., Pluym, M., *et al.* (2008) Demonstration of the iron-regulated surface determinant (Isd) heme transfer pathway in *Staphylococcus aureus*. *J. Biol. Chem.*, **283**, 28125–28136.

Nambu, S., Matsui, T., Goulding, C.W., *et al.* (2013) A new way to degrade heme: the *Mycobacterium tuberculosis* enzyme MhuD catalyzes heme degradation without generating CO. *J. Biol. Chem.*, **288**, 10101–10109.

Navarathna, D.H. and Roberts, D.D. (2010) *Candida albicans* heme oxygenase and its product CO contribute to pathogenesis of candidemia and alter systemic chemokine and cytokine expression. *Free Radic. Biol. Med.*, **49**, 1561–1573.

Neilands, J.B. (1952) A crystalline organo-iron pigment from a rust fungus (*Ustilago sphaerogena*). *J. Am. Chem. Soc.*, **74**, 4846–4847.

Noinaj, N. and Buchanan, S.K. (2014) Structural insights into the transport of small molecules across membranes. *Curr. Opin. Struct. Biol.*, **27C**, 8–15.

Noinaj, N., Easley, N.C., Oke, M., *et al.* (2012a) Structural basis for iron piracy by pathogenic *Neisseria*. *Nature*, **483**, 53–58.

Noinaj, N., Buchanan, S.K. and Cornelissen, C.N. (2012b) The transferrin-iron import system from pathogenic *Neisseria* species. *Mol. Microbiol.*, **86**, 246–257.

Noinaj, N., Cornelissen, C.N. and Buchanan, S.K. (2013) Structural insight into the lactoferrin receptors from pathogenic *Neisseria*. *J. Struct. Biol.*, **184**, 83–92.

Noto, J.M. and Cornelissen, C.N. (2008) Identification of TbpA residues required for transferrin-iron utilization by *Neisseria gonorrhoeae*. *Infect. Immun.*, **76**, 1960–1969.

Novick, R.P. (2003) Mobile genetic elements and bacterial toxinoses: the superantigen encoding pathogenicity islands of *Staphylococcus aureus*. *Plasmid*, **49**, 93–105.

Novick, R.P. and Subedi, A. (2007) The SaPIs: mobile pathogenicity islands of *Staphylococcus*. *Chem. Immunol. Allergy*, **93**, 42–57.

Oakhill, J.S., Sutton, B.J., Gorringe, A.R. and Evans, R.W. (2005) Homology modelling of transferrin-binding protein A from *Neisseria meningitidis*. *Protein Eng. Des. Sel.*, **18**, 221–228.

Oelschläger, T.A., Zhang, D., Schubert, S., *et al.* (2003) The high-pathogenicity island is absent in human pathogens of *Salmonella enterica* subspecies I but present in isolates of subspecies III and VI. *J. Bacteriol.*, **185**, 1107–1111.

Oglesby, A.G., Farrow, J.M., III, Lee, J.H., *et al.* (2008) The influence of iron on *Pseudomonas aeruginosa* physiology: a regulatory link between iron and quorum sensing. *J. Biol. Chem.*, **283**, 15558–15567.

Oldham, M.L., Khare, D., Quiocho, F.A., Davidson, A.L. and Chen, J. (2007) Crystal structure of a catalytic intermediate of the maltose transporter. *Nature*, **450**, 515–521.

Olinger, J., Song, K.B., Antelmann, H, *et al.* (2006) Role of the Fur regulon in iron transport in *Bacillus subtilis*. *J. Bacteriol.*, **188**, 3664–3673.

Olsson, C., Olofsson, T., Ahrné, S. and Molin, G. (2003) The *Yersinia* HPI is present in *Serratia liquefaciens* isolated from meat. *Lett. Appl. Microbiol.*, **37**, 275–280.

Pallen, M.J., Beatson, S.A. and Bailey, C.M. (2005) Bioinformatics analysis of the locus for enterocyte effacement provides novel insights into type-III secretion. *BMC Microbiol.*, **5**, 9.

Pendrak, M.I., Chao, M.P., Yan, S.S. and Roberts, D.D. (2004) Heme oxygenase in *Candida albicans* is regulated by hemoglobin and is necessary for metabolism of exogenous heme and hemoglobin to alpha-biliverdin. *J. Biol. Chem.*, **279**, 3426–3433.

Poole, K., Neshat, S., Krebes, K. and Heinrichs, D.E. (1993) Cloning and nucleotide sequence analysis of the ferripyoverdine receptor gene fpvA of *Pseudomonas aeruginosa*. *J. Bacteriol.*, **175**, 4597–4604.

Posey, J.E. and Gherardini, F.C. (2000) Lack of a role for iron in the Lyme disease pathogen. *Science*, **288**, 1651–1653.

Pradel, E. and Locht, C. (2001) Expression of the putative siderophore receptor gene bfrZ is controlled by the extracytoplasmic-function sigma factor BupI in *Bordetella bronchiseptica*. *J. Bacteriol.*, **183**, 2910–2917.

Pressler, U., Staudenmaier, H., Zimmermann, L. and Braun, V. (1988) Genetics of the iron dicitrate transport system of *Escherichia coli*. *J. Bacteriol.*, **170**, 2716–2724.

Purdy, G.E. and Payne, S.M. (2001) The SHI-3 iron transport island of *Shigella boydii* 0-1392 carries the genes for aerobactin synthesis and transport. *J. Bacteriol.*, **183**, 4176–4182.

Quiocho, F.A. and Ledvina, P.S. (1996) Atomic structure and specificity of bacterial periplasmic receptors for active transport and chemotaxis: variation of common themes. *Mol. Microbiol.*, **20**, 17–25.

Rakin, A., Urbitsch, P. and Heesemann, J. (1995) Evidence for two evolutionary lineages of highly pathogenic *Yersinia* species. *J. Bacteriol.*, **177**, 2292–2298.

Rakin, A., Schneider, L. and Podladchikova, O. (2012) Hunger for iron: the alternative siderophore iron scavenging systems in highly virulent *Yersinia*. *Front. Cell. Infect. Microbiol.* **2**, 151.

Ramanan, N. and Wang, Y. (2000) A high-affinity iron permease essential for *Candida albicans* virulence. *Science*, **288**, 1062–1064.

Ratliff, M., Zhu, W., Deshmukh, R., Wilks, A. and Stojiljkovic I. (2001) Homologues of neisserial heme oxygenase in gram-negative bacteria: degradation of heme by the product of the pigA gene of *Pseudomonas aeruginosa*. *J. Bacteriol.*, **183**, 6394–6403.

Ravel, J. and Cornelis, P. (2003) Genomics of pyoverdine-mediated iron uptake in pseudomonads. *Trends Microbiol.*, **11**, 195–200.

Reniere, M.L., Ukpabi, G.N., Harry, S.R., *et al.* (2010) The IsdG-family of haem oxygenases degrades haem to a novel chromophore. *Mol. Microbiol.*, **75**, 1529–1538.

Rossi, M.S., Paquelin, A., Ghigo, J.M. and Wandersman, C. (2003) Haemophore-mediated signal transduction across the bacterial cell envelope in *Serratia marcescens*: the inducer and the transported substrate are different molecules. *Mol. Microbiol.*, **48**, 1467–1480.

Runyen-Janecky, L.J., Reeves, S.A., Gonzales, E.G. and Payne, S.M. (2003) Contribution of the *Shigella flexneri* Sit, Iuc, and Feo iron acquisition systems to iron acquisition in vitro and in cultured cells. *Infect. Immun.*, **71**, 1919–1928.

Saha, R., Saha, N., Donofrio, R.S. and Bestervelt, L.L. (2012) Microbial siderophores: a mini review. *J. Basic Microbiol.*, **53**, 303–317.

Schalk, I.J. (2008) Metal trafficking via siderophores in Gram-negative bacteria: specificities and characteristics of the pyoverdine pathway. *J. Inorg. Biochem.*, **102**, 1159–1169.

Schalk, I.J., Kyslik, P., Prome, D., *et al.* (1999) Copurification of the FpvA ferric pyoverdin receptor of *Pseudomonas aeruginosa* with its iron-free ligand: implications for siderophore-mediated iron transport. *Biochemistry*, **38**, 9357–9365.

Schalk, I.J., Yue, W.W. and Buchanan, S.K. (2004) Recognition of iron-free siderophores by TonB-dependent iron transporters. *Mol. Microbiol.*, **54**, 14–22.

Schubert, S., Cuenca, S., Fischer, D. and Heesemann, J. (2000) High-pathogenicity island of *Yersinia pestis* in enterobacteriaceae isolated from blood cultures and urine samples: prevalence and functional expression. *J. Infect. Dis.*, **182**, 1268–1271.

Schubert, S., Dufke, S., Sorsa, J. and Heesemann, J. (2004) A novel integrative and conjugative element (ICE) of *Escherichia coli*: the putative progenitor of the *Yersinia* high pathogenicity island. *Mol. Microbiol.*, **51**, 837–848.

Schrettl, M., Bignell, E., Kragl, C., *et al.* (2007) Distinct roles for intra- and extracellular siderophores during *Aspergillus fumigatus* infection. *PLoS Pathog.*, **3**, 1195–1207.

Stintzi, A., Barnes, C., Xu, J. and Raymond, K.N. (2000) Microbial iron transport via a siderophore shuttle: a membrane ion transport paradigm. *Proc. Natl Acad. Sci. USA*, **97**, 10691–10696.

Sievert, D.M., Ricks, P., Edwards, J.R., *et al.* (2013) Antimicrobial-resistant pathogens associated with healthcare-associated infections: summary of data reported to the National Healthcare Safety Network at the Centers for Disease Control and Prevention, 2009–2010. *Infect. Control Hosp. Epidemiol.*, **34**, 1–14.

Singh, P.K., Parsek, M.R., Greenberg, E.P. and Welsh, M.J. (2002) A component of innate immunity prevents bacterial biofilm development. *Nature*, **417**, 552–555.

Soares, S.C., Abreu, V.A., Ramos, R.T., *et al.* (2012) PIPS: pathogenicity island prediction software. *PLoS One*, **7**, e30848.

Speciali, C.D., Dale, S.E., Henderson, J.A., Vinés, E.D. and Heinrichs, D.E. (2006) Requirement of *Staphylococcus aureus* ATP-binding cassette-ATPase FhuC for iron restricted growth and evidence that it functions with more than one iron transporter. *J. Bacteriol.*, **188**, 2048–2055.

Spirig, T., Weiner, E.M. and Clubb, R.T. (2011) Sortase enzymes in Gram-positive bacteria. *Mol. Microbiol.*, **82**, 1044–1059.

Steere, A.N., Byrne, S.L., Chasteen, N.D. and Mason, A.B. (2012) Kinetics of iron release from transferrin bound to the transferrin receptor at endosomal pH. *Biochim. Biophys. Acta*, **1820**, 326–333.

Stintzi, A., Barnes, C., Xu, J. and Raymond, K.N. (2000) Microbial iron transport via a siderophore shuttle: a membrane ion transport paradigm. *Proc. Natl Acad. Sci. USA*, **97**, 10691–10696.

Stojiljkovic. I. and Perkins-Balding, D. (2002) Processing of heme and heme-containing proteins by bacteria. *DNA Cell Biol.*, **21**, 281–295.

Tiedemann, M.T., Heinrichs, D.E. and Stillman, M.J. (2012) Multiprotein heme shuttle pathway in *Staphylococcus aureus*: iron-regulated surface determinant cog-wheel kinetics. *J. Am. Chem. Soc.*, **134**, 16578–16585.

Todd, B. (2006) Beyond MRSA: VISA and VRSA: what will ward off these pathogens in health care facilities? *Am. J. Nurs.*, **106**, 28–30.

Tongen, K.L., Jung, W.H., Sham, A.P., Lian, T. and Kronstad, J.W. (2007) The iron- and cAMP-regulated gene SIT1 influences ferrioxamine B utilization, melanization and cell wall structure in *Cryptococcus neoformans*. *Microbiology*, **153**, 29–41.

Traxler, M.F., Seyedsayamdost, M.R., Clardy, J. and Kolter, R. (2012) Interspecies modulation of bacterial development through iron competition and siderophore piracy. *Mol. Microbiol.*, **86**, 628–644.

Troxell, B. and Hassan, H.M. (2013) Transcriptional regulation by Ferric Uptake Regulator (Fur) in pathogenic bacteria. *Front. Cell. Infect. Microbiol.*, **3**, 59.

Visca, P., Leoni, L., Wilson, M.J. and Lamont, I.L. (2002) Iron transport and regulation, cell signalling and genomics: lessons from *Escherichia coli* and *Pseudomonas*. *Mol. Microbiol.*, **45**, 1177–1190.

Visca, P., Imperi, F. and Lamont, I.L. (2007) Pyoverdine siderophores: from biogenesis to biosignificance. *Trends Microbiol.*, **15**, 22–30.

Wallner, A., Blatzer, M., Schrettl, M., *et al.* (2009) Ferricrocin, a siderophore involved in intra- and trans-cellular iron distribution in *Aspergillus fumigatus*. *Appl. Environ. Microbiol.*, **75**, 4194–4196.

Wandersman, C. (2010) Iron uptake and homeostasis in microorganisms, in *Haem Uptake and Iron Extraction by Bacteria* (eds P. Cornelis and S.C. Andrews), Claister Academic Press, Norfolk.

Wandersman, C. and Stojiljkovic, I. (2000) Bacterial heme sources: the role of heme, hemoprotein receptors and hemophores. *Curr. Opin. Microbiol.*, **3**, 215–220.

Wandersman, C. and Delepelaire, P. (2004) Bacterial iron sources: from siderophores to Hemophores. *Annu. Rev. Microbiol.*, **58**, 611–647.

Wandersman, C. and Delepelaire, P. (2012) Haemophore functions revisited. *Mol. Microbiol.*, **85** (4), 618–631.

Wang, Y. and Newman, D.K. (2008) Redox reactions of phenazine antibiotics with ferric (hydr)oxides and molecular oxygen. *Environ. Sci. Technol.*, **42**, 2380–2386.

Wang, Y., Wilks, J.C., Danhorn, T., *et al.* (2011) Phenazine-1-carboxylic acid promotes bacterial biofilm development via ferrous iron acquisition. *J. Bacteriol.*, **193**, 3606–3617.

Warner, R.J., Williams, P.H., Bindereif, A. and Neilands, J.B. (1981) ColV plasmid-specific aerobactin synthesis by invasive strains of *Escherichia coli*. *Infect. Immun.*, **33**, 723–730.

Weinberg, E.D. (1978) Iron and infection. *Microbiol. Rev.*, **42**, 45–66.

Weinberg, E.D. (1990) Cellular iron metabolism in health and disease. *Drug Metab. Rev.*, **22**, 531–579.

Weinberg, E.D. (2007) Antibiotic properties and applications of lactoferrin. *Curr. Pharm. Des.*, **13**, 801–811.

Weinberg, E.D. (2009) Iron availability and infection. *Biochim. Biophys. Acta*, **1790**, 600–605.

Welch, R.A., Burland, V., Plunkett, G., III, *et al.* (2002) Extensive mosaic structure revealed by the complete genome sequence of uropathogenic *Escherichia coli*. *Proc. Natl Acad. Sci. USA*, **99**, 17020–17024.

Weissman, Z. and Kornitzer, D. (2004) A family of *Candida* cell surface haem-binding proteins involved in haemin and haemoglobin-iron utilization. *Mol. Microbiol.*, **53**, 1209–1220.

Weissman, Z., Shemer, R., Conibear, E. and Kornitzer, D. (2008) An endocytic mechanism for haemoglobin-iron acquisition in *Candida albicans*. *Mol. Microbiol.*, **69**, 201–217.

Wilks, A. and Ikeda-Saito M. (2014) Heme utilization by pathogenic bacteria: Not all pathways lead to biliverdin. *Acc. Chem. Res.*, **47**, 2291–2298.

Williams, P.H. (1979) Novel iron uptake system specified by ColV plasmids: an important component in the virulence of invasive strains of *Escherichia coli*. *Infect. Immun.*, **26**, 925–932.

Williams, P.H. and Warner, P.J. (1980) ColV plasmid-mediated, colicin V-independent iron uptake system of invasive strains of *Escherichia coli*. *Infect. Immun.*, **29**, 411–416.

Winkelmann, G. (2007) Ecology of siderophores with special reference to the fungi. *Biometals*, **20**, 379–392.

Wolff, N., Izadi-Pruneyre, N., Couprie, J., *et al.* (2008) Comparative analysis of structural and dynamic properties of the loaded and unloaded hemophore HasA: functional implications. *J. Mol. Biol.*, **376**, 517–525.

Worlitzsch, D., Tarran, R., Ulrich, M., *et al.* (2002) Effects of reduced mucus oxygen concentration in airway *Pseudomonas* infections of cystic fibrosis patients. *J. Clin. Invest.*, **109**, 317–325.

Woo, J.S., Zeltina, A., Goetz, B.A. and Locher, K.P. (2012) X-ray structure of the *Yersinia pestis* heme transporter HmuUV. *Nat. Struct. Mol. Biol.*, **19**, 1310–1315.

Wooldridge, K.G. and Williams, P. (1993) Iron uptake mechanisms of pathogenic bacteria. *FEMS Microbiol. Rev.*, **12**, 325–348.

Yapar, N. (2014) Epidemiology and risk factors for invasive candidiasis. *Ther. Clin. Risk Manag.*, **10**, 95–105.

Yokoto, K., Shimada, H., Kamaguchi, A. and Sakaguchi, O. (1997) Studies on the toxin of *Aspergillus fumigatus*. VII. Purification and some properties of hemolytic toxin (asp-hemolysin) from culture filtrates and mycelia. *Microbiol. Immunol.*, **21**, 11–22.

Yu, C. and Genco, C.A. (2012) Fur-mediated global regulatory circuits in pathogenic *Neisseria* species. *J. Bacteriol.*, **194**, 6372–6381.

Yue, W.W., Grizot, S. and Buchanan S.K. (2003) Structural evidence for iron-free citrate and ferric citrate binding to the TonB-dependent outer membrane transporter FecA. *J. Mol. Biol.*, **332**, 353–368.

Zaharik, M.L., Gruenheid, S., Perrin, A.J. and Finlay, B.B. (2002) Delivery of dangerous goods: type III secretion in enteric pathogens. *Int. J. Med. Microbiol.*, **291**, 593–603.

Zawadzka, A.M., Kim, Y., Maltseva, N., *et al.* (2009a) Characterization of a *Bacillus subtilis* transporter for petrobactin, an anthrax stealth siderophore. *Proc. Natl Acad. Sci. USA*, **106**, 21854–21859.

Zawadzka, A.M., Abergel, R.J., Nichiporuk, R., Andersen, U.N. and Raymond, K.N. (2009b) Siderophore-mediated iron acquisition systems in *Bacillus cereus*: Identification of receptors for anthrax virulence-associated petrobactin. *Biochemistry*, **48**, 3645–3657.

Zhu, W., Wilks, A. and Stojiljkovic, I. (2000) Degradation of heme in gram-negative bacteria: the product of the hemO gene of *Neisseriae* is a heme oxygenase. *J. Bacteriol.*, **182**, 6783–6790.

5

Iron Uptake by Plants and Fungi

5.1 Iron Uptake by Plants

5.1.1 Introduction

Mineral nutrition in plants is an important factor in both growth and development and, as a consequence, in crop productivity. Since plants are sessile organisms, they need to have appropriate strategies in order to obtain essential metal micronutrients from soils of varying compositions (Marschner, 1995). Like mammals, most plants have a circulatory system which enables them to take up nutrients and water from the soil through their roots and to transport it upwards through the lignified xylem vessels in the xylem sap to the shoots and leaves. The evaporation of water from the leaves (transpiration) creates the force that pulls the xylem sap upwards. Sugars produced by photosynthesis in the leaves are transported in the phloem sap to the roots and other parts of the plant. Iron transport from the soil to the leaves is illustrated schematically in Figure 5.1.

Iron is an essential nutrient for plants, being required for respiration, photosynthesis and a number of other important functions that include nitrogen fixation and DNA synthesis. However, iron is also involved in key enzymes of plant hormone synthesis, such as lipooxygenases and ethylene-forming enzymes. Iron is one of the three nutrients that most commonly limit plant growth but, unlike the other two limiting nutrients – nitrogen and phosphorus – iron deficiency is not easily remedied by fertilisers because the added iron becomes unavailable in the form of insoluble iron hydroxides. Despite the fact that iron represents 4–5% of the total solid mineral composition of soils, it is generally present in soils in a poorly soluble form, and its bioavailability is further decreased at the neutral and alkaline pH values found in semi-arid, calcareous (calcium carbonate rich) soils.[1]

---

[1] These are estimated to represent over one-third of the world's surface area, and to account for 44 million acres of cropland in the United States.

Iron Metabolism – From Molecular Mechanisms to Clinical Consequences, Fourth Edition. Robert Crichton.
© 2016 John Wiley & Sons, Ltd. Published 2016 by John Wiley & Sons, Ltd.

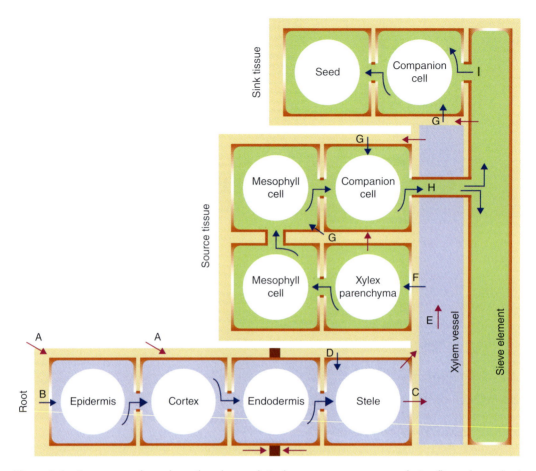

Figure 5.1   *Fe transport from the soil to the seed. Red arrows represent speculative flow of apoplastic Fe; blue arrows indicate Fe movement into symplastic space. After initial diffusion from the soil (A), Fe is imported into epidermal or cortex cells (B). Once in the cytoplasm, Fe moves through symplastic passages to the stele and then is exported into a xylem vessel (C). Apoplastic leakage is blocked by the Casparian strip (shown in brown boxes). Fe precipitates in root apoplast is reabsorbed under Fe-deficiency (D). Fe is transported to the shoot through the transpiration stream (E) and imported into the leaf cytoplasm (F). Fe precipitates in the shoot apoplast are remobilised on demand of sink tissues (G). Fe moves through symplastic passages from a source tissue to a sink tissue via phloem loading (H) and unloading (I). Reproduced with permission from Elsevier from Kim, S.A. and Guerinot, M.L. (2007) Mining iron: iron uptake and transport in plants.* FEBS Lett., **581**, *2273–2280*

Insufficient iron uptake leads to symptoms of iron deficiency, such as interveinal chlorosis in leaves and a reduction of crop yields. Plants need to maintain iron at a concentration of between 10^{-9} and 10^{-4} M to achieve optimal growth (Guerinot and Yi, 1994), yet in well-aerated soils at physiological pH the concentrations of free Fe^{3+} and Fe^{2+} are less than 10^{-15} M, at least six orders of magnitude below that required for optimal growth (Marschner, 1995). One-third of the world's cultivated soils are calcareous and considered to be iron-deficient, which often limits plant growth (Mori, 1999). The poor solubility of iron in the soil and the demand for iron are the primary cause of iron-deficiency chlorosis in plants, and without active mechanisms for extracting iron from the soil most plants would therefore exhibit symptoms of iron deficiency. However, since the solubility of iron in soils will also be affected by the redox potential and pH, it is clear that in flooded or waterlogged acidic soils, where O_2 availability is low, Fe^{2+} can attain high concentrations and become toxic to the plants by producing reactive oxygen free radicals such as $OH^{\bullet}$. These can of course damage cellular components, leading to a loss of cellular integrity and eventually cell death, as is discussed in Chapter 13.

The immobility of plants also results in large differences of iron availability in their immediate environment. On account of iron's poor bioavailability on the one hand, and its potential toxicity on the other hand, plant cells must carefully regulate iron uptake, and as we will see later, iron uptake and homeostasis are tightly regulated at both the transcriptional and posttranscriptional level. These responses are mediated by signals, many of which are still not well characterised but which result in the control of iron uptake by the roots, long-distance iron transport between roots and shoots, in sensing the iron status of the leaves and signalling it to the roots, in subcellular iron distribution, and in detoxifying and buffering iron when it is in excess.

5.1.2 Genome Sequencing

Since the last edition of this book, progress in the genome sequencing of plants has been fulgurant (Bolger *et al.*, 2014). The initial determination of the complete genome of the flowering plant *Arabidopsis thaliana* (Arabidopsis Genome Initiative, 2000) was followed rapidly by the sequence of the rice genome (Yu *et al.*, 2002; Goff *et al.*, 2002), representing the first fully sequenced and annotated crop plant genome to be established, and this has been followed by a steadily increasing number of crop genomes.

The initial approach was to use overlapping bacterial artificial chromosome (BAC) clones, which represent the minimal number of overlaps to cover each arm of the chromosome (Figure 5.2). The BAC sequences were then assembled and arranged to create a very high-quality genome sequence. In the next phase of genome sequencing, whole-genome shotgun strategies (WGS) were used, whereby the genome was randomly fragmented into smaller pieces which were subsequently reassembled, often resulting in a more fragmented genome sequence. Among the genomes sequenced by WGS were two grapevine sequences, one of an inbred line (Jaillon *et al.*, 2007) and the other of a heterozygous genotype used for wine production (Velasco *et al.*, 2007). This opened the way for the identification of genetic factors which affect wine quality, and also enabled the production of genotypes that will withstand the huge amounts of fungicide required prior to harvesting, while maintaining the individuality of the grapevine cultivars (Bolger *et al.*, 2014). Subsequently, the so-called Next Generation Sequencing (NGS) approach was introduced, culminating first in the woodland strawberry genome sequence (Shulaev *et al.*, 2011), and later by genomes such as Chinese cabbage (Wang *et al.*, 2011), potato (Potato Genome Consortium, 2011), banana (d'Hondt *et al.*, 2012), chickpea (Varshney *et al.*, 2013), orange (Xu *et al.*, 2013), pigeonpea (Varshney *et al.*, 2012) and watermelon (Guo *et al.*, 2013), and even the very much larger genome of spruce (Nystedt *et al.*, 2013) (see Figure 5.3 for a timeline putting the genome sequences into chronological order).

NGS has been less successful, however, in sequencing of the Triticeae – large cereal genomes such as barley, rye and wheat – which are important crops for animal feed and human nutrition (Feullet *et al.*, 2012). Not only are their genomes much larger than mammalian or other crop genomes, but 80–90% of the genomes consist of repetitive sequences distributed throughout the genome. Recently, considerable progress has been made in establishing the genomes of the Triticeae using the third method (shown in Figure 5.2), namely chromosome sorting (Mayer *et al.*, 2011). This involves the purification of individual chromosomes, which are subsequently used as

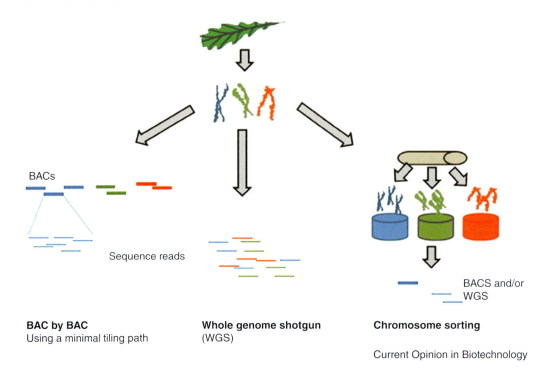

BACs

Sequence reads

BACS and/or
WGS

BAC by BAC
Using a minimal tiling path

Whole genome shotgun
(WGS)

Chromosome sorting

Current Opinion in Biotechnology

Figure 5.2 *DNA sequencing and assembly strategies. For BAC by BAC sequencing (left panel), the genome is split into a minimal tiling path consisting of BACs which are then sequenced. In WGS (middle panel) the whole genome is sheared, sequenced and assembled. A relatively new technique, chromosome sorting (right panel), is used to reduce the genomic complexity. The purified chromosomes can then be used for BAC by BAC or WGS sequencing. Reproduced with permission from Elsevier from Bolger, M.E., Weisshaar, B., Scholz, U., et al. (2014) Plant genome sequencing – applications for crop improvement. Curr. Opin. Biotechnol., 26, 31–37*

a template for shotgun sequencing, NGS or the construction of BAC libraries. Combining this with the systematic exploitation of conserved synteny with the model grasses rice (*Oryza sativa*), sorghum (*Sorghum bicolor*) and *Brachypodium distachyon* has enabled the assembly of 21 766 barley (*Hordeum vulgare*) genes in a putative linear order (Mayer *et al.*, 2011). This approach, pioneered in barley, has since been applied to rye-grass (Pfeifer *et al.*, 2013), wheat (Hernandez *et al.*, 2012), and rye (Martis *et al.*, 2013).

5.1.2.1 *Quantitative Trait Loci*

A quantitative trait locus (QTL) is a stretch of DNA that contains or is linked to the genes that underlie a quantitative trait. As increasing numbers of genome sequences become available they will be used for QTL mapping of desirable traits, even when only a few sequences are available (Bolger *et al.*, 2014), and a few examples are presented here A major QTL for rice grain production was found to be a cytokinin oxidase (Ashikari *et al.*, 2005), and this was later shown to be under the control of the zinc-finger transcription factor DST (Li *et al.*, 2013) which had previously been shown to regulate drought and salinity tolerance in rice (Huang *et al.*, 2009). A few other examples are shown in Figure 5.3 (summarised in Bolger *et al.*, 2014). Genome sequences have helped to

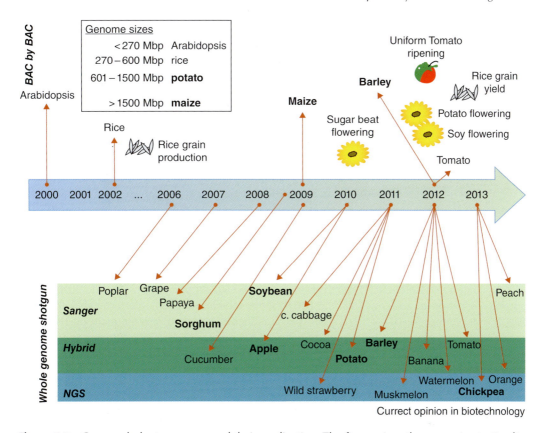

Figure 5.3 *Crop and plant genomes and their application. The figure gives the approximate timeline of when crop genomes were sequenced, along with the underlying techniques and sequencing strategy used (see Figure 5.1). Hybrid strategies which use BAC by BAC and WGS are indicated by the placement of a genome twice. Also note that the distinction between pure NGS and hybrid sequencing is sometimes arbitrary, as many genome projects rely on previously generated Sanger sequences. In addition, some major applications are marked by symbols: Grains for an improvement in grain quality; a flower for flowering time; and a tomato for a tomato ripening trait. Reproduced with permission from Elsevier from Bolger, M.E., Weisshaar, B., Scholz, U., et al. (2014) Plant genome sequencing – applications for crop improvement.* Curr. Opin. Biotechnol., **26**, *31–37*

identify genes involved in crop yield. The determination of the tomato genome (Tomato Genome Consortium, 2012) allowed the identification of an esterase responsible for differences in volatile ester content in different tomato species (Goulet *et al.*, 2012), while a gene which determines chlorophyll distribution in unripe fruits was identified as the uniformly ripening locus in tomato (Powell *et al.*, 2012). The control of flowering and maturation time is an important agronomical trait for adaptation to different photoperiod regimes and geographic latitude. The soybean genome was used to unravel the maturity locus E1, which has a major impact on flowering time (Xia *et al.*, 2012), the potato genome sequence helped in the identification of a transcription factor regulating plant maturity and life cycle (Kloosterman *et al.*, 2013), while the sugar beet genome was used to determine the biology of its flowering time control (Pin *et al.*, 2010). Finally, in a large genomewide association study in rice, flowering time was one of the many identified traits for which a QTL was found (Huang *et al.*, 2012).

With increasing demand to support and accelerate progress in breeding for novel traits, the plant research community faces the need to provide quantitative analyses of plant structure and functions relevant for traits that help plants better adapt to low-input agriculture and resource-limited environments. Developments to overcome the current bottleneck constituted by plant phenotyping, focusing on traits that will assist in selecting genotypes with increased resource use efficiency, have been recently reviewed (Fiorani and Schurr, 2013), and should lead to an even faster identification of many more QTLs. This, in turn, will undoubtedly stimulate breeding to produce crops of improved quality (Bolger *et al.*, 2014).

5.1.3   Iron Acquisition by the Roots of Plants

In the absence of iron stress – that is, in iron-sufficient conditions – all plant roots reduce Fe(III) chelates and transport the resulting Fe(II) through the plasma membrane via low-affinity iron transport systems (Bienfait, 1985; Briat *et al.*, 1995). However, physiological responses to iron deficiency stress, which result in increased iron acquisition, can be classified into two different strategies (Marschner and Römheld, 1994) (Figure 5.4). Nongraminaceous plants, such as *Arabidopsis thaliana*, use the *Strategy I* response, involving the induction of three activities under low iron conditions (Römheld, 1987): (i) H$^+$-ATPases, which extrude protons into the rhizosphere[2] to lower the pH of the soil, thus making Fe(III) more soluble; (ii) inducible ferric chelate reductases (FROs) reduce Fe(III) to Fe(II); (iii) Fe(II) is then transported into the plant by IRT1, the major iron transporter of the plant root. In contrast, the grasses such as rice (Takagi *et al.*, 1984) use the *Strategy II* response, which relies on the chelation of Fe(III) rather than reduction. Phytosiderophores are released into the soil where they chelate Fe(III) and are then internalised in the iron-bound state via specific transporters (Curie *et al.*, 2001).

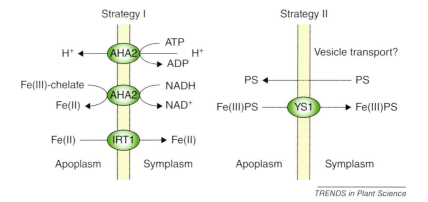

Figure 5.4   *Mechanisms of iron uptake by higher plants. In Strategy I plants (e.g. Arabidopsis, pea and tomato), Fe(III) chelates are reduced before the Fe(II) ion is transported across the plasma membrane. Strategy II plants (e.g. barley, maize and rice) release siderophores capable of solubilising external Fe(III) and then transport the Fe(III) siderophore complex into the cell. AHA2 is a P-type H$^+$-ATPase, FRO2 is the Fe(III) chelate reductase, IRT1 is a Fe(II) transporter, and YS1 is the transporter of the phytosiderophore (PS)–Fe complex. Reproduced with permission from Elsevier from Schmidt, W. (2003) Iron solutions: acquisition strategies and signaling pathways in plants.* Trends Plant Sci., **8**, *188–193*

---

[2] The part of the soil enclosing and influenced by the roots of a plant. It encloses a symbiotic microcosm in which microorganisms co-habitate with the plant roots, each supplying the other with nutrients that the partner cannot manufacture.

5.1.3.1 Non-graminaceous Plants

All non-graminaceous plants (Figure 5.4) use the reduction-based Strategy I to acquire Fe (Kim and Guerinot, 2007; Kobayashi and Nishizawa, 2012). In iron-deficient conditions, protons are released by root plasma membrane proton pumps driven by the hydrolysis of ATP. The low pH increases iron solubility, since for every one unit drop in pH the solubility of Fe(III) increases 1000-fold (Olsen *et al.*, 1981). These P-type ATPases are members of the autoinhibited H$^+$ P-type ATPase (AHA) family (Santi *et al.*, 2005; Santi and Schmidt, 2008). *Arabidopsis* has 11 such AHAs, and an analysis of loss-of-function mutants suggests that rhizosphere acidification in response to Fe deficiency is chiefly mediated by AHA2 (Santi and Schmidt, 2009), whereas AHA1 most likely functions in a housekeeping role and AHA7 is possibly involved in the differentiation of rhizodermic cells. The *CsHA1* gene is induced by iron deficiency and is thought to function in Strategy 1 responses in cucumber (Santi *et al.*, 2005).

Following acidification, Fe^{3+} is reduced to Fe^{2+} at the root surface in a process which has been well documented in several plant species, including *Arabidopsis* (Yi and Guerinot, 1996), pea (Waters *et al.*, 2002), tomato (Li *et al.*, 2004), as well as in the green algae *Chlamydomonas reinhardtii* (Eckhardt and Buckhout, 1998). The *Arabidopsis* gene *FRO2* was the first plant metalloreductase gene to be cloned (Robinson *et al.*, 1999), and was shown to complement the phenotype of an *frd1* (*ferric chelate reductase defective*) *Arabidopsis* mutant, establishing that *FRO2* encodes the root surface ferric chelate reductase. FRO2 was identified based on its sequence similarity to the yeast ferric reductase, FRE1, as well as to the gp91phox subunit of the human NADPH oxidase, which is involved in the production of reactive oxygen species (ROS) to protect against invading pathogens (Robinson *et al.*, 1999; Vignais, 2002). As expected, FRO2 is expressed in the root epidermis and is strongly induced by iron deficiency (Connolly *et al.*, 2003). FRO2 belongs to a superfamily of flavocytochromes which transport electrons across membranes, with intramembrane binding sites for haem (four His residues which are predicted to bind two haems) and cytoplasmic binding sites for nucleotide cofactors (FAD and NADPH) that donate and transfer electrons. The transmembrane topology is different from that obtained by theoretical predictions and appears to contain eight transmembrane helices, four of which build up the highly conserved core of the protein. This core is present in the entire flavocytochrome *b* family. The large water-soluble domain of FRO2, which contains NADPH, FAD and oxidoreductase sequence motifs, was located on the inside of the membrane (Schagerlöf *et al.*, 2006). By analogy with the human phagocytic NADPH oxidase gp91phox and yeast ferric chelate reductases such as FRE1 and FRP1, it is proposed that FRO2 transfers electrons from cytosolic donors to FAD, and then through two consecutive haem groups to single-electron acceptors (Fe^{3+} chelate) on the opposite face of the membrane. However, although the plant flavocytochrome *b* family is well characterised with respect to its function, the molecular mechanism of electron transfer remains uncertain (Lüthje *et al.*, 2013).

The FRO family in *Arabidopsis* contains eight members (Wu *et al.*, 2005; Mukherjee *et al.*, 2006), and although FRO2 seems to be solely responsible for the reduction of ferric chelates in the rhizosphere, the other seven FRO proteins are believed to function as metalloreductases involved in the reduction of iron and copper. Copper concentrations are not reduced in *frd1* mutants, suggesting that FRO2 is not involved in physiological reduction of Cu. Recent studies have shown that FRO4 and FRO5 act redundantly to reduce Cu at the root surface (Bernal *et al.*, 2012). It remains unclear whether FRO4 and FRO5 are involved in Fe homeostasis, although the expression of *FRO5* is induced under iron deficiency (Wu *et al.*, 2005; Mukherjee *et al.*, 2006). *FRO6* is expressed at high levels in leaves (Mukherjee *et al.*, 2006), and overexpression of *FRO6* in leaves can facilitate the reduction of iron in leaves (Li *et al.*, 2011). FRO6 expression is controlled in a light-dependent manner, as the *FRO6* promoter contains several light-responsive elements and etiolated *FRO6-GUS* seedlings exhibit no *FRO6* promoter activity (Feng *et al.*, 2006). Together, these data suggest that FRO6 may function to reduce iron in leaves when light is available, perhaps to enable the assembly of new photosynthetic complexes (Jain *et al.*, 2014).

Significant amounts of iron are required for chloroplast and mitochondrial function as a cofactor for haem and Fe–S proteins. Indeed, the vast majority of iron in leaves is located within the chloroplasts. FRO7 localises to the chloroplast, and chloroplasts prepared from *fro7* loss-of-function mutants have 75% less Fe(III) chelate reductase activity and contain 33% less iron per microgram of chlorophyll than wild-type chloroplasts. This decreased iron content is presumably responsible for the observed defects in photosynthetic electron transport. When germinated in alkaline soil, *fro7* seedlings show severe chlorosis and die without setting seed unless watered with high levels of soluble iron (Jeong *et al.*, 2008). The importance of a reduction-based mechanism for iron acquisition by chloroplasts is supported by recent studies in sugar beet (Solti *et al.*, 2012).

FRO3 and FRO8 have been predicted to localise to mitochondrial membranes in *Arabidopsis* (Jeong and Connolly, 2009), and a mitochondrial proteomics study has placed FRO8 at the mitochondrial membrane (Heazlewood *et al.*, 2004), although neither has been functionally characterised. The expression patterns of *FRO3* and *FRO8* are largely non-overlapping, suggesting that they do not function redundantly (Jain and Connolly, 2013). However, the picture with regard to the role and distribution of ferric reductases in mitochondrial iron homeostasis remains unclear (Nouet *et al.*, 2011; Vigani *et al.*, 2013; Jain *et al.*, 2014). It is certainly worth pointing out that currently there is no evidence for a concrete role for a metalloreductase in mitochondria in any organism, despite the observation that the yeast metalloreductase FRE5 localises to mitochondria (Sickmann *et al.*, 2003).

Once ferric iron has been reduced, Fe^{2+} is transported into the root by the ferrous Fe(II) transporter IRT1 (Eide *et al.*, 1996; Vert *et al.*, 2002), a member of the ZIP (ZRT, *I*RT-like *p*rotein) metal transporter family. The family name comes from the yeast Zrt1 protein and the *Arabidopsis thaliana* Irt1 proteins, the first identified members of a family of Zn transporters which are found at all levels of phylogeny (Guerinot, 2000; Eide, 2004, 2006). The loss-of-function mutant *irt1* exhibits a severe Fe deficiency phenotype with chlorotic symptoms and growth arrest which can be specifically rescued by Fe resupply, but not by other metals (Vert *et al.*, 2002). IRT1 is expressed specifically in response to iron starvation in epidermal cells of iron-deficient roots and localises to the plasma membrane, suggesting that it is the major iron transporter of the plant root (Vert *et al.*, 2002). The analysis of plants which overexpress IRT1 shows that it is only present in iron-deficient roots, implying that its expression is controlled post-transcriptionally (Kerkeb *et al.*, 2008). The *IRT1* gene codes for a predicted protein of 339 amino acids (Eide *et al.*, 1996), with eight transmembrane domains like other members of the ZIP family (Guerinot *et al.*, 2000) and has four HisGly repeats, constituting potential metal-binding domains in the intracellular loop between transmembrane domains 3 and 4. It appears likely that IRT1 is a broad-range metal ion transporter in plants, transporting manganese, zinc and cobalt in addition to iron. The iron-induced turnover of IRT1, analogous to that of ZRT1 (Gitan and Eide, 2000), a yeast Zn transporter, involves the ubiquitination of one of two Lys residues situated in the intracellular loop of IRT1 between transmembrane domains 3 and 4 (Kerkeb *et al.*, 2008; Shin *et al.*, 2013).

There are some 16 ZIP metal transporters in *Arabidopsis* (Mäser *et al.*, 2001), of which the most similar in amino acid sequence to IRT1, IRT2, is expressed in the external layers of iron-deficient roots (Vert *et al.*, 2001). However, *irt2* plants show no signs of iron deficiency, and its overexpression cannot compensate for the loss of IRP1, suggesting that it plays some other role than IRT1. Orthologues of IRT1 have been found in other Strategy I plants such as tomato and pea (Eckhardt *et al.*, 2001; Cohen *et al.*, 2004), and have also been found in rice, a Strategy II plant (as discussed below). IRTI shows low selectivity when expressed in yeast, transporting Zn, Mn, Co, Ni and Cd as well as Fe (Kobayashi and Nishizawa, 2012). Other divalent metal transporters such as NRAMP1 (DMT1) have been implicated in iron uptake from soil, although its role seems marginal and its specific contribution remains unclear (Cailliatte *et al.*, 2010).

Reduction-based Fe acquisition is suppressed by high pH and the presence of bicarbonates. Many crop species with reduction-based Fe acquisition, such as soybean (*Glycine max*) or potato (*Solanum tuberosum*), are often cultivated on calcareous soils, which represent approximately one-third of the world's soils (Chen and Barak, 1982), yet they appear to overcome the problem of low Fe solubility and impeded Fe reducibility in high pH soils. It is assumed that Strategy I plants induce additional mechanisms to assist and/or complement the reduction-based Fe acquisition machinery. Iron chelators, such as caffeic acid from soybeans and tomatoes, pistidic acid from pigeon peas, or alfafuran from alfalfa, had been reported to be secreted from roots (reviewed in Mori, 1998). Indeed, root secretion of phenolic compounds has long been hypothesised to be a component of the reduction strategy of Fe acquisition in non-graminaceous plants. It has been shown that Fe deficiency stimulates the exudation of organic compounds, such as phenolics, organic acids, sugars and flavins (Römheld and Marschner, 1983; Mori, 1999; Welkie, 2000; Jin *et al.*, 2007; Carvalhais *et al.*, 2011; Rodríguez-Celma *et al.*, 2011). Recently, it has been shown that Fe-deficient *Arabidopsis* plants produce and release fluorescent phenolic compounds derived from the phenylpropanoid biosynthetic pathway into the growth media (Fourcroy *et al.*, 2013; Rodríguez-Celma *et al.*, 2013), and the ABCG37 (PDR9) ABC transporter was shown to be involved in the secretion of scopoletin (Fourcroy *et al.*, 2013). Subsequently, metabolome analysis has identified scopoletin and other coumarins in root exudates under iron-deplete conditions (Schmidt *et al.*, 2014), and feruloyl-CoA hydroxylase 1 has been shown to be necessary for the biosynthesis of these fluorescent coumarins, some of which (e.g. esculetin, 6,7-dihydroxycoumarin) are iron chelators (Schmid *et al.*, 2014). Since the protocatechuic effluxers PEZ1 (Phenolics Efflux Zero 1) and PEZ2 are involved in solubilising precipitated apoplasmic iron in the plant stele of rice (Ishimaru *et al.*, 2011; Bashir *et al.*, 2011a), it has been suggested that non-gramminaceous counterparts may be involved in Strategy 1 plants (Kobayashi and Nishizawa (2012).

In iron deficiency the induction of proton-extruding H^+-ATPase and ferric reductase activity coincides with the spatial and temporal alteration of root morphology (Schmidt, 2003). Iron deficiency increases not only the quantity of transporters facing the rhizosphere but also the exchange surface of the root system and its foraging capacity (Arahou and Diem, 1997; Schikora and Schmidt, 2001; Schmidt *et al.*, 2000). Iron limitation promotes lateral root elongation of the root system architecture in zones where Fe is available. This process requires the plant hormone auxin and the AUX1 auxin influx transporter (Giehl *et al.*, 2012). Iron deficiency also triggers the formation of ectopic root hairs at positions normally occupied by non-hair cells in an ethylene-dependent and auxin-dependent manner (Schmidt *et al.*, 2000), and leads to bifurcated root hairs with two tips. This phenotype requires the ubiquitin-conjugating enzyme UBC13 (Li and Schmidt, 2010), although the precise molecular events are unknown.

5.1.3.2 *Graminaceous Plants*

Graminaceous plants (grasses) such as corn, wheat and rice respond to iron deficiency by the chelation-based Strategy II, which involves releasing phytosiderophores (Figure 5.4) to chelate poorly soluble iron from soils by the formation of Fe(III)–phytosiderophore (Fe–PS) complexes. The Fe–PS complexes are then taken up at the root plasma membrane via specific Fe–PS transporters. Phytosiderophores chelate and solubilise soil iron efficiently at high pH values and high concentrations of bicarbonate whereas, as noted earlier, the combination of low Fe solubility and impeded Fe reducibility in high-pH soils inhibits the mobilisation of iron by Strategy I plants. This ecological advantage of Strategy II plants favours grasses over non-graminaceous species in bicarbonate-buffered soils (Mori, 1999).

Nicotianamine (NA), the key intermediate in the generation of phytosiderophores, is synthesised (Figure 5.5) from three molecules of *S*-adenosyl methionine (SAM), and involves two carboxypropyl group transfers and one azetidine ring formation, with the release of three

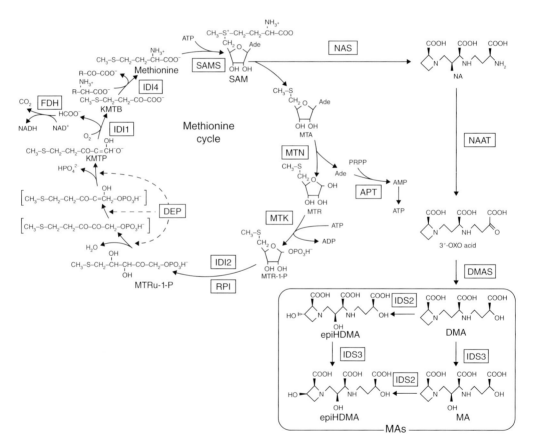

Figure 5.5 *Outline of the biosynthesis of nicotianamine in graminaceous and non-graminaceous plants, and its conversion to deoxymugineic acid (DMA) in graminaceous plants and the conversion of DMA to other phytosiderophores. Reproduced with permission from Springer Science + Business Media from Nozoye, T., Inoue, H., Takahashi, M., et al. (2007) The expression of iron homeostasis-related genes during rice germination.* Plant Mol. Biol., **64**, *35–47*

molecules of 5′-methylthioadenosine (5MTA). All three reactions are catalysed by the enzyme nicotianamine synthase (Herbik *et al.*, 1999; Higuchi *et al.*, 1999; Ling *et al.*, 1999). NA is present not only in grasses but is also found in all plants where, as we will see shortly, it participates in the trafficking of metal ions – notably iron – within the plant (Higuchi *et al.*, 2001; Takahashi *et al.*, 2003). NA is capable of forming complexes with manganese (Mn), Fe(II), cobalt (Co), zinc (Zn), nickel (Ni) and copper (Cu) in increasing order of affinity (Anderegg and Ripperger, 1989).

In graminaceous plants, NA is the precursor of phytosiderophores (Figure 5.5), which are essential in acquiring iron from the soil. They are all members of the family of so-called mugineic acids (MAs), including mugineic acid (MA) itself, together with 3-epihydroxy-2′-deoxymugeneic acid (epiHDMA), 3-epihydroxy-mugeneic acid (epiHMA) and 2′-deoxymugineic acid (DMA) (Figure 5.5). NA is converted first to a phytosiderophore, DMA, by a transamination catalysed by NAAT, followed by a reduction step catalysed by deoxymugineic acid synthase (DMAS) (Mori and Nishizawa, 1987; Bashir *et al.*, 2006), amino transfer and subsequent reduction (Figure 5.5). Only gramminaceous plants possess the *NAAT* and *DMAS* genes, and so whilst all plants produce NA only Graminae can transform NA into PS. DMA is the precursor of the other MAs. Consecutive hydroxylation steps catalysed by two dioxygenases, IDS2 and IDS3 (Nakanishi *et al.*, 2000), convert DMA to the other phytosiderophores, MA, epiHDMA and epiHMA (Figure 5.5). Each of the grasses produces its own sets of MAs, the production and secretion of which is increased in response to iron deficiency. Some plants, such as rice, wheat and corn, produce DMA in only relatively small amounts, and are therefore particularly susceptible to iron stress. Barley, in contrast, secretes large amounts of many types of PS and is therefore more tolerant to iron-deficient conditions (Bashir *et al.*, 2006).

Following their synthesis in response to iron stress, the phytosiderophores are secreted into the rhizosphere (see Figure 5.4), where they complex and solubilise Fe(III). The Fe(III)–phytosiderophore is then transported by a high-affinity uptake system specific for Fe(III)–phytosiderophores into the epidermal cells of iron-deficient roots. *Yellow stripe 1* (*ys1*) and *ys3* are recessive mutants of maize (*Zea mays* L.) that show typical symptoms of Fe deficiency, that is, interveinal chlorosis of the leaves. Whereas (as discussed below), the *ys1* mutant is defective in the Fe(III)–phytosiderophore transporter YS1, and is therefore unable to take up Fe(III)–phytosiderophore complexes, the *ys3* mutant has been shown to be defective in phytosiderophore secretion even though phytosiderophore synthesis is not compromised (Basso *et al.*, 1994). Evidence has been presented that, in rice and barley, the *TOM1* gene encodes a putative efflux transporter, which mediates the efflux of DMA when expressed in *Xenopus* oocytes, and is expressed in the root cells of rice (Nozoye *et al.*, 2011). More recently, it has been suggested that a homolog of TOM1 in maize may in fact be involved in the *ys3* phenotype (Nozoye *et al.*, 2013).

Maize YS1 is the founding member of a family of membrane transporters called YS1-like (YSL), which function in root Fe–phytosiderophore uptake from the soil (Curie *et al.*, 2001; Schaaf *et al.*, 2004; Murata *et al.*, 2006; Curie *et al.*, 2009). The *ZmYS1* gene encodes a protein that is an integral membrane protein with 12 putative transmembrane domains and is distantly related to the Oligopeptide Transporter (OPT) family of proteins (Curie *et al.*, 2001; Yen *et al.*, 2001).

Rice is atypical because it absorbs iron using features of both Strategy I and II plants. In addition to the PS system, rice has Fe^{2+} transporters, OsIRT1 and OsIRT2, which are predominantly expressed in roots, and are induced in iron deficiency (Ishimaru *et al.*, 2006). In the wetland paddy field cultures of rice, the equilibrium of Fe^{3+}/Fe^{2+} is shifted in favour of Fe^{2+} due to the low levels of oxygen. Rice thus appears to have evolved and adapted to its growth habitat where oxygen is low due to flooding, thus favouring the uptake of iron in its Fe(II) form (Thomine and Vert, 2013).

5.1.4 Long-distance Iron Transport

Confronted with the double hazards of poor solubility and high reactivity of iron (the potential notably for generation of reactive oxygen species; see Chapter 13), the translocation of iron inside the plant must be associated with suitable iron chelators and correct control of redox states. The translocation of Fe in plants involves various steps (see Figure 5.1) which include: symplastic transport to pass through the Casparian strip; xylem loading, transport and unloading; xylem to phloem transfer; phloem loading, transport and unloading; and movement towards the site of demand and retranslocation from source or senescing tissue (Kim and Guerinot, 2007). Once iron enters the symplast of the root, where it must be bound to chelators in order to maintain its solubility, it diffuses through different intracellular compartments along a diffusion gradient into the stele. Iron in the soil is taken up from the root surface through the epidermis and cortex to the endodermis, the innermost layer of cells of the cortex (see Figure 5.1). The Casparian strip, a ring-like cell-wall modification in the root endodermis of vascular plants, generates a paracellular barrier that is analogous to the tight junctions between animal cells and which prevents the passive movement of ions into the stele. To move from the cortex to the xylem at the Casparian band, iron must move through the plasma membrane of the endodermis and then through symplastic passages to the stele, from which it is exported into the vessels of the xylem for distribution. Iron is then transported to the shoots through the transpiration stream and imported into the leaf cytoplasm; it can also be transported through symplastic passages from a source tissue (e.g. leaves) to a sink tissue (e.g. seeds) via phloem loading and unloading (Kim and Guerinot, 2007). Because the xylem consists of dead cells which transport water and minerals to the leaves, whereas the phloem consists of living cells transporting food to the growing parts and storage organs of the plant, it is assumed that xylem loading requires efflux transporters whereas phloem loading requires influx transporters. The way in which iron moves through the plant is described in greater detail in the following paragraphs.

The principal iron chelators which are thought to be involved in the long-distance transport of iron are citrate (Brown and Chaney, 1971; Tiffin, 1966), NA (Hell and Stephan, 2003; Takahashi *et al.*, 2003) and, in Strategy II plants, mugenic acids (Aoyama *et al.*, 2009; Kakei *et al.*, 2009).

Citrate has been thought to play the dominant role in the transport of iron in xylem sap (Brown and Chaney, 1971; Kim and Guerinot, 2007; Conte and Walker, 2011). Citrate is not the only chelator in the xylem. As we saw above, in Strategy II plants the PEZ1 and PEZ2 efflux phenolics (notably protocatechuic acid and caffeic acid) into rice xylem sap, facilitating the solubilisation of precipitated apoplasmic Fe inside the stele (Bashir *et al.*, 2011a; Ishimaru *et al.*, 2011). NA and DMA are found in the xylem sap under iron-deficient conditions, suggesting that they may also be involved in iron migration through the xylem (Kakei *et al.*, 2009; Wada *et al.*, 2007), although their stability at the xylem pH of 5.5 is low (Rellán-Alvarez *et al.*, 2008).

Two proteins have been implicated in the transport of citrate and iron out of the root stele and into the apoplastic space of the xylem, namely Ferric Reductase Defective (FRD3) and Ferroportin 1 (FPN1) (Durrett *et al.*, 2007; Morrissey *et al.*, 2009; Yokosho *et al.*, 2009; Roschzttardtz *et al.*, 2011).

FRD3, an *Arabidopsis* transporter of the multidrug and toxin efflux (MATE) family, has been shown to facilitate citrate efflux into the xylem (Durrett *et al.*, 2007). In addition to its expression in the root stele, a more general role for FRD3 in iron localisation and homeostasis throughout plant development in *Arabidopsis* has been proposed (Green and Rogers, 2004; Roschzttardtz *et al.*, 2011). An FRD-like gene in rice, *OsFRDL1*, also encodes a citrate effluxer required for efficient Fe translocation (Yokosho *et al.*, 2009), and two soybean genes have been identified and characterised with similar sequence and function to AtFRD3 (Rogers *et al.*, 2009).

Iron release from the symplast into the apoplastic space (see Figure 5.1), and thence to the xylem vesicles, is not well understood. Since FRD3, FRDL1 and PES1 are thought to efflux Fe-chelating molecules without bound iron, an iron transporter is necessary to efflux Fe into the xylem. It seems likely that a plant analogue of the mammalian Fe export protein ferroportin (FPN, IREG1) which is involved in iron absorption by intestinal enterocytes and in Fe recycling in macrophages (discussed in detail in Chapters 6 and 10), is the most promising candidate. There are two closely related orthologues in *Arabadopsis*, namely AtFPN1(AtIREG1) and AtFPN2 (AtIREG2). AtFPN1 localises to the plasma membrane and is expressed in the stele, suggesting a role in vascular loading (Morrissey *et al.*, 2009), whereas AtFPN2 localises to the vacuolar membrane of root epidermal cells, is involved in iron-dependent nickel detoxification (Schaaf *et al.*, 2006), and is expressed in the two outermost layers of the root in response to iron deficiency, suggesting a role in buffering metal influx. Consistent with these roles, *fpn2* has a diminished iron-deficiency response, whereas *fpn1 fpn2* has an elevated iron-deficiency response (Morrissey *et al.*, 2009).

The transpiration flow in xylem vessels is not adequate to supply the iron requirements of developing organs such as the apex, seeds and root tips, such that iron remobilisation takes place from older leaves to younger leaves via phloem sap transport. The pH of the phloem is alkaline (>7), which means that in order to remain soluble, iron – both Fe(II) and Fe(III) – must be firmly bound to chelators. Citrate cannot achieve this, whereas NA can, binding Fe(II) and Fe(III) with almost equal affinity: of particular importance is the fact that the Fe(II)–NA complex is very stable at the alkaline pH of the phloem sap (von Wiren *et al.*, 1999). Evidence for the importance of NA in iron circulation within plants has come essentially from two mutants where NA production is impaired: the tomato *chloronerva* (*chl*) mutant, which has a loss of function in its unique *NAS* gene, and a tobacco transgenic plant, which overexpresses the Strategy II gene NAAT, which consumes NA. In both of these mutants the lack of NA resulted in chlorosis, sterility, and a lack of iron to reach the intraveinal areas of leaves and, more generally, the young growing tissues which are essentially fed by the phloem (Takahashi *et al.*, 2003). Studies on the quadruple *nas4x-2* mutant of *Arabidopsis thaliana*, which cannot synthesise NA, have indicated that NA facilitates the transport of Fe from the phloem to sink organs, as well as for pollen development and pollen tube growth (Schuler *et al.*, 2012).

The major transporters of iron in the phloem are therefore NA and, in grasses, DMA (Mori *et al.*, 1991; Schmidke and Stephan, 1995; Inoue *et al.*, 2003, 2008; Koike *et al.*, 2004; Bashir *et al.*, 2006). The possibility that iron might bind to higher-molecular-weight peptide ligands inside the phloem (Schmidke *et al.*, 1999) has led to a number of candidates being proposed to fulfil such a function. In castor bean *Ricinus communis*, an 11 kDa iron transport protein (ITP) has been shown to bind Fe(III) in the phloem (Kruger *et al.*, 2002), and is presumed to transport Fe(III). It is a member of the large family of the late embryogenesis proteins known as dehydrins. More recent candidates include the cell wall arabinogalactan protein 24 (AtAGP24) which, like ITP, has a His-rich motif with a putative metal-binding function (Ellis *et al.*, 2010), and its homolog in barley, HvHRA1, which has 13 His-rich domains and increases the seed iron, zinc and copper contents when it is overexpressed (Aizat *et al.*, 2011). The existence of AGPs has also been documented in the xylem stream of *Brassica oleracea* (Ligat *et al.*, 2011). OPT3, previously classified as an oligopeptide transporter, has been shown to be a plasma membrane transporter capable of transporting transition ions *in vitro*, and which in *Arabidopsis thaliana* loads iron into the phloem, facilitates iron recirculation from the xylem to phloem, and regulates both shoot-to-root iron signalling and iron redistribution from mature to developing tissues (Zhai *et al.*, 2014).

We have already encountered the YSL family involved in facilitating the uptake of Fe(III)–DMA from the rhizosphere. YS1, the founding member of this family is induced in both root and shoots in response to iron deficiency (Curie *et al.*, 2001), which implies that it may also play an important role in iron translocation inside the plant. Members of the YSL family are also present in Strategy I plants which do not synthesise phytosiderophores, and it is thought that these non-graminaceous YSL transporters are involved in the translocation of iron and other metals chelated by NA (Curie *et al.*, 2009). AtYSL1 and AtYSL2 are thought to play redundant roles in the translocation of Fe and other metals (Le Jean *et al.*, 2005; Waters *et al.*, 2006; Curie *et al.*, 2009; Chu *et al.*, 2010), and AtYSL2 may also be involved in the lateral movement of metals (DiDonato *et al.*, 2004; Schaaf *et al.*, 2005; Curie *et al.*, 2009).

Rice, which has some of the characteristics of a Strategy I plant, has no less than 18 YSL members (OsYSL1–18), some of which function as influx transporters. YSL2 transports Fe(II)–NA and Mn(II)–NA, but not Fe(III)–MA (Koike *et al.*, 2004), and seems to be responsible for the long-distance translocation of NA-chelated Fe and Mn into sink tissues, including leaves and grains (Koike *et al.*, 2004; Ishimaru *et al.*, 2010). OsYSL15 is involved in both the root absorption of Fe(III)-DMA and the internal translocation of Fe for long-distance transport and seedling growth (Inoue *et al.*, 2009; Lee *et al.*, 2009), while the Fe(III)–DMA OsYSL18 is expressed in restricted parts of the plant, particularly in reproductive tissues and the phloem of laminar joints, suggesting a role in fertilisation and phloem Fe transport (Aoyama *et al.*, 2009). Fe(III)–DMA supplied to barley roots is mostly translocated via the xylem to older leaves, but via the phloem to the youngest leaves (Tsukamoto *et al.*, 2009), underlining the importance of Fe transfer from xylem to phloem in laminar joints (Kobayashi and Nishizawa, 2012). Like OsYSL15, the DMA effluxer TOM1 and the Fe(II) transporter OsIRT1 are also expressed in vascular tissues in rice (Ishimaru *et al.*, 2006; Nozoye *et al.*, 2011) suggesting their involvement in Fe translocation inside the plant.

In the final analysis, Fe must be transported from the roots to the photosynthetic electron transport chain in the leaves which have the highest demand, as well as to the reproductive organs, and to the seeds where iron is stored to support embryogenesis (Grillet *et al.*, 2014a; Roschztardtz *et al.*, 2013). Before reaching the chloroplasts and mitochondria, iron must be offloaded from the xylem, distributed to the different tissues, and transported across the plasma membrane (PM) of sink cells. In the Strategy I plant, *Arabidopsis* (Grillet *et al.*, 2014a), iron from the roots is translocated to the shoots through the xylem as ferric citrate. After reduction to Fe(II), it is transported into shoot and leaf cells by an IRT-like transporter. The reduction step may involve a PM-bound ferric reductase of the FRO family, photoreduction, and/or extracellular ascorbate. Although the ferric reductase AtFRO6 is the most highly expressed member of the FRO family in *Arabidopsis* shoots (Wu *et al.*, 2005; Mukherjee *et al.*, 2006) and is located in the PM (Jeong *et al.*, 2008), *fro6* knockout lines do not display any phenotype (Jeong and Connolly, 2009). Since other family members are either not expressed in shoots, or are localised in intracellular compartments, this implies that a FRO-independent mechanism must exist. This might involve the photoreduction of ferric citrate, which is known to occur rapidly accompanied by the degradation of citrate and a rise in pH. A viable alternative strategy may involve the efflux of ascorbate (Grillet *et al.*, 2014b). *In vitro* transport experiments on isolated pea embryos using radiolabelled ^{55}Fe demonstrated that this ascorbate-mediated reduction is an obligatory step for the uptake of Fe(II). The ascorbate efflux activity was also measured in *Arabidopsis* embryos, suggesting that this new iron transport system may be generic to dicotyledonous plants. The transport of Fe(II) is probably carried out by the PM-localised ArIRT3, which is produced in large amounts in the xylem and in mesophyll cells (Lin *et al.*, 2009), and has been shown to be involved in iron uptake in *Arabidopsis* (Shanmugam *et al.*, 2011).

5.2 Iron Metabolism and Homeostasis in Plants

5.2.1 New Tools in Plant Research

Arabidopsis thaliana, because of its small size, rapid life cycle and simple genome, has been a model system for decades. Since sequencing of the *A. thaliana* genome in 2000 (Arabidopsis Genome Initiative, 2000) in the following 'post-genomic' era, many different types of new 'omics' data have become available to *Arabidopsis* researchers (Lu and Last, 2008), and beyond that to the wider plant research community (Deshmukh *et al.*, 2014). These include, among others, genomics, transcriptomics, proteomics, phenomics, metabolomics and ionomics. However, considering the interaction of the many thousands of molecular components within plant cells and tissues which form the regulatory networks and the biochemical complexes which control organ growth and development, the current research challenge is to make sense of the avalanche of -omics information about these components and their relationships. This requires integrative-omic analyses (Radomiljac *et al.*, 2013; Deshmukh *et al.*, 2014), and clearly *systems biology* provides an optimum method to analyze these complex data sets and reveal new biological insights (Eckardt and Bennett, 2012) (Systems biology is an interdisciplinary field of study that focuses on complex interactions within biological systems, using a holistic approach instead of the more traditional reductionist approach to biological and biomedical research.)

The increasing use of systems biology approaches, bringing together high-throughput biochemical, genetic and molecular approaches to generate large-scale and high-resolution proteomics, metabolomics, interactomics, transcriptomics and translatomics data to generate *predictive models* (Bassel *et al.*, 2012) can be expected to enhance the present understanding of iron metabolism and homeostasis, including the identification of the proper localisation and availability of Fe (Samira *et al.*, 2013). The *models* of course remain *models* until they are supplemented by the kind of old-fashioned biochemical and physiological spadework that readers of previous editions will recognise as one of the author's old-fashioned convictions. My despair at the number of colleagues, even biochemists and synthetic organic chemists, who spend their working days (usually relatively short by the standards of previous generations) in front of their computer screens, grows from year to year. If only *in silico* could replace real practical experimentation, we could all go home and leave it to what I am tempted to call '*la biologie imaginaire*'.

Despite these reservations, large-scale datasets have been produced which can be used in combination to make testable and predictive models of Fe homeostasis (Schmidt and Buckhout, 2011; Ivanov *et al.*, 2012). Most of these modelling efforts involve coexpression systems which can, at best, predict regulatory relationships between transcription factors and their targets and identify genes which may be involved in these networks. Some caution is required in the interpretation of data (Samira *et al.*, 2013): (i) the identification of network nodes can be confounded by redundancy, rendering single mutant studies futile – this could be alleviated by microRNA (miRNA) approaches which target gene families; (ii) more accurate predictive models require spatial resolution; (iii) metabolic flux data, which could provide the greatest predictive power for generating models of Fe homeostasis is difficult to obtain in plant systems (Bassel *et al.*, 2012; Sweetlove and Ratcliffe, 2011); (iv) inclusion of the metabolic rates of key enzymes, such as H^+-ATPases, ferric reductases and PEPcarboxylase (which forms oxaloacetate from phosphoenolpyruvate (PEP) for metabolism by the tricarboxylic acid cycle in plants), could generate models which couple Fe uptake, translocation and assimilation with metabolic pathways such as photosynthesis and respiration.

Histochemical methods and advanced ionic quantification techniques have resulted in high-resolution elemental maps at specific time points allowing the visualisation and determination of

Fe and other metals at cellular and subcellular resolution (reviewed in Samira *et al.*, 2013). The use of such methods has already increased the present understanding of where Fe is localised in plants and what transporters and ligands contribute to this localisation. A systematic analysis of Fe distribution in roots, leaves and reproductive organs of *A. thaliana*, using wild-type and mutant genotypes affected in iron transport and storage, has been carried out with the Perls/DAB Fe staining procedure (Roschzttardtz *et al.*, 2013). Techniques such as synchrotron X-ray fluorescence microtomography (Lombi and Susini, 2009; Lombi *et al.*, 2011) or micro-PIXE (Roschzttardtz *et al.*, 2011; Cvitanich *et al.*, 2010), which have already given promising results with plant samples (Schnell-Ramos *et al.*, 2013), could be used on known regulatory, signalling and metabolic mutants, combined with large-scale datasets, to build more inclusive, dynamic Fe homeostasis models (Samira *et al.*, 2013).

5.2.2 Intracellular Iron Metabolism

Once iron has entered a cell, it is delivered to appropriate intracellular compartments such as chloroplasts, mitochondria or vacuoles, where it may be integrated into iron-containing proteins for functional utilisation, or stored to prevent the cytotoxicity which is the consequence of iron accumulating in excess. Iron transport to chloroplasts involves Permease In Chloroplasts 1 (PIC1) (Duy *et al.*, 2007, 2011), whereas the Mitochondrial Iron Transporter (MIT) is involved in the uptake of cytoplasmic iron into mitochondria (Bashir *et al.*, 2011a,b). The main cellular storage compartments are the vacuoles, which acquire iron through the Vacuolar Iron Transporter 1 (VIP1) (Kim, S.A. *et al.*, 2006). By far the largest pool of iron in plant cells is in the chloroplast, which contains 80–90% of cellular iron (Terry and Abadia, 1986; Hänsch and Mendel, 2008). That chloroplasts are a major sink compartment for iron comes as no surprise, since each chain of the photosynthetic electron transfer pathway in the thylakoid membrane contains as many as 22 Fe atoms in both haem and iron–sulphur cluster proteins (see Chapter 8). Iron starvation particularly affects photosystem I (PSI), which contains 12 iron atoms per monomer. It also causes chlorosis due to a reduction in chlorophyll synthesis, possibly because the enzyme catalysing the biosynthesis step between Mg-protoporphyrin IX monomethyl ester and protochlorophyllide requires two iron atoms (Moseley *et al.*, 2000; Tottey *et al.*, 2003). The ubiquitous iron storage protein ferritin is also located in the chloroplasts (Briat *et al.*, 2010a,b), and plant ferritins are also found in mitochondria as well as in non-photosynthetic plastids (Seckback, 1982; van der Mark *et al.*, 1982; Zancani *et al.*, 2004; Briat *et al.*, 2010a,b; Zhao, 2010). This is in marked contrast to mammalian ferritins which are found in the cytoplasm, reflecting that plant ferritins are synthesised as a higher-molecular-weight precursor, with a transit peptide which directs it to the plastids. *Arabidopsis thaliana* has four ferritin genes (*AtFer1–4*), of which only FER1 exists as a 28-kDa mature subunit in leaves where it is the most highly expressed ferritin; FER3 and FER4 exist in leaves only as a 26.5-kDa processed subunit, while FER2 is the only subunit present in seeds (Ravet *et al.*, 2009). Most dicotyledonous genomes have three or more ferritin genes, and graminaceous plants have only two (Strozycki *et al.*, 2010). Whereas mammalian ferritins are assembled from two types of subunit, plant ferritins are homopolymers with different isoforms resulting from post-transcriptional processing, and plant ferritin synthesis is regulated at the level of transcription, in contrast to the translational control of mammalian ferritin expression (Briat *et al.*, 2010a,b). It has been concluded that, while there are strong links between plant ferritins and protection against oxidative stress, their putative iron-storage function to furnish iron during various development processes is unlikely to be essential (Briat *et al.*, 2010b). A more detailed discussion of the structure and function of plant ferritins can be found, together with a more general account of ferritins, in Chapter 9.

In conditions of iron overload, although iron can be stored in the apoplast, much of the iron storage is ensured by the vacuole or within the plastids. As indicated earlier, VIT1 appears to transport iron into the vacuole. Vit1 mutants show poor germination and an aberrant localisation of Fe in seeds, while AtFPN2, the Fe-deficiency-induced tonoplast transporter of Ni and Co into the vacuole in the detoxification of root epidermal cells (Morrissey *et al.*, 2009; Schaaf *et al.*, 2006), might also be involved in Fe transport into the vacuole (Morrissey *et al.*, 2009).

The retrieval of Fe from the vacuole is less clear. In the NA-less tomato chloronerva mutant, insoluble Fe(III)-phosphate precipitates are detected in the vacuoles of leaf cells, suggesting that NA is required to maintain vacuolar iron in a soluble state (Becker *et al.*, 1995). This prompts speculation that members of the *YSL* gene family might be localised to the vacuolar membrane, and involved in the re-translocation of Fe–NA into the cytosol. Both AtYSL4 and AtYSL6 proteins were identified in the proteome of *Arabidopsis* vacuoles (Jaquinod *et al.*, 2007), where they might be expected to act, on the basis of the activity of ZmYS1 as a H^+/metal complex symporter (Schaaff *et al.*, 2004) in vacuolar iron export.

Members of the natural resistance-associated macrophage protein (Nramp) gene family play an important role in divalent metal ion transport in mammals (as is described in greater detail in Chapters 6 and 8). The *Arabidopsis* proteins AtNramp3 and AtNramp4 are able to complement the phenotype of a metal uptake-deficient yeast strain (Curie *et al.*, 2000; Thomine *et al.*, 2000), and both Nramp3 and Nramp4 localise to the vacuolar membrane in *Arabidopsis* (Curie *et al.*, 2000; Lanquar *et al.*, 2005) and are upregulated in response to iron deficiency. Seeds of the double knockout *Arabidopsis* mutant *AtNramp3 AtNramp4* contain wild-type levels of iron, yet the seedlings display retarded root growth and cotyledon greening during seed germination under low iron, apparently due to an inability to retrieve iron from vacuolar stores (Lanquar *et al.*, 2005). The implication is clear that vacuoles are an important iron storage site and that remobilisation of vacuolar iron during germination is crucial for seedling development when the supply of iron in the rhizosphere is low.

5.2.3 Plant Iron Homeostasis

Since iron levels need to be maintained at an optimum level for function inside the plant cell in an aerobic environment, while minimizing the dangers of iron-mediated oxidative stress, plant iron homeostasis is extremely tightly regulated. Current views on the regulators of iron homeostasis are outlined in the following text. Recent reviews on the topic are available by Kobayashi and Nishizawa (2012, 2014), Hindt and Guerinot (2012), Darbani *et al.* (2013), as well as articles in the edition of *Frontiers in Plant Science* edited by Vigani *et al.* (2013).

Figure 5.6 outlines, schematically, the iron-deficiency response in plants, beginning with the induction of a number of transcription factors (Figure 5.6a). The first of these to be identified was the basic helix-loop-helix protein FER (iron-deficiency response) in tomato (Ling *et al.*, 2002) which targets the *Nramp1*, *Irt1* and *Fro1* (Bereczky *et al.*, 2003; Li *et al.*, 2004) genes. The functional homolog in *Arabidopsis*, *AtFIT* (FER-like iron deficiency-induced factor) increases its expression fourfold in iron deficiency, and in addition to being a positive regulator of its own gene it regulates *Nramp1*, *Fro2*, *Nas1* (NA synthase 1) and *Fpn2* (ferroportin 2) genes and IRT protein expression (Colangelo and Guerinot, 2004; Jakoby *et al.*, 2004). The turnover of FIT by the ubiquitination/26S proteosome system appears to be crucial for the iron-deficiency response (Sivitz *et al.*, 2011), whereas nitric oxide (NO) seems to stabilise the FIT protein (Meiser *et al.*, 2011; Sivitz *et al.*, 2011). A rapid and constitutive degradation of IRT1 allows plants to respond quickly to changing conditions to maintain Fe homeostasis. AtIRT1 degradation involves the

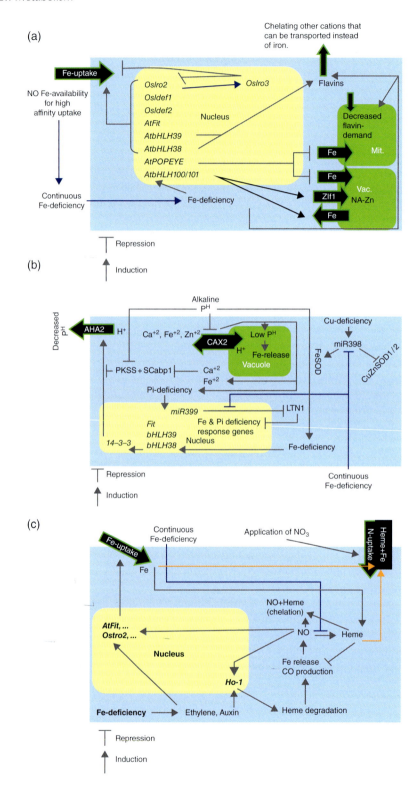

ubiquitination of Lys146 and Lys 171, located in the intracellular loop of the protein (Kerkeb *et al.*, 2008), although endocytosis seems to involve only the monoubiquitinated protein (Barberon *et al.*, 2011). The RING E3 ubiquitin ligase which is involved has been recently identified (Shin *et al.*, 2013).

ArFIT1 interacts with two other basic helix-loop-helix (bHLH) proteins, AtbHLH38 and AtbHLH39 (Yuan *et al.*, 2008), whose overexpression in tobacco enhances riboflavin secretion (Vorweiger *et al.*, 2007; Higa *et al.*, 2008), which is a typical Fe deficiency response in some plant species. Fe deficiency also leads to changes in the mitochondrial electron transfer pathways involving use of the alternative NAD(P)H dehydrogenases, complex III and IV pathway (Figure 5.7) rather than the use of flavin- and iron-rich Complexes I and II (Higa *et al.*, 2010). This is accompanied by the *de novo* synthesis of riboflavin and hydrolysis of FMN, which leads to increased riboflavin secretion (Higa *et al.*, 2012), thereby protecting the plant from an overaccumulation of zinc and other toxic metal ions under iron-deficiency conditions (Lin *et al.*, 2009).

Two other members of the subgroup of 1b bHLH genes, AtbHLH100 and ArbHLH101, are also strongly induced in iron deficiency in both roots and leaves (Wang *et al.*, 2007; Sivitz *et al.*, 2012), and are involved in the upregulation of genes which include *Zif1*, the iron deficiency-inducible Zinc Induced Facilitator 1, ZIF1, which sequesters zinc and also NA inside vacuoles (Haydon *et al.*, 2012). Because plant iron transporters are often Fe(II) chelators, they cannot readily discriminate against other divalent metal ions, unlike the Fe(III) systems of bacteria. Yet another bHLH transcription factor, POPEYE (PYE), also appears to be involved in regulating the expression of known iron homeostasis genes. PYE interacts with PYE homologues, including IAA-Leu Resistant3 (ILR3), another bHLH transcription factor that is involved in metal ion homeostasis, which in turn interacts with a third protein, BRUTUS (BTS), a putative E3 ligase protein, with metal ion-binding and DNA-binding domains, which negatively regulates the response to iron deficiency (Long *et al.*, 2010). The corresponding regulatory response to iron deficiency in rice is orchestrated by OsIRO2 (Ogo *et al.*, 2006, 2007, 2011).

The secretion of protons into the rhizosphere in Strategy I plants is an important part of their iron uptake strategy, and the proton pump AHA2 is the main protagonist (Santi and Schmidt, 2009). In response to iron deficiency, ArFIT induces a 14-3-3 protein (Figure 5.6b) which activates AHA2 (Colangelo and Guerinot, 2004; Jahn *et al.*, 1997). The 14-3-3 protein can also upregulate FIT in

---

Figure 5.6 *The iron-deficiency response. (a) Iron deficiency induces a number of transcription factors, e.g., OsIRO2 and AtFIT, to upregulate the uptake mechanisms, to downregulate the consumption pathways like restructuring of the electron transfer chains inside mitochondria in order to decrease the demand for riboflavin and iron, and to utilise the iron reserves trapped inside vacuoles. (b) AHA2 is one of the Strategy I components that secretes protons into the rhizosphere. Iron-deficiency response induces the protein 14-3-3, which activates the proton pump AHA2. Alkaline pH conditions also activate the proton pump by repressing the expression of PKS5 and by calcium-mediated blocking of the interaction between PKS5 and SCabp. This follows the downregulation of CAX2, which can increase the cytoplasmic levels of calcium, iron and zinc and reduce the vacuolar pH. (c) Upstream in the iron deficiency, signalling hormones such as auxin and ethylene are key players. Auxin induces haem degradation resulting in iron release and NO production with a positive feedback on haem degradation. NO, in parallel with ethylene, induces the transcription factors, e.g., OsIRO2 and AtFIT, involved in the iron- deficiency response. Induction of iron uptake increases haem production with a negative feedback effect on NO production. Haem also has the capacity to scavenge NO. Reproduced with permission from Elsevier from Darbani, B., Briat, J.F., Holm, P.B., et al. (2013) Dissecting plant iron homeostasis under short and long-term iron fluctuations.* Biotechnol. Adv., **31**, 1292–1307

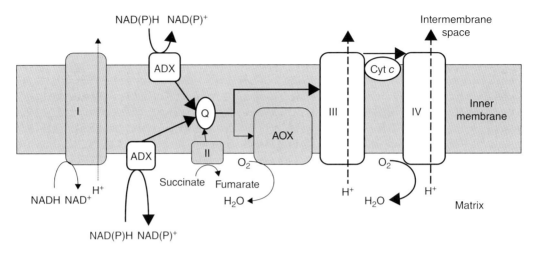

Figure 5.7 *Possible major mitochondrial electron transfer chains operating under conditions in which riboflavin secretion is occurring. Possible major proteins involved and electron flows are shown in bold squares/ellipsoids and bold arrows, respectively. Q, ubiquinone; Cyt c, cytochrome c. Reproduced from Higa, A., Mori, Y. and Kitamura, Y. (2010) Iron deficiency induces changes in riboflavin secretion and the mitochondrial electron transport chain in hairy roots of* Hyoscyamus albus. *J. Plant Physiol.,* **167**, *870–878*

an NO-dependent manner (Yang *et al.*, 2013). A Ser/Thr protein kinase, PKS5 is a negative regulator of AHA2 by phosphorylating Ser931 in the C-terminal regulatory domain of AHA2, thereby inhibiting the interaction of AHA2 with 14-3-3 (Fuglsang *et al.*, 2007). PKS5 needs to bind a calcium-binding protein SCaBP (calcineurin B-like protein) in order to phosphorylate and negatively regulate AHA2 and hence to mediate cytoplasmic pH homeostasis (Fuglsang *et al.*, 2007; Yang *et al.*, 2010). The downregulation at high pH of the Ca^{2+}/H^+ calcium exchanger CAX2, which can also transport other cations such as Fe^{2+} and Zn^{2+} (Kim, C.K., 2006), increases cellular iron as well as Ca^{2+}, decreasing the expression of PKS5 by blocking its interaction with SCaBP and releasing the 14-3-3 protein to activate AHA2. The repression of CAX proteins decreases the vacuole pH, which increases iron release from phytate. In addition, it can induce phosphorus deficiency response by an induction of the microRNA miR399, which in rice downregulates Leaf Tip Necrosis 1 (OsLTN1) which would repress phosphorus and iron deficiency response genes (Hu *et al.*, 2011). Continuous iron deficiency represses uptake mechanisms, and also copper and phosphorus deficiency responses. This means that a repression of iron uptake mechanisms would favour non-iron enzymes, such as CuZnSOD, instead of FeSOD (Darbani *et al.*, 2013).

Finally, in the iron-deficiency pathway, signalling hormones such as auxin and ethylene are key players (Chen *et al.*, 2010; Lingam *et al.*, 2011) (Figure 5.6c). Fe deficiency leads to increased auxin synthesis in *Arabidopsis*, which leads to an enhanced expression of *FIT* and *FRO2* (Chen *et al.*, 2010). Auxin clearly plays a role in the root morphology response to Fe deficiency (Schmidt, 2003), and it has been shown that a localised iron supply triggers lateral root elongation in *Arabidopsis* by altering the AUX1-mediated auxin distribution (Giehl *et al.*, 2012). Auxin upregulates haem oxygenase (Xuan *et al.*, 2008), resulting in the release of iron and CO, and the increased levels of CO stimulate the iron-deficiency response through NO (Kong *et al.*, 2010). NO itself is clearly involved in responses to both iron deficiency and iron overload (Arnaud *et al.*, 2006). Ethylene induces transcription factors involved in the iron-deficiency response, such as

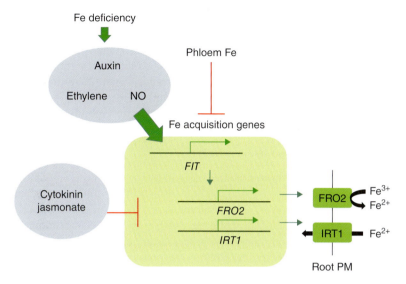

Figure 5.8 *Model of hormone and small molecule effects on regulation of the Strategy I Fe deficiency response. Auxin, ethylene and NO have been implicated as positive regulators of the Fe acquisition genes FIT, FRO2, and IRT1, while cytokinin and jasmonate have been demonstrated to negatively regulate FRO2 and IRT1 in a FIT-independent manner. Fe from the phloem is thought to serve as a negative regulator of Fe deficiency gene expression. Reproduced from Hindt, M.N. and Guerinot, M.L. (2012) Getting a sense for signals: regulation of the plant iron deficiency response.* Biochim. Biophys. Acta, **1823**, *1521–1530*

OsIRO2 and AtFIT (Garcia *et al.*, 2010; Wu *et al.*, 2011), as does NO. It is proposed that the interaction between the ethylene-insensitive 3 (EIN3)/ethylene-insensitive 3-like 1 (EIL1) and FIT is the mechanism used to accumulate the FIT protein through alleviating its degradation (Lingam *et al.*, 2011). The induction of iron uptake increases haem production with a negative feedback effect on NO production. Haem also has the capacity to scavenge NO. When iron is restricted, haem will not be synthesised and the uptake mechanisms will be turned down. Iron and haem utilisation by the nitrogen uptake pathway explain why NO_3 application increases the iron content of plants. Induction of the nitrogen uptake pathway by NO_3 decreases freely available iron and haem concentrations inside the cell, and leads to the induction of an iron-deficiency response (Darbani *et al.*, 2013).

In addition to the positive regulation of the iron acquisition genes *FIT*, *FRO2* and *IRT1* by auxin, ethylene and NO, there are two other classes of plant hormones, namely cytokinins (Seguela *et al.*, 2008) and jasmonates (Maurer *et al.*, 2011), which have been demonstrated to negatively regulate *FRO2* and *IRT1* in a FIT-independent manner (Figure 5.8). Cytokinins (CKs) are hormones known to control growth and developmental processes (Sakakibara, 2006), while jasmonates are oxylipin-based mobile plant hormones which act systemically and belong to a category of stress hormones which are known to act in response to various stimuli, such as wounding, insect attack or ultraviolet light (Shah, 2009; Wasternack and Kombrink, 2010).

Fe deficiency could be effectively ameliorated by promoting nutritious foods, using Fe supplements, and fortifying food with Fe; however, these strategies are not easy to implement in practice, especially for poor families with limited financial resources (Haas *et al.*, 2005). Fe deficiency could also be mitigated by increasing the Fe content and bioavailability of food grains, such as wheat and rice (Schroeder *et al.*, 2013). Recently, three approaches were combined to increase the Fe content of rice seeds (Bashir *et al.*, 2013): (i) enhancing iron storage in grains via expression of the Fe storage protein ferritin: (ii) enhancing Fe translocation from roots to seeds through overproduction of the iron chelator, NA; and (iii) enhancing Fe flux into the endosperm through the overexpression *of OsYSL2*, the gene responsible for the long-distance translocation of NA-chelated Fe into sink tissues, including leaves and grains. The Fe concentration of polished seeds of field grown rice increased to fourfold that of wild-type plants.

5.2.4 Diurnal Regulation of Iron Homeostasis

Expression of the genes involved in iron homeostasis in plants is subjected, like many other processes, to diurnal fluctuations. Indeed, metal ion homeostasis in general is controlled by circadian rhythms (Chen *et al.*, 2013; Hong *et al.*, 2013; Salomé *et al.*, 2013). In conditions of iron need, the iron uptake mechanisms are upregulated while the availability of the intracellular iron stores is increased at the beginning of the day, and these processes are progressively downregulated in the course of the day (Figure 5.9). A reciprocal pattern of expression is observed in genes involved in iron sequestration. The synthesis and secretion of mugenic acid also peaks with the arrival of daylight (Nagasaka *et al.*, 2000; Nozoye *et al.*, 2004; Takagi *et al.*, 1984).

The delightfully named *TIME FOR COFFEE* (*TIC*) gene, which encodes a nuclear regulator of the circadian clock (Ding *et al.*, 2007; Hall *et al.*, 2003), regulates iron overload-responsive genes (notably plant ferritins). TIC represses the expression of *AtFer1, 3* and *4* ferritin genes under low-iron conditions, and its activity requires light and light/dark cycles (Duc *et al.*, 2009). The *Arabidopsis* protein kinase AKIN10 is a metabolic sensor targeting a remarkably broad array of genes that orchestrate transcription networks, promote catabolism and suppress anabolism (Baena-Gonzalez *et al.*, 2007; Baena-Gonzalez and Sheen, 2008), including TIC. It has been suggested (Darbani *et al.*, 2013) that when it is activated, AKIN10 could act together with TIC to repress the expression of *AtFer1, 3* and *4* genes. The interaction between TIC and AKIN10 can be inhibited by PRL1 (Pleiotropic Response Locus 1), which results in the derepression of *AtFer1, 3* and *4* genes (Baruah *et al.*, 2009; Duc *et al.*, 2009). AKIN10 participates in diurnal regulation by starch degradation and mobilisation, repressing the sucrose synthase genes and itself being inactivated by sucrose (Baena-Gonzalez *et al.*, 2007; Fragoso *et al.*, 2009). NO quickly accumulates in the plastids after iron treatment and ferritin mRNA turnover occurs 9–12 h after derepression by NO (Arnaud *et al.*, 2006). NO acts downstream of iron and upstream of a PP2A-type phosphatase to promote an increase in AtFer1 mRNA level (Figure 5.9). Once darkness falls, ferritin expression is repressed through AKIN10 and TIC, and once again the signal is initiated in the chloroplast, where the demand for iron is high during daylight.

The plant hormones auxin, ethylene and abscissic acid (ABA) also intervene in iron homeostasis (Briat *et al.*, 2010a), and it is not surprising to find that hormone levels are connected with dark/light fluctuations; indeed, high levels of sugars induce ABA, and ethylene can inhibit this induction (Gazzarini and McCourt, 2001). The following model has therefore been proposed (Darbani *et al.*, 2013): at the end of the day, an increased sugar level results in a high level of ABA which can induce *Fer2* gene expression. During iron shortage at the end of the night, as a consequence of the iron-deficiency response, ethylene production blocks ABA induction leading to a deactivation of *Fer2* induction.

So, as indicated in Figure 5.9, as dawn breaks, light initiates photosynthesis, which induces starch and sucrose assimilation. Signalling pathways, which may be both sucrose-dependent and -independent, involving PRL1-mediated inhibition of the interaction between TIC and AKIN10,

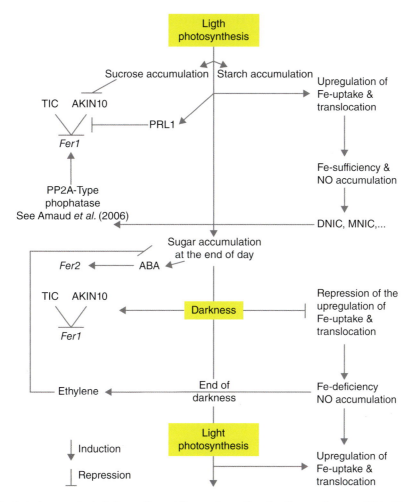

Figure 5.9 *Iron homeostasis follows diurnal fluctuations. For details, see the text. ABA: Abscissic acid; DNIC: Di-nitrosyl-iron complex; MNIC: Mono-nitrosyl-iron complex. Reproduced with permission from Elsevier from Darbani B., Briat, J.F., Holm, P.B., et al. (2013) Dissecting plant iron homeostasis under short and long-term iron fluctuations.* Biotechnol. Adv., **31**, 1292–1307

derepress *Fer1* isoform expression thereby increasing the FER1/FER2 ratio. As we will see in greater detail in Chapter 9, FER1 is the best isoform to take up and mobilise the incoming iron for photosynthesis, whereas the FER2 isoform is best suited for iron storage. As iron begins to accumulate as a consequence of the upregulation of light-induced iron uptake and translocation, the NO level rises forming iron nitrosyl complexes such as DNIC and MNIC. This initiates a signalling pathway to further enhance the *Fer1* expression mediated by a PP2A-type phosphatase (Arnaud *et al.*, 2006). As daylight wanes, sugar accumulation results in ABA biosynthesis, inducing *Fer2* expression, while in parallel the interaction of TIC and AKIN10 can once again repress Fer1 expression, and the altered ratio of FER1/FER2 enhances the storage capacity of ferritin. At the end of the night, ABA synthesis is repressed by ethylene, resulting in Fer2 repression, while induction of the iron uptake mechanisms described earlier swing into operation as daylight once again appears.

5.3 Iron Uptake, Metabolism and Homeostasis in Fungi

5.3.1 Introduction

As a genetically tractable unicellular eukaryote, the budding yeast *Saccharomyces cerevisiae* is an extremely attractive model system for the study of genes involved in fungal iron uptake, and has served until recently as the paradigm for fungal iron metabolism. This is easily explained by the organism's short generation time, the ease with which relatively large amounts of biomass can be grown relatively inexpensively on defined media, and the fact that it was the first complete eukaryote genome to be sequenced (since then a great many more fungal genomes have been sequenced). Its genome is small (6043 genes), yeast favours homologous recombination (unlike mammals), and it is comparatively easy to inactivate specific genes. Finally, it emerges that not only do many of the mechanisms involved in iron uptake and metabolism in higher eukaryotes have homologous systems in yeast, but that many of the genes involved in iron acquisition in yeast have homologous genes in higher eukaryotes which are frequently able to rescue yeast mutants defective in iron acquisition and metabolism.

However, unlike most filamentous fungi and a handful of yeasts such as *Schizosaccharomyces pombe* (Schrettl *et al.*, 2004; Haas *et al.*, 2008), *S. cerevisiae* is not able to synthesise siderophores although, as we will see, it can take up iron bound to siderophores produced by other microorganisms. Also, only *Saccharomyces* and related species of yeast rely on Aft1-like transcription factors to control iron homeostasis. Other fungal species, such as *S. pombe*, *C. albicans*, and *Aspergillus* spp. rely on iron-regulated transcriptional repressors of the GATA and CCAAT-box binding families (Labbe *et al.*, 2007; Schrettl and Haas, 2011).

While iron metabolism has been most extensively studied in *Saccharomyces cerevisiae*, much work has been carried out at the molecular level in other fungal species, including *S. pombe*, *Aspergillus fumigatus*, *Aspergillus nidulans*, *C. albicans*, and *Cryptococcus neoformans* (Philpott *et al.*, 2012; Cyert and Philpott, 2013). In the following, a brief description is provided of the uptake systems that are widely used by non-pathogenic fungi (the specific iron uptake pathways used by fungal pathogens were discussed in Chapter 4), before considering fungal iron metabolism and homeostasis.

Just as with bacteria, fungi possess multiple transport systems for iron (for reviews, see Philpott, 2006; Philpott *et al.*, 2012; Cyert and Philpott, 2013). At present, essentially three systems are known (Figure 5.10), which are described in detail below:

i. A high-affinity, reductive iron transport system which involves the initial reduction of Fe^{3+} to Fe^{2+} by plasma membrane reductases, followed by uptake of the Fe^{2+} by a complex consisting of the proteins coded by the *FET3* gene (a ferroxidase) and the *FTR1* gene (an Fe(III) permease).
ii. Low-affinity ferrous iron transport systems which have been characterised at the molecular level in *S. cerevisiae*, but not in any other fungal species. The permeases involved transport not only ferrous iron but also other divalent metals such as copper and zinc (Kaplan and Kaplan, 2009).
iii. Nonreductive transport systems able to mediate the uptake of iron from iron–siderophore complexes either synthesised and secreted by the fungi themselves, or produced by other organisms in their environment.

These different systems come into operation under different conditions of environmental and growth requirements.

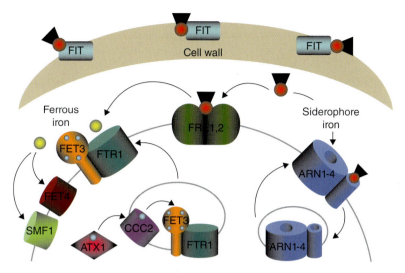

Figure 5.10 *Iron uptake systems of* S. cerevisiae. *The plasma membrane of yeast is surrounded by a porous cell wall that protects the cell from osmotic lysis and excludes larger macromolecules. The FIT mannoproteins of the cell wall facilitate retention of siderophore–iron in the cell wall, but are not required for siderophore uptake. Many siderophores likely cross the cell wall through nonspecific pores. Siderophore-bound iron can be reduced and released from the siderophore by the FRE reductases. Ferric iron salts and low-affinity chelates are also reduced by the FRE reductases prior to uptake. Reduced iron can then be taken up through either the high-affinity ferrous iron transporter (the Fet3p and Ftr1p complex) or through low-affinity transporters (Fet4, Smf1). Fet3p is a ferroxidase that requires copper for function. Fet3p does not become functional until it is loaded with copper intracellularly through the activities of the copper chaperone Atx1p and the copper transporter Ccc2p. Although the Fet3p/Ftr1p complex mediates the uptake of much of the iron released from siderophores, there is also another uptake route. Intact siderophore–iron chelates can be taken up via members of the ARN transporter family. The Arn transporter binds the ferric siderophore and the transporter– siderophore complex undergoes endocytosis prior to translocation of the ferric siderophore chelate across the membrane. Reprinted with permission from Elsevier from Philpott, C.C. (2006) Iron uptake in fungi: a system for every source.* Biochim. Biophys. Acta, **1763**, 636–645

5.3.2 High- and Low-affinity Iron Uptake Pathways

Before the yeast cell can take up any iron, in whatever form it presents itself, the iron must cross the cell wall. In fungi, the cell wall is a dynamic structure composed of a lattice of glucans and chitin, to which is covalently attached to an outer layer of mannoproteins, the composition of which can change considerably under different growth conditions. This will affect the passage of nutrients through the cell wall to the periplasmic space and the plasma membrane. In *S. cerevisiae*, iron depletion induces very high levels of expression of three cell wall mannoproteins, *Fit1p*, *Fit2p* and *Fit3p* (Facilitator of *i*ron *t*ransport) (Protchenko *et al.*, 2001). These proteins enhance retention of the siderophores in the cell wall and increase the uptake of siderophore iron at the cell surface, but their precise mechanism of action is unknown.

In early studies it was shown that iron uptake in *S. cerevisiae* involves a reductive step (Lesuisse *et al.*, 1987), and that there were at least two iron-reducing enzymes one of which was subsequently purified to homogeneity (Lesuisse *et al.*, 1990). *Saccharomyces cerevisiae* has two cell surface reductases, both members of the FRE family of metalloreductases, designated FRE1 and

FRE2, which account for the majority of cell surface reductase activity (Dancis *et al.*, 1990, 1992; Georgatsou and Alexandraki, 1994; Lesuisse and Labbe, 1994; Hassett and Kosman, 1995; Georgatsou *et al.*, 1997). Both are required for growth on a media containing low concentrations of ferric salts. FRE1 has a sequence homology to the large subunit, gpP1phox of the NADPH oxidase localised in the plasma membrane of human phagocytic cells (Chanock *et al.*, 1994). FRE1 is thought to be a transmembrane flavocytochrome b_{558} electron transfer protein, with NADPH- and FAD-binding domains at its cytosolic face, and a pair of intramembrane haems which transfer electrons one at a time to Fe(III) at the external surface of the cell (Shatwell *et al.*, 1996). Although *FRE1* and *FRE2* encode essentially all of the metalloreductase activity on the plasma membrane of yeast cells, seven more genes with significant homology to *FRE2* have been found within the yeast genome (Georgatsou and Alexandraki, 1999; Martins *et al.*, 1998); their possible role in iron uptake is not established. *FRE1, 2, 3, 4, 5* and *6* are transcribed in conditions of iron depletion, whereas *FRE1* and *FRE7* are transcribed when cells are copper-depleted. The expression of the two remaining unnamed *FRE* family members (YGL160W and YLR047C) is not affected by iron or copper status. Fre3p and Fet4p have weak activity in the reduction of ferric siderophores (Yun *et al.*, 2001). Fre5 has been localised to the mitochondria (Sickman *et al.*, 2003), although its function is unknown, and Fre6P seems instead to be involved in iron efflux from the yeast vacuole (Rees and Thiele, 2007; Singh *et al.*, 2007).

As is outlined in Figure 5.10, in yeast (and probably most other fungi[3]), environmental Fe(III) is mobilised by reduction to Fe^{2+} by surface metalloreductases such as Fre1p and Fre2p, after which the Fe^{2+} is taken up by the high-affinity transport system. This consists of the multicopper ferroxidase Fet3p (Askwith *et al.*, 1994), which oxidises the Fe^{2+} to Fe^{3+}, with the Fe^{3+} produced by Fet3p being transferred directly to the Fe^{3+} permease Ftr1p (Stearman *et al.*, 1996) for transfer across the plasma membrane (de Silva *et al.*, 1995, 1997; Hassett *et al.*, 1998a,b) by a classic metabolite channelling mechanism.

The link between copper and iron in mammalian iron metabolism will be described in more detail in Chapter 13. Clearly, the copper–iron link also exists in *S. cerevisiae*, since copper is required for the activity of the ferroxidase-dependent, high-affinity iron uptake complex in the yeast plasma membrane.

Fet3p shows extensive homology with the family of multicopper oxidases (MCOs), including ascorbate oxidase, laccase and ceruloplasmin (reviewed in Kosman, 2010), which couple the oxidation of substrates with the four-electron reduction of molecular oxygen to water. This represents a cumulative, even vaguely cooperative, process where the enzymes oxidise their substrates sequentially, storing the abstracted electrons until, when the fourth electron has been removed from the substrate, they attack the dioxygen molecule in a concerted fashion, without the release of reactive oxygen species, and transform it into two molecules of water. Like all MCOs, Fet3p has three spectroscopically different forms of copper (Hassett *et al.*, 1998b; Blackburn *et al.*, 2000; Machonkin *et al.*, 2001; Palmer *et al.*, 2002) – one Type 1 copper, one Type 2 copper, and one dinuclear Type 3 copper cluster, in which the unpaired electrons on the two cupric ions in the cluster are spin-coupled. The Type 2 and Type 3 coppers are assembled in a trinuclear copper centre. The oxidation of Fe^{2+} takes place at the Type 1 copper site, while dioxygen is reduced to water at the trinuclear cluster (Solomon *et al.*, 1996; Palmer *et al.*, 2002). The four copper atoms necessary for oxidase activity are inserted into Fet3p by the microsomal copper transporter Ccc2p (Dancis *et al.*, 1994). Ccc2p transports copper, delivered from the cytoplasm by the copper chaperone Atx1p (Lin

---

[3]An exception seems to be *Aspergillus nidulans*, which does not express a reductive system of iron uptake; as a consequence no orthologues of *FET3* or *FTR1* are found in the genome (Eisendle *et al.*, 2003).

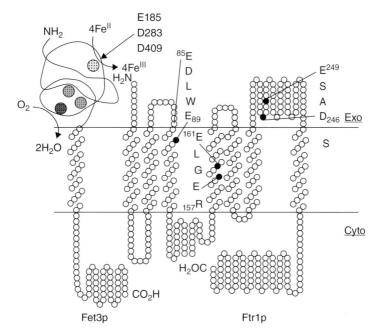

Figure 5.11 *Structural models of Fet3p and Ftr1p in the yeast plasma membrane. Fet3p has a single transmembrane domain, and Ftr1p has seven domains; the proteins share an* N_{exo}/C_{cyt} *topology. Fet3p residues E185, D283, and D409 at this enzyme's type 1 copper ferroxidase site contribute to Fe trafficking from Fet3p to Ftr1p, as do Ftr1p residues. Reprinted with permission from Kwok, E.Y., Severance, S. and Kosman, D.J. (2006a) Evidence for iron channeling in the Fet3p–Ftr1p high-affinity iron uptake complex in the yeast plasma membrane.* Biochemistry, **45**, 6317–6327; © 2006, American Chemical Society

et al., 1997), across the lumen of post-Golgi vesicles (Yuan *et al.*, 1995), as described in more detail in Chapter 14.

The topology and orientation (Figure 5.11) of Fet3p, a type 1 membrane protein with a single transmembrane domain, is amino-terminal extracellular and carboxy- terminal intracellular, with the MCO activity located within the 555-amino acid residue extracellular domain (de Silva *et al.*, 1997; Hassett *et al.*, 1998b). The three-dimensional structure of the extracellular ferroxidase domain of Fet3p has been determined (Taylor *et al.*, 2005) (PDB accession code 1zpu). Both substrate oxidation and oxygen reduction are performed by copper ions in different sites. MCOs contain at least four copper ions, which are arranged in a type 1, blue mononuclear copper centre and a trinuclear copper cluster consisting of a type 2 copper ion and a dinuclear type 3 centre (Figure 5.12a). The substrate is oxidised by the T1 site, which then shuttles electrons to the trinuclear cluster, where the dioxygen reduction takes place. Thus, the T2 and the T3 centres represent a functional unit in which the T3 site exhibits unique electron transfer activity. The structure of the multinuclear metal site of reduced Fet3p (PDB accession code 1zpu) with its characteristic type 1, type 2 and type 3 copper ions is shown in Figure 5.13 (Zaballa *et al.*, 2010).

Whereas most MCOs exhibit broad specificity towards organic substrates, Fet3p functions exclusively as a ferroxidase (de Silva *et al.*, 1995), like the mammalian MCOs ceruloplasmin and hephaestin. Combining the X-ray data with Markus theory has helped to determine which characteristic amino acid residues of Fep3p confer its specificity for Fe^{2+} as its electron transfer partner

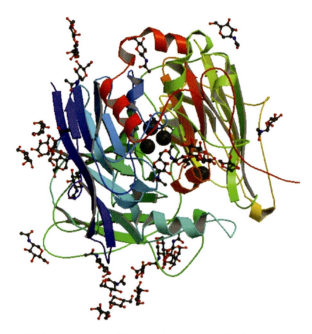

Figure 5.12 *Ribbon diagram of* S. cerevisiae *Fet3p (PDB accession code 1zpu)*

rather than some other substrate. It is concluded (Stoj *et al.*, 2006; Quintanar *et al.*, 2007) that D283, E185 and D409 in Fet3p provide an Fe(II) binding site (Figure 5.13b) which actually favours ferric iron, thus reducing the reduction potential of the bound Fe(II) in comparison to that of aqueous ferrous iron, and providing a thermodynamically more robust driving force for electron transfer. In addition, E185 and D409 constitute parts of the electron transfer pathway from the bound Fe(II) to the protein's type 1 Cu(II). This electronic coupling relies on hydrogen bonds from the carboxylate OD2 atom of each residue to the NE2 NH group of the two histidine ligands at the type 1 copper site. These two acidic residues and this hydrogen bond network appear to distinguish the fungal ferroxidase from a fungal laccase, since the specificity that Fet3p has for Fe(II) is completely lost in a Fet3pE185A/D409A mutant, while this double mutant functions kinetically better as a laccase (but not a very efficient one).

The ferroxidase step is necessary for high-affinity iron uptake, since Fet3p mutants lacking oxidase activity do not support iron transport (Wang *et al.*, 2003), and ferric iron does not function as a substrate for the Fet3p/Ftr1p complex. However, as pointed out earlier, Fet3p contains only a single transmembrane domain in its carboxyl terminus (de Silva *et al.*, 1995), and cannot be an ion channel. The identification of the *FTR1* gene, which encodes a protein with potential iron-binding sites (Stearman *et al.*, 1996) resolved this dilemma. Ftr1p has seven membrane-spanning helices (see Figure 5.11) with an overall orientation N-terminal out, C-terminal in (Severance *et al.*, 2004), and two putative iron-binding motifs REXLE in transmembrane domains; the mutation of any one of these inactivates iron transport.

Fet3p and Ftr1p are the only plasma membrane proteins required for high-affinity iron transport (Stearman *et al.*, 1996; Askwith and Kaplan, 1997), and biochemical and genetic data suggest that they form a complex in the plasma membrane (Stearman *et al.*, 1996; Yuan *et al.*, 1997; Severance *et al.*, 2004). In much the same way as iron binding to transferrin and iron incorporation into ferritin requires the oxidation of ferrous to ferric iron (see Chapters 6 and 8), iron permeation into

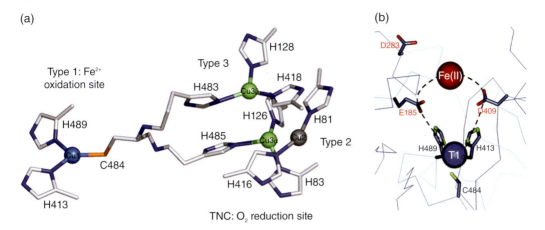

(a)

Type 1: Fe²⁺ oxidation site

Type 3

H128

H418

H483

H489

H126

H485

H81

H416

H83

Type 2

C484

H413

TNC: O₂ reduction site

(b)

D283

Fe(II)

E185

D409

H489　T1　H413

C484

Figure 5.13　*(a) Multinuclear metal site of reduced Fet3p (PDB accession code 1zpu). Type 1, type 2 and type 3 copper ions are shown as blue, grey and green spheres, respectively. The figure was rendered with PyMol version 0.97 (DeLano Scientific). Reprinted from Zaballa, M.E., Ziegler, L., Kosman, D.J. and Vila, A.J. (2010) NMR study of the exchange coupling in the trinuclear cluster of the multicopper oxidase Fet3p. J. Am. Chem. Soc.,* **132***, 11191–11196; © 2010, American Chemical Society. (b) Proposed Fe(II) binding and electron transfer site in Fet3p. The iron-binding residues E185, D283 and D409 are shown relative to the T1 copper site. Residues that coordinate the T1 copper (blue) include H413, C484 and H489. The crystal structure indicates that the OD2 carboxylate oxygen atoms of E185 and D409 are hydrogen-bonded to the NE2 NH groups of H489 and H413, respectively. The dashed arrows indicate the electron transfer pathways from the Fe(II) species to the T1 copper. The two carboxylate–imidazole hydrogen bonds are essential components of these pathways. Reprinted with permission from Stoj, C.S., Augustine, A.J., Zeigler, I., Solomon, E.I. and Kosman, D.J. (2006) Structural basis of the ferrous iron specificity of the yeast ferroxidase, Fet3p.* Biochemistry*,* **45***, 12741– 12749; © 2006, American Chemical Society*

the cell through Ftr1p is absolutely coupled to ferroxidation by Fet3p. It is proposed that the Fe(III) produced by Fet3p does not equilibrate with the bulk phase, but is transferred directly to Ftr1p for permeation by a classic metabolite channelling mechanism (Figure 5.14). Metabolite or substrate channelling[4] is a common feature of multifunctional enzymes. The transfer of Fe³⁺ from Fet3p to Ftr1p is nondissociative, and probably involves a series of ligand-exchange reactions, with a number of residues in both proteins associated with the trafficking process (for a more extensive discussion, see the articles by Kwok *et al.*, 2006a, b).

When yeast have ready access to iron, particularly as Fe²⁺, the high-affinity systems are not expressed and iron uptake takes place via low-affinity, low-specificity transporters of Fe²⁺, which can also transport other divalent cations. Three members of the Nramp family of divalent metal ion transporters, Smf1p, Smf2p and Smf3p (which we will encounter in greater detail in Chapter 7) are expressed in most yeasts (Portnoy *et al.*, 2000). Smf1p and Smf2p are essentially Mn²⁺ transporters (Portnoy *et al.*, 2000; Culotta *et al.*, 2005), although they can also transport Fe²⁺ (Cohen *et al.*, 2000). Smf3p localises to the vacuolar membrane and is proposed to help mobilise vacuolar iron

---

[4]Substrate channelling is the process of direct transfer of an intermediate between the active sites of two enzymes that catalyse sequential reactions in a biosynthetic pathway (for reviews see Srere, 1987; Ovadi, 1991).

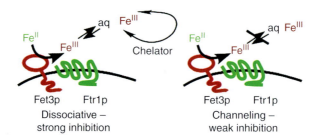

Figure 5.14 *Cartoon representing the effect of iron chelators in dissociative and channelling models of transfer of Fe(III) from Fet3p to Ftr1p. Reprinted with permission from Kwok, E.Y., Severance, S. and Kosman, D.J. (2006a) Evidence for iron channeling in the Fet3p–Ftr1p high-affinity iron uptake complex in the yeast plasma membrane.* Biochemistry, **45**, 6317–6327; © 2006, American Chemical Society

stores (Portnoy *et al.*, 2000). The role of the *SMF* gene family in iron transport in yeast is still unclear, although they may be responsible for some part of iron uptake (Portnoy *et al.*, 2002).

A second type of low-affinity, low-specificity ferrous iron transporter encoded by the *FET4* gene (Dix *et al.*, 1994, 1997) has been identified in *S. cerevisiae*, but not in other fungi. Like the Smf family of transporters, Fet4 has a relatively low substrate specificity, supporting the low-affinity uptake of other divalent metals such as cadmium, cobalt, copper, manganese and zinc (Hassett *et al.*, 2000; Portnoy *et al.*, 2001; Waters and Eide, 2002), which can result in increased metal sensitivity (Li and Kaplan, 1998). *FET4* expression and/or activity are influenced by a number of factors, including iron, zinc and oxygen (Waters and Eide, 2002).

5.3.3 Siderophore-mediated Iron Uptake

Most fungi synthesise and secrete siderophores, and express a nonreductive iron uptake system that is specific for ferric siderophores (Hsiang and Baillie, 2005). The biosynthesis of fungal siderophores, primarily hydroxamates, is well understood from molecular genetic studies in *Ustilago maydis* and *Aspergillus* sp. (Haas, 2003, 2014). The principal families of fungal siderophores are ferrichromes, fusarinines, coprogens and rhodotorulic acid. Ferric sidero-phores are taken up by plasma membrane permeases of the ARN/SIT subfamily[5] of the major facilitator superfamily (MFS) (Nelissen *et al.*, 1997; Pao *et al.*, 1998). These facilitators are composed of a single polypeptide chain predicted from homology modelling to contain 14 transmembrane domains, which most probably act as proton symporters energised by the plasma membrane potential.

Many fungi express transporters for siderophores which they are incapable of synthesizing or secreting themselves, but which are produced by other species of fungi or even by bacteria. SIT-mediated iron uptake is universally conserved in the fungal kingdom, even in species not producing siderophores, such as *S. cerevisiae*, *Candida* spp. and *C. neoformans*. More than half of the genes which are activated in *S. cerevisiae* during iron deprivation are directly or indirectly involved in the uptake of iron chelates.

The first evidence for the existence of a siderophore transport system in *S. cerevisiae* was the observation that ferrioxamine B (FOB) is efficiently taken up by cells with defective reductive

---

[5] The nomenclature in this area is incredibly complicated – the ARN nomenclature results from the fact that mRNAs for these facilitators were detected in a microarray as Aft1p-regulated (Yun *et al.*, 2000a); hence, **ARN** stands for *A*ft1p*R*egulo*N*. The *SIT* notation – *S*iderophore *I*ron *T*ransport – is probably more appropriate.

transport of iron (Lesuisse and Labbe, 1989). *Saccharomyces cerevisiae* expresses four ferri-siderophore transporters of the Arn/Sit family, capable of taking up ferri-siderophores released into the environment by other fungi and bacteria (Lesuisse *et al.*, 1998; Heymann *et al.*, 1999, 2000a,b; Yun *et al.*, 2000a,b). Each transporter exhibits specificity for a subset of siderophores: Sit1p/Arn3p for ferrioxamine B (a hydroxamate-type siderophore produced by various *Streptomyces* species), Arn1p for ferrichromes, Taf1p/Arn2p for TAFC, Enb1p/Arn4p for enterobactin (a catecholate-type siderophore produced by various Enterobacteriaceae) (Haas, 2014). In addition to the uptake of ferrioxamine B by Arn3p, another pathway was found involving the reduction and release of iron from the ferrisiderophore by the membrane ferrireductases, followed by uptake via the Fet3p/Ftr1p system (Yun *et al.*, 2000a). While the reductive system can take up iron efficiently from ferric siderophores when siderophore levels are high, at lower concentrations the uptake occurs primarily through specific siderophore transporters (Lesuisse *et al.*, 2001).

The intracellular release of iron from siderophores is probably mediated by special reductases, although this remains a matter of debate (Moore *et al.*, 2003). Subsequent to uptake, the ester bonds of triacylfusarine and fusarine–iron complexes are hydrolyzed in the cytosol respectively by the esterases EstB and SidJ (Kragl *et al.*, 2007; Grundlinger *et al.*, 2013), which belong to two different protein families. EstB is homologous to the bacterial siderophore-degrading enzyme Fes, which is involved in the release of iron from enterobactin (Brickman and McIntosh, 1992). The release of iron from siderophores is also facilitated by low pH, so special acidic compartments of the cell, such as vacuoles, may also be involved. The details of intracellular ferrisiderophore trafficking, iron release from ferrisiderophores and iron distribution following release remain unclear (reviewed in Haas, 2003, 2014). The intracellular fate of siderophores is an important element in the present understanding of the fundamental aspects of iron metabolism.

Under conditions of iron deficiency, after transcription and translation of the *ARN/SIT* family of siderophore transporters, the proteins proceed along the secretory pathway to the *trans*-Golgi network (TGN). When siderophore substrates for Arn1 and Arn3 are not available outside the cell they are sorted at the TGN into vesicles destined for degradation in the vacuolar lumen, bypassing the plasma membrane (Kim *et al.*, 2002; Froissard *et al.*, 2007). This sorting process requires recognition by clathrin adaptor proteins at the TGN, followed by ubiquitination and sorting into luminal vesicles of the multivesicular body, which are then degraded in the lumen of the vacuole (Kim *et al.*, 2007; Erpapazoglou *et al.*, 2008; Deng *et al.*, 2009). However, when siderophore substrates for Arn1 or Arn3 are present outside the cell, even at very low concentrations, the substrates entering the endosome through fluid phase endocytosis bind to a receptor domain on the transporter, which redirects the transporter into vesicles destined for the plasma membrane (Moore *et al.*, 2003; Kim *et al.*, 2005; Froissard *et al.*, 2007; Erpapazoglou *et al.*, 2008; Deng *et al.*, 2009). Thus, the Arn1 and Arn3 transporters are not expressed at the surface of yeast unless the cells are both iron-deficient and their specific siderophore substrates are available for uptake.

5.3.4 Intracellular Iron Metabolism

The mitochondria are not only the energy powerhouse of the cell but are also the site of the biosynthesis of both haem and iron–sulphur clusters (discussed in greater detail in Chapter 8). Many, but not all, of the proteins which contain haem and iron–sulphur clusters are located in the mitochondria, which makes the mitochondria a focal point for the coordination of intracellular iron metabolism. Yeast strains with a deletion in the gene *YFH1* (which corresponds to the human protein, frataxin, deficient in Friedreich's ataxia, and is discussed in more detail in Chapter 15) accumulate excess iron in mitochondria and demonstrate mitochondrial damage (Radisky *et al.*, 1999).

The excess mitochondrial iron produces increased amounts of hydroxyl radical, which in turn damages mitochondrial proteins, lipids and DNA. The damage to mitochondrial DNA generates respiratory-incompetent yeast, termed *petites*, which can survive because they regenerate cytosolic NADH by fermentation. Although the ATP yield is much less than by respiration, their survival strategy lies in fermentation, which Louis Pasteur described as '*la vie sans air*' (life without air). Mitochondrial iron metabolism will be discussed in Chapter 8.

To date, no ferritin-like iron storage proteins similar to those found in bacteria, plants, animals and almost every other living organism (see Chapter 6) have been reported in yeast. Scrutiny of the *S. cerevisiae* genome fails to reveal any gene with convincing homology to consensus sequences for ferritins. Yet, yeast cells can grow in iron-depleted media for several generations, which would imply that they must have some form of iron storage as well as mobilisation (Philpott and Protchenko, 2008). Where then is the iron stored in *S. cerevisiae*? The vacuole in fungi is a dynamic organelle which provides a storage depot for newly arrived nutrients, is the site of macromolecular degradation and nutrient recycling, and with regard to metal metabolism is associated with the handling of copper, iron, manganese and zinc, in addition to magnesium and calcium. Growth of *S. cerevisiae* on an iron-rich medium leads to iron accumulation as ferric(poly)phosphate predominantly in the vacuole (Raguzzi *et al.*, 1988), which can subsequently be used for mitochondrial haem synthesis.

In *S. cerevisiae*, the vacuolar iron importer Ccc1 transfers iron from the cytosol to the vacuole under iron-replete conditions (Li *et al.*, 2001). When *S. cerevisiae* cells undergo a transition from iron sufficiency to iron deficiency, export of iron from the vacuole to the cytosol is mediated by an oxidase–permease complex consisting of Fet5 and Fth1. The complex is functionally similar to the Fet3–Ftr1 heteromeric iron transport complex at the cell surface (Spizzo *et al.*, 1997; Urbanowski and Piper, 1999; Stearman *et al.*, 1996). This of course presupposes that there is a reductase which can supply the Fe^{2+} to the oxidase–permease complex, and it has been proposed that Fre6p plays this role (Singh *et al.*, 2007). In *S. pombe*, Pcl1 exhibits homology to *S. cerevisiae* Ccc1, and is thought to store iron in the vacuole in a manner similar to that of Ccc1 in *S. cerevisiae*. However, although the vacuolar iron importers seem similar in both yeasts, the proteins that mediate vacuolar iron export appear to be very different because of a lack of *S. pombe* homologues to the *S. cerevisiae* Fth1 and Fet5 proteins (Pouliot *et al.*, 2010). Likewise, other filamentous fungi such as *Aspergillus nidulans*, *Aspergillus fumigatus* and *Ustilago maydis* do not possess Fth1 orthologues (Haas *et al.*, 2008). It is suggested that the vacuolar transmembrane protein Abc3 may mobilise stored iron from the vacuole to the cytosol (Pouliot *et al.*, 2010), as may similar ABC transporters in the other fungi mentioned above (Labbé *et al.*, 2013).

In a recent study (Singh *et al.*, 2007) it was shown that the two efflux pathways represented by Smf3p and the ferroxidase/permease proteins, Fet5p and Fth1p, are equally efficient in trafficking iron out of the vacuole, and that Fre6p supplies Fe(II) to both efflux systems, while Fre7p plays no role in iron efflux from the vacuole. Demonstrating a role for a vacuolar metalloreductase in iron efflux supports the model that iron in the vacuole is stored in the ferric state.

In *S. cerevisiae*, ferric-ferrichrome is found in the cytosol where it seems to represent an iron storage molecule (Moore *et al.*, 2003). In some fungi that synthesise intracellular siderophores which are not secreted, iron is transferred from internalised siderophores to the intracellular siderophores for storage.

5.3.5 Iron Homeostasis

Iron homeostasis in *S. cerevisiae* for the most part involves transcriptional and post-transcriptional regulation of genes involved in iron uptake (Outten and Albetel, 2013). In response to iron deficiency, the major iron-dependent transcriptional activator Aft1 (Yamaguchi-Iwai *et al.*, 1995, 1996;

Shakoury-Elizeh *et al.*, 2004) and to a lesser extent its paralogue Aft2 (Blaiseau *et al.*, 2001; Rutherford *et al.*, 2001, 2003; Courel *et al.*, 2005), move to the nucleus where they activate genes encoding functions for iron uptake, vacuolar iron transport and mitochondrial iron metabolism. Aft1 and Aft2 bind to overlapping and separate DNA sequences through a consensus upstream activation sequence (PyPuCACCC). Nuclear localisation of the Aft1 (and presumably Aft2) is controlled by the cellular iron status (Figure 5.15). In iron-starved cells, Aft1 accumulates in the nucleus, while under iron-replete conditions Aft1 is shuttled to the cytosol by the nuclear exportin Msn5 (Yamaguchi-Iwai *et al.*, 1995, 2002; Ueta *et al.*, 2007). However, it has now been demonstrated that Msn5-mediated export is not required for the inhibition of Aft1 activity, since the transcriptional activity of Aft1p is suppressed under iron-replete conditions in the Δmsn5 strain, although Aft1p remains in the nucleus (Ueta *et al.*, 2012). Aft1p dissociates from its target promoters under iron-replete conditions due to an interaction between Aft1p and the monothiol glutaredoxins Grx3p

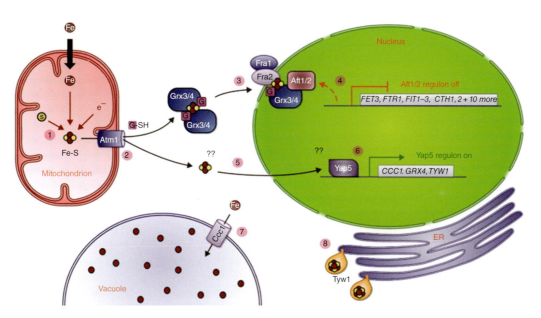

Figure 5.15 *Fe–S clusters are essential for transcriptional regulation by Aft1/2 and Yap5 during iron sufficiency in S. cerevisiae. (1) During conditions of iron sufficiency, Fe–S clusters are synthesised in mitochondria via integration of iron, sulphur, and redox control pathways. (2) An unknown substrate produced by the mitochondrial ISC machinery is exported out to the cytosol by the transporter Atm1. Glutathione (GSH) is also required for export of this signal. (3) Grx3 and Grx4, which form GSH-ligated, Fe–S-bridged complexes, are proposed to relay this signal to Aft1/2 in conjunction with Fra2 and Fra1. (4) Interaction of Grx3/4 with Aft1/2 promotes dissociation of the transcriptional activators from their target DNA, leading to deactivation of Aft1/2-regulated genes. (5) Meanwhile, the mitochondria ISC-dependent signal exported by Atm1 is also relayed to Yap5 via as-yet-unidentified factor(s). (6) This signal stimulates Yap5 activation of its target genes including CCC1, GRX4, and TYW1. (7) Increased expression of CCC1 stimulates iron import and sequestration in the vacuole, (8) while increased expression of TYW1 promotes iron sequestration as protein-bound Fe–S clusters. Increased Grx4 protein levels may also act as an iron sink in addition to ensuring Aft1/2 inactivation. Reprinted with permission from Elsevier from Outten, C.E. and Albetel, A.N. (2013) Iron sensing and regulation in Saccharomyces cerevisiae: Ironing out the mechanistic details. Curr. Opin. Microbiol., 16, 662–668*

(a)

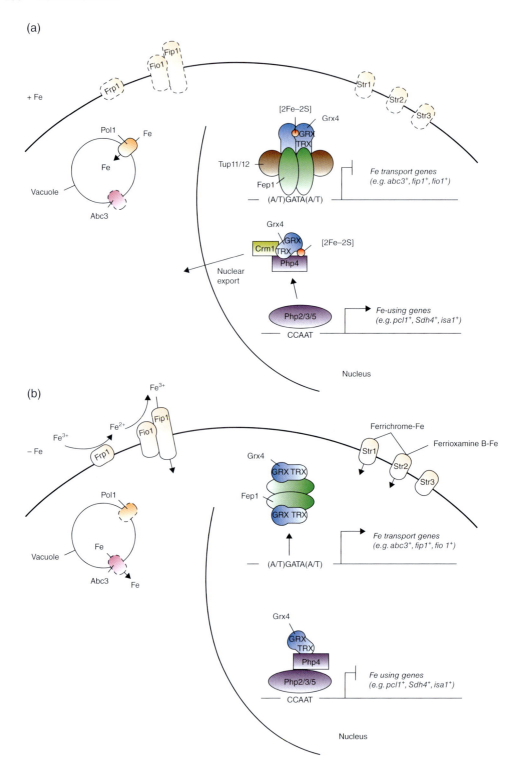

(b)

and Grx4p. Grx3 and Grx4 are known to form [2Fe–2S] cluster-binding complexes which, together with the cytosolic proteins Fra1 and Fra2, transmit an inhibitory signal to Aft1/2 that is dependent on the synthesis of mitochondrial Fe–S clusters (Rutherford *et al.*, 2005; Kumánovics *et al.*, 2008; Li *et al.*, 2009, 2011; Mühlenhoff *et al.*, 2010). The mitochondrial transporter Atm1p, which plays crucial roles in the delivery of iron–sulphur clusters from the mitochondria to the cytoplasm and nucleus, is required not only for iron binding to Grx3p but also for the dissociation of Aft1p from its target promoters. These results suggest that iron binding to Grx3p and Grx4p is a prerequisite for the suppression of Aft1p (Ueta *et al.*, 2012). As we will see in Chapter 8, all of these results support the previous observations that the mitochondrial iron–sulphur cluster assembly machinery is involved in cellular iron sensing (Figure 5.15). Previous studies by Lill and coworkers demonstrated that iron binding to Grx3/4 *in vivo* requires components of the mitochondrial Fe–S cluster (ISC) assembly machinery but not cytosolic Fe–S cluster assembly factors (Mühlenhoff *et al.*, 2010). Atm1 is proposed to export an unknown sulphur-containing substrate from the mitochondria which is used to build and/or insert Fe–S clusters into cytosolic proteins (reviewed in Lill *et al.*, 2012).

The transcriptional activator, Yap5 was first identified as an iron-responsive transcriptional activator that regulates vacuolar iron storage (Li *et al.*, 2008) by activating the expression of the vacuolar importer Ccc1 for iron storage under overload conditions. The mitochondrial ISC-dependent signal exported by Atm1 is also relayed to Yap5 via as-yet unidentified factor(s), and this stimulates Yap5 activation of its target genes including *CCC1*, and the Fe–S cluster binding proteins *GRX4*, and *TYW1* (Li *et al.*, 2011; Pimentel *et al.*, 2012) (Figure 5.15). Yap5 also appears to respond to the level of Fe–S clusters through a mechanism that does not appear to involve the glutaredoxins (Li *et al.*, 2012).

Figure 5.16 *A proposed model for the iron-dependent control of gene expression in S. pombe. (a) Under iron-replete conditions, Fep1 specifically interacts with GATA elements within the iron transport genes, repressing target gene transcription with the help of the corepressor Tup11 or Tup12. In this context, the TRX domain of Grx4 interacts with the C-terminal region of Fep1, whereas the GRX domain of Grx4 coordinates an iron–sulphur cluster ([2Fe–2S]) (red circle). In this conformation, the N terminus of Fep1 is available for DNA binding. Under iron-sufficient conditions, the GRX domain of Grx4 can also interact with Php4, leading to its inactivation. The inactivation of Php4 results in its release from the Php2/Php3/Php5 heterotrimer complex and its subsequent export from the nucleus to the cytoplasm by exportin Crm1. The absence of Php4 enables genes encoding iron-using proteins to be expressed through the CCAAT-binding core complex that is composed of Php2, Php3 and Php5. Under high-iron conditions, the pcl1⁺-encoded vacuolar transporter is expressed, whereas the transcription of abc3⁺, frp1⁺, fio1⁺, fip1⁺, str1⁺, str2⁺ and str3⁺ is repressed. (b) Under low-iron conditions, the GRX domain of Grx4 associates with Fep1 through its N terminus, blocking its interaction with chromatin and subsequently preventing its repressive effect on iron acquisition gene expression. In contrast, under the same conditions the GRX domain of Grx4 dissociates from the C-terminal region of Php4, resulting in the ability of Php4 to bind the Php2/Php3/Php5 heterotrimeric complex, thus repressing the transcription of iron-using genes, including pcl1⁺, sdh4⁺ and isa1⁺. When iron is scarce, Fe^{3+} is reduced to Fe^{2+} by the Frp1 cell surface reductase. Fe^{2+} is oxidised to Fe^{3+} by the Fio1 ferroxidase and then transported across the plasma membrane by the Fip1 permease. Siderophore-iron transporters Str1, Str2 and Str3 are active as well as Abc3, which transports stored iron from the vacuole to the cytoplasm. Protein colour codes are: Fep1 in green; Tup11/12 in brown; Grx4 in blue; Crm1 in yellow; Php2/3/4/5 in purple; Frp1, Fio1, Fip1, and Str1/2/3 in beige; Pcl1 in orange and Abc3 in pink. (Reprinted with permission from Elsevier from Labbé, S., Khan, M.G. and Jacques, J.F. (2013) Iron uptake and regulation in Schizosaccharomyces pombe. Curr. Opin. Microbiol., 16, 669–676*

At the post-transcriptional level the mRNA-binding proteins, Cth1 and Cth2, are induced by Aft1 and Aft2. The mRNAs targeted by Cth1 and Cth2 encode proteins involved in respiration, the TCA cycle, haem biosynthesis, amino acid, sterol, and fatty acid metabolism, and mitochondrial Fe–S cluster biogenesis (Philpott *et al.*, 2012). Although the targets of Cth1 and Cth2 are well-characterised, the details of how and where Cth1/Cth2 recognise and traffic their mRNA targets are nebulous, although shuttling of Cth2 between the nucleus and cytosol is important for its function in iron regulation (Vergara *et al.*, 2011).

Overall, the studies in *S. cerevisiae* highlight the importance of Fe–S clusters as key sensory molecules to monitor intracellular iron conditions, as well as revealing details of communication between vacuoles and mitochondria in response to perturbations in iron regulation and mitochondrial Fe–S biogenesis (Outten and Albatel, 2013).

In contrast to the iron-responsive activators of transcription in *S. cerevisiae*, *S. pombe* employs a GATA-type repressor, Fep1, to repress iron transport functions in iron-replete conditions. When iron is replete, Fep1 is upregulated and represses the expression of several genes, including those encoding products of the reductive, nonreductive and vacuolar iron transport systems (Pelletier, *et al.*, 2002, 2003; Pouliot *et al.*, 2010). Fep1 interacts with its target genes through recognition of the *cis*-acting element (A/T)GATA(A/T). However, like Aft1 and Aft2, Fep1 is regulated via an interaction with a monothiol glutaredoxin, Grx4. In particular, Grx4 appears to be an inhibitory binding partner for Fep1 when cells are shifted from iron sufficiency to iron depletion (Jbel *et al.*, 2011; Kim *et al.*, 2011). Whereas bacteria and *S. cerevisiae* use small RNAs and RNA-binding proteins respectively to bind specific mRNAs and to trigger their degradation, upon iron limitation *S. pombe* functions through a heteromeric DNA-binding complex that acts at the transcriptional level (Puig *et al.*, 2005; Mercier *et al.*, 2006; Labbé *et al.*, 2007; Desnoyers *et al.*, 2013; Martinez-Pastor *et al.*, 2013). Instead, this regulation occurs via a CCAAT-binding protein complex consisting of the core proteins Php2, Php3 and Php5, and the negative regulatory subunit Php4 (Mercier *et al.*, 2006, 2008). Whereas the expression of *Php2*, *Php3* and *Php5* genes is constitutive, the expression of *Php4* is induced in iron starvation and repressed in iron repletion (Mercier *et al.*, 2006). When iron is replete, Php4 expression is turned off by Fep1, and the protein is also exported from the nucleus to the cytoplasm in a process that is dependent on Grx4 and the exportin Crm1 (Mercier and Labbé, 2009). A compelling regulatory model (Figure 5.16) postulates that Grx4 binds an Fe–S cluster under the high-iron condition and interacts with Php4, leading to dissociation from the CCAAT complex and export from the nucleus. Under low-iron conditions, Grx4 dissociates from Php4 thereby allowing the protein to act with the CCAAT complex to repress the expression of iron-using functions (Labbé *et al.*, 2013).

References

Aizat, W.M., Preuss, J.M., Johnson, A.A., Tester, M.A. and Schultz, C.J. (2011) Investigation of a His-rich arabinogalactan-protein for micronutrient biofortification of cereal grain. *Physiol. Plant.*, **143**, 271–286.

Anderegg, G. and Ripperger, H. (1989) Correlation between metal complex formation and biological activity of nicotianamine analogues. *J. Chem. Soc. Chem. Commun.*, **10**, 647–650.

Aoyama, T., Kobayashi, T., Takahashi, M. (2009) OsYSL18 is a rice iron(III)-deoxymugineic acid transporter specifically expressed in reproductive organs and phloem of lamina joints. *Plant Mol. Biol.*, **70**, 681–692.

Arabidopsis Genome Initiative (2000) Analysis of the genome sequence of the flowering plant *Arabidopsis thaliana*. *Nature*, **408**, 796–815.

Arahou, M. and Diem, H.G. (1997) Iron deficiency induces cluster (proteoid) root formation in *Casuarina glauca*. *Plant Soil*, **196**, 71–79.

Arnaud, N., Murgia, I., Boucherez, J., et al. (2006) An iron-induced nitric oxide burst precedes ubiquitin-dependent protein degradation for *Arabidopsis* AtFer1 ferritin gene expression. *J. Biol. Chem.*, **281**, 23579–23588.

Ashikari, M., Sakakibara, H., Lin, S., *et al.* (2005) Cytokinin oxidase regulates rice grain production. *Science*, **309**, 741–745.

Askwith, C. and Kaplan, J. (1997) An oxidase-permease-based iron transport system in *Schizosaccharomyces pombe* and its expression in *Saccharomyces cerevisiae*. *J. Biol. Chem.*, **272**, 401–405.

Askwith, C., Eide, D., Van Ho, A. *et al.* (1994) The FET3 gene of *S. cerevisiae* encodes a multicopper oxidase required for ferrous iron uptake. *Cell*, **76**, 403–410.

Baena-Gonzalez, E. and Sheen, J. (2008) Convergent energy and stress signaling. *Trends Plant Sci.*, **13**, 474–482.

Baena-Gonzalez, E., Rolland, F., Thevelein, J.M. and Sheen, J. (2007) A central integrator of transcription networks in plant stress and energy signaling. *Nature*, **448**, 938–942.

Barberon, M., Zelazny, E., Robert, S., *et al.* (2011) Monoubiquitin-dependent endocytosis of the iron-regulated transporter 1 (IRT1) transporter controls iron uptake in plants. *Proc. Natl Acad. Sci. USA*, **108**, E450–E458.

Baruah, A., Simková, K., Apel, K. and Laloi, C. (2009) *Arabidopsis* mutants reveal multiple singlet oxygen signaling pathways involved in stress response and development. *Plant Mol. Biol.*, **70**, 547–563.

Bashir, K., Inoue, H., Nagasaki, S., *et al.* (2006) Cloning and characterization of deoxymugineic acid synthase genes from graminaceous plants. *J. Biol. Chem.*, **281**, 32395–32402.

Bashir, K., Ishimaru, Y., Shimo, H., *et al.* (2011a) The rice mitochondrial iron transporter is essential for plant growth. *Nat. Commun.*, **2**, 322.

Bashir, K., Ishimaru, Y. and Nishizawa, N.K. (2011b) Identification and characterization of the major mitochondrial Fe transporter in rice. *Plant Signal. Behav.*, **6**, 1591–1593.

Bashir, K., Nozoye, T., Ishimaru, Y., Nakanishi, H. and Nishizawa, N.K. (2013) Exploiting new tools for iron bio-fortification of rice. *Biotechnol. Adv.*, **31**, 1624–1633.

Bassel, G.W., Gaudinier, A., Brady, S.M., *et al.* (2012) Systems analysis of plant functional, transcriptional, physical interaction, and metabolic networks. *Plant Cell*, **24**, 3859–3875.

Basso, B., Bagnaresi, P., Bracale, M. and Soave, C. (1994) The yellow-stripe-1 and -3 mutants of maize: nutritional and biochemical studies. *Maydica*, **39**, 97–105.

Becker, R., Fritz, E. and Manteuffel, R. (1995) Subcellular localization and characterization of excessive iron in the nicotianamine-less tomato mutant chloronerva. *Plant Physiol.*, **108**, 269–275.

Bereczky, Z., Wang, H.Y., Schubert, V., Ganal M. and Bauer, P. (2003) Differential regulation of nramp and irt metal transporter genes in wild type and iron uptake mutants of tomato. *J. Biol. Chem.*, **278**, 24697–24704.

Bernal, M., Casero, D., Singh, V., *et al.* (2012) Transcriptome sequencing identifies SPL7-regulated copper acquisition genes FRO4/FRO5 and the copper dependence of iron homeostasis in *Arabidopsis*. *Plant Cell*, **24**, 738–761.

Bienfait, H.F. (1985) Regulated redox processes at the plasmalemma of plant root cells and their function in iron uptake. *J. Bioenerg. Biomembr.*, **17**, 73–83.

Blackburn, N.J., Ralle, M., Hassett, R. and Kosman, D.J. (2000) Spectroscopic analysis of the trinuclear cluster in the Fet3 protein from yeast, a multinuclear copper oxidase. *Biochemistry*, **39**, 2316–2324.

Blaiseau, P.L., Lesuisse, E. and Camadro, J.M. (2001) Aft2p, a novel iron-regulated transcription activator that modulates, with Aft1p, intracellular iron use and resistance to oxidative stress in yeast. *J. Biol. Chem.*, **276**, 34221–34226.

Bolger, M.E., Weisshaar, B., Scholz, U., *et al.* (2014) Plant genome sequencing – applications for crop improvement. *Curr. Opin. Biotechnol.*, **26**, 31–37.

Briat, J.-F., Fobis-Loisy, I., Grignon, N., *et al.* (1995) Cellular and molecular aspects of iron metabolism in plants. *Biol. Cell*, **84**, 69–81.

Briat, J.-F., Duc, C., Ravet, K. and Gaymard, F. (2010a) Ferritins and iron storage in plants. *Biochim. Biophys. Acta*, **1800**, 806–814.

Briat, J.-F., Ravet, K., Arnaud, N., Duc, C., *et al.* (2010b) New insights into ferritin synthesis and function highlight a link between iron homeostasis and oxidative stress in plants. *Ann. Bot.*, **105**, 811–822.

Brickman, T.J. and McIntosh, M.A. (1992) Overexpression and purification of ferric enterobactin esterase from *Escherichia coli*. Demonstration of enzymatic hydrolysis of enterobactin and its iron complex. *J. Biol. Chem.*, **267**, 12350–12355.

Brown, J.C. and Chaney, R.L. (1971) Effect of iron on the transport of citrate into the xylem of soybeans and tomatoes. *Plant Physiol.*, **47**, 836-840.

Cailliatte, R., Schikora, A., Briat, J.F., Mari, S. and Curie, C. (2010) High-affinity manganese uptake by the metal transporter NRAMP1 is essential for *Arabidopsis* growth in low manganese conditions. *Plant Cell*, **22**, 904–917.

Carvalhais, L.C., Dennis, P.G., Fedoseyenko, D., *et al.* (2011) Root exudation of sugars, amino acids, and organic acids by maize as affected by nitrogen, phosphorus, potassium, and iron deficiency. *J. Plant Nutr. Soil Sci.*, **174**, 3–11.

Chanock, S.J., el Benna, J., Smith, R.M. and Babior, B.M. (1994) The respiratory burst oxidase. *J. Biol. Chem.*, **269**, 24519–24522.

Chen, W.W., Yang, Y., Shin, J.L., *et al.* (2010) Nitric oxide acts downstream of auxin to trigger root ferric-chelate reductase activity in response to iron deficiency in *Arabidopsis*. *Plant Physiol.*, **154**, 810–819.

Chen, Y. and Barak, P. (1982) Iron nutrition of plants in calcareous soils. *Adv. Agron.*, **35**, 217–240.

Chen, Y.Y., Wang, Y., Shin, L.J., *et al.* (2013) Iron is involved in maintenance of circadian period length in *Arabidopsis*. *Plant Physiol.* 10.1104/112.212068.

Chu, H.H., Chiecko, J., Punshon, T., *et al.* (2010) Successful reproduction requires the function of *Arabidopsis* Yellow Stripe-Like1 and Yellow Stripe-Like3 metal nicotianamine transporters in both vegetative and reproductive structures. *Plant Physiol.*, **154**, 197–210.

Cohen, A., Nelson, H. and Nelson, N. (2000) The family of SMF metal ion transporters in yeast cells. *J. Biol. Chem.*, **275**, 33388–33394.

Cohen, C.K., Garvin, D.F. and Kochian, L.V. (2004) Kinetic properties of a micronutrient transporter from *Pisum sativum* indicate a primary function in Fe uptake from the soil. *Planta*, **218**, 784–792.

Colangelo, E.P. and Guerinot, M.L. (2004) The essential basic helix-loop-helix protein FIT1 is required for the iron deficiency response. *Plant Cell*, **16**, 3400–3412.

Connolly, E.L., Campbell, N.H., Grotz, N., *et al.* (2003). Overexpression of the FRO2 ferric chelate reductase confers tolerance to growth on low iron and uncovers posttranscriptional control. *Plant Physiol.*, **133**, 1102–1110.

Conte, S.S. and Walker, E.L. (2011) Transporters contributing to iron trafficking in plants. *Mol. Plant*, **4**, 464–476.

Courel, M., Lallet, S., Camadro J.M. and Blaiseau, P.L. (2005) Direct activation of genes involved in intracellular iron use by the yeast iron-responsive transcription factor Aft2 without its paralog Aft1. *Mol. Cell. Biol.*, **25**, 6760–6771.

Culotta, V.C., Yang, M. and Hall, M.D. (2005) Manganese transport and trafficking: lessons learned from *Saccharomyces cerevisiae*. *Eukaryot. Cell*, **4**, 1159–1165.

Curie, C., Alonso, J.M., Le Jean, M., *et al.* (2000) Involvement of NRAMP1 from *Arabidopsis thaliana* in iron transport. *Biochem. J.*, **347**, 749–755.

Curie, C., Panaviene, Z., Loulergue, C., *et al.* (2001). Maize *yellow stripe1* encodes a membrane protein directly involved in Fe(III) uptake. *Nature*, **409**, 346–349.

Curie, C., Cassin, G., Couch, D., *et al.* (2009) Metal movement within the plant: contribution of nicotianamine and yellow stripe 1-like transporters. *Ann Bot.*, **103**, 1–11.

Cvitanich, C., Przybyłowicz, W.J., Urbanski, D.F., *et al.* (2010) Iron and ferritin accumulate in separate cellular locations in Phaseolus seeds. *BMC Plant Biol.*, **10**, 26.

Cyert, M.S. and Philpott, C.C. (2013) Regulation of cation balance in *Saccharomyces cerevisiae*. *Genetics*, **193**, 677–713.

Dancis, A., Klausner, R.D., Hinnebusch, A.G. and Barriocanal, J.G. (1990) Genetic evidence that ferric reductase is required for iron uptake in *Saccharomyces cerevisiae*. *Mol. Cell. Biol.*, **10**, 2294–2301.

Dancis, A., Roman D.G., Anderson, G.J., *et al.* (1992) Ferric reductase of *Saccharomyces cerevisiae*: molecular characterization, role in iron uptake, and transcriptional control by iron. *Proc. Natl Acad. Sci. USA*, **89**, 3869–3873.

Dancis, A., Yuan, D.S., Haile, D., *et al.* (1994) Molecular characterization of a copper transport protein in *S. cerevisiae*: an unexpected role for copper in iron transport. *Cell*, **76**, 393–402.

Darbani, B., Briat, J.F., Holm, P.B., *et al.* (2013) Dissecting plant iron homeostasis under short and long-term iron fluctuations. *Biotechnol. Adv.*, **31**, 1292–1307.

Deng, Y., Guo, Y., Watson, H., *et al.* (2009) Gga2 mediates sequential ubiquitin independent and ubiquitin-dependent steps in the trafficking of ARN1 from the trans Golgi network to the vacuole. *J. Biol. Chem.*, **284**, 23830–23841.

Deshmukh, R., Sonah, H., Patil, G., *et al.* (2014) Integrating omic approaches for abiotic stress tolerance in soybean. *Front Plant Sci.*, **5**, 244.

de Silva, D.M., Askwith, C.C., Eide, J. and Kaplan, J. (1995) The FET3 gene product required for high affinity iron transport in yeast is a cell surface ferroxidase. *J. Biol. Chem.*, **270**, 1098–1101.

de Silva, D., Davis-Kaplan, S., Fergestad, J. and Kaplan, J. (1997) Purification and characterization of Fet3 protein, a yeast homologue of ceruloplasmin. *J. Biol. Chem.*, **272**, 14208–14213.

Desnoyers, G., Bouchard, M.P. and Massé, E. (2013) New insights into small RNA dependent translational regulation in prokaryotes. *Trends Genet.*, **29**, 92–98.

D'Hont, A., Denoeud, F., Aury, J.M., *et al.* (2012) The banana (*Musa acuminata*) genome and the evolution of monocotyledonous plants. *Nature*, **488**, 213–217.

DiDonato, R.J., Jr, Roberts, L.A., Sanderson, T., Eisley, R.B. and Walker, E.L. (2004) *Arabidopsis* Yellow Stripe-Like2 (YSL2): a metal-regulated gene encoding a plasma membrane transporter of nicotianamine–metal complexes. *Plant J.*, **39**, 403–414.

Ding, Z., Millar, A.J., Davis, A.M. and Davis, S.J. (2007) TIME FOR COFFEE encodes a nuclear regulator in the *Arabidopsis thaliana* circadian clock. *Plant Cell*, **19**, 1522–1536.

Dix, D.R., Bridgham, J.T., Broderius, M.A., Byersdorfer, C.A. and Eide, D.J. (1994) The FET4 gene encodes the low affinity Fe(II) transport protein of *Saccharomyces cerevisiae*. *J. Biol. Chem.*, **269**, 26092–26099.

Dix, D.R., Bridgham, J.T., Broderius, M.A. and Eide, D.J. (1997) Characterization of the FET4 protein of yeast. Evidence for a direct role in the transport of iron. *J. Biol. Chem.*, **272**, 11770–11777.

Durrett, T.P., Gassmann, W. and Rogers, E.E. (2007) The FRD3-mediated efflux of citrate into the root vasculature is necessary for efficient iron translocation. *Plant Physiol.*, **144**, 197–205.

Duc, C., Cellier, F., Lobréaux, S., Briat, J.F. and Gaymard, F. (2009) Regulation of iron homeostasis in *Arabidopsis thaliana* by the clock regulator time for coffee. *J. Biol. Chem.*, **284**, 36271–36281.

Duy, D., Wanner, G., Meda, A.R., *et al.* (2007) PIC1, an ancient permease in *Arabidopsis* chloroplasts, mediates iron transport. *Plant Cell*, **19**, 986–1006.

Duy, D., Stübe, R., Wanner, G. and Philippar, K. (2011) The chloroplast permease PIC1 regulates plant growth and development by directing homeostasis and transport of iron. *Plant Physiol.* **155**, 1709–1722.

Eckardt, N.A. and Bennett, M. (2012) In silico plant biology comes of age. *Plant Cell*, **24**, 3857–3858.

Eckhardt, U. and Buckhout, T.J. (1998) Iron assimilation in *Chlamydomonas reinhardtii* involves ferric reduction and is similar to Strategy I higher plants. *J. Exp. Bot.*, **9**, 1219–1226.

Eckhardt, U., Mas Marques, A. and Kochian, L.V. (2001) Two iron-regulated cation transporters from tomato complement metal uptake-deficient yeast mutants. *Plant Mol. Biol.*, **45**, 437–448.

Eide, D.J. (2004) The SLC39 family of metal ion transporters. *Pflugers Arch.*, **447**, 796–800.

Eide, D.J. (2006) Zinc transporters and the cellular trafficking of zinc. *Biochim. Biophys. Acta*, **1763**, 711–722.

Eide, D., Broderius, M., Fett, J. and Guerinot, M.L. (1996) A novel iron-regulated metal transporter from plants identified by functional expression in yeast. *Proc. Natl Acad. Sci. USA*, **93**, 5624–5628.

Eisendle, M., Oberegger, H., Zadra, I. and Haas, H. (2003) The siderophore system is essential for viability of *Aspergillus nidulans*: functional analysis of two genes encoding l-ornithine N-5-monooxygenase (sidA) and a non-ribosomal peptide synthetase (sidC). *Mol. Microbiol.*, **49**, 359–375.

Ellis, M., Egelund, J., Schultz, C.J. and Bacic, A. (2010) Arabinogalactan-proteins: key regulators at the cell surface? *Plant Physiol.*, **153**, 403–419.

Erpapazoglou, Z., Froissard, M., Nondier, I., *et al.* (2008) Substrate- and ubiquitin dependent trafficking of the yeast siderophore transporter Sit1. *Traffic*, **9**, 1372–1391.

Feng, H., An, F., Zhang, S., *et al.* (2006) Light-regulated, tissue-specific, and cell differentiation-specific expression of the *Arabidopsis* Fe(III)-chelate reductase gene AtFRO6. *Plant Physiol.*, **140**, 1345–1354.

Fiorani, F. and Schurr, U. (2013) Future scenarios for plant phenotyping. *Annu. Rev. Plant Biol.*, **64**, 267–291.

Fourcroy, P., Sisó-Terraza, P., Sudre, D., *et al.* (2013) Involvement of the ABCG37 transporter in secretion of scopoletin and derivatives by *Arabidopsis* roots in response to iron deficiency. *New Phytol.*, **201**, 155–167.

Fragoso, S., Espíndola, L., Páez-Valencia, J., *et al.* (2009) SnRK1 isoforms AKIN10 and AKIN11 are differentially regulated in *Arabidopsis* plants under phosphate starvation. *Plant Physiol.*, **149**, 1906–1916.

Froissard, M., Belgareh-Touzé, N., Dias, M., *et al.* (2007) Trafficking of siderophore transporters in *Saccharomyces cerevisiae* and intracellular fate of ferrioxamine B conjugates. *Traffic*, **8**, 1601–1616.

Fuglsang, A.T., Guo, Y., Cuin, T.A., *et al.* (2007) *Arabidopsis* protein kinase PKS5 inhibits the plasma membrane H$^+$-ATPase by preventing interaction with 14-3-3 protein. *Plant Cell*, **19**, 1617–1634.

Garcia, M.J., Lucena, C., Romera, F.J., Alcántara, E. and Pérez-Vicente, R. (2010) Ethylene and nitric oxide involvement in the up-regulation of key genes related to iron acquisition and homeostasis in *Arabidopsis*. *J. Exp. Bot.*, **61**, 3885–3899.

Gazzarini, S. and McCourt, P. (2001) Genetic interactions between ABA, ethylene and sugar signaling pathways. *Curr. Opin. Plant Biol.*, **4**, 387–391.

Giehl, R.F., Lima, J.E. and von Wiren, N. (2012) Localized iron supply triggers lateral root elongation in *Arabidopsis* by altering the AUX1-mediated auxin distribution. *Plant Cell*, **24**, 33–49.

Gitan, R.S. and Eide, D.J. (2000) Zinc-regulated ubiquitin conjugation signals endocytosis of the yeast ZRT1 zinc transporter. *Biochem. J.*, **346**, 329–336.

Georgatsou, E. and Alexandraki, D. (1994) Two distinctly regulated genes are required for ferric reduction, the first step of iron uptake in *Saccharomyces cerevisiae*. *Mol. Cell. Biol.*, **14**, 3065–3073.

Georgatsou, E. and Alexandraki, D. (1999) Regulated expression of the *Saccharomyces cerevisiae* Fre1p/Fre2p Fe/Cu reductase related genes. *Yeast*, **15**, 573–584.

Georgatsou, E., Mavrogiannis, L.A., Fragiadakis, G.S. and Alexandraki, D. (1997) The yeast Fre1p/Fre2p cupric reductases facilitate copper uptake and are regulated by the copper-modulated Mac1p activator. *J. Biol. Chem.*, **272**, 13786–13792.

Goff, S.A., Ricke, D., Lan, T.H., *et al.* (2002) A draft sequence of the rice genome (*Oryza sativa* L. ssp. *japonica*). *Science*, **296**, 92–100.

Goulet, C., Mageroy, M.H., Lam, N.B., *et al.* (2012) Role of an esterase in flavor volatile variation within the tomato clade. *Proc. Natl Acad. Sci. USA*, **109**, 19009–19014.

Green, L.S. and Rogers, E.E. (2004) FRD3 controls iron localization in *Arabidopsis*. *Plant Physiol.*, **136**, 2523–2531.

Grillet, L., Mari, S. and Schmidt, W. (2014a) Iron in seeds – loading pathways and subcellular localization. *Front. Plant Sci.*, **4**, 535.

Grillet, L., Ouerdane, L., Flis, P., *et al.* (2014b) Ascorbate efflux as a new strategy for iron reduction and transport in plants. *J. Biol. Chem.*, **289**, 2515–2525.

Guerinot, M.L. and Yi, Y. (1994) Iron: Nutritious, noxious, and not readily available. *Plant Physiol.*, **104**, 815–820.

Guerinot, M.L. (2000) The ZIP family of metal transporters. *Biochim. Biophys. Acta*, **1465**, 190–198.

Guo, S., Zhang, J., Sun, H., *et al.* (2013) The draft genome of watermelon (*Citrullus lanatus*) and resequencing of 20 diverse accessions. *Nat. Genet.*, **45**, 51–58.

Gründlinger, M., Gsaller, F., Schrettl, M., Lindner, H. and Haas, H. (2013) *Aspergillus fumigatus* SidJ mediates intracellular siderophore hydrolysis. *Appl. Environ. Microbiol.*, **79**, 7534–7536.

Haas, H. (2003) Molecular genetics of fungal siderophore biosynthesis and uptake: the role of siderophores in iron uptake and storage. *Appl. Microbiol. Biotechnol.*, **62**, 316–330.

Haas, H. (2014) Fungal siderophore metabolism with a focus on *Aspergillus fumigatus*. *Nat. Prod. Rep.*, **31**, 1266–1276.

Haas, J.D., Beard, J.L., Murray-Kolb, L.E., *et al.* (2005) Iron-biofortified rice improves the iron stores of nonanemic Filipino women. *J. Nutr.*, **135**, 2823–2830.

Haas, H., Eisendle, M. and Turgeon, B.G. (2008) Siderophores in fungal physiology and virulence. *Annu. Rev. Phytopathol.*, **46**, 149–187.

Hall, A., Bastow, R.M., Davis, S.J, *et al.* (2003) The TIME FOR COFFEE gene maintains the amplitude and timing of *Arabidopsis* circadian clocks. *Plant Cell*, **15**, 2719–2729.

Hänsch, R. and Mendel, R.R. (2008) Physiological functions of mineral micronutrients (Cu, Zn, Mn, Fe, Ni, Mo, B, Cl). *Curr. Opin. Plant Biol.*, **12**, 259–266.

Hassett, R.F. and Kosman, D.J. (1995) Evidence for Cu(II) reduction as a component of copper uptake by *Saccharomyces cerevisiae*. *J. Biol. Chem.*, **270**, 128–134.

Hassett, R.F., Romeo, A.M. and Kosman, D.J. (1998a) Regulation of high affinity iron uptake in the yeast *Saccharomyces cerevisiae*. Role of dioxygen and Fe. *J. Biol. Chem.*, **273**, 7628–7636.

Hassett, R.F., Yuan, D.S. and Kosman, D.J. (1998b) Spectral and kinetic properties of the Fet3 protein from *Saccharomyces cerevisiae*, a multinuclear copper ferroxidase enzyme. *J. Biol. Chem.*, **273**, 23274–23282.

Hassett, R., Dix, D.R., Eide, D.J. and Kosman, D.J. (2000) The Fe(II) permease Fet4p functions as a low affinity copper transporter and supports normal copper trafficking in *Saccharomyces cerevisiae*. *Biochem. J.*, **351** (Pt 2), 477–484.

Haydon, M.J., Kawachi, M., Wirtz, M., *et al.* (2012) Vacuolar nicotianamine has critical and distinct roles under iron deficiency and for zinc sequestration in *Arabidopsis*. *Plant Cell*, **24**, 724–737.

Heazlewood, J.L., Tonti-Filippini, J.S., Gout, A.M., *et al.* (2004) Experimental analysis of the *Arabidopsis* mitochondrial proteome highlights signaling and regulatory components, provides assessment of targeting prediction programs, and indicates plant-specific mitochondrial proteins. *Plant Cell*, **16**, 241–256.

Hell, R. and Stephan, U.R. (2003) Iron uptake, trafficking and homeostasis in plants. *Planta*, **216**, 541–551.

Herbik, A., Koch, G., Mock, H.P., *et al.* (1999) Isolation, characterization and cDNA cloning of nicotianamine synthase from barley. A key enzyme for iron homeostasis in plants. *Eur. J. Biochem.*, **265**, 231–239.

Hernandez, P., Martis, M., Dorado, G., *et al.* (2012) Next-generation sequencing and syntenic integration of flow-sorted arms of wheat chromosome 4A exposes the chromosome structure and gene content. *Plant J.*, **69**, 377–386.

Heymann, P., Ernst, J.F. and Winkelmann, G. (1999) Identification of a fungal triacetylfusarinine C siderophore transport gene (*TAF1*) in *Saccharomyces cerevisiae* as a member of the major facilitator superfamily. *Biometals*, **12**, 301–306.

Heymann, P., Ernst, J.F. and Winkelmann, G. (2000a) Identification and substrate specificity of a ferrichrome-type siderophore transporter (Arn1p) in *Saccharomyces cerevisiae*. *FEMS Microbiol. Lett.*, **186**, 221–227.

Heymann, P., Ernst, J.F. and Winkelmann, G. (2000b) A gene of the major facilitator superfamily encodes a transporter for enterobactin (Enb1p) in *Saccharomyces cerevisiae*. *Biometals*, **13**, 65–72.

Higa, A., Miyamoto, E., ur Rahman, L. and Kitamura, Y. (2008) Root tip-dependent, active riboflavin secretion by *Hyoscyamus albus* hairy roots under iron deficiency. *Plant Physiol. Biochem.*, **46**, 452–460.

Higa, A., Mori, Y. and Kitamura, Y. (2010) Iron deficiency induces changes in riboflavin secretion and the mitochondrial electron transport chain in hairy roots of *Hyoscyamus albus*. *J. Plant Physiol.*, **167**, 870–878.

Higa, A., Khandakar, J., Mori, Y. and Kitamura Y. (2012) Increased de novo riboflavin synthesis and hydrolysis of FMN are involved in riboflavin secretion from *Hyoscyamus albus* hairy roots under iron deficiency. *Plant Physiol. Biochem.*, **58**, 166–173.

Higuchi, K., Suzuki, K., Nakanishi, H., *et al.* (1999) Cloning of nicotianamine synthase genes, novel genes involved in the biosynthesis of phytosiderophores. *Plant Physiol.*, **119**, 471–480.

Higuchi, K., Tani, M., Nakanishi, H., *et al.* (2001) The expression of a barley *HvNAS1* nicotianamine synthase gene promoter-*gus* fusion gene in transgenic tobacco is induced by Fe-deficiency in roots. *Biosci. Biotechnol. Biochem.*, **65**, 1692–1696.

Hindt, M.N. and Guerinot, M.L. (2012) Getting a sense for signals: regulation of the plant iron deficiency response. *Biochim. Biophys. Acta*, **1823**, 1521–1530.

Hong, S., Kim, S.A., Guerinot, M.L. and McClung, C.R. (2013) Reciprocal interaction of the circadian clock with the Fe homeostasis network in *Arabidopsis thaliana*. *Plant Physiol.*, **161**, 893–903.

Hsiang, T. and Baillie, D.L. (2005) Comparison of the yeast proteome to other fungal genomes to find core fungal genes. *J. Mol. Evol.*, **60**, 475–483.

Hu, B., Zhu, C., Li, F., *et al.* (2011) LEAF TIP NECROSIS1 plays a pivotal role in the regulation of multiple phosphate starvation responses in rice. *Plant Physiol.*, **156**, 1101–1115.

Huang, X.Y., Chao, D.Y., Gao, J.P., *et al.* (2009) A previously unknown zinc finger protein, DST, regulates drought and salt tolerance in rice via stomatal aperture control. *Genes Dev.*, **23**, 1805–1817.

Huang, X., Zhao, Y., Wei, X., *et al.* (2012) Genome-wide association study of flowering time and grain yield traits in a worldwide collection of rice germplasm. *Nat. Genet.*, **44**, 32–39.

Inoue, H., Higuchi, K., Takahashi, M., *et al.* (2003) Three rice nicotianamine synthase genes, *OsNAS1*, *OsNAS2*, and *OsNAS3*, are expressed in cells involved in long-distance transport of iron and differentially regulated by iron. *Plant J.*, **36**, 366–381.

Inoue, H., Takahashi, M., Kobayashi, M., *et al.* (2008) Identification and localisation of the rice nicotianamine aminotransferase gene *OsNAAT1* expression suggests the site of phytosiderophore synthesis in rice. *Plant Mol. Biol.*, **66**, 193–203.

Inoue, H., Kobayashi, T., Nozoye, T., *et al.* (2009) Rice OsYSL15 is an iron-regulated iron(III)-deoxymugineic acid transporter expressed in the roots and is essential for iron uptake in early growth of the seedlings. *J. Biol. Chem.*, **284**, 3470–3479.

Ishimaru, Y., Suzuki, M., Tsukamoto, T., *et al.* (2006) Rice plants take up iron as a Fe^{3+}-phytosiderophore and as Fe^{2+}. *Plant J.*, **45**, 335–346.

Ishimaru, Y., Masuda, H., Bashir, K., *et al.* (2010) Rice metal-nicotianamine transporter, OsYSL2, is required for the long-distance transport of iron and manganese. *Plant J.*, **62**, 379–390.

Ishimaru, Y., Kakei, Y., Shimo, H., *et al.* (2011) A rice phenolic efflux transporter is essential for solubilizing precipitated apoplasmic iron in the plant stele. *J. Biol. Chem.*, **286**, 24649–24655.

Ivanov, R., Brumbarova, T. and Bauer, P. (2012) Fitting into the harsh reality: regulation of iron-deficiency responses in dicotyledonous plants. *Mol. Plant*, **5**, 27–42.

Jahn, T. Fuglsang, A.T., Olsson, A., *et al.* (1997) The 14-3-3 protein interacts directly with the C-terminal region of the plant plasma membrane H(+)-ATPase. *Plant Cell*, **9**, 1805–1814.

Jaillon, O., Aury, J.M., Noel, B., *et al.*, (2007) The grapevine genome sequence suggests ancestral hexaploidization in major angiosperm phyla. *Nature*, **449**, 463–467.

Jain, A. and Connolly, E.L. (2013) Mitochondrial iron transport and homeostasis in plants. *Front. Plant Sci.*, **4**, 348.

Jain, A., Wilson, G.T. and Connolly, E.L. (2014) The diverse roles of FRO family metalloreductases in iron and copper homeostasis. *Front. Plant Sci.*, **5**, 100.

Jakoby, M., Wang, H.Y., Reidt, W., Weisshaar, B. and Bauer, P. (2004) FRU(BHLH029) is required for induction of iron mobilization genes in *Arabidopsis thaliana*. *FEBS Lett.*, **577**, 528–534.

Jaquinod, M., Villiers, F., Kieffer-Jaquinod, S., *et al.* (2007) A proteomics dissection of *Arabidopsis thaliana* vacuoles isolated from cell culture. *Mol. Cell. Proteomics*, **6**, 394–412.

Jbel, M., Mercier, A. and Labbé, S. (2011) Grx4 monothiol glutaredoxin is required for iron limitation-dependent inhibition of Fep1. *Eukaryot. Cell*, **10**, 629–645.

Jeong, J. and Connolly, E.L. (2009) Iron uptake mechanisms in plants: function of the FRO family of ferric reductases. *Plant Sci.*, **176**, 709–714.

Jeong, J., Cohu, C., Kerkeb, L., *et al.* (2008) Chloroplast Fe(III) chelate reductase activity is essential for seedling viability under iron limiting conditions. *Proc. Natl Acad. Sci. USA*, **105**, 10619–10624.

Jin, C.W., You, G.Y., He, Y.F., *et al.* (2007) Iron deficiency-induced secretion of phenolics facilitates the reutilization of root apoplastic iron in red clover. *Plant Physiol.*, **144**, 278–285.

Kakei, Y., Yamaguchi, I., Kobayashi, T., *et al.* (2009) A highly sensitive, quick and simple quantification method for nicotianamine and 2'-deoxymugineic acid from minimum samples using LC/ESI-TOF-MS achieves functional analysis of these components in plants. *Plant Cell Physiol.* **50**, 1988–1993.

Kaplan, C.D. and Kaplan, J. (2009) Iron acquisition and transcriptional regulation. *Chem. Rev.*, **109**, 4536–4552.

Kerkeb, L., Mukherjee, I., Chatterjee, I., *et al.* (2008) Iron-induced turnover of the *Arabidopsis* IRON-REGULATED TRANSPORTER1 metal transporter requires lysine residues. *Plant Physiol.*, **146**, 1964–1973.

Kim, C.K., Han, J.S., Lee, H.S., *et al.* (2006) Expression of an *Arabidopsis* CAX2 variant in potato tubers increases calcium levels with no accumulation of manganese. *Plant Cell Rep.*, **25**, 1226–1232.

Kim, H.J., Lee, K.C. and Roe, J.H. (2011) Multi-domain CGFS-type glutaredoxin Grx4 regulates iron homeostasis via direct interaction with a repressor Fep1 in fission yeast. *Biochem. Biophys. Res. Commun.*, **408**, 609–614.

Kim, S.A. and Guerinot, M.L. (2007) Mining iron: iron uptake and transport in plants. *FEBS Lett.*, **581**, 2273–2280.

Kim, S.A., Punshon, T., Lanzirotti, A., *et al.* (2006) Localization of iron in *Arabidopsis* seed requires the vacuolar membrane transporter VIT1. *Science*, **314**, 1295–1298.

Kim, Y., Yun, C.W. and Philpott, C.C. (2002) Ferrichrome induces endosome to plasma membrane cycling of the ferrichrome transporter, Arn1p, in *Saccharomyces cerevisiae*. *EMBO J.*, **21**, 3632–3642.

Kim, Y., Lampert, S.M. and Philpott, C.C. (2005) A receptor domain controls the intracellular sorting of the ferrichrome transporter, ARN1. *EMBO J.*, **24**, 952–962.

Kim, Y., Deng, Y. and Philpott, C.C. (2007) GGA2- and ubiquitin-dependent trafficking of Arn1, the ferrichrome transporter of *Saccharomyces cerevisiae*. *Mol. Biol. Cell*, **18**, 1790–1802.

Kloosterman, B., Abelenda, J.A., Gomez Mdel, M., *et al.* (2013) Naturally occurring allele diversity allows potato cultivation in northern latitudes. *Nature*, **495**, 246–250.

Kobayashi, T. and Nishizawa, N.K. (2012) Iron uptake, translocation, and regulation in higher plants. *Annu. Rev. Plant Biol.*, **63**, 131–152.

Kobayashi, T. and Nishizawa, N.K. (2014) Iron sensors and signals in response to iron deficiency. *Plant Sci.*, **224**, 36–43.

Koike, S., Inoue, H., Mizuno, D., *et al.* (2004) OsYSL2 is a rice metal-nicotianamine transporter that is regulated by iron and expressed in the phloem. *Plant J.*, **39**, 415–424.

Kong, W.W., Zhang, L.P., Guo, K., Liu, Z.P. and Yang, Z.M. (2010) Carbon monoxide improves adaptation of *Arabidopsis* to iron deficiency. *Plant Biotechnol. J.*, **8**, 88–99.

Kosman, D.J. (2010) Multicopper oxidases: a workshop on copper coordination chemistry, electron transfer, and metallophysiology. *J. Biol. Inorg. Chem.*, **15**, 15–28.

Kragl, C., Schrettl, M., Abt, B., *et al.* (2007) EstB-mediated hydrolysis of the siderophore triacetylfusarinine C optimizes iron uptake of *Aspergillus fumigatus*. *Eukaryot. Cell*, **6**, 1278–1285.

Kruger, C., Berkowitz, O., Stephan, U.W. and Hell, R. (2002) A metal-binding member of the late embryogenesis abundant protein family transports iron in the phloem of *Ricinus communis* L. *J. Biol. Chem.*, **277**, 25062–25069.

Kumánovics, A., Chen, O.S., Li, L., *et al.* (2008) Identification of FRA1 and FRA2 as genes involved in regulating the yeast iron regulon in response to decreased mitochondrial iron-sulfur cluster synthesis. *J. Biol. Chem.*, **283**, 10276–10286.

Kwok, E.Y., Severance, S. and Kosman, D.J. (2006a) Evidence for iron channeling in the Fet3p-Ftr1p high-affinity iron uptake complex in the yeast plasma membrane. *Biochemistry*, **45**, 6317–6327.

Kwok, E.Y., Stoj, C.S., Severance, S. and Kosman, D.J. (2006b) An engineered bifunctional high-affinity iron uptake protein in the yeast plasma membrane. *J. Inorg. Biochem.*, **100**, 1053–1060.

Labbé, S., Pelletier, B. and Mercier, A. (2007) Iron homeostasis in the fission yeast *Schizosaccharomyces pombe*. *Biometals*, **20**, 523–537.

Labbé, S., Khan, M.G. and Jacques, J.F. (2013) Iron uptake and regulation in *Schizosaccharomyces pombe*. *Curr. Opin. Microbiol.*, **16**, 669–676.

Lanquar, V., Lelièvre, F., Bolte, S., *et al.* (2005) Mobilization of vacuolar iron by AtNRAMP3 and AtNRAMP4 is essential for seed germination on low iron. *EMBO J.*, **24**, 4041–4051.

Le Jean, M., Schikora, A., Mari, S., Briat, J.F. and Curie C. (2005) A loss-of-function mutation in AtYSL1 reveals its role in iron and nicotianamine seed loading. *Plant J.*, **44**, 769–782.

Lee, S., Chiecko, J.C., Kim, S.A., *et al.* (2009) Disruption of OsYSL15 leads to iron inefficiency in rice plants. *Plant Physiol.*, **150**, 786–800.

Lesuisse, E. and Labbe, P. (1989) Reductive and non-reductive mechanisms of iron assimilation by the yeast *Saccharomyces cerevisiae*. *J. Gen. Microbiol.*, **135**, 257–263.

Lesuisse, E., Raguzzi, F. and Crichton, R.R. (1987) Iron uptake by the yeast *Saccharomyces cerevisiae*: involvement of a reduction step. *J. Gen. Microbiol.*, **133**, 3229–3236.

Lesuisse, E., Crichton, R.R. and Labbe, P. (1990) Iron-reductases in the yeast *Saccharomyces cerevisiae*. *Biochim. Biophys. Acta*, **1038**, 253–259.

Lesuisse, E., Simon-Casteras, M. and Labbe, P. (1998) Siderophore-mediated iron uptake in *Saccharomyces cerevisiae*: the SIT1 gene encodes a ferrioxamine B permease that belongs to the major facilitator superfamily. *Microbiology*, **144**, 3455–3462.

Lesuisse, E., Blaiseau, P.-L., Dancis, A. and Camadro, J.-M. (2001) Siderophore uptake and use by the yeast *Saccharomyces cerevisiae*. *Microbiology*, **147**, 289–298.

Li, H., Mapolelo, D.T., Dingra, N.N., *et al.* (2009) The yeast iron regulatory proteins Grx3/4 and Fra2 form heterodimeric complexes containing a [2Fe–2S] cluster with cysteinyl and histidyl ligation. *Biochemistry*, **48**, 9569–9581.

Li, H., Mapolelo, D.T., Dingra, N.N., *et al.* (2011) Histidine 103 in Fra2 is an iron–sulfur cluster ligand in the [2Fe–2S] Fra2-Grx3 complex and is required for *in vivo* iron signaling in yeast. *J. Biol. Chem.*, **286**, 867–876.

Li, L. and Kaplan, J. (1998) Defects in the yeast high-affinity iron transport system result in increased metal sensitivity because of the increased expression of transporters with a broad transition metal specificity. *J. Biol. Chem.*, **273**, 22181–22187.

Li, L., Chen, O.S., McVey Ward, D. and Kaplan, J. (2001) CCC1 is a transporter that mediates vacuolar iron storage in yeast. *J. Biol. Chem.*, **276**, 29515–29519.

Li, L., Cheng, X. and Ling, H.-Q. (2004) Isolation and characterization of Fe(III)-chelate reductase gene LeFRO1 in tomato. *Plant Mol. Biol.*, **54**, 125–136.

Li, L., Bagley, D., Ward, D.M. and Kaplan, J. (2008) Yap5 is an iron-responsive transcriptional activator that regulates vacuolar iron storage in yeast. *Mol. Cell. Biol.*, **28**, 1326–1337.

Li, L., Miao, R., Bertram, S., *et al.* (2012) A role for iron–sulfur clusters in the regulation f transcription factor Yap5-dependent high iron transcriptional responses in yeast. *J. Biol. Chem.*, **287**, 35709–35721.

Li, S., Zhao, B., Yuan, D., *et al.* (2013) Rice zinc finger protein DST enhances grain production through controlling Gn1a/OsCKX2 expression. *Proc. Natl Acad. Sci. USA*, **110**, 3167–3172.

Li, W. and Schmidt, W. (2010) A lysine-63-linked ubiquitin chain-forming conjugase, UBC13, promotes the developmental responses to iron deficiency in *Arabidopsis* roots. *Plant J.*, **6**, 330–343.

Ligat, L., Lauber, E., Albenne, C., *et al.* (2011) Analysis of the xylem sap proteome of *Brassica oleracea* reveals a high content in secreted proteins. *Proteomics*, **11**, 1798–1813.

Lill, R., Hoffmann, B., Molik, S., *et al.* (2012) The role of mitochondria in cellular iron-sulfur protein biogenesis and iron metabolism. *Biochim. Biophys. Acta*, **1823**, 1491–1508.

Lin, S.J., Pufahl, R.A., Dancis, A., *et al.* (1997) A role for the *Saccharomyces cerevisiae ATX1* gene in copper trafficking and iron transport. *J. Biol. Chem.*, **272**, 9215–9220.

Lin, Y.F., Liang, H.M., Yang, S.Y., *et al.* (2009) *Arabidopsis* IRT3 is a zinc-regulated and plasma membrane localized zinc/iron transporter. *New Phytol.*, **182**, 392–404.

Ling, H.Q., Koch, G., Baumlein, H. and Ganal, M.W. (1999) Map-based cloning of *chloronerva*, a gene involved in iron uptake of higher plants encoding nicotianamine synthase. *Proc. Natl Acad. Sci. USA*, **96**, 7098–7103.

Ling, H.Q., Bauer, P., Bereczky, Z., Keller, B. and Ganal, M. (2002) The tomato fer gene encoding a bHLH protein controls iron-uptake responses in roots. *Proc. Natl Acad. Sci. USA*, **99**, 13938–13943.

Lingam, S., Mohrbacher, J., Brumbarova, T., *et al.* (2011) Interaction between the bHLH transcription factor FIT and ETHYLENE INSENSITIVE3/ETHYLENE INSENSITIVE3-LIKE1 reveals molecular linkage between the regulation of iron acquisition and ethylene signaling in *Arabidopsis. Plant Cell*, **23**, 1815–1829.

Lombi, E. and Susini, J. (2009) Synchrotron-based techniques for plant and soil science: opportunities, challenges and future perspectives. *Plant Soil*, **320**, 1–35.

Lombi, E., de Jonge, M.D., Donner, E., *et al.* (2011) Fast X-ray fluorescence microtomography of hydrated biological samples. *PLoS One*, **6**, e20626.

Long, T.A., Tsukagoshi, H., Busch, W., *et al.* (2010) The bHLH transcription factor POPEYE regulates response to iron deficiency in *Arabidopsis* roots. *Plant Cell*, **22**, 2219–2236.

Lu, Y. and Last, R.L. (2008) Web-based *Arabidopsis* functional and structural genomics resources. *Arabidopsis Book*, **6**, e0118.

Lüthje, S., Möller, B., Perrineau, F.C. and Wöltje, K. (2013) Plasma membrane electron pathways and oxidative stress. *Antioxid. Redox Signal.*, **18**, 2163–2183.

Machonkin, T.E., Quintanar, L., Palmer, A.E., *et al.* (2001) Spectroscopy and reactivity of the type 1 copper site in Fet3p from *Saccharomyces cerevisiae*: correlation of structure with reactivity in the multicopper oxidases. *J. Am. Chem. Soc.*, **123**, 5507–5517.

Marschner, H. (1995) *Mineral Nutrition of Plants*. Academic Press, Boston, pp. 889.

Marschner, H. and Römheld, V. (1994) Strategies of plants for acquisition of iron. *Plant Soil*, **165**, 375–388.

Martinez-Pastor, M.T., Vergara, S.V., Puig, S. and Thiele DJ. (2013) Negative feedback regulation of the yeast CTH1 and CTH2 mRNA binding proteins is required for adaptation to iron deficiency and iron supplementation. *Mol. Cell. Biol.*, **33**, 2178–2187.

Martins, L.J., Jensen, L.T., Simons, J.R., *et al.* (1998) Metalloregulation of FRE1 and FRE2 homologs in *Saccharomyces cerevisiae. J. Biol. Chem.*, **273**, 23716–23721.

Martis, M.M., Zhou, R., Haseneyer, G., *et al.* (2013) Reticulate evolution of the rye genome. *Plant Cell*, **25**, 3685–3698.

Mäser, P., Thomine, S., Schroeder, J.I., *et al.* (2001) Phylogenetic relationships within cation transporter families of *Arabidopsis. Plant Physiol.*, **126**, 1646–1667.

Maurer, F., Mueller, S. and Bauer, P. (2011) Suppression of Fe deficiency gene expression by jasmonate. *Plant Physiol. Biochem.*, **49**, 530–536.

Mayer, K.F., Martis, M., Hedley, P.E., *et al.* (2011) Unlocking the barley genome by chromosomal and comparative genomics. *Plant Cell*, **23**, 1249–1263.

Meiser, J., Lingam, S. and Bauer, P. (2011) Posttranslational regulation of the iron deficiency basic helix-loop-helix transcription factor FIT is affected by iron and nitric oxide. *Plant Physiol.*, **157**, 2154–2166.

Mercier, A. and Labbé, S. (2009) Both Php4 function and subcellular localization are regulated by iron via a multistep mechanism involving the glutaredoxin Grx4 and the exportin Crm1. *J. Biol. Chem.*, **28**, 20249–20262.

Mercier, A., Pelletier, B. and Labbé, S. (2006) A transcription factor cascade involving Fep1 and the CCAAT-binding factor Php4 regulates gene expression in response to iron deficiency in the fission yeast *Schizosaccharomyces pombe. Eukaryot. Cell*, **5**, 1866–1881.

Mercier, A., Watt, S., Bähler, J. and Labbé, S. (2008) Key function for the CCAAT-binding factor Php4 to regulate gene expression in response to iron deficiency in fission yeast. *Eukaryot. Cell*, **7**, 493–508.

Moore, R.E., Kim, Y. and Philpott, C.C. (2003) The mechanism of ferrichrome transport through Arn1p and its metabolism in *Saccharomyces cerevisiae. Proc. Natl Acad. Sci. USA*, **100**, 5664–5669.

Mori, S. (1998) Iron transport in Graminaceous Plants, in *Metal Ions in Biological Systems* (eds A. Sigel and H. Sigel), **35**, 215–38.

Mori, S. (1999) Iron acquisition by plants. *Curr. Opin. Plant Biol.*, **2**, 250–253.

Mori, S. and Nishizawa, N.K. (1987) Methionine as a dominant precursor of phytosiderophores in graminae plants. *Plant Cell Physiol.*, **28**, 1081–1092.

Mori, S., Nishizawa, N., Hayashi, H., *et al.* (1991) Why are young rice plants highly susceptible to iron deficiency? *Plant Soil*, **130**, 143–156.

Morrissey, J., Baxter, I.R., Lee, J., *et al.* (2009) The ferroportin metal efflux proteins function in iron and cobalt homeostasis in *Arabidopsis*. *Plant Cell*, **21**, 3326–3338.

Moseley, J., Quinn, J., Eriksson, M. and Merchant, S. (2000) The *Crd1* gene encodes a putative di-iron enzyme required for photosystem I accumulation in copper deficiency and hypoxia in *Chlamydomonas reinhardtii*. *EMBO J.*, **19**, 2139–2151.

Mühlenhoff, U., Molik, S., Godoy, J.R., *et al.* (2010) Cytosolic monothiol glutaredoxins function in intracellular iron sensing and trafficking via their bound iron-sulfur cluster. *Cell Metab.*, **12**, 373–385.

Mukherjee, I., Campbell, N.H., Ash, J.S. and Connolly, E.L. (2006) Expression profiling of the *Arabidopsis* ferric chelate reductase (FRO) gene family reveals differential regulation by iron and copper. *Planta*, **223**, 1178–1190.

Murata, Y., Ma, J.F., Yamaji, N., *et al.* (2006) A specific transporter for iron(III) phytosiderophore in barley roots. *Plant J.*, **46**, 563–572.

Nagasaka, S., Takahashi, M., Nakanishi-Itai, R., *et al.* (2000) Time course analysis of gene expression over 24 hours in Fe-deficient barley roots. *Plant Mol. Biol.*, **69**, 621–631.

Nakanishi, H., Yamaguchi, T., Sasakuma, T., *et al.* (2000) Two dioxygenase genes, Ids3 and Ids2, from *Hordeum vulgare* are involved in the biosynthesis of mugineic acid family phytosiderophores. *Plant Mol. Biol.*, **44**, 199–207.

Nelissen, B., de Wachter, R. and Goffeau, A. (1997) Classification of all putative permeases and other membrane plurispanners of the major facilitator superfamily encoded by the complete genome of *Saccharomyces cerevisiae*. *FEMS Microbiol. ev.*, **21**, 113–134.

Nouet, C., Motte, P. and Hanikenne, M. (2011) Chloroplastic and mitochondrial metal homeostasis. *Trends Plant Sci.*, **16**, 395–404.

Nozoye, T., Itai, R.N., Nagasaka, S., *et al.* (2004) Diurnal changes in the expression of genes that participate in phytosiderophore synthesis in rice. *Soil Sci. Plant Nutr.*, **50**, 1125–1131.

Nozoye, T., Inoue, H., Takahashi, M., *et al.* (2007) The expression of iron homeostasis-related genes during rice germination. *Plant Mol. Biol.*, **64**, 35–47.

Nozoye, T., Nagasaka, S., Kobayashi, T., *et al.* (2011) Phytosiderophore efflux transporters are crucial for iron acquisition in graminaceous plants. *J. Biol. Chem.*, **28**, 5446–5454.

Nozoye, T., Nakanishi, H. and Nishizawa, N.K. (2013) Characterizing the crucial components of iron homeostasis in the maize mutants ys1 and ys3. *PLoS One*, **8**, e62567.

Nystedt, B., Street, N.R., Wetterbom, A., *et al.* (2013) The Norway spruce genome sequence and conifer genome evolution. *Nature*, **497**, 579–584.

Ogo, Y., Itai, R.N., Nakanishi, H., *et al.* (2006) Isolation and characterization of IRO2, a novel iron-regulated bHLH transcription factor in graminaceous plants. *J. Exp. Bot.*, **57**, 2867–2878.

Ogo, Y., Itai, R.N., Nakanishi, H., *et al.* (2007) The rice bHLH protein OsIRO2 is an essential regulator of the genes involved in Fe uptake under Fe-deficient conditions. *Plant J.*, **51**, 366–377.

Ogo, Y., Itai, R.N., Kobayashi, T., *et al.* (2011) OsIRO2 is responsible for iron utilization in rice and improves growth and yield in calcareous soil. *Plant Mol. Biol.*, **75**, 593–605.

Olsen, R.A., Clark, R.B. and Bennett, J.H. (1981) The enhancement of soil fertility by plant roots. *Am. Scientist*, **69**, 378–384.

Outten, C.E. and Albetel, A.N. (2013) Iron sensing and regulation in *Saccharomyces cerevisiae*: Ironing out the mechanistic details. *Curr. Opin. Microbiol.*, **16**, 662–668.

Ovadi, J. (1991) Physiological significance of metabolic channelling. *J. Theor. Biol.*, **152**, 1–22.

Palmer, A.E., Quintanar, L., Severance, S., *et al.* (2002) Spectroscopic characterization and O_2 reactivity of the trinuclear Cu cluster of mutants of the multicopper oxidase Fet3p. *Biochemistry*, **41**, 6438–6448.

Pao, S.S., Paulsen, I.T. and Saier, M.H., Jr (1998) Major facilitator superfamily. *Microbiol. Mol. Biol. Rev.*, **62**, 1–34.

Pelletier, B., Beaudoin, J., Mukai, Y. and Labbé, S. (2002) Fep1, an iron sensor regulating iron transporter gene expression in *Schizosaccharomyces pombe*. *J. Biol. Chem.*, **277**, 22950–22958.

Pelletier, B., Beaudoin, J., Philpott, C.C. and Labbé, S. (2003) Fep1 represses expression of the fission yeast *Schizosaccharomyces pombe* siderophore-iron transport system. *Nucleic Acids Res.*, **31**, 4332–4344.

Pfeifer, M., Martis, M., Asp, T., *et al.* (2013) The perennial ryegrass GenomeZipper: targeted use of genome resources for comparative grass genomics. *Plant Physiol.*, **161**, 571–582.

Philpott, C.C. (2006) Iron uptake in fungi: a system for every source. *Biochim. Biophys. Acta*, **1763**, 636–645.

Philpott, C.C. and Protchenko O. (2008) Response to iron deprivation in *Saccharomyces cerevisiae*. *Eukaryot Cell.*, **7**, 20–27.

Philpott, C.C., Leidgens, S. and Frey, A.G. (2012) Metabolic remodeling in iron-deficient fungi. *Biochim. Biophys. Acta*, **1823**, 1509–1520.

Pimentel, C., Vicente, C., Menezes, R.A, *et al.* (2012) The role of the Yap5 transcription factor in remodeling gene expression in response to Fe bioavailability. *PLoS One*, **7**, e37434.

Pin, P.A., Benlloch, R., Bonnet, D., *et al.* (2010) An antagonistic pair of ft homologs mediates the control of flowering time in sugar beet. *Science*, **330**, 1397–1400.

Portnoy, M.E., Liu, X.F. and Culotta, V.C. (2000) *Saccharomyces cerevisiae* expresses three functionally distinct homologues of the nramp family of metal transporters. *Mol. Cell. Biol.*, **20**, 7893–7902.

Portnoy, M.E., Schmidt, P.J., Rogers, R.S. and Culotta, V.C. (2001) Metal transporters that contribute copper to metallochaperones in *Saccharomyces cerevisiae*. *Mol. Genet. Genomics*, **265**, 873–882.

Portnoy, M.E., Jensen, L.T. and Culotta, V.C. (2002) The distinct methods by which manganese and iron regulate the Nramp transporters in yeast. *Biochem. J.*, **362**, 119–124.

Potato Genome Sequencing Consortium (2011) Genome sequence and analysis of the tuber crop potato. *Nature*, **475**, 189–195.

Pouliot, B., Jbel, M., Mercier, A. and Labbé, S. (2010) abc3+ encodes an iron-regulated vacuolar ABC-type transporter in *Schizosaccharomyces pombe*. *Eukaryot. Cell.* **9**, 59–73.

Powell, A.L.T., Nguyen, C.V., Hill, T., *et al.* (2012) Uniform ripening encodes a golden 2-like transcription factor regulating tomato fruit chloroplast development. *Science*, **336**, 1711–1715.

Protchenko, O., Ferea, T., Rashford, J., *et al.* (2001) Three cell wall mannoproteins facilitate the uptake of iron in *Saccharomyces cerevisiae*. *J. Biol. Chem.*, **276**, 49244–49250.

Puig, S., Askeland, E. and Thiele, D.J. (2005) Coordinated remodeling of cellular metabolism during iron deficiency through targeted mRNA degradation. *Cell*, **120**, 99–110.

Quintanar, L., Stoj, C., Taylor, A.B., *et al.* (2007) Shall we dance? How a multicopper oxidase chooses its electron transfer partner. *Acc. Chem. Res.*, **40**, 445–452.

Radisky, D.C., Babcock, M.C. and Kaplan, J. (1999) The yeast frataxin homologue mediates mitochondrial iron efflux. Evidence for a mitochondrial iron cycle. *J. Biol. Chem.*, **274**, 4497–4499.

Radomiljac, J.D., Whelan, J. and van der Merwe, M. (2013) Coordinating metabolite changes with our perception of plant abiotic stress responses: emerging views revealed by integrative-omic analyses. *Metabolites*, **3**, 761–786.

Raguzzi, F., Lesuisse, E. and Crichton, R.R. (1988) Iron storage in *Saccharomyces Cerevisiae*. *FEBS Lett.*, **231**, 253–258.

Ravet, K., Touraine, B., Boucherez, J., *et al.* (2009) Ferritins control interaction between iron homeostasis and oxidative stress in *Arabidopsis*. *Plant J.*, **57**, 400–412.

Rees, E.M. and Thiele, D.J. (2007) Identification of a vacuole-associated metalloreductase and its role in Ctr2-mediated intracellular copper mobilization. *J. Biol. Chem.*, **282**, 21629–21638.

Rellán-Alvarez, R., Abadía, J. and Alvarez-Fernández, A. (2008) Formation of metal nicotianamine complexes as affected by pH, ligand exchange with citrate and metal exchange. A study by electrospray ionization time-of-flight mass spectrometry. *Rapid Commun. Mass Spectrom.*, **22**, 1553–1562.

Robinson, N.J., Procter, C.M., Connolly, E.L. and Guerinot, M.L. (1999) A ferric-chelate reductase for iron uptake from soils. *Nature*, **397**, 694–697.

Rodríguez-Celma, J., Vázquez-Reina, S., Orduna, J., *et al.* (2011) Characterization of flavins in roots of Fe-deficient strategy I plants, with a focus on *Medicago truncatula*. *Plant Cell Physiol.*, **52**, 2173–2189.

Rodríguez-Celma, J., Lin, W.D., Fu, G.M., *et al.* (2013) Mutually exclusive alterations in secondary metabolism are critical for the uptake of insoluble iron compounds by *Arabidopsis* and *Medicago truncatula*. *Plant Physiol.*, **162**, 1473–1485.

Rogers, E.E., Wu, X., Stacey, G. and Nguyen, H.T. (2009) Two MATE proteins play a role in iron efficiency in soybean. *J. Plant Physiol.*, **166**, 1453–1459.

Römheld, V. (1987). Different strategies for iron acquisition in higher plants. *Physiol. Plant.*, **70**, 231–234.

Römheld, V. and Marschner, H. (1986) Evidence for a specific uptake system for iron phytosiderophores in roots of grasses. *Plant Physiol.*, **80**, 175–180.

Roschzttardtz, H., Séguéla-Arnaud, M., Briat, J.F., Vert, G. and Curie, C. (2011) The FRD3 citrate effluxer promotes iron nutrition between symplastically disconnected tissues throughout *Arabidopsis* development. *Plant Cell*, **23**, 2725–2737.

Roschzttardtz, H., Conéjéro, G., Divol, F., *et al.* (2013) New insights into Fe localization in plant tissues. *Front. Plant Sci.*, **4**, 350. doi: 10.3389/fpls.2013.00350.

Rutherford, J.C., Jaron, S., Ray, E., *et al.* (2001) A second iron-regulatory system in yeast independent of Aft1p. *Proc. Natl Acad. Sci. USA*, **98**, 14322–14327.

Rutherford, J.C., Jaron, S. and Winge, D.R. (2003) Aft1p and Aft2p mediate iron responsive gene expression in yeast through related promoter elements. *J. Biol. Chem.*, **278**, 27636–27643.

Rutherford, J.C., Ojeda, L., Balk, J., *et al.* (2005) Activation of the iron regulon by the yeast Aft1/Aft2 transcription factors depends on mitochondrial but not cytosolic iron sulfur protein biogenesis. *J. Biol. Chem.*, **280**, 10135–10140.

Sakakibara, H. (2006) Cytokinins: activity, biosynthesis, and translocation. *Annu. Rev. Plant Biol.*, **57**, 431–449.

Salomé, P.A., Oliva, M., Weigel, D. and Krämer, U. (2013) Circadian clock adjustment to plant iron status depends on chloroplast and phytochrome function. *EMBO J.*, **32**, 511–523.

Samira, R., Stallmann, A., Massenburg, L.N. and Long, T.A. (2013) Ironing out the issues: integrated approaches to understanding iron homeostasis in plants. *Plant Sci.*, **210**, 250–259.

Santi, S. and Schmidt, W. (2008) Laser microdissection-assisted analysis of the functional fate of iron deficiency-induced root hairs in cucumber. *J. Exp. Bot.*, **59**, 697–704.

Santi, S. and Schmidt, W. (2009) Dissecting iron deficiency-induced proton extrusion in *Arabidopsis* roots. *New Phytol.*, **183**, 1072–1084.

Santi, S., Cesco, S., Varanini, Z. and Pinton, R. (2005) Two plasma membrane H(+)-ATPase genes are differentially expressed in iron-deficient cucumber plants. *Plant Physiol. Biochem.*, **43**, 287–292.

Schaaff, G., Ludewig, U., Erenoglu, B.E., *et al.* (2004) ZmYS1 functions as a proton coupled symporter for phytosiderophore- and nicotianamine-chelated metals. *J. Biol. Chem.*, **279**, 9091–9096.

Schaaf, G., Schikora, A., Häberle, J., *et al.* (2005) A putative function for the *Arabidopsis* Fe-Phytosiderophore transporter homolog AtYSL2 in Fe and Zn homeostasis. *Plant Cell Physiol.*, **46**, 762–774.

Schaaf, G., Honsbein, A. and Meda, A.R. (2006) AtIREG2 encodes a tonoplast transport protein involved in iron-dependent nickel detoxification in *Arabidopsis thaliana* roots. *J. Biol. Chem.*, **281**, 25532–25540.

Schagerlöf, U., Wilson, G., Hebert, H., Al-Karadaghi, S. and Hägerhäll C. (2006) Transmembrane topology of FRO2, a ferric chelate reductase from *Arabidopsis thaliana*. *Plant Mol. Biol.*, **62**, 215–221.

Schikora, A. and Schmidt, W. (2001) Iron stress-induced changes in root epidermal cell fate are regulated independently from physiological responses to low iron availability. *Plant Physiol.*, **125**, 1679–1687.

Schmid, N.B., Giehl, R.F., Döll, S., *et al.* (2014) Feruloyl-CoA 6'-hydroxylase-dependent coumarins mediate iron acquisition from alkaline substrates in *Arabidopsis*. *Plant Physiol.*, **164**, 160–172.

Schmidke, I. and Stephan, U.W. (1995) Transport of metal micronutrients in the phloem of castor bean (*Ricinus communis*) seedlings. *Physiol. Plant.*, **95**, 147–153.

Schmidke, I., Kruger, C., Frommichen, R., Scholz, G. and Stephan, U. (1999) Phloem loading and transport characteristics of iron in interaction with plant-endogenous ligands in castor bean seedlings. *Physiol. Plant.*, **106**, 82–89.

Schmidt, H., Günther, C., Weber, M., *et al.* (2014) Metabolome analysis of *Arabidopsis thaliana* roots identifies a key metabolic pathway for iron acquisition. *PLoS One*, **9**, e102444.

Schmidt, W. (2003) Iron solutions: acquisition strategies and signaling pathways in plants. *Trends Plant Sci.*, **8**, 188–193.

Schmidt, W. and Buckhout, T.J. (2011) A hitchhiker's guide to the *Arabidopsis* ferrome. *Plant Physiol. Biochem.*, **49**, 462–470.

Schmidt, W., Tittel, J. and Schikora, A. (2000) Role of hormones in the induction of iron deficiency responses in *Arabidopsis* roots. *Plant Physiol.*, **122**, 1109–1118.

Schnell Ramos, M., Khodja, H., Mary, V. and Thomine, S. (2013). Using μ PIXE for quantitative mapping of metal concentration in *Arabidopsis thaliana* seeds. *Front. Plant Sci.*, **4**, 168.

Schrettl, M. and Haas, H. (2011) Iron homeostasis – Achilles' heel of *Aspergillus fumigatus*? *Curr. Opin. Microbiol.*, **14**, 400–405.

Schrettl, M., Winkelmann, G. and Haas, H. (2004) Ferrichrome in *Schizosaccharomyces pombe* – an iron transport and iron storage compound. *Biometals*, **17**, 647–654.

Schroeder, J.I., Delhaize, E., Frommer, W.B., *et al.* (2013) Using membrane transporters to improve crops for sustainable food production. *Nature*, **497**, 60–66.

Schuler, M., Rellán-Álvarez, R., Fink-Straube, C., Abadía, J. and Bauer, P. (2012) Nicotianamine functions in the phloem-based transport of iron to sink organs, in pollen development and pollen tube growth in *Arabidopsis*. *Plant Cell*, **24**, 2380–2400.

Seckback, J.J. (1982) Ferreting out the secret of plant ferritin – a review. *J. Plant Nutr.*, **5**, 369–394.

Seguela, M., Briat, J.-F., Vert, G. and Curie, C. (2008) Cytokinins negatively regulate the root iron uptake machinery in *Arabidopsis* through a growth-dependent pathway. *Plant J.*, **55**, 289–300.

Severance, S., Chakraborty, S. and Kosman, D.J. (2004) The Ftr1p iron permease in the yeast plasma membrane: orientation, topology and structure–function relationships, *Biochem. J.*, **380**, 487–496.

Shah, J. (2009) Plants under attack: systemic signals in defence. *Curr. Opin. Plant Biol.*, **12**, 459–464.

Shakoury-Elizeh, M., Tiedeman, J., Rashford, J., *et al.* (2004) Transcriptional remodeling in response to iron deprivation in *Saccharomyces cerevisiae*. *Mol. Biol. Cell*, **15**, 1233–1243.

Shanmugam, V., Lo, J.C., Wu, C.L., *et al.* (2011) Differential expression and regulation of iron-regulated metal transporters in *Arabidopsis halleri* and *Arabidopsis thaliana* – the role in zinc tolerance. *New Phytol.*, **190**, 125–137.

Shatwell, K.P., Dancis, A., Cross, A.R., *et al.* (1996) The FRE1 ferric reductase of *Saccharomyces cerevisiae* is a cytochrome b similar to that of NADPH oxidase. *J. Biol. Chem.*, **271**, 14240–14244.

Shin, L.J., Lo, J.C., Chen, G.H., *et al.* (2013) IRT1 degradation factor1, a ring E3 ubiquitin ligase, regulates the degradation of iron-regulated transporter1 in *Arabidopsis*. *Plant Cell*, **25**, 3039–3051.

Shulaev, V., Sargent, D.J., Crowhurst, R.N., *et al.* (2011) The genome of woodland strawberry (*Fragaria vesca*). *Nat. Genet.*, **43**, 109–116.

Sickmann, A., Reinders, J., Wagner, Y., *et al.* (2003) The proteome of *Saccharomyces cerevisiae* mitochondria. *Proc. Natl Acad. Sci. USA*, **100**, 13207–13212.

Singh, A., Kaur, N. and Kosman, D.J. (2007) The metalloreductase Fre6p in Fe-efflux from the yeast vacuole. *J. Biol. Chem.*, **282**, 28619–28626.

Sivitz, A., Grinvalds, C., Barberon, M., Curie, C. and Vert, G. (2011) Proteasome mediated turnover of the transcriptional activator FIT is required for plant iron-deficiency responses. *Plant J.*, **66**, 1044–1052.

Sivitz, A.B., Hermand, V., Curie, C. and Vert, G. (2012) *Arabidopsis* bHLH100 and bHLH101 control iron homeostasis via a FIT-independent pathway. *PLoS One*, **7**, e44843.

Solomon, E.I., Sundaram, U.M. and Machonkin, T.E. (1996) Multicopper oxidases and oxygenases. *Chem. Rev.*, **96**, 2563–2606.

Solti, A., Kovács, K., Basa, B., *et al.* (2012) Uptake and incorporation of iron in sugar beet chloroplasts. *Plant Physiol. Biochem.*, **52**, 91–97.

Spizzo, T., Byersdorfer, C., Duesterhoeft, S. and Eide, D. (1997) The yeast FET5 gene encodes a FET3-related multicopper oxidase implicated in iron transport. *Mol Gen Genet.*, **256**, 547–556.

Srere, P.A. (1987) Complexes of sequential metabolic enzymes. *Annu. Rev. Biochem.*, **56**, 89–124.

Stearman, R., Yuan, D.S., Yamaguchi-Iwai, Y., *et al.* (1996) A permease-oxidase complex involved in high-affinity iron uptake in yeast. *Science*, **271**, 1552–1557.

Stoj, C.S., Augustine, A.J., Zeigler, I., *et al.* (2006) Structural basis of the ferrous iron specificity of the yeast ferroxidase, Fet3p. *Biochemistry*, **45**, 12741–12749.

Strozycki, P.M., Szymanski, M., Szczurek, A., Barciszewski, J. and Figlerowicz, M. (2010) A new family of ferritin genes from *Lupinus luteus* – comparative analysis of plant ferritins, their gene structure, and evolution. *Mol. Biol. Evol.*, **27**, 91–101.

Sweetlove, L.J. and Ratcliffe, R.G. (2011) Flux-balance modeling of plant metabolism. *Front Plant Sci.*, **2**, 38.

Takagi, S., Nomoto, K. and Takemoto, T. (1984). Physiological aspect of mugineic acid, a possible phytosiderophore of graminaceous plants. *J. Plant Nutr.*, **7**, 469–477.

Takahashi, M., Terada, Y. and Nakai, I. (2003) Role of nicotianamine in the intracellular delivery of metals and plant reproductive development. *Plant Cell*, **15**, 1263–1280.

Taylor, A.B., Stoj, C.S., Ziegler, L., *et al.* (2005) The copper-iron connection in biology: structure of the metallo-oxidase Fet3p. *Proc. Natl Acad. Sci. USA*, **102**, 15459–15464.

Terry, N. and Abadia, J. (1986) Function of iron in chloroplasts. *J. Plant Nutr.*, **9**, 609–646.

Tiffin, O.L. (1966) Iron translocation II. *Citrate/iron ratios in plant stem exudates*. *Plant Physiol.*, **41**, 515–518.

Thomine, S. and Vert, G. (2013) Iron transport in plants: better be safe than sorry. *Curr. Opin. Plant Biol.*, **16**, 322–327.

Thomine, S., Wang, R., Ward, J.M., *et al.* (2000) Cadmium and iron transport by members of a plant metal transporter family in *Arabidopsis* with homology to Nramp genes. *Proc. Natl Acad. Sci. USA*, **97**, 4991–4996.

Tomato Genome Consortium (2012) The tomato genome sequence provides insights into fleshy fruit evolution. *Nature*, **485**, 635–641.

Tottey, S., Block, M.A., Allen, M., *et al.* (2003) *Arabidopsis* CHL27, located in both envelope and thylakoid membranes, is required for the synthesis of protochlorophyllide. *Proc. Natl Acad. Sci. USA*, **100**, 16119–16124.

Tsukamoto, T., Nakanishi, H., Uchida, H., *et al.* (2009) ^{52}Fe translocation in barley as monitored by a positron-emitting tracer imaging system (PETIS): evidence for the direct translocation of Fe from roots to young leaves via phloem. *Plant Cell Physiol.*, **50**, 48–57.

Ueta, R., Fujiwara, N., Iwai, K. and Yamaguchi-Iwai, Y. (2007) Mechanism underlying the iron-dependent nuclear export of the iron-responsive transcription factor Aft1p in *Saccharomyces cerevisiae*. *Mol. Biol. Cell*, **18**, 2980–2990.

Ueta, R., Fujiwara, N., Iwai, K. and Yamaguchi-Iwai, Y. (2012) Iron-induced dissociation of the Aft1p transcriptional regulator from target gene promoters is an initial event in iron-dependent gene suppression. *Mol. Cell. Biol.*, **32**, 4998–5008.

Urbanowski, J.L. and Piper, R.C. (1999) The iron transporter Fth1p forms a complex with the Fet5 iron oxidase and resides on the vacuolar membrane. *J. Biol. Chem.*, **274**, 38061–38070.

van der Mark, F., van den Briel, M.L., van Oers, J.W. and Bienfait, H.F. (1982) Ferritin in bean leaves with constant and changing iron status. *Planta*, **156**, 341–344.

Varshney, R.K., Chen, W., Li, Y., *et al.* (2012) Draft genome sequence of pigeonpea (*Cajanus cajan*), an orphan legume crop of resource-poor farmers. *Nat. Biotechnol.*, **30**, 83–89.

Varshney, R.K., Song, C., Saxena, R.K., *et al.* (2013) Draft genome sequence of chickpea (*Cicer arietinum*) provides a resource for trait improvement. *Nat. Biotechnol.*, **31**, 240–246.

Velasco, R., Zharkikh, A., Troggio, M., *et al.* (2007) A high-quality draft consensus sequence of the genome of a heterozygous grapevine variety. *PLoS One*, **19** (2), e1326.

Vergara, S.V., Puig, S. and Thiele, D.J. (2011) Early recruitment of AU-rich element containing mRNAs determines their cytosolic fate during iron deficiency. *Mol. Cell. Biol.*, **31**, 417–429.

Vert, G., Briat, J.-F. and Curie, C. (2001) *Arabidopsis* IRT2 gene encodes a root-periphery iron transporter. *Plant J.*, **26**, 181–189.

Vert, G., Grotz, N., Dédaldéchamp, F., *et al.* (2002) IRT1, an *Arabidopsis* transporter essential for iron uptake from the soil and for plant growth. *Plant Cell*, **14**, 1223–1233.

Vigani, G., Zocchi, G., Bashir, K., Philippar, K. and Briat, J.F. (2013) Signals from chloroplasts and mitochondria for iron homeostasis regulation. *Trends Plant Sci.*, **18**, 305–311.

Vignais, P.V. (2002) The superoxide-generating NADPH oxidase: structural aspects and activation mechanism. *Cell. Mol. Life Sci.*, **59**, 1428–1459.

Von Wiren, N., Klair, S., Bansal, S., *et al.* (1999) Nicotianamine chelates both FeIII and FeII. Implications for metal transport in plants. *Plant Physiol.*, **119**, 1107–1114.

Vorweiger, A., Gryczka, C., Czihal, A., *et al.* (2007) Iron assimilation and transcription factor controlled synthesis of riboflavin in plants. *Planta*, **226**, 147–158.

Wada, Y., Yamaguchi, I., Takahashi, M., *et al.* (2007) Highly sensitive quantitative analysis of nicotianamine using LC/ESI-TOF-MS with an internal standard. *Biosci. Biotechnol. Biochem.*, **71**, 435–441.

Wang, H.Y., Klatte, M., Jakoby, M., *et al.* (2007) Iron deficiency-mediated stress regulation of four subgroup Ib BHLH genes in *Arabidopsis thaliana*. *Planta*, **226**, 897–908.

Wang, T.P., Quintanar, L., Severance, S., *et al.* (2003) Targeted suppression of the ferroxidase and iron trafficking activities of the multicopper oxidase Fet3p from *Saccharomyces cerevisiae*. *J. Biol. Inorg. Chem.*, **8**, 611–620.

Wang, X., Wang, H., Wang, J., *et al.* (2011) The genome of the mesopolyploid crop species *Brassica rapa*. *Nat. Genet.*, **43**, 1035–1039.

Wasternack, C. and Kombrink, E. (2010) Jasmonates: structural requirements for lipid derived signals active in plant stress responses and development. *ACS Chem. Biol.*, **5**, 63–77.

Waters, B.M. and Eide, D.J. (2002) Combinatorial control of yeast FET4 gene expression by iron, zinc and oxygen. *J. Biol. Chem.*, **277**, 33749–33757.

Waters, B.M., Blevins, D.G. and Eide, D.J. (2002) Characterization of FRO1, a pea ferric-chelate reductase involved in root iron acquisition. *Plant Physiol.*, **129**, 85–94.

Waters, B.M., Chu, H.H., Didonato, R.J., *et al.* (2006) Mutations in *Arabidopsis* yellow stripe-like1 and yellow stripe-like3 reveal their roles in metal ion homeostasis and loading of metal ions in seeds. *Plant Physiol.*, **141**, 1446–1458.

Welkie, G.W. (2000) Taxonomic distribution of dicotyledonous species capable of root excretion of riboflavin under iron deficiency. *J. Plant Nutr.*, **23**, 1819–1831.

Wu, H., Li, L., Du, J., *et al.* (2005) Molecular and biochemical characterization of the Fe(III) chelate reductase gene family in *Arabidopsis thaliana*. *Plant Cell Physiol.*, **46**, 1505–1514.

Wu, J., Wang, C., Zheng, L., *et al.* (2011) Ethylene is involved in the regulation of iron homeostasis by regulating the expression of iron-acquisition-related genes in *Oryza sativa*. *J. Exp. Bot.*, **62**, 667–674.

Xia, Z., Watanabe, S., Yamada, T., *et al.* (2012) Positional cloning and characterization reveal the molecular basis for soybean maturity locus e1 that regulates photoperiodic flowering. *Proc. Natl Acad. Sci. USA*, **109**, E2155–E2164.

Xu, Q., Chen, L.L., Ruan, X., *et al.* (2013) The draft genome of sweet orange (*Citrus sinensis*). *Nat. Genet.*, **45**, 59–66.

Xuan, W., Zhu, F.Y., Xu, S., *et al.* (2008) The heme oxygenase/carbon monoxide system is involved in the auxin-induced cucumber adventitious rooting process. *Plant Physiol.*, **148**, 881–893.

Yamaguchi-Iwai, Y., Dancis, A. and Klausner, R.D. (1995) AFT1: a mediator of iron regulated transcriptional control in *Saccharomyces cerevisiae*. *EMBO J.*, **14**, 1231–1239.

Yamaguchi-Iwai, Y., Stearman, R., Dancis, A. and Klausner R.D. (1996) Iron-regulated DNA binding by the AFT1 protein controls the iron regulon in yeast. *EMBO J.*, **15**, 3377–3384.

Yamaguchi-Iwai, Y., Ueta, R., Fukunaka, A. and Sasaki, R. (2002) Subcellular localization of Aft1 transcription factor responds to iron status in *Saccharomyces cerevisiae*. *J. Biol. Chem.*, **277**, 18914–18918.

Yang, J.L., Chen, W.W., Chen, L.Q., *et al.* (2013) The 14-3-3 protein GENERAL REGULATORY FACTOR11 (GRF11) acts downstream of nitric oxide to regulate iron acquisition in *Arabidopsis thaliana*. *New Phytol.*, **197**, 815–824.

Yang, Y., Qin, Y., Xie, C., *et al.* (2010) The *Arabidopsis* chaperone J3 regulates the plasma membrane H+-ATPase through interaction with the PKS5 kinase. *Plant Cell*, **22**, 1313–1332.

Yen, M.R., Tseng, Y.H. and Saier, M.H., Jr (2001) Maize Yellow Stripe1, an iron phytosiderophore uptake transporter, is a member of the oligopeptide transporter (OPT) family. *Microbiology*, **147**, 2881–2883.

Yi, Y. and Guerinot, M.L. (1996) Genetic evidence that induction of root Fe(III) chelate reductase activity is necessary for iron uptake under iron deficiency. *Plant J.*, **10**, 835–844.

Yokosho, K., Yamaji, N., Ueno, D., Mitani, N. and Ma, J.F. (2009) OsFRDL1 is a citrate transporter required for efficient translocation of iron in rice. *Plant Physiol.*, **149**, 297–305.

Yu, J., Hu, S., Wang, J., *et al.* (2002) A draft sequence of the rice genome (*Oryza sativa* L. ssp. *indica*). *Science*, **296**, 79–92.

Yuan, D.S., Stearman, R., Dancis, A., *et al.* (1995) The Menkes/Wilson disease gene homologue in yeast provides copper to a ceruloplasmin-like oxidase required for iron uptake. *Proc. Natl Acad. Sci. USA*, **92**, 2632–2636.

Yuan, D.S., Dancis, A. and Klausner, R.D. (1997) Restriction of copper export in *Saccharomyces cerevisiae* to a late Golgi or post-Golgi compartment in the secretory Pathway. *J. Biol. Chem.*, **272**, 25787–25793.

Yuan, Y., Wu, H., Wang, N., *et al.* (2008) FIT interacts with AtbHLH38 and AtbHLH39 in regulating iron uptake gene expression for iron homeostasis in *Arabidopsis*. *Cell Res.*, **18**, 385–397.

Yun, C.W., Ferea, T., Rashford, J., *et al.* (2000a) Desferrioxamine-mediated iron uptake in *Saccharomyces cerevisiae*. *Evidence for two pathways of iron uptake. J. Biol. Chem.*, **275**, 10709–10715.

Yun, C.W., Tiedeman, J.S., Moore, R.E. and Philpott, C.C. (2000b) Siderophore-iron uptake in *Saccharomyces cerevisiae*. Identification of ferrichrome and fusarinine transporters. *J. Biol. Chem.*, **275**, 16354–16359.

Yun, C.W., Bauler, M., Moore, R.E., Klebba, P.E. and Philpott, C.C. (2001) The role of the FRE family of plasma membrane reductases in the uptake of siderophore-iron in *Saccharomyces cerevisiae*. *J. Biol. Chem.*, **276**, 10218–10223.

Zaballa, M.E., Ziegler, L., Kosman, D.J. and Vila, A.J. (2010) NMR study of the exchange coupling in the trinuclear cluster of the multicopper oxidase Fet3p. *J. Am. Chem. Soc.*, **132**, 11191–11196.

Zancani, M., Peresson, C., Biroccio, A., *et al.* (2004) Evidence for the presence of ferritin in plant mitochondria. *Eur. J. Biochem.*, **271**, 3657–3664.

Zhao, G. (2010) Phytoferritin and its implications for human health and nutrition. *Biochim. Biophys. Acta*, **1800**, 815–823.

Zhai, Z., Gayomba, S.R., Jung, H.I., *et al.* (2014) OPT3 Is a phloem-specific iron transporter that is essential for systemic iron signaling and redistribution of iron and cadmium in *Arabidopsis*. *Plant Cell*, **26**, 2249–2264.

6

Cellular Iron Uptake and Export in Mammals

6.1 The Transferrins

6.1.1 Introduction

The transferrins are a family of iron-binding proteins which were initially found in the physiological fluids of many vertebrates. Their original identification in egg white by serendipity, is a good illustration of the *Oxford English Dictionary* definition of the word – '…the faculty of making happy and unexpected discoveries by accident' (Roberts, 1989). Ovotransferrin, originally called conalbumin, was first purified from six litres of the whites of freshly laid eggs by Osborne and Campbell (1900), although it was only identified as the antimicrobial agent of egg white (Alderton *et al.*, 1946) nearly a half-century later. During the Second World War, while working for the US Army Medical Corps in the search for the component of raw egg white which protected a polyvalent bacteriophage lysate effective against dysentery from the effects of desiccation (Schade and Caroline, 1944a), Arthur Schade made the serendipitous observation that egg white had a profound bacteriostatic effect, which was abolished by the addition of iron (Schade and Caroline, 1944b). The iron-binding protein of human serum whose antibacterial properties were also abolished by iron, initially called siderophilin, quickly followed (Schade and Caroline, 1946), as did the 'red protein' of pig plasma (Laurell and Ingelman, 1947). The name transferrin was then proposed (Holmberg and Laurell, 1947), and has been used ever since as the generic name for proteins of this family. The iron-binding protein of human milk, usually referred to as lactoferrin, was discovered later (Groves, 1960; Johansson, 1960; Montreuil *et al.*, 1960).

The initial discovery of the transferrins was made possible by their potent antibacterial activities – by depriving bacteria of iron they contribute to the defence of mammalian cells against infection. However, the specific role of transferrin (often referred to as serotransferrin, STF) in vertebrates in

Iron Metabolism – From Molecular Mechanisms to Clinical Consequences, Fourth Edition. Robert Crichton.
© 2016 John Wiley & Sons, Ltd. Published 2016 by John Wiley & Sons, Ltd.

the transport of iron from sites of absorption (the gastrointestinal tract) and haem degradation (the reticuloendothelial system) to sites of utilisation (for erythropoeisis, and incorporation into iron-containing proteins) and storage (in ferritin) became apparent later.

6.1.2 The Transferrin Family

Transferrins are monomeric glycoproteins that are probably ubiquitous in all multicellular animals. The structure of most family members includes two lobes, each with a potential iron-binding domain; however, molecules with one and three lobes have also been found. Transferrins are best known for their ability to sequester and transport non-haem iron, but some homologues have evolved quite different functions, and many are employed in immune response activities (Lambert, 2012). The domains of the bilobal proteins are homologous, with approximately 30% sequence identity between them, and probably arose as the result of an intragenic recombination event occurring in an ancestral gene with a single lobe (Park *et al.*, 1985). Multiple gene duplication events produced the range of family members known today.

Since detailed information will be presented on serotransferrin subsequently, which will be referred to as transferrin in later sections, some other members of the transferrin family will be briefly described here. These are listed in Table 6.1, while their domain architecture is illustrated in Figure 6.1.

Table 6.1 *Characteristics of transferrin family members*

Protein	Gene	No. of lobes	Iron binding	Tissues	Taxonomic groups
Transferrin	*TF*	2	Yes	Liver, serum, brain, pancreas, bone marrow	Mammals
Ovotransferrin	*OTF*	2	Yes	Serum, egg yolk	Birds, reptiles
Lactoferrin	*LTF*	2	Yes	Milk, saliva, tears, bile, other secretions	Mammals
Inhibitor of carbonic anhydrase	*ICA*	2	No	Serum (expressed in liver)	Mammals; pseudogene in primates
Melanotransferrin	*MFI2*	2	N-lobe only	Melanomas, saliva, sweat, liver, intestine	Vertebrates; all metazoans?
Saxiphilin	*SAX*	2	No	Serum	*Rana* (bullfrog)
Otolith matrix protein 1	*OMP1*	1	No	Otolith organ	Fish
Major yolk protein	*MYP*	2	Yes?	Digestive tract and gonads; hepatic caecum, hindgut, ovary	Hemichordates; Cephalachordates
Toposome	*TOP*	2	Yes?	Digestive tract and gonads	Sea urchins
Ciona TF1 (mono)	*TF*	1	Yes	Plasma	Urochordates
Ciona TF2 (bi)	*TF?*	2	?	?	Urochordates
Sea urchin MTF	*MTF?*	2	?	Intestines?	Hemichordates
Pacifastin	*PAC*	3	Yes	Hepatopancreas and haemocytes	Crustaceans
Insect TF	*TF*	2	Yes	Haemolymph (expressed in fat body), ovaries	Insects
Triplicated transferrins	*TTF*	3	Yes	Plasma membrane	Halotolerant algae
IDI-100	*IDI-100*	2	No	Plasma membrane	Halotolerant algae

Reprinted with permission from Elsevier from Lambert, L.A. (2012) Molecular evolution of the transferrin family and associated receptors. *Biochim. Biophys. Acta,* **1820**, 244–255.

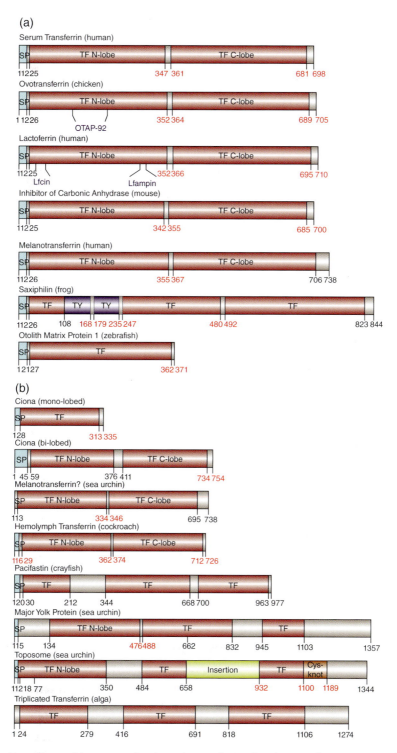

Figure 6.1 *Domain architecture of selected transferrin family members. (a) Vertebrates. (b) Invertebrates (and algae). SP = signal peptide; TF = transferrin domain; TY = thyroglobulin repeat; WAP = whey acidic protein domain. Image created with DOG 2.0 (Ren* et al., *2009). Reprinted with permission from Elsevier from Lambert, L.A. (2012) Molecular evolution of the transferrin family and associated receptors.* Biochim. Biophys. Acta, **1820**, 244–255

Ovotransferrin (OTF), which is the transferrin orthologue in birds and reptiles, composes 12% of avian egg white protein, and is expressed in the liver and oviduct. It appears to serve both an iron transport (in serum) and an antimicrobial (in egg yolk) function in birds, perhaps bridging an evolutionary gap between iron transport and an iron-withdrawing role as a protection against infections. Chicken OTF and chicken serum transferrins are known to be derived from the same gene (Thibodeau *et al.*, 1978; Jeltsch and Chambon, 1982; Ciuraszkiewicz *et al.*, 2006). Transferrin orthologues are also found in amphibians and fish, where they function as serum iron transporters.

Lactoferrin (LTF) is distinct from the other classes of transferrins both on account of its high isoelectric point (above 8.0) and its much tighter iron binding (Pakdaman *et al.*, 1998; MacGillivray and Mason, 2002). It is likely that its principal role is as an iron scavenger, preventing the proliferation of invading microorganisms (Baker *et al.*, 1987; Aguila *et al.*, 2001). LTF is expressed by cells of the mucosal epithelia and by polymorphonuclear granulocytes, and is found in a number of secreted fluids including milk and colostrum, saliva, tears, bile, respiratory pathway fluids, vaginal secretions, and seminal fluid (see reviews by Teng, 2010; Adlerova *et al.*, 2008), and also accumulates in amyloid deposits in the cornea and brain (Nilsson and Dobson, 2003; Leveugle *et al.*, 1994). The targeted disruption of the mouse LTF gene shows that it does not play a major role in the regulation of iron homeostasis (Ward *et al.*, 2003), but this may simply reflect the fact that in mice, rats and rabbits the major iron-binding protein of milk is STF (Lee *et al.*, 1987; Escalante *et al.*, 1993). Unlike serum transferrin, LTF cannot bind to either of the two transferrin receptors, TFR1 or TFR2. It does, however, bind to a number of receptors from many unrelated protein families (reviewed in Lambert, 2012).

Melanotransferrin (MTF or tumour-bound antigen 97) is a cell-surface glycoprotein, anchored to the membranes of melanocytes and other cells by a glycosyl–phosphatidylinositol linkage, which was first isolated from human melanomas, and identified by sequence homology as a member of the transferrin family (Rose *et al.*, 1986). It is widely expressed in many normal tissues, including salivary glands, sweat glands, liver, intestine and umbilical cord (Suryo Rahmanto *et al.*, 2007). MTF has two transferrin domains, and is bound to cell membranes via a GPI anchor, although a secreted form is also found at low levels in the bloodstream. Elevated levels of MTF are found in most melanomas, and it has been shown that surface expression of MTF increases the capacity of melanoma cells to cross the blood–brain barrier and form metastases (Rolland *et al.*, 2009). MTF genes are found in all vertebrates; orthologues are also present in tunicates and sea urchins (Lambert, 2012). Despite its ability to bind iron, MTF cannot bind either TFR1 or TFR2 (Kawabata *et al.*, 2004b; Food *et al.*, 2002), although it has been shown to bind plasminogen (Demeule *et al.*, 2003). The high expression of melanotransferrin in several disease states, particularly malignant melanoma, remains intriguing and may have clinical significance. Although the exact physiological functions of MTF remain elusive, a growing number of roles have been attributed to the protein, including iron transport/metabolism, angiogenesis, proliferation, cellular migration and tumorigenesis (Suryo Rahmanto *et al.*, 2012).

A number of other vertebrate transferrin-like proteins have been identified by sequence homology, although most of them do not appear to play a role in iron metabolism. A glycoprotein inhibitor of carbonic anhydrase (ICA) was identified in pig serum, which has 63% homology with porcine STF (Wuebbens *et al.*, 1997), and its X-ray structure revealed that, although it does not bind iron, both lobes were in the closed conformation usually associated with presence of iron in the cleft (see later in the chapter), making the structure most similar to diferric pig TF (Eckenroth *et al.*, 2010). While ICA is expressed in some mammals, it is an inactivated pseudogene in humans and does not appear to be present in marsupials, birds, or other vertebrates (Lambert and Mitchell, 2007). Saxitoxin is a trialkyl tetrahydropurine neurotoxin produced by a number of aquatic microorganisms, and the bilobal transferrin orthologue saxiphilin, found in the plasma of the North American bullfrog, binds saxitoxin with a K_d of 0.35 nM. It does not bind iron (Li *et al.*, 1993) and seems to have a rather limited distribution among vertebrates (Llewellyn *et al.*, 1997). Otoliths or earstones are calcareous bodies formed from calcium carbonate and proteins which are found in the inner ear of vertebrates and some invertebrates. One component, otolith matrix protein-1 (OMP-1), contains a single transferrin domain, although the iron-binding ligands are absent, and it has only been found in fish (Murayama *et al.*, 2000).

Originally thought to be restricted to vertebrates, transferrin-like proteins have been found in all metazoan (nonparasitic multicellular animals) classes examined to date (reviewed in Lambert, 2012); the invertebrate transferrin family members are listed in Table 6.1. Two transferrin homologues have been identified in the urochordate, *Ciona intestinalis*, a mono-lobal protein that binds Fe(III) (Tinoco *et al.*, 2008; Uppal *et al.*, 2008) and a bilobal protein (GenBank ID: XP_002120780) which has yet to be characterised. A similar, mono-lobed protein was found earlier in the ascidians *Pyura stolonifera* (Martin *et al.*, 1984) and *Halocynthia roretzi* (GenBank ID: BAB16119) (Abe *et al.*, 2001). The *Pyura stolonifera* protein was able to deliver iron to rat reticulocytes for incorporation into haem (Martin *et al.*, 1984). MTF-like sequences are predicted for the sea urchin (*Strongylocentrotus purpuratus*: GenBank ID: XP_001194989) and the sea cucumbers (*Holothuria glaberrima*: GenBank ID: ACS74869 and *Apostichopus japonicus*: GenBank ID: ADO66732).

Many studies have been carried out on transferrin in insects (reviewed in Dunkov and Georgieva, 2006; Geiser and Winzerling, 2012). Insect transferrin can have one or two lobes similar to mammalian Tsf, and can bind iron in one or both, although the most commonly studied bilobal insect transferrins shows greatest homology to mammalian serotransferrin. However, to date no orthologues of the vertebrate transferrin receptors have been reported in any insects. If insect transferrins do function as iron transporters, then the manner in which the iron enters the target cells remains to be determined (Lambert, 2012). The iron-binding ligands identified for the lobes of mammalian blood transferrin are generally conserved in the lobes of insect transferrins that have an iron-binding site. The fat body is the likely source of insect haemolymph transferrin. Although transferrin mRNA is expressed in several tissues in many insects, the fat body is the likely source of haemolymph transferrin. Insect transferrin is a vitellogenic protein that is downregulated by Juvenile Hormone, and serves a role in transporting iron to eggs in some insects, while transferrin found in eggs appears to come from the female. In addition to its role in iron delivery, transferrin also functions to reduce oxidative stress and to enhance survival from infection.

The major yolk protein in sea urchins, classified as a vitellogenin, has been shown to be an iron-binding, transferrin-like protein (Unuma *et al.*, 2001, 2003; Brooks and Wessel, 2002), which may be involved in shuttling iron to developing germ cells. This protein is produced in both the ovary and testis, in the coelomic fluid, and the intestines of both sexes (Brooks and Wessel, 2002; Unuma *et al.*, 2010). Major yolk protein orthologues have also been identified in the sea cucumber (Ramírez-Gómez *et al.*, 2008; Fujiwara *et al.*, 2009). In at least two sea urchins the major yolk protein sequence has either been modified, or duplicated and modified, to form another homolog, the toposome, a modified calcium-binding, iron-less transferrin, the first member of a new class of cell adhesion proteins (Noll *et al.*, 2007). The N-lobe transferrin domains of the toposomes reported for the sea urchins *Paracentrotus lividus* and *Tripneustes gratilla* share a strong identity with the major yolk proteins. This new member of the transferrin family shows special features (Figure 6.2), which explain its evolutionary adaptation to development and adhesive function in sea urchin embryos: (i) a protease-inhibiting WAP domain; (ii) a 280-amino acid cysteine-less insertion in the C-terminal lobe; and (iii) a 240-residue C-terminal extension with a modified cystine knot motif found in multisubunit external cell surface glycoproteins. Proteolytic removal of the N-terminal

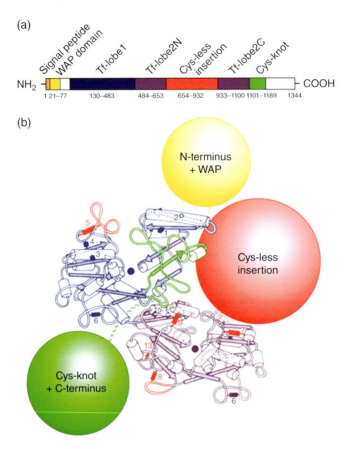

Figure 6.2 *Toposome domain structure in linear and 3D representation. (a) Linear domain structure of the toposome precursor. The various domains are illustrated in different colours, with the beginning and end indicated by the numbers of the corresponding amino acids of the* T. gratilla *toposome precursor. (b) 3D diagram of* T. gratilla *toposome precursor modified from that of lactoferrin (Baker et al., 1987). α-helices are shown as cylinders, β-strands as arrows, position of iron atoms for ferric Tfs as solid circles, disulphide bridges (numbered according to Williams, 1982) as solid bars. The N-terminal half (N-lobe) is at the top, the C-terminal half (C-lobe) at the bottom, and their relative orientations are related to a twofold screw axis. The three coloured spheres illustrate the two additions and the insertion shown linearly in panel (A), estimated under conditions of globular chain folding. The attachment points to the canonical transferrin framework are shown by stippled double lines. The external small loop and the large loop, including an α-helix and β-strand (in green) correspond to the variable sequence predicted to be the epitope for Fabs capable of dissociating embryos into single cells. The loops in red are not present in toposomes, and the disulphide bridges marked in red are missing because one or both cysteines are absent in toposomes. Reprinted with permission from Elsevier from Noll, H., Alcedo, J., Daube, M., et al. (2007) The toposome, essential for sea urchin cell adhesion and development, is a modified iron-less calcium-binding transferrin. Dev. Biol.,* **310***, 54–70*

WAP domain generates the mature toposome present in the oocyte. The modified cystine knot motif stabilises cell-bound trimers upon Ca-dependent dissociation of hexamer-linked cells.

Pacifastin, a proteinase inhibitor from crayfish is a heterodimer composed of two covalently linked subunits, the larger of which contains three transferrin lobes, two of which seem to be active for iron binding (Liang *et al.*, 1997). The halotolerant unicellular green alga *Dunaliella salina* is outstanding in its ability to withstand extremely high salinities. It has a 150 kDa transferrin-like protein in its plasma membrane, which is involved in iron uptake and relies on the presence of bicarbonate/carbonate anions (Fisher *et al.*, 1997, 1998). Unlike animal transferrins, it contains three, rather than two, internal repeats and a COOH-terminal extension including an acidic amino acid cluster. A multicopper ferroxidase has been shown to localise with the triplicated transferrin, and may function to enhance iron uptake (Paz *et al.*, 2007). A second, 100-kDA transferrin-like protein with two TF domains has also been identified, but does not appear to bind iron (Schwarz *et al.*, 2003).

6.1.3 Structure of Transferrins

All members of the transferrin family are glycoproteins of molecular weight around 80 kDa, composed of a single polypeptide chain of about 680 amino acid residues. The structures of three serum transferrins, six lactotransferrins and two ovotransferrins have been determined (reviewed in Mizutani *et al.*, 2012), and representative structures of the human serum apotransferrin (Wally *et al.*, 2006), human apolactoferrin (Anderson *et al.*, 1990) and apo-ovotransferrin (Kurokawa *et al.*, 1999) are presented in Figure 6.3. All three transferrins consist of two homologous, globular lobes (N- and C-lobes) connected by a short loop region, and have one iron-binding site in each lobe. Each of the lobes includes two similarly sized domains, domain 1 and domain 2 (domains N1 and N2 in the N-lobe and domains C1 and C2 in the C-lobe), and the two iron-binding sites are located within the inter-domain clefts of each lobe (N1 and N2; C1 and C2). Domain 2 (N2 and C2) consists of a contiguous polypeptide segment, but domain 1 is comprised of two polypeptide segments interrupted by domain 2. Thus, for example in lactoferrin, domain N1 contains residues 1–91 and 250–332, and domain C1 contains residues 343–434 and 594–691, respectively (Figure 6.3c). Domains N2 and C2 and the loop-region consist of residues 92–249, 435–593, and 333–342. The N-terminal lobe is on the right and the C-terminal lobe on the left. The lobe and domain architectures are well conserved in all of the reported structures of transferrins (Mizutani *et al.*, 2012). The same fold has been found in all members of the family for which X-ray structures have been determined.

In LTF, the two lobes are joined by a short, three-turn α-helix (Figure 6.3b) and, at the C terminus, by a final helix which again makes contact between the lobes. In transferrins and ovotransferrins, this inter-lobe peptide is irregular and flexible. All four domains have a similar super-secondary structure consisting of a central core of five or six irregularly twisted, mostly parallel β-sheets of similar topology, with α-helices packed on either side of them. There are two antiparallel β-strands (89–94 and 244–249), which run behind the iron-binding site, forming a flexible hinge between the two domains. This allows the domains to open and close upon metal binding and metal release, as we will see later. Within each lobe there are disulfide bridges, six in the N lobe and ten in the C lobe. Many of these disulfide bridges are conserved in other transferrins, but since none of them cross from one lobe to the other this explains how single half-molecules can be isolated from many species of transferrin by proteolytic cleavage of the peptide which joins the N and C lobes, or generated by recombinant DNA methods.

Depending on their metal ion status, transferrins can adopt one of two conformational states – either open or closed – which are illustrated for LTF in Figure 6.4 (Baker and Baker, 2012). In the diferric state (Fe_2LTF), two Fe^{3+} ions are bound, together with the synergistically bound carbonate ion, and the two domains of each lobe are fully closed over the bound metal ion (Figure 6.4a). This closed metal-bound form is highly stable and relatively rigid as the metal ions lock the domains

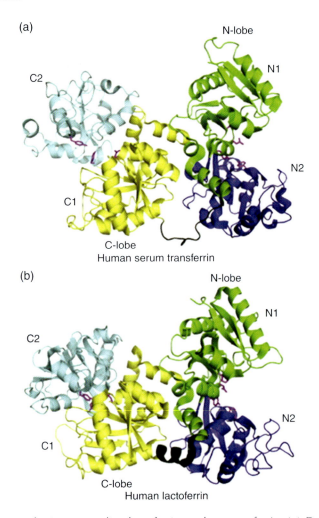

(a)

N-lobe

N1

C2

N2

C1

C-lobe
Human serum transferrin

(b)

N-lobe

N1

C2

N2

C1

C-lobe
Human lactoferrin

Figure 6.3 *Serum transferrin, mammalian lactoferrin, and ovotransferrin. (a) Domains N1 (residues 4–94 and 246–328), C1 (340–425 and 582–679), N2 (95–245) and C2 (426–581) of apo human serum transferrin (PDB: 2HAV) are shown in green, blue, yellow and cyan, respectively, in cartoon form. (b) Domains N1 (residues 1–91 and 250–332), C1 (343–434 and 594–691), N2 (92–249) and C2 (435–593) of apo human lactoferrin (PDB: 1CB6) are shown in green, blue, yellow and cyan, respectively. (c) Domains N1 (residues 1–91 and 247–332), C1 (343–429 and 589–686), N2 (92–246) and C2 (430–588) of apo ovotransferrin (PDB: 1AIV) are shown in green, blue, yellow and cyan, respectively. Loops connecting two lobes are shown in black. Iron-binding residues, Asp, two Tyr and His, are shown in magenta as stick models. Reprinted with permission from Elsevier from Mizutani, K., Toyoda, M. and Mikami, B. (2012) X-ray structures of transferrins and related proteins. Biochim. Biophys. Acta, **1820**, 203–211*

together, and is characteristic of all metal-bound Lfs, including complexes with other transition metal ions such as Cu^{2+} and Mn^{3+} and non-biological ions such as Al^{3+} and Ce^{4+} (Smith *et al.*, 1992, 1994; Kumar *et al.*, 2000; Mizutani *et al.*, 2005). In contrast, in its apo state LTF adopts an open form in which the two domains of each lobe are opened wide. In the structure in Figure 6.4b the N-lobe is in its open form, whereas the C-lobe is still closed although no iron is bound.

(c)

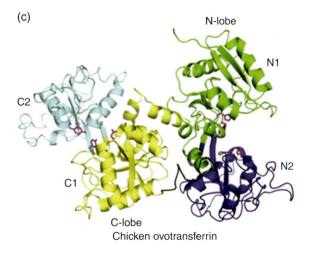

Chicken ovotransferrin

Figure 6.3   *(Continued)*

That substantial conformational changes occur upon uptake and release of Fe^{3+} in all three transferrins was already clear from small-angle X-ray solution scattering (SAXS) studies. The proteins were assumed to form open and closed conformations in the apo- and holo-forms, respectively (Grossmann *et al.*, 1992, 1993; Mecklenburg *et al.*, 1997). X-ray crystallographic studies then confirmed this for both lobes of ovotransferrin (Kurokawa *et al.*, 1995, 1999), of human serum transferrin (Wally *et al.*, 2006) and of goat lactoferrin (Kumar *et al.*, 2002), and for the N-lobes of human lactoferrin (Anderson *et al.*, 1989, 1990) and serum transferrin (Jeffrey *et al.*, 1998; MacGillevray *et al.*, 1998). The domain motion in these transferrin lobes follows a common structural mechanism which was first proposed for the lactoferrin N-lobe (Anderson *et al.*, 1989, 1990). The domains 1 and 2 rotate by around 50° as rigid bodies with a translation of 2.1 Å around a screw-axis which passes through the two interdomain β-strands (89–94 and 244–249), with both strands displaying a hinge-like motion. From high-resolution studies on hen ovotransferrin (Mizutani *et al.*, 2001) it was shown the conformational change in the first β-strand (89–94) was more complex. It was also shown that the screw-axis passes through inter-domain van der Waals contacts in the N-lobe, or a disulfide bond in the C-lobe which exists at the corresponding position to the van der Waals contacts (Mizutani *et al.*, 2001, 2012). The van der Waals contacts and the disulfide bond are significantly distant from the inter-domain β-strands (about 15 Å), and the van der Waals contacts in the N-lobe (or the disulfide bond in the C-lobe) help the precise hinge motion of domains around the β-strands as an alternative hinge. The disulfide bond in the C-lobe is well conserved in all of the serum transferrins, ovotransferrins and lactoferrins.

Metal binding and release are thus associated with large-scale conformational changes in which the domains close over the bound metal ion, or open to release it (Anderson *et al.*, 1990; Gerstein *et al.*, 1993). There is strong evidence that the apo-protein is in some sort of dynamic equilibrium between open and closed states (Baker *et al.*, 2002; Baker, 1994). Although X-ray crystallography cannot usually monitor dynamic processes, when an equilibrium exists in solution crystal formation can trap one out of multiple species present in solution. Thus, crystallographic analyses have variously visualised apo-LTFs with both lobes open (Khan *et al.*, 2001; Baker *et al.*, 2002), both closed (Sharma *et al.*, 1999), and one open, one closed (Anderson *et al.*, 1990), showing that the apo-form is flexible, alternating between open and closed forms.

(a)

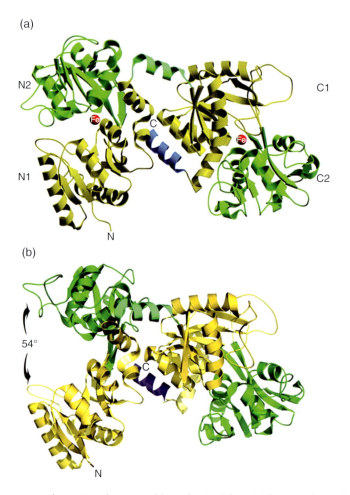

(b)

Figure 6.4 *The two conformational states of lactoferrin (Lf). (a) The iron-bound form, Fe$_2$Lf. The N-lobe is on the left, with its two domains N1 (gold) and N2 (green) closed over the bound iron atom (red sphere), while the C-lobe is on the right with its two domains C1 (gold) and C2 (green) also closed over the iron atom. The α-helix that joins the two lobes is shown in turquoise, and the C-terminal helix in blue. (b) The iron-free form, apo-Lf. In this structure the N-lobe is in its open form, with the two domains having moved apart through a rigid-body domain movement. This movement corresponds to a relative rotation of 54° around a hinge at the back of the iron-binding site. In this structure the C-lobe is still closed although no iron is bound, while in other apoLf structures it is found in open conformations, like that of the N-lobe. Reproduced with permission from NRC Research Press from Baker, H.M. and Baker, E.N. (2012) A structural perspective on lactoferrin function.* Biochem. Cell Biol., **90**, *320–328*

We have already indicated that the present-day transferrrins resulted from gene fusion and dupli-cation (Park *et al.*, 1985). It was originally proposed, based on the comparison of eight transferrin sequences, that the MTF sequences were the oldest vertebrate transferrins and that the SFT/MFT duplication occurred sometime before the split between birds and mammals, some 300 million years ago (Baldwin, 1993). Subsequently, the alignment of 71 full-length transferrin sequences from 51 different species (Lambert *et al.*, 2005), many of them derived from genome sequencing projects, suggested that this duplication took place much earlier (more than 580 million years ago).

Since then, the MTF lobes have changed relatively little. The authors also concluded that the LTF duplication occurred more recently (less than 125 million years ago) and that the LTF sequences showed a comparatively fast rate of change compared to either MTF or STF sequences. Continued analysis of the way in which the relatively ancient transferrin gene has evolved, acquiring new functions along the way and optimizing these functions under selective pressure over relatively long time scales, promises to bring an even greater understanding of the mysterious processes of evolution.

This is thrown into perspective by the observation (which has been delayed until now) that bacterial periplasmic binding proteins in *Neisseria* and *Haemophilus* (Nowalk *et al.*, 1994; Bruns *et al.*, 1997), which transport iron across the periplasm of Gram-negative pathogens (see Chapter 4), are also members of the transferrin family together with a number of other periplasmic binding proteins (PBPs). The PBPs transport a wide variety of nutrients, including sugars, amino acids and ions, across the periplasm from the outer to the inner (plasma) membrane in bacteria (see Chapter 3). Iron binding by transferrins (see below) requires concomitant binding of a carbonate anion, which is located at the N terminus of a helix, and this corresponds to the site at which anions are specifically bound in bacterial periplasmic sulphate and phosphate-binding proteins (Pflugrath and Quiocho, 1988; Luecke and Quiocho, 1990). This led to the suggestion that the transferrins could have arisen by divergent evolution and subsequent duplication from an anion-binding precursor common to the transferrins and the PBPs (Baker *et al.*, 1987) that existed prior to the divergence of prokaryotes and eukaryotes, about 1500 million years ago.

And to add even more spice to this tasty dish, comes the observation that the periplasmic protein which is involved in iron uptake in *Bordetella pertussis* (the bacterium responsible for whopping cough) has the ability not only to bind iron directly but also to bind iron–siderophore complexes (Banerjee *et al.*, 2014).

6.1.4 Transferrin Iron Binding

Transferrins are able to bind tightly, but reversibly, two Fe^{3+} ions with concomitant binding of two carbonate anions, as was first established for human serotransferrin (Schade *et al.*, 1949). The metal and coordinating anion sites in both lobes are well-conserved in all vertebrates; however, the dynamics of iron binding and release differs between the lobes (Zak and Aisen, 2003). Physiologically, the synergistic anion is carbonate, although a number of other anions can serve as bridging ligands between the protein and the metal ion *in vitro* (Schlabach and Bates, 1975; Gumerov and Kaltashov, 2001; Harris, 2012). The role of the bridging anion may be to prevent water from binding in the coordination sphere of the metal, locking the metal firmly to the protein and avoiding hydrolysis. *In vitro*, iron can be released from serum transferrin by acidification (Surgenor *et al.*, 1949).

The canonical hexadentate iron-binding sites in transferrins, shown in Figure 6.5 for the N lobe of human lactoferrin, consists of four protein ligands (two Tyr, one His and one Asp), plus two oxygen atoms from the synergistically bound CO_3^{2-} anion. Together, they form a nearly ideal octahedral metal coordination sphere, with tight Fe^{3+} binding $K_d = 10^{-19}$ to 10^{-20} M^{-1} (Aisen *et al.*, 1978; Pakdaman *et al.*, 1998). In contrast, the estimated binding constant of Fe^{2+} is of the order of 10^3 M^{-1} (Harris, 1986). Four of the six iron-coordination sites are supplied by protein ligands (one Asp, two Tyr and one His), and the other two by a bidentate carbonate anion (Figure 6.5). Of the four iron-binding residues, Asp and His are located in domain 1 (N1 or C1), and the two Tyr in domain 2 (N2 or C2) (one of the Tyr ligands is proximate to one of the two β-sheets connecting the two domains). All of the four iron-binding residues (Asp, two Tyr and His) and the anion-binding sites of both the N and C lobes of all transferrins (serum transferrins, ovotransferrins and lactoferrins) so far

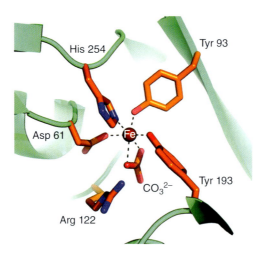

Figure 6.5 *The canonical iron-binding site for transferrins. Shown here for the N-lobe site of human lactoferrin, this site includes two tyrosine side chains (Tyr93 and Tyr193), one aspartic acid (Asp61), one histidine (His254), plus a bidentate-bound carbonate ion that forms a bridge between the metal ion and an arginine residue (Arg122) at the N terminus of an α-helix on domain N2. Reproduced with permission from NRC Research Press from Baker, H.M. and Baker, E.N. (2012) A structural perspective on lactoferrin function.* Biochem. Cell Biol., **90**, 320–328

characterised are highly conserved, with only one exception – in some insect transferrins His is substituted by Gln (Baker *et al.*, 2001) – and apparently optimised for the binding of Fe^{3+} and CO_3^{2-}.

The 3+ charge on the ferric Fe(III) ion is matched by the three anionic ligands Asp60, Tyr92 and Tyr192 (the fourth, His253 is neutral), while the charge on the carbonate anion is almost matched by the positive charge on Arg121 and the N-terminal dipole of helix 5. This explains why the synergistic anion is necessary for iron binding, since it effectively neutralises the positive charge in the putative binding pocket and supplies two oxygen ligands to bind the metal.

Pioneering studies on the crystal structure of ferric lactoferrin (Anderson *et al.*, 1987, 1989; Haridas *et al.*, 1995) were responsible for establishing how the carbonate anion was coordinated as a bidentate ligand to the ferric ion and was anchored into its binding site by hydrogen bonds. This was verified by equivalent structures for serum transferrin (Bailey *et al.*, 1988) and ovotransferrin (Kurokawa *et al.*, 1995). Figure 6.6 shows the interactions that bind the carbonate in the $Fe–CO_3–$ Tf complex. In addition to the two coordinate bonds to the ferric ion (2.19 and 2.06 Å), it is held in place by two hydrogen bonds to the side chain of Arg124 (2.60 and 2.74 Å), one hydrogen bond to the side chain of Thr120 (2.71 Å), and hydrogen bonds to the amide NH groups of Gly125 and Ala126 (both 2.83 Å) at the N terminus of helix 5. The structure also shows a solvent-filled cavity adjacent to the iron, which could account for the ability to accommodate synergistic anions with a bulky substituent (Anderson *et al.*, 1989). The carbonate-binding residues are well conserved in both lobes of serum transferrin, lactoferrin and ovotransferrin, except for Met in the place of Thr in the N-lobe of goat lactoferrin (Kumar *et al.*, 2002) and Ala for Gly in the C-lobe of horse lactoferrin (Sharma *et al.*, 1999).

The requirement for a synergistic carbonate to form a stable $M–CO_3–Tf$ ternary complex applies to other metal ions as well (Chasteen, 1977). The only exceptions appear to be the binding of vanadyl (VO^{2+}) (Casey and Chasteen, 1980) and vanadate ($H_2VO_4^-$ at physiological pH) (Harris and Carrano, 1984), where an oxo group on the vanadium may act as a replacement for the carbonate

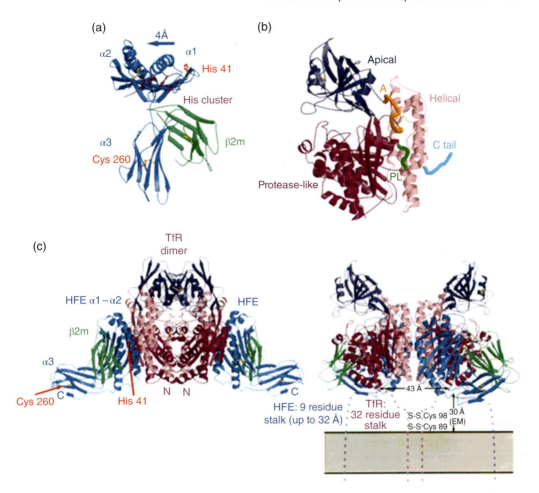

Figure 6.6 *Ribbon diagrams of HFE, TfR and HFE–TfR structures. (a) HFE (PDB code 1A6Z). Residues substituted in HH mutations (Cys260 and His41) and a cluster of histidines (residues 87, 89, 94 and 123) are highlighted. An arrow indicates the inward displacement of α1 domain helix as compared with the analogous class I MHC helix. (b) TfR monomer from homodimer structure (made using coordinates provided by C.M. Lawrence and S.C. Harrison). A, apical loop (residues 312–328); PL, protease-like loop (residues 469–476); C tail, C-terminal tail (residues 750–760). (c) Two views of the HFE–TfR structure related by a 90° rotation about the vertical axis. Chain termini nearest the predicted transmembrane region (C terminus for HFE heavy chain; N terminus for TfR) are labelled (left). The membrane bilayer is represented by a grey box (right). Reproduced with permission from Nature Publishing Group from Bennett, M.J., Lebron, J.A. and Bjorkman, P.J. (2000) Crystal structure of the hereditary haemochromatosis protein HFE complexed with transferrin receptor. Nature,* **403***, 46–53*

anion. Although carbonate is considered to be the physiological anion, in the absence of carbonate other anions – particularly small carboxylic acids such as oxalate – can also function as synergistic anions (Schlabach and Bates, 1975; Dubach *et al.*, 1991), and crystal structures with other anions, such as oxalate, have been reported (Baker *et al.*, 1996; Halbrooks *et al.*, 2004). Other inorganic anions bind to apotransferrin (Harris, 1985; Harris *et al.*, 1990; Cheng *et al.*, 1995), but do not act in a synergistic manner to promote metal binding (Schlabach and Bates, 1975; Foley and Bates,

1988). Anions can also bind to allosteric sites, called KISAB sites (kinetically significant anion binding site on ferric transferrin), and can alter the rates of iron release from transferrin to different chelating agents (Baldwin, 1980; Baldwin and de Sousa, 1981; Harris and Bali, 1988;. Kretchmar and Raymond, 1988; Egan *et al.*, 1992; reviewed in Evans *et al.*, 2012; Harris, 2012). Iron release from diferric-transferrin will be discussed later in the chapter, in an *in vivo* context.

6.1.5 Binding of other Metals by Transferrin

Since in human serum, transferrin is normally about 30% saturated with iron, it can potentially bind and transport other metal ions. While it is unlikely to be involved in the serum transport of essential divalent metal ions, such as Ca^{2+}, Co^{2+}, Cu^{2+}, Mg^{2+}, or Zn^{2+}, transferrin may play a physiological role in the transport of Mn, as Mn^{3+}, and has been postulated to play a significant role in transporting metal ions of potential therapeutic significance, such as Ti^{4+}, VO^{2+} (V^{4+}), Cr^{3+}, Ru^{3+}, and Bi^{3+}, as well as being a carrier for gallium and indium in tumour diagnosis. However, it may also play a role in carrying potentially toxic Al^{3+} and actinides, including Pu^{4+}, to tissues (reviewed in Vincent and Love, 2012).

Interest in titanium compounds as drugs arises from the use of titanocene dichloride (Cp_2TiCl_2 where Cp is the cyclopentadiene anion) as an anticancer compound (Abeysinghe and Harding, 2007), and although specific binding of titanium to transferrin was demonstrated (Sun *et al.*, 1998) the lack of success of clinical trials with potential titanium-based anticancer agents suggests that Ti-transferrin has limited therapeutic significance. However, the increasing use of titanium in prosthetics devices will probably lead to more interest in toxicological studies of effects of high levels of titanium in the bloodstream (Vincent and Love, 2012).

Vanadium does not appear to be an essential trace element for mammals, but it has potential pharmacological interest for the treatment of type 2 diabetes as long as its toxic side effects can be avoided. A number of vanadium chelates have been developed (Willsky *et al.*, 2001; Liboiron *et al.*, 2006; Kiss *et al.*, 2009; Sanna *et al.*, 2009a,b, 2010a,b; Jakusch *et al.*, 2009), of which the best studied is bis(maltolato)oxovanadium(IV), which have been shown to possess biological activity *in vivo* as insulin mimetics. Like insulin, vanadate administration results in the movement of transferrin receptors to the cell membrane, which results in the incorporation of more iron into the cell (Fantus *et al.*, 1995; Tang *et al.*, 1998) and theoretically this should also increase vanadium transport into the cells. In the bloodstream, VO^{2+} binds to transferrin as VO^{2+}-transferrin and $(VO^{2+})_2$-transferrin, regardless of whether V^{3+}, V^{4+}, or V^{5+} sources are injected into the bloodstream (Sabbioni *et al.*, 1978; Harris *et al.*, 1984). The formation constants indicate tight binding of VO^{2+}. VO^{2+} from VO^{2+}-transferrin delivered to cells apparently can be incorporated into ferritin (Sabbioni *et al.*, 1980; Chasteen *et al.*, 1986; Sabbioni and Marafante, 1991). Whether the tightrope between adverse and beneficial effects can be walked would appear to be seriously in doubt (Vincent and Love, 2012).

While chromium has generally been believed to be an essential trace element for approximately 50 years, recent research has not supported such a role for the metal (Vincent, 2014). In fact, a recent study has convincingly refuted the earlier nutritional studies on which the proposed status of chromium as essential is based (Di Bona *et al.*, 2011).

Interest in ruthenium complexes and their interaction with transferrin comes from the testing of the complexes as anticancer agents over the last two decades (Bergamo and Sava, 2011; Levina *et al.*, 2009; Hartinger *et al.*, 2008). Two ruthenium(III) complexes, namely trans-imidazolium[tetrachlorobis(imidazole)–ruthenate(III)], $HIm[RuIm_2Cl_4]$ (known as KP418) and trans-indazolium[tetrachlorobis(indazole)–ruthenate(III)], $HInd[RuInd_2Cl_4]$ (known as KP1019) have been extensively studied and shown to exhibit high anticancer activity in a colorectal carcinoma model in rats

(Hartinger *et al.*, 2008; Kratz *et al.*, 1996). Both complexes bind to transferrin, KP1019 with greater specificity than KP418. However, at the molar ratio of proteins in blood – that is, a ten-fold excess of albumin over transferrin – KP1019 binds to albumin more strongly than to transferrin, with almost all of the ruthenium (98–99%) in the albumin fraction (Polec-Pawlak *et al.*, 2006). This leaves the role of transferrin in the undoubted anticancer activity of these ruthenium drugs rather uncertain.

Mn is an essential trace element for mammals, although excess manganese is toxic to the nervous system. While Mn^{3+}-transferrin has been implicated in manganese transport, the significance of this is poorly understood. We will discuss the interactions between manganese and iron in Chapter 14.

Radionuclides of both indium and gallium are extensively used in nuclear medicine, and it has been clearly established that both metal ions are bound by transferrin. Since rapidly dividing cells (e.g. cancer cells) overexpress transferrin receptors, short-lived radiotracers bound to transferrin (by binding to the transferrin receptor) can have a certain diagnostic value. However, evidence suggests that indium-bound transferrin is not internalised, whereas gallium–transferrin is, allowing the imaging of certain tumours. The problems of aluminium toxicity will be discussed further in Chapter 14, as will the potential transport of actinides in mammalian systems by transferrin.

6.2 Cellular Iron Uptake

6.2.1 The Transferrin Receptors

Early studies with doubly labelled transferrin established that whereas iron is rapidly cleared from the circulation, the protein recycles many times – in humans the half-life of transferrin is about 7.6 days, whereas that of transferrin-bound iron is around 1.7 h (Katz, 1961). It can be estimated that the transferrin molecule undergoes more than 100 cycles of iron binding, transport and release, before it is finally removed from the circulation. Further, it was shown that the treatment of reticulocytes with trypsin abolished iron uptake, suggesting that there was a membrane receptor for transferrin (Jandl *et al.*, 1959). This led to the proposal of a plasma-to-cell cycle for transferrin (Jandl and Katz, 1963) in which the iron-loaded transferrin released its iron within the cell, where it remained, while the apotransferrin was released back to the circulation in search of more iron. Before discussing the present understanding of the transferrin-to-cell cycle, details of the transferrin receptors are presented.

In essentially all proliferating, differentiating and haemoglobin-synthesizing mammalian cells, iron uptake from transferrin is mediated by transferrin receptors (TfRs). Two TfRs have been described: the first, and much more extensively characterised, TfR1, is expressed by all iron-requiring cells, and is much more abundant than the more recently characterised second receptor, TfR2. Orthologues of TfR1 are found in all vertebrates, but not in hemichordates, tunicates and insects (Lambert, 2012). TfR1 and TfR2 are members of a larger family which includes glutamate carboxypeptidase II, N-acetylated α-linked acidic dipeptidases-like protein, as well as at least three other genes (Lambert and Mitchell, 2007).

TfR1 is expressed as a homodimer on the surface of almost every cell type in humans. In humans, the gene for the TfR1 is located on the long arm of the same chromosome 3, as are the genes for transferrin, melanotransferrin and ceruloplasmin (Rabin *et al.*, 1985). In common with other type II transmembrane proteins, TfR1 does not have a cleavable signal sequence, and during its synthesis it is inserted into the rough endoplasmic reticulum with the N terminus facing the cytoplasm (Zerial *et al.*, 1986). The subunit, a disulfide-linked transmembrane polypeptide of 760 amino acid residues, has three asparagine-linked glycans and one threonine-linked glycan. It consists of a short amino-terminal cytoplasmic domain (residues 1–61), a single-pass hydrophobic transmembrane region (residues 62–89), which is presumed to contain the signal for translocation across the plasma membrane of the cell (Zerial *et al.*, 1986), and a large extracellular portion (ectodomain, residues 89–760), which contains a binding site for the transferrin molecule. Electron cryomicroscopy shows that the transferrin receptor has a globular, extracellular structure separated from the membrane by a stalk of about 3.0 nm (Fuchs *et al.*, 1998). The stalk includes the residues immediately following the transmembrane region, including the oxygen-linked glycan and two intermolecular disulfide bonds which link the two subunits, one formed by Cys89 and one by Cys98 of each subunit, located in the extracellular domain of the protein close to the cell membrane (Jing and Trowbridge, 1987). The intermolecular disulfides are not required for dimerisation (Alvarez *et al.*, 1989). The extracellular domain can be isolated by trypsin digestion (Turkewitz *et al.*, 1988) as a soluble fragment containing residues 121–760; it is not disulfide-linked, yet it is a dimer which binds two molecules of transferrin with normal affinity. A similar fragment is found as a normal component of human serum, where its level is inversely correlated with body iron stores (see Chapter 10).

Like several other genes involved in iron transport and regulation (e.g. DMT1 and ferritin), the TFR1 mRNA contains untranslated iron-responsive elements (IREs). When iron concentrations are low, iron regulatory proteins (IRPs) bind to the IREs, stabilizing the transcript and increasing expression, whereas when iron is abundant the IRPs no longer bind to the IREs and this results in a rapid degradation of the TFR1 mRNA. At the promoter level, TFR1 expression is upregulated by anaemia and hypoxia and downregulated in conditions of iron-overload.

The crystal structure of the ectodomain of the human TfR1 has been determined as unbound TfR1 (PDB: 1CX8; Lawrence *et al.*, 1999), in a complex with human HFE (haemochromatosis protein) (PDB: 1DE4; Bennett *et al.*, 2000) and in a complex with Machupo virus glycoprotein (PDB: 3KAS; Abraham, 2010). All three structures reveal the transferrin receptor monomer to be made up of three distinct domains, organised in such a way that the dimer itself is butterfly-shaped (Figure 6.6). The likely orientation of the dimer with respect to the plasma membrane is indicated. The first, protease-like domain contains residues 122–188 and 384–606, and has a fold similar to carboxy or aminopeptidase (Chevrier *et al.*, 1996), consisting of a central, seven-stranded mixed β-sheet with flanking helices. The second, apical domain, contains residues 189–383, and can best be described as a β-sandwich in which the two sheets are splayed apart, with an α-helix (α1-2) running along the open edge. The apical domain is inserted between the first and second strands of the central β-sheet in the protease-like domain. The third, helical domain contains residues 607–760, and is essentially a four-helix bundle (like ferritin; see Chapter 8), with a large loop-like insert between two of the helices, which has contacts with both the apical and the protease-like domains, as well as with its counterpart across the molecular twofold axis. The helical domain seems to be particularly important for receptor dimerisation, since it contacts each of the three domains in the dimer partner.

The TfR1 homodimer can bind two molecules of Fe_2-Tf and bring them into the cell through endocytosis of the complex. The interaction between the partners is species-specific: human TfR1 does not bind bovine or goat Tf (Kawabata *et al.*, 2004b). Using cryoelectron microscopy, a density map of the TfR–Tf complex at subnanometer resolution was produced, and a 7.5 Å model of the human TF–TfR1 complex model was obtained by fitting crystal structures of diferric Tf and the receptor ectodomain into the map (Cheng *et al.*, 2004). The map shows the TFR1 helical domain binding the TF C-domain, while the TfR1 protease-like domain is in contact with the Tf N-lobe

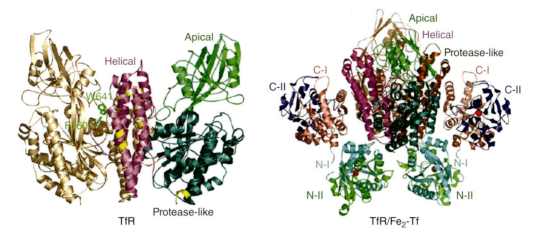

Figure 6.7 *Structure of the TfR homodimer alone (Lawrence et al., 1999; left) and bound to Fe₂-Tf (Cheng et al., 2004; right). One of the TfR chains is brown and the other is colour-coded to differentiate the three domains. The positions of residues contributing significantly to Fe₂-Tf binding (Giannetti et al., 2003) are highlighted in yellow, and the side chains of residues specific for binding apo-Tf (W641 and F760) are highlighted in green*

(Giannetti *et al.*, 2003; Cheng *et al.*, 2004). When Tf binds the receptor, its N-lobe moves by about 9 Å with respect to its C-lobe. The structure of the TfR–Tf complex is shown in Figure 6.7. A single particle reconstruction for the complex in its iron-free form, the apo-transferrin (apoTf)–TfR complex has also been obtained, although the authors were unable to improve the resolution of the apoTf–TfR density map beyond 16 Å, most likely because of the significant structural variability of Tf in its iron-free state (Cheng *et al.*, 2004). The density map does, however, support the model for the apoTf–TfR previously proposed (Giannetti *et al.*, 2003), based on the FeTf–TfR complex structure, and suggests that receptor-bound apoTf prefers to adopt an open conformation. Subsequently, the identification of TfR and Tf residues critical for TfR-facilitated iron release (Figure 6.8), yet distant from a Tf iron-binding site, demonstrates that TfR transmits long-range conformational changes and stabilises the conformation of apo-Tf to accelerate iron release from Fe-Tf (Giannetti *et al.*, 2005).

Isothermal titration calorimetry of Tf N-lobe mutants has shown that a cluster of residues in Tf (142–145) is important for interaction specifically with human TfR1 (Mason *et al.*, 2009). One of these, Pro142, is well conserved in all mammalian Tf and OTF sequences. The other three (Arg143, Lys144 and Pro145) are conserved in primates, rodents, and pigs; the TfR1 molecules of these groups have all been shown to bind human TfR1, while species which lack this motif cannot (Wally *et al.*, 2006; Mason *et al.*, 2009). In the TfR1 helical domain an RGD motif (646–648), which is also present in mammalian, bird, reptile and amphibian TfR1 (Lambert, 2012), is part of the binding site for both human Tf and HFE (Dubljevic *et al.*, 1999; Bennett *et al.*, 2000), Human TfR1 has been reported to bind the ferritin H chain (Li *et al.*, 2010), although quite what physiological significance this might have is unclear.

TfR2 is a paralogue of human TfR1, its gene located on chromosome 7q22, which binds diferric transferrin (Fe₂-Tf) and mediates iron uptake of Tf-bound iron (Kawabata *et al.*, 1999). However, the affinity of TfR2 for Fe₂-Tf is significantly lower (K_D ~30 nM) (Kawabata *et al.*, 2000; West *et al.*, 2000) than TfR1, it has no IREs in its mRNA, is only slightly upregulated in iron overload (Kawabata

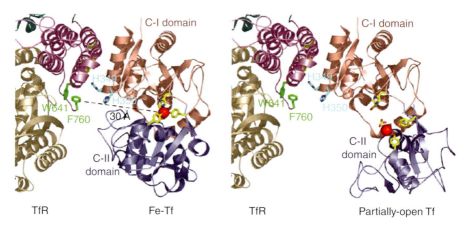

Figure 6.8 *Predicted TfR/Tf Interfaces. Close-up of predicted interactions at the interface between TfR (brown and magenta) and the C-lobes of iron-loaded Tf (left) and a partially open Tf (right) (salmon and blue) (based on the structure of an open form of iron-loaded camel lactoferrin) (Khan et al., 2001) to represent structural changes that might occur during opening of the Tf C-lobe to release the bound iron ion. TfR residues F760 and W641 are highlighted in green, Tf residues H349 and H350 are in cyan, and residues coordinating the bound iron in Tf are in yellow. A dashed line drawn between TfR residue F760 (green) and the iron atom in Tf (red) (predicted distance of ~30 Å) bisects the C-I/C-II domain boundary in the Tf C-lobe. The left panel is drawn from PDB code 1SUV (Cheng et al., 2004), and the right panel was generated by superimposing the C-I domain of the open form of iron-bound camel lactoferrin (Khan et al., 2001) (right panel) on the counterpart regions of the Fe_2-Tf molecule in the electron microscopic structure of the Fe_2–Tf/TfR complex. Reproduced with permission from Elsevier from Giannetti, A.M., Halbrooks, P.J., Mason, A.B. et al. (2005) The molecular mechanism for receptor-stimulated iron release from the plasma iron transport protein transferrin.* Structure, **13**, *1613–1623*

et al., 2000), and TfR2 orthologues are found only invertebrates (Lambert and Mitchell, 2007). TfR1 knockout mutation in the mouse leads to defective erythropoiesis and neurologic development showing that TfR2 cannot compensate for TfR1, perhaps reflecting its absence of expression in a number of tissues (Fleming *et al.*, 2000). A truncation mutation in TfR2 is associated with a rare form of hereditary haemochromatosis (type 3, HFE3, described in Chapter 9), an iron overload disorder characterised by excessive dietary iron absorption and iron deposition in liver and other parenchymal tissues (Camaschella *et al.*, 2000). The analogous mutation or knockout of *TfR2* in mice reproduces the disease phenotype (Fleming *et al.*, 2002; Wallace *et al.*, 2005), demonstrating that TfR2 is required for normal systemic iron homeostasis. It has been shown that TfR2 is a component of the erythropoietin receptor complex and is required for efficient erythropoiesis (Forejtnikova *et al.*, 2010).

6.2.2 The Transferrin to Cell Cycle and Iron Release

Whether they are haemoglobin-synthesizing immature erythroid cells, placental tissues, rapidly dividing cells, both normal and malignant, all cells obtain most of the iron that they require via receptor-mediated uptake from transferrin. The plasma iron pool (essentially transferrin-bound iron) in humans is normally only 30% saturated, so that the bulk of the transferrin lacks iron at one or both sites. It is, therefore, of great importance that the transferrin receptor can distinguish between Fe_2-Tf, the two Fe-Tfs and apotransferrin at the plasma membrane. Rabbit apotransferrin is bound by TrF1 with only one-twenty-fifth of the affinity of Fe_2-Tf, whilst the two monomeric forms bind six to seven times less tightly (Young *et al.*, 1984).

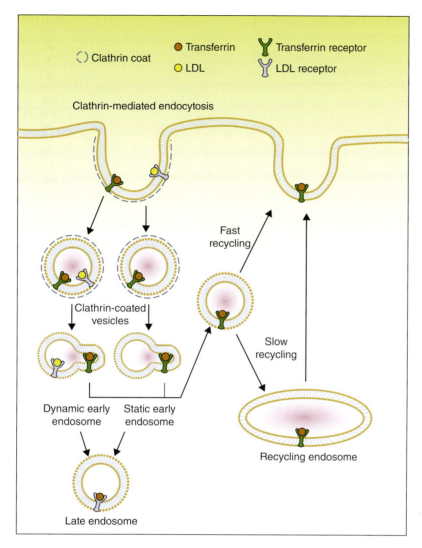

Figure 6.9 *An overall diagram of Tf trafficking. Tf is internalised via clathrin-mediated endocytosis and taken up into clathrin-coated vesicles. After the uncoating of clathrin, Tf can be found in both populations of static and dynamic early endosomes, as Tf shows no preference for either population. LDL, which follows the degradation pathway, is trafficked preferentially to dynamic early endosomes. Tubulation occurs in both populations of early endosomes, and proceeds to separate from early endosomes and traffic Tf to recycling pathways. A fast recycling route takes Tf directly back to the plasma membrane. A slower recycling route delivers Tf first to the perinuclear recycling compartment before Tf is trafficked back to the cell surface. Reprinted with permission from Elsevier from Mayle, L.M., Le, A.M. and Kamei, D.T. (2012) The intracellular trafficking pathway of transferrin.* Biochim. Biophys. Acta, ***1820***, *264–281*

After binding to its receptor at the plasma membrane, in a step which does not require energy, the diferric transferrin receptor complex invaginates into a clathrin-coated pit (Figure 6.9). Clathrin molecules assemble into a basket-like network on the cytoplasmic side of the membrane, and this assembly process starts to shape the membrane into a vesicle. A small GTP-binding protein, called dynamin, assembles around the neck of each deeply invaginated coated pit. The dynamin then hydrolyzes its bound GTP, causing the ring to constrict, so as to pinch off the vesicle from the membrane. This constitutes a coated vesicle, a membranous sac encased in a polyhedral frame-work of clathrin together with associated coat proteins, some of which – the adaptins – not only bind the coat to the vesicle membrane but also help to select ligand molecules for transport. After budding is complete, the clathrin and coat proteins are removed, resulting in the formation of smooth-surfaced vesicles. These naked transport vesicles can then fuse with the target membranes of endosomes. Fusion of the two membranes delivers the vesicle contents into the interior of the endosome, and adds the vesicle membrane to the endosomal membrane.

When ligands, such as holo-Tf, are internalised through clathrin-mediated endocytosis, as shown in Figure 6.9, the endocytosed ligands are sorted (reviewed in Mayle *et al.*, 2012) along the trafficking pathway into three main populations of early, late, and recycling endosomes (Gruenberg and Stenmark, 2004). Ligand sorting begins at the cell surface, separating ligands into two distinct populations of early endosomes with different maturation kinetics: *dynamic* or *static* (Lakadamyali *et al.*, 2006; Leonard *et al.*, 2008). The *dynamic* population of early endosomes matures quickly into late endosomes: ligands destined for degradation, such as low-density lipoprotein (LDL), are preferentially trafficked to this population (Lakadamyali *et al.*, 2006), whereas slower-maturing endosomes comprise the *static* population. Tf follows the recycling pathway, and although it indiscriminately enters both populations of early endosomes (Lakadamyali *et al.*, 2006), since the population of static early endosomes is much greater than of dynamic early endosomes, Tf becomes enriched in the static population of early endosomes. This pre-early endosomal sorting process is the first step in the segregation of cargo destined for degradation from those intended to be recy-cled back to the cell surface. Both populations of early endosomes then undergo a second sorting process, initiated by the development of tubular formations, in order to direct any cargo intended for recycling to the recycling pathway. Since Tf is contained within both dynamic and static early endosomes, these tubular formations function to traffic Tf to the recycling pathways from both populations of early endosomes. Ligands intended for degradation remain in the early endosomes, which then mature into late endosomes that subsequently proceed toward the degradation pathway involving lysosomes.

The interior of the endosome compartment is maintained at a pH of around 5.5–6.0 by the action of an ATP-dependent proton pump in the endosomal membrane, which pumps protons into the endosomal lumen from the cytosol. The endosomal compartment acts as the main sorting station in the inward endocytic pathway. The acidic environment of the endosome plays a crucial role in the sorting process by causing many receptors to release their bound ligand. These early endosomes, containing transferrin bound to its receptor, are rapidly sorted to deflect them from lysosomal degradation.

The mildly acidic pH values within the early endosome facilitates the release of Fe^{3+} from the hTF–TfR complex to an as yet unidentified biological iron chelator in a receptor-mediated manner; when it is bound to its receptor, iron release is facilitated compared to that from diferric-transferrin alone (Bali and Aisen, 1991, 1992; Bali *et al.*, 1991; Sipe and Murphy, 1991). While still within the endosome, Fe^{3+} must be reduced to Fe^{2+} by a ferrireductase, most probably Steap3 (Ohgami *et al.*, 2005), and is then transported across the endosomal membrane into the cytosol by the divalent metal transporter, DMT1 (Gunshin *et al.*, 1997). It has been proposed that in certain cell types the transmembrane metal ion transporter Zip 14 may also be involved in the transport of Fe^{2+} out of the endosome (Zhao *et al.*, 2010). Because apoTf retains a high affinity for its receptor at acidic pH values (unlike most other protein ligands), it remains bound to it at the endosomal pH, which facilitates correct sorting and recycling back to the plasma membrane (Dautry-Varsat *et al.*, 1983). There, at the slightly alkaline extracellular pH (7.4), apoTf is released or displaced by Fe$_2$hTf from the receptor (Leverence *et al.*, 2010) to go off into the circulation in search of iron. This constitutes the transferrin-to-cell cycle (Figure 6.10) which, given the high affinity of apotransferrin for the receptor at acidic pH values and its low affinity at pH 7.4, functions in one direction only, namely to take iron into cells that have transferrin receptors. The detail of how this process is achieved is discussed in greater detail below, with particular attention to implications from the 3.22 Å resolution crystal structure of a monoferric N-lobe hTf/TfR complex (Eckenroth *et al.*, 2011).

The first question concerns the preferential binding of Fe$_2$hTf by TfR at pH 7.4, and the crystal structure of the monoferric N-lobe hTF/TFR complex (3.22 Å resolution) identifies two binding

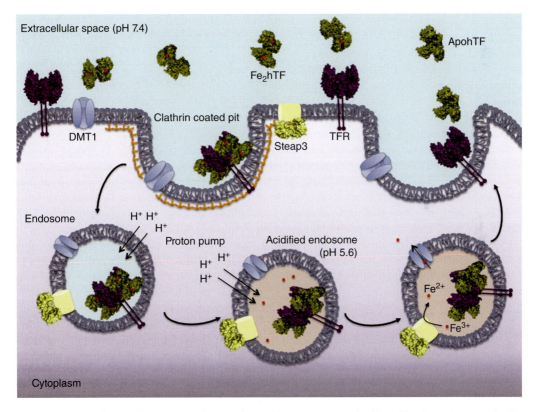

Figure 6.10 *Endocytic hTF–TFR cycle. Iron-bound hTF (green) in the blood binds to the specific TFR (purple) with nanomolar affinity at the cell surface (pH 7.4). The hTF–TFR complex is endocytosed in a clathrin-coated pit. Within the endosome, the pH is lowered to ~5.6 causing iron to be released from hTF to an (as yet) unidentified chelator. Fe^{3+} is reduced to Fe^{2+} by the ferrireductase Steap3 (yellow) within the endosome. The Fe^{2+} can then be transported out of the endosome via the divalent metal transporter DMT1 (blue) for use throughout the cell. The apohTF remains tightly bound to the TFR at pH 5.6 and is recycled back to the cell surface. Upon exposure to the slightly basic pH (7.4), apohTF is released or displaced from the TFR and is free to bind more Fe^{3+}. Reprinted with permission from Elsevier from Steere, A.N., Byrne, S.L., Chasteen, N.D., et al. (2012) Kinetics of iron release from transferrin bound to the transferrin receptor at endosomal pH. Biochim. Biophys. Acta,* **1820***, 326–339*

motifs in the N lobe and one in the C lobe of hTF (Eckenroth *et al.*, 2011). Binding of Fe$_N$hTf to TfR involves three primary interaction motifs. The regions of the N1 and N2 subdomains that contact TfR (helical and protease-like domains, respectively) are located on either side of the hinge region of the N lobe. The C lobe of hTf only contacts the TfR (helical domain) through the C1 subdomain, and there is no evidence to support the involvement of the C2 subdomain in binding to TfR.

The N1/TfR interface accounts for approximately 57% of the total contact surface area between the N lobe and TfR, and the contacts are more extensive than suggested by the cryoelectron microscopy model. Yet, there is no clear pattern of conservation of the residues in this motif (Wally *et al.*, 2006) which could account for the specificity of the interaction between the N1 subdomain of hTf and TfR. Eckenroth *et al.* (2011) suggested that the requirement for specific residues is somewhat obviated by the presence of backbone interactions. This is consistent with the observation that the mutation of either TfR residue Asn662 or Glu664, both of which are seen to make contact with TfR, did not significantly affect binding of Fe$_2$hTf or apohTF to the TfR, as measured by surface plasmon resonance (Giannetti *et al.*, 2003). In the N2 subdomain, two Pro residues (142 and 145) in the first loop of hTF (139–145) contact Asp125 and Tyr123 in the TfR, while two residues in the second hTF loop (154–167), Asp166 and Phe167, also contact Tyr123 in TfR. The importance of three of the four residues in the first loop (142–145, referred to as the PRKP loop) in the binding of the N2 subdomain has been unequivocally established (Mason *et al.*, 2009), and conservation of this region of hTf correlates with the ability of a given Tf to specifically bind to the human TfR (Wally *et al.*, 2006). All four residues of this loop were proposed to make contact with Leu122–Tyr123–Trp124–Asp125 of the sTfR in 7.5 Å structure (Cheng *et al.*, 2004).

The interaction of the C1 domain of hTf with TfR will not be discussed here. However, it should be noted that in the canonical RGD (Arg646, Gly647, and Asp648) sequence previously shown to be critical for hTf binding (Giannetti *et al.*, 2005), no obvious interactions with hTF and TFR residues Gly647 or Asp648 are observed and Arg646 in TfR is not within realistic H-bonding distance of hTF. As with the N1 motif, the side chain to backbone and van der Waals interactions may account for the limited conservation of C1 residues among Tfs (Wally *et al.*, 2006).

Pioneering insights into the role of the TfR on the kinetics of iron release from hTf at the endosomal pH of 5.6 came from the Aisen laboratory (Bali and Aisen, 1991, 1992; Bali *et al.*, 1991). Notably, these authors showed that in the absence of TfR, iron is released first from the N-lobe followed by the C-lobe; however, it was also suggested that the presence of TfR reversed this order (Bali and Aisen, 1991, 1992). Subsequent studies utilizing a time-based, steady-state tryptophan fluorescence technique clearly demonstrated that TfR enhanced the rate of iron release from the C-lobe of hTF at pH 5.6 (Zak and Aisen, 2003). Specifically, polyethylene glycol (PEG) precipitation studies with TfR led to the initial suggestion that TfR hinders iron release from hTF at pH 7.4 while facilitating iron release from hTF at pH 5.6 (Bali *et al.*, 1991). Crucially, it was noted the absolute requirement for an iron chelator, even at low pH, to achieve reasonable rates of iron removal from hTF – that is, to remove 50% of iron from an hTF–TFR complex at pH 5.6 in the absence of an iron chelator – required hours (Zak and Aisen, 2003).

Understanding the detailed mechanism of iron release from each lobe of hTf during receptor-mediated endocytosis is extremely challenging because of the active participation not only of the transferrin receptor (TfR), as well as Tf lobe–lobe interactions, but also the salt concentration, the requirement for a chelator, and the endosomal pH. The capture and unambiguous assignment of *all* of the kinetic events associated with iron release by the use of stopped-flow spectrofluorimetry, in the presence and absence of TfR, in an extraordinary *tour de force*, has now unequivocally established the decisive role of TfR in promoting efficient and balanced iron release from *both* lobes of hTf during one endocytic cycle. For the first time, the four microscopic rate constants required to accurately describe the kinetics of iron removal have been reported for hTF, with and without TfR (Byrne *et al.*, 2010a).

In summary, the stopped-flow spectrofluorimetric study confirms that, in the absence of sTfR, iron is almost exclusively released first from the N-lobe and then slowly from the C-lobe, with 95% of the iron being removed from the diferric protein through the upper kinetic pathway of Figure 6.11a. In contrast, at pH 5.6 and corroborating previous findings (Bali and Aisen, 1991, 1992), in the stopped-flow studies TfR enhances the rate of iron release from the C-lobe (from seven- to 11-fold) and slows the rate of iron release from the N-lobe (from six- to 15-fold), making them more equivalent and producing an increase in the net rate of iron removal from Fe_2hTF (Byrne *et al.*, 2010a). sTfR induces a switch in the order of iron release, such that the C-lobe preferentially releases its iron, followed by the N-lobe (Figure 6.11b, lower pathway) However, the situation is more complex, and in reality iron release through the upper pathway of Figure 6.11b is reduced from 96% in the absence of receptor to approximately 35% in its presence. Therefore, both the upper and the lower pathways play important roles in the efficient removal of iron from Fe_2hTF in the presence of sTfR.

The crystal structure of a monoferric N-lobe hTf/TfR complex has allowed the identification of both global and site-specific conformational changes within the TfR. Specifically, movements at

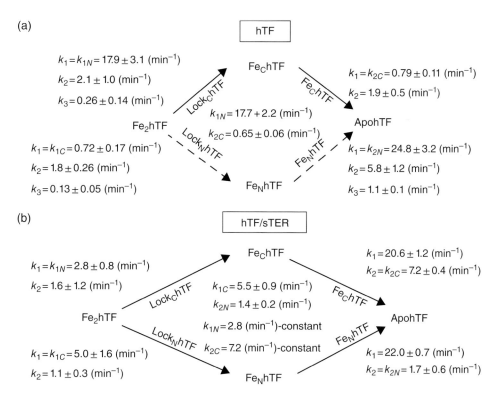

Figure 6.11 *Pathways of iron release ± sTFR. (a) Iron release pathways of Fe_2hTF in the absence of the sTFR. (b) Iron release pathways of Fe_2hTF in the presence of sTFR. Reproduced with permission from Elsevier from Byrne, S.L., Chasteen, N.D., Steere, A.N. and Mason, A.B. (2010a) The unique kinetics of iron release from transferrin: the role of receptor, lobe-lobe interactions, and salt at endosomal pH. J. Mol. Biol.,* **396**, *130–140*

the TFR dimer interface appear to prime the TfR to undergo pH-induced movements that alter the hTf/TfR interaction. Iron release from each lobe then occurs by distinctly different mechanisms. The binding of His349 to the TfR (strengthened by protonation at low pH) controls iron release from the C-lobe, whereas the displacement of one N-lobe binding motif, in concert with the action of the dilysine trigger, elicits iron release from the N-lobe. One binding motif in each lobe remains attached to the same α-helix in the TfR throughout the endocytic cycle. Collectively, the structure elucidates how the TfR accelerates iron release from the C-lobe, slows it from the N-lobe, and stabilises the binding of apohTF for return to the cell surface (Eckenroth *et al.*, 2011).

Iron release from the C-lobe of hTf in the absence of the TfR is extremely slow and unaffected by the N-lobe (Bali *et al.*, 1991). The C-lobe features a triad of residues (Lys534–Arg632–Asp634) that appear to control the rate of iron release in the absence of TfR (Halbrooks *et al.*, 2005; James *et al.*, 2009). However, as we saw earlier, iron release from the C-lobe in the presence of TfR is much faster and proceeds by a different mechanism (Byrne *et al.*, 2010a). The driving force here is His349, and the critical role of His349 is clearly demonstrated by the H349A mutant in the Fe_2hTF–TFR complex where the rate constant is reduced 12-fold (Steere *et al.*, 2011). Based on the cryoelectron microscopy-determined structure, it was predicted that a hydrophobic patch (TfR residues Trp641 and Phe760) interacts with His349 and stimulates iron release by stabilizing the apohTf–TfR complex (Giannetti *et al.*, 2003), whereas because of a 5 Å shift of helix α-1 of the C-lobe in the new structure, His349 actually lies in the intersection between the two TfR monomers forming the N-terminal cap of hTf helix α-1. Its role as a pH-inducible switch responsible for iron release from the C-lobe in the presence of the TfR (Giannetti *et al.*, 2005; Steere *et al.*, 2011) can be explained as follows. At pH 7.5, His349 interacts with at least two residues in the C-terminal portion of the TfR, including Asp757 and Asn758, and potentially with Phe760. It is proposed that in wild-type hTf, protonation of His349 at pH 5.6 converts an interaction with either Phe760 or Asp757, which causes a conformational change in the C-lobe and accelerates iron release from this lobe (Eckenroth *et al.*, 2011).

In the absence of the TfR, iron release from the N-lobe relies on a pair of lysines (Lys206 and Lys296 – the 'dilysine trigger') on opposing sides of the binding cleft which form a hydrogen bond at neutral pH, and their protonation at endosomal pH literally triggers cleft opening (He *et al.*, 1998). Iron release from the N-lobe is further accelerated by the binding of anions to Arg143, a recently identified kinetically significant anion binding (KISAB) site in the PRKP loop in the N2 subdomain (Byrne *et al.*, 2010b). The attachment of both the N1 and N2 subdomains to TfR limits access to this KISAB site, hinders cleft opening, and results in a rate of iron release that is six- to 15-fold slower than in the absence of the TFR (Byrne *et al.*, 2010a). Since the N1 and C1 subdomains maintain their positions relative to each other in both rabbit Fe_2Tf and human apoTf structures, the N2 subdomain must clearly disengage from TfR to allow the cleft to open. It is suggested that a pH-induced movement of the TfR may help destabilise binding of the N2 subdomain, which is relatively weak. Rearrangement of the PRKP loop in the N-lobe then pulls the N2 subdomain away from the TfR, allowing the cleft to open and release iron (Eckenroth *et al.*, 2011).

6.2.3 Iron Uptake from other Sources

Iron in the plasma can also be transported in other forms than transferrin-bound iron, as haem iron, as ferritin or, in conditions of iron overload, as another species designated non-transferrin-bound iron (NTBI). Ferritin represents only a tiny amount of iron, since the iron content of plasma ferritin is low and the normal plasma ferritin levels are less than 300 μg l^{-1}.

The release of haem proteins, particularly haemoglobin, into extracellular fluids during haemolysis and tissue damage is potentially hazardous due to the reactivity of free haem, which can generate toxic free radicals (Sadrzadeh *et al.*, 1984) and, as seen in Chapter 4, can also serve as a major source of iron for invading bacterial pathogens. The release of haemoglobin into plasma is a physiological phenomenon associated with intravascular haemolysis. While senescent erythrocytes are normally engulfed by macrophages, nonetheless, intravascular haemolysis due to normal 'wear and tear' on the erythrocytes accounts for at least 10% of red cell breakdown in normal individuals (Garby and Noyes, 1959). After release into plasma, tetrameric haemoglobin dissociates into αβ dimers, and is instantly captured by the acute-phase protein haptoglobin in a virtually irreversible reaction (Shim *et al.*, 1965). These stable haptoglobin–haemoglobin complexes are rapidly cleared through high-affinity binding to the macrophage scavenger receptor CD163 (Kristiansen *et al.*, 2001). The CD163 receptor binds and internalises the resultant high-affinity haptoglobin–haemoglobin complex, but binds neither free haemoglobin nor free haptoglobin (Kristiansen *et al.*, 2001). Uptake of the haemoglobin–haptoglobin complex is followed by the destruction of both haemoglobin and haptoglobin, confirming the role of CD163 as a scavenger receptor in tissue macrophages, thereby preventing haemoglobin toxicity while also playing a role in the recycling of iron (Kristiansen *et al.*, 2001). The crystal structure of the porcine haptoglobin–haemoglobin complex has been determined to 2.9 Å resolution (Andersen *et al.*, 2012).

Haem arising from the degradation of haemoglobin, myoglobin and of enzymes with haem prosthetic groups can also be present in plasma. Protection from haem is ensured by haemopexin (Hpx), a 60 kDa serum protein which binds haem with very high affinity (K_d <1 pM; Hrkal *et al.*, 1974) and delivers the haem to target cells such as liver hepatocytes via specific receptors. By sequestering free haem, Hpx provides a backup mechanism for the clearance of haemoglobin by haptoglobin. Internalisation of the haem–haemopexin complex releases haem for intracellular degradation by haem oxygenase, stimulates intracellular protective mechanisms, including the induction of haem oxygenase 1 and the anti-apoptotic transcription factor NF-κB. In this way, haem binding and transport by Hpx provides protection against both extracellular and intracellular damage by free haem, limits access to haem by pathogenic organisms, and conserves iron by recycling the haem iron. The haem–Hpx complex is internalised by CD91 receptor-mediated endocytosis, and the haem is then released into hepatic parenchymal cells. Like apotransferrin, Hpx is recycled back into the circulation for re-use after delivering haem intracellularly (Smith and Morgan, 1979, 1981; Smith and Hunt, 1990). Human albumin also has multiple low-affinity binding sites for haem (Smith and Neuschatz, 1983). Haemopexin is composed of two homologous domains, each consisting of about 200 amino acids linked by a 20-residue linker (Morgan and Smith, 1984; Takahashi *et al.*, 1985). From the crystal structure it is clear that both domains have the same fold, each comprising an unusual arrangement of four β-sheet modules, like the blades of a four-bladed β-propeller (Paoli *et al.*, 1999). In the haem–Hpx complex the haem is bound between the N- and C-terminal β-propeller domains in a pocket which is bounded by the interdomain linker peptide. The two domains associate with one edge of the C-terminal domain packed against the face of the N-terminal domain, in the vicinity of the central tunnel opening. The mechanism of haem release from Hpx, like the release of iron from transferrin, takes place in the acidic pH environment of the endosome following receptor-mediated endocytosis, although little is known about the influence of the receptor. It is likely that the mechanism involves (as in the case of transferrin) a transition from the tight association of the rigid domains seen in the crystal structure of the haem–Hpx structure to a flexible open form (Baker and Baker, 2012). The four-bladed β-propeller fold that is typical of Hpx-like proteins is widespread in viruses, prokaryotes and eukaryotes, and most recently was found in fungi (Ota *et al.*, 2013).

Non-transferrin-bound iron (NTBI) was first discovered by Hershko *et al.* (1978), and will be discussed in greater detail in Chapter 11 (for a review see Brissot *et al.*, 2012). It is found in serum if the transferrin saturation exceeds 45% (Brissot *et al.*, 2012) and its chemical nature remains to be determined. It is mostly taken up by the liver (Wheby and Jones, 1963), and in perfused liver single-pass experiments have shown the iron uptake of NTBI to range between 58% and 75% (Brissot *et al.*, 1985). The pathway of NTBI uptake also remains largely problematic. The obvious candidate would appear to be DMT1, as appears from studies on normal hepatocytes (Shindo *et al.*, 2006) and hepatic cells from HFE knockout mice (Chua *et al.*, 2004), but mice which lack DMT1 can still accumulate hepatic iron (Gunshin *et al.*, 2005), indicating that at least one alternative transferrin-independent uptake pathway must exist.

There are a number of other candidates for NTBI uptake. These include the Zn^{2+} transporter Zrt-Irt-like protein 14 (ZIP14) (Liuzzi *et al.*, 2006; Zhao *et al.*, 2010), and L-type voltage-dependent Ca^{2+} channels, which are known to mediate transferrin-independent iron entry into cardiomyocytes in iron overload (Oudit *et al.*, 2003); these may also play a role in iron delivery to neuronal cells (Gaasch *et al.*, 2007). It has been shown that calcium channel blockers such as nifedipine mobilise liver iron and enhance urinary excretion in iron-loaded mice, probably by increasing DMT1-mediated iron transport (Ludwiczek *et al.*, 2007). Ferric siderophore-mediated iron uptake by lipocalin 2-dependent endocytosis (Kaplan, 2002) via the SLC22A17 lipocalin receptor has been observed in cultured kidney cells (Devireddy *et al.*, 2005), but the physiological relevance of this pathway remains uncertain as lipocalin 2 knockout mice develop normally. Serum ferritin can be taken up by the Scara5 (scavenger receptor class A, member 5) and TIM-2 (T-cell immunoglobulin and mucin domain-containing 2) ferritin receptors (Li *et al.*, 2009; Chen *et al.*, 2005; Han *et al.*, 2011). Incidentally, as the name implies, DMT1 transports divalent metal ions so it is likely that a plasma membrane uptake system would also require an as yet unidentified ferrireductase.

6.3   Cellular Iron Export

In the absence of a regulated mechanism for iron excretion in humans, only iron acquisition can be regulated, and therefore (as will be seen in later chapters) both iron deficiency and iron overload represent major problems in systemic iron homeostasis. Nonetheless, iron must be transferred from one tissue to another, and four tissues play a critical role in this aspect of cellular iron homeostasis, namely the intestine and the placenta, which are responsible for the net transfer of iron to the rest of the organism, whereas macrophages and parenchymal tissues such as hepatocytes are involved in iron recycling. Erythrocytes contain most of the iron in vertebrates in the form of haemoglobin, and when they reach the end of their defined life span they are cleared from the circulation by macrophages. After phagocytosis, the erythrocytes are degraded in lysosomes, haem is released, iron extracted by haem oxygenase, and the iron is released for storage or exportation. As will be seen later, the major source of iron which enters the plasma daily comes from the macrophages, which recycle iron from the erythrophagocytosis of effete erythrocytes, whereas intestinal iron absorption normally accounts for only about one-thirtieth of total plasma iron turnover.

In order to recycle iron, tissues such as liver and the macrophages must have an export pathway, and that is represented unequivocally by ferroportin, the unique protein that is capable of exporting iron from the cells (Kaplan and Ward, 2102). Ferroportin1/IREG1/MTP1, the product of the *SLC40A1* gene, was independently identified by three different laboratories in 2000 and shown to play a role in the export of iron from a number of different types of cell (McKie *et al.*, 2000; Donovan *et al.*, 2000; Abboud and Haile, 2000).

In the search for the cause of autosomal recessive mutations in the hypochromic zebrafish mutant *weissherbst*[1] (*weh*), Donovan *et al.* (2000) not only isolated and characterised ferroportin but later also showed that in mutant embryos the iron content of intestinal cells and macrophages was increased, suggesting a transport defect (Fraenkel *et al.*, 2005. This was confirmed in mice with a targeted deletion in the *fpn* gene (Donovan *et al.*, 2005), thus also establishing the essential role of Fpn in early embryonic development. Mice with a deletion of *Fpn1 in utero* were viable, and accumulated iron in enterocytes, macrophages and hepatocytes, consistent with an essential role for Fpn in cellular iron export (Donovan *et al.*, 2005). Curiously, mice with a targeted deletion of Fpn1 in macrophages showed only a relatively mild anaemia (Zhang *et al.*, 2011), as did mice with the flatiron (ffe) mutation, which prevents wild-type Fpn from localizing to the cell surface (Zohn *et al.*, 2007). One explanation for this is that macrophages can export iron via the Feline Leukemia Virus C Receptor (FLVCR) transporter (Keel *et al.*, 2008), which might compensate for the loss of Fpn (Ward and Kaplan, 2012).

Fpn1 is a multidomain, transmembrane protein which is expressed in cells that play critical roles in mammalian iron metabolism, including placental syncytiotrophoblasts, duodenal enterocytes, hepatocytes and reticuloendothelial macrophages. Its expression is responsive to iron and inflammatory stimuli, and its mRNA possesses an iron responsive element (IRE) in the 5′-untranslated region (UTR) which could bind iron regulatory proteins and might confer iron-dependent regulation. Ferroportin (Ward and Kaplan, 2012) is also regulated at the level of expression of its mRNA, and as will be seen in Chapter 10, above all by its interaction with the key regulator of iron homeostasis, hepcidin, for which it can essentially be considered to be the plasma membrane receptor (Ganz and Nemeth, 2006; Nemeth and Ganz, 2006).

The structure of ferroportin has not been determined to date, but the 12 transmembrane domain model first proposed by Liu *et al.* (2005) has been most often used as a model (Wallace *et al.*, 2010). While there is agreement that the amino-terminus is cytosolic, the location of the carboxy-terminus is unclear, as is the question of whether it is a monomer or a dimer (reviewed in Ward and Kaplan, 2012). Likewise, very little is known about the mechanism by which Fpn mediates iron transport. Mutations in the ferroportin gene may affect either regulation of the protein's transporter function or the ability of hepcidin to regulate iron efflux. Using a combination of functional analysis and theoretical modelling, a model was proposed for this (Wallace *et al.*, 2010) in which mutations clustered according to phenotype. Gain-of-function mutations were associated with a hypothetical channel through the axis of ferroportin, whereas loss-of-function variants were located at the membrane/cytoplasm interface. More recently, an approach based on comparative modelling has led to the construction of a model of the three-dimensional (3D) structure of ferroportin (Figure 6.12) by homology to the crystal structure of a Major Facilitator Superfamily member (EmrD) (Le Gac *et al.*, 2013). This model predicts atomic details for the organisation of ferroportin transmembrane helices, and is in agreement with the current understanding of ferroportin function and its interaction with hepcidin. *In-vitro* experiments have been used to demonstrate that this model can be used to identify novel critical amino acids. Figure 6.13 shows the model of the amino acids participating in the ferroportin pore. In particular, Trp42, which is localised within the extracellular end of the ferroportin pore, is likely to be involved in both the iron export function and in the mechanism of inhibition by hepcidin.

---

[1] The zebra fish has been a rich source for the identification of genes involved in haematopoiesis and iron metabolism. In addition to *weissherbst*, these include *chardonnay* (DMT1), *chianti* (TfR1), *dracula* (ferrochelatase), *riesling* (spectrin β), *sauternes* (δ-aminlaevulinate synthase), *weissherbst* (ferroportin), *yquem* (uroporphyrinogen decarboxylase) and *zinfandel* (globin locus) (de Jong and Zon, 2005).

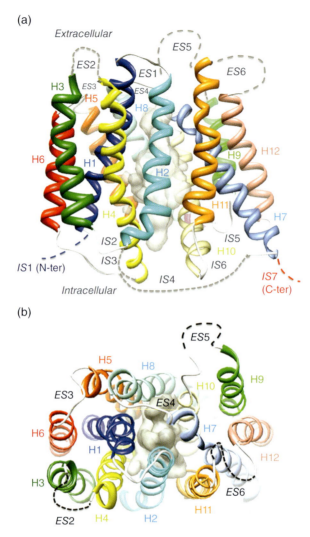

Figure 6.12 *Ribbon representation of the model of the human ferroportin 3D structure based on the EmrD experimental 3D structure. The model is shown viewed from the membrane plane (a, side view) and from the extracellular side (b, top view). The structure is organised into equivalent domains, each possessing six helices (helices H1–H6 and H7–H12) and organised as two, three-helix bundles. Ribbons are rainbow-coloured (from blue to red) in the two halves to highlight the duplication and the equivalent helices. The loops are designated as extracellular and intracellular segments (ES and IS, respectively), with the nonmodelled loops represented as dashed lines. The solvent-accessible surface of residues participating in the pore is shown, which is displayed at the interface of the two subdomains (also see Figure 6.13). Reproduced with permission from John Wiley & Sons from Le Gac, G., Ka, C., Joubrel, R., et al. (2013) Structure–function analysis of the human ferroportin iron exporter (SLC40A1): effect of hemochromatosis type 4 disease mutations and identification of critical residues.* Hum. Mutat., **34**, 1371–1380*

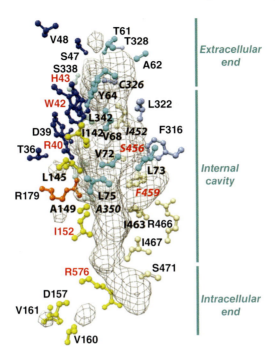

Figure 6.13 *Amino acids participating in the ferroportin pore. Amino acid residues (side chains) participating in the pore and their solvent-accessible surface (meshes) are shown. Amino acid residues are coloured according to the colours of the different helices, as depicted in Figure 6.12. The labels of amino acids observed behind the meshes are in italics (details of the labels of amino acids chosen for further experimental characterisation are shown in red). Reproduced with permission from John Wiley & Sons from Le Gac, G., Ka, C., Joubrel. R., et al. (2013) Structure–function analysis of the human ferroportin iron exporter (SLC40A1): effect of hemochromatosis type 4 disease mutations and identification of critical residues. Hum. Mutat., **34**, 1371–1380*

The substrate for Fpn is presumed to be Fe^{2+}, essentially based on the observation that iron transport requires the activity of an extracellular ferroxidase. The connection between Fe and Cu will be explored in greater detail in Chapter 14, and an interesting history of the relationship can be found in Fox (2003). Early animal studies established that copper-deficient animals were also iron-deficient, and that the copper-containing ferroxidase ceruloplasmin (Cp) was required to release iron from macrophages and hepatocytes (Gubler *et al.*, 1952; McDermott *et al.*, 1968; Osaki *et al.*, 1971; Frieden and Hsieh, 1976). Vulpe *et al.* (1999) then identified the Cp homologue hephaestin as the gene defective in sex-linked anaemia in mice. Hephaestin is a membrane-bound multicopper oxidase which is highly expressed in the intestine. The anaemia is a consequence of defective iron export from the intestine, due to the absence of hephaestin. Hephaestin, Cp and the curiously named zyklopen – a newcomer present in placenta and mammary gland, with an expression pattern distinct from that of Cp and hephaestin (Chen *et al.*, 2012) – are all members of the multicopper oxidase family of proteins. They join the orthologous ferroxidase Fet3p in fungi and algae, whose key role in the high-affinity iron uptake system in *Saccharomyces cerevisiae* was described in the previous chapter.

Ceruloplasmin clearly plays a key role in the mobilisation of iron from cells, and it appears that this is its principal physiological role.[2] As will be reviewed in Chapter 15, the genetic absence or mutation of ceruloplasmin (aceruloplasminaemia) results in an accumulation of iron in tissues such as the liver and brain. Indeed, it has been suggested that *in vivo* ceruloplasmin plays a custodial role, mediating the release of Fe^{2+} from cells and ensuring that it is subsequently incorporated into apotransferrin in the Fe^{3+} form (Lindley, 1996), while obviating the danger of releasing 'free' Fe^{2+}, which could potentially lead to the production of the highly toxic hydroxyl radical ($OH^{\bullet}$) (see Chapter 13).

As the multicopper ferroxidases are discussed in greater detail in Chapter 14 (for reviews, see Quintanar *et al.*, 2007; Vashchenko and MacGillivray, 2013), at this point their involvement in iron incorporation into apotransferrin, and whether apotransferrin interacts directly with ceruloplasmin, will be only briefly addressed. The reaction catalysed by the multicopper ferroxidases involves the oxidation of four atoms of Fe^{2+} to Fe^{3+}, oxidizing the iron atoms one at a time and storing the electrons until, when the fourth electron has been abstracted, the stored electrons can reduce molecular oxygen to water in a concerted reaction:

$$4Fe^{2+} + 4H^{+} + O_2 \rightarrow 4Fe^{3+} + 2H_2O$$

It might be asked why it is necessary to involve a multicopper enzyme in a process which, at pH 7.4 will occur spontaneously. Two very good reasons can be advanced. First, as pointed out earlier, the reaction carried out by the oxidases does not generate oxygen radicals, in contrast to the spontaneous oxidation of iron. Second, at low oxygen concentrations the non-enzymatic oxidation of iron is slow whereas, because of their high affinity for oxygen, the oxidases dramatically increase the rate of reaction (Sarkar *et al.*, 2003).

Cp has six plastacyanin domains (Figure 6.14), with type 1 copper in domains 4 and 6 and a trinuclear cluster situated between domains 1 and 6. The three-copper domain is critical not only to the catalytic activity of Cp, but also because it holds together the N- and C-terminal domains of holoCp (Vachette *et al.*, 2002). From X-ray studies on crystals of human ceruloplasmin soaked in metal salts, ferrous-binding sites have been identified in the vicinity of two of the type I mononuclear copper sites in domains 4 and 6 (Lindley *et al.*, 1997). One of these potential ferroxidase centres consists of one His and three carboxylates (Figure 6.15), with His940, Glu935 and Asp1025 contributed by domain 6 and Glu25 by domain 2. This site has similarities with the ferroxidase sites in H chain ferritins (see Chapter 7), and is also similar to the ferroxidase site in Fet3p (Taylor *et al.*, 2005). Near-infrared magnetic circular dichroism (MCD) studies have shown that the Fe^{2+} is hexacoordinate, suggesting the presence of two water molecules as additional iron ligands (Quintanar *et al.*, 2007). Glu272 is hydrogen-bonded to His1046, one of the copper ligands in domain 2, and is predicted to participate in electron transfer to the type 1 copper site in domain 2. The functionality of iron-binding sites in domains 4 and 6 has been confirmed in mutagenesis studies (Brown *et al.*, 2004).

As to whether apotransferrin interacts directly with ceruloplasmin, it has been shown that both apo- and holotransferrin interact with Cp with a dissociation constant of 15 μM (Ha-Duong *et al.*, 2010). In a more recent study from the same group (Eid *et al.*, 2014), the oxidation kinetics of Fe^{2+} by Cp has been studied in great detail, and it is proposed that the oxidisation of Fe^{2+} occurs first at the divalent iron-binding site in domain 6, and subsequently at the corresponding site in domain 4,

---

[2] Ceruloplasmin has seen numerous roles attributed to it, including that of copper transport in serum, a role which it certainly does not play, since patients with aceruloplasminaemia have unperturbed copper metabolism.

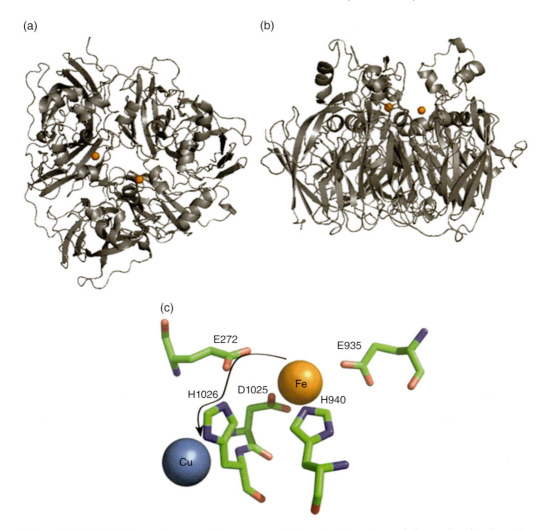

Figure 6.14 *(a) Ribbon diagram of human ceruloplasmin. Top view of the molecule along the pseudo-three-fold axis. (b) Side view of ceruloplasmin almost perpendicular to the pseudo-three-fold axis with the putative iron binding site. (c) Iron-binding site in domain 6 of ceruloplasmin. Residues E272, E935, H940 and D1025 represent iron ligands, residue H1026 is a ligand of type 1 copper in domain 6. The arrow shows the putative electron transfer path from the iron atom to the adjacent type 1 copper atom. Figures were generated using Pymol software (PDB ID 1KCW, Schrödinger, Portland, OR, USA). From Vashchenko, G. and MacGillivray, R.T. (2013) Multi-copper oxidases and human iron metabolism. Nutrients, 5, 2289–2313. This is an open access article distributed under the* Creative Commons Attribution License

punctuated by the transfer of the first iron to be oxidised to a holding site somewhere nearer to the surface. In a Cp-apoTf adduct, both Fe^{3+} are transferred from the holding sites to the appropriate sites on Tf (Figure 6.15).

Overlapping peptide libraries for human ceruloplasmin have been probed with a number of different lactoferrins to identify putative lactoferrin-binding regions on human ceruloplasmin, and three predominantly acidic lactoferrin-binding peptides – located in domains 2, 5 and 6 of human

Ceruloplasmin-transferrin

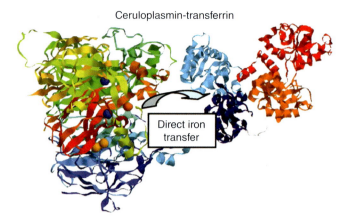

Direct iron transfer

Figure 6.15 *Fe³⁺ is transferred after Fe²⁺ uptake and oxidation by ceruloplasmin to the C-lobe of transferrin in a protein–protein adduct. This adduct is in a permanent state of equilibrium with all the metal-free or bounded ceruloplasmin and transferrin species present in the medium. Reproduced with permission from Elsevier from Eid, C., Hémadi, M., Ha-Duong, N.T. and El Hage Chahine, J.M. (2014) Iron uptake and transfer from ceruloplasmin to transferrin.* Biochim. Biophys. Acta, ***1840***, *1771–1781*

ceruloplasmin – were identified. The docking software identified a complex such that the N-lobe of human apo-lactoferrin interacts with the catalytic ferroxidase centre on human ceruloplasmin (White *et al.*, 2012). Whilst the present author's opinion of *in-silico* studies has already been made clear, it should respectfully be pointed out that the role of lactoferrin in normal iron metabolism is marginal, and the reader should left to draw their own conclusions concerning the relevance of this research in a physiological context.

References

Abboud, S. and Haile, D.J. (2000) A novel mammalian iron-regulated protein involved in intracellular iron metabolism. *J. Biol. Chem.*, **275**, 19906–19912.

Abe, Y., Nagata, R., Hasunuma, Y. and Yokosawa, H. (2001) Isolation, characterization and cDNA cloning of a one-lobed transferrin from the ascidian *Halocynthia roretzi. Comp. Biochem. Physiol. B*, **128**, 73–79.

Abeysinghe, P.M. and Harding, M.M. (2007) Antitumour bis(cyclopentadienyl) metal complexes: titanocene and molybdocene dichloride and derivatives. *Dalton Trans.*, **28**, 3474–3482.

Abraham, J., Corbett, K.D., Farzan, M., Choe, H. and Harrison, S.C. (2010) Structural basis for receptor recognition by New World hemorrhagic fever arenaviruses. *Nat. Struct. Mol. Biol.*, **17**, 438–444.

Adlerova, L., Bartoskova, A. and Faldyna, M. (2008) Lactoferrin a review. *Vet. Med.*, **53**, 457–468.

Aguila, A., Herrera, A.G., Morrison, D., et al. (2001) Bacteriostatic activity of human lactoferrin against *Staphylococcus aureus* is a function of its iron-binding properties and is not influenced by antibiotic resistance. *FEMS Immunol. Med. Microbiol.*, **31**, 145–152.

Aisen, P., Leibman, A. and Zweir, J. (1978) Stoichiometric and site characteristics of the binding of iron to human transferrin. *J. Biol. Chem.*, **253**, 1930–1937.

Alderton, G., Ward, W.H. and Ferold, H.L. (1946) Identification of the bacteria-inhibiting iron-binding protein of egg white as conalbumin. *Arch. Biochem. Biophys.*, **11**, 9–12.

Alvarez, E., Girones, N. and Davis, R.J. (1989) Intermolecular disulfide bonds are not required for the expression of the dimeric state and functional activity of the transferrin receptor. *EMBO J.*, **6**, 2231–2240.

Andersen, C.B., Torvund-Jensen, M., Nielsen, M.J., et al. (2012) Structure of the haptoglobin-haemoglobin complex. *Nature*, **489**, 456–459.

Anderson, B.F., Baker, H.M., Dodson, E.J., et al. (1987) Structure of human lactoferrin: crystallographic analysis and refinement at 3.2 Å. *Proc. Natl Acad. Sci. USA*, **84**, 1769–1773.

Anderson, B.F., Baker, H.M., Norris, G.E., *et al.* (1989) Structure of human lactoferrin: crystallographic structure analysis and refinement at 2.8 Å resolution. *J. Mol. Biol.*, **209**, 711–734.

Anderson, B.F., Baker, H.M., Norris, G.E., Rumball, S.V. and Baker, E.N. (1990) Apolactoferrin structure demonstrates ligand-induced conformational change in transferrins. *Nature*, **344**, 784–787.

Bailey, S., Evans, R.W., Garratt, R.C., *et al.* (1988) Molecular structure of serum transferrin at 3.3 Å resolution. *Biochemistry*, **27**, 5804–5812.

Baker, E.N. (1994) Structure and reactivity of transferrins. *Adv. Inorg. Chem.*, **41**, 389–463.

Baker, E.N., Rumball, S.V. and Anderson, B.F. (1987) Transferrins: insights into structure and function from studies on lactoferrin. *Trends Biochem. Sci.*, **12**, 350–353.

Baker, E.N., Baker, H.M. and Kidd RD. (2002) Lactoferrin and transferrin: functional variations on a common structural framework. *Biochem. Cell Biol.*, **80**, 27–34.

Baker, H.M. and Baker, E.N. (2012) A structural perspective on lactoferrin function. *Biochem. Cell Biol.*, **90**, 320–328.

Baker, H.M., Anderson, B.F., Brodie, A.M., *et al.* (1996) Anion binding by transferrins: importance of second-shell effects revealed by the crystal structure of oxalate-substituted diferric lactoferrin. *Biochemistry*, **34**, 14879–14884.

Baker, H.M., Mason, A.B., He, Q.-Y., *et al.* (2001) Ligand variation in the transferrin family: the crystal structure of the H249Q mutant of the human transferrin N-lobe as a model for iron binding in insect transferrins. *Biochemistry*, **40**, 11670–11675.

Baldwin, D.A. (1980) The kinetics of iron release from human transferrin by EDTA. *Effects of salts and detergents. Biochim. Biophys. Acta*, **623**, 183–198.

Baldwin, D.A. and de Sousa, D.M.R. (1981) The effect of salts on the kinetics of iron release from N-terminal and C-terminal monoferrictransferrins. *Biochem. Biophys. Res. Commun.*, **99**, 1101–1107.

Baldwin, G.S. (1993) Comparison of transferrin sequences from different species. *Comp. Biochem. Physiol. B*, **106**, 203–218.

Bali, P.K. and Aisen, P. (1991) Receptor-modulated iron release from transferrin: differential effects on N- and C-terminal sites. *Biochemistry*, **30**, 9947–9952.

Bali, P.K. and Aisen, P. (1992) Receptor-induced switch in site-site cooperativity during iron release by transferrin. *Biochemistry*, **31**, 3963–3967.

Bali, P.K., Zak, O. and Aisen, P. (1991) A new role for the transferrin receptor in the release of iron from transferrin. *Biochemistry*, **30**, 324–328.

Banerjee, S., Weerasinghe, A.J., Parker Siburt, C.J., *et al.* (2014) *Bordetella pertussis* FbpA binds both unchelated iron and iron siderophore complexes. *Biochemistry*, **53**, 3952–3960.

Bennett, M.J., Lebron, J.A. and Bjorkman, P.J. (2000) Crystal structure of the hereditary haemochromatosis protein HFE complexed with transferrin receptor. *Nature*, **403**, 46–53.

Bergamo, A. and Sava, G. (2011) Ruthenium anticancer compounds: myths and realities of the emerging metal-based drugs. *Dalton Trans.* **40**, 7817–7823.

Brissot, P., Wright, T.L,. Ma, W.L. and Weisiger, R.A. (1985) Efficient clearance of non-transferrin-bound iron by rat liver. Implications for hepatic iron loading in iron overload states. *J. Clin. Invest.*, **76**, 1463–1470.

Brissot, P., Ropert, M., Le Lan, C. and Loréal, O. (2012) Non-transferrin bound iron: a key role in iron overload and iron toxicity. *Biochim. Biophys. Acta*, **1820**, 403–410.

Brooks, J.M. and Wessel, G.M. (2002) The major yolk protein of sea urchins is endocytosed by a dynamin-dependent mechanism. *Biol. Reprod.*, **71**, 705–713.

Brown, J.X., Buckett, P.D. and Wessling-Resnick, M. (2004) Identification of small-molecule inhibitors that distinguish between non-transferrin bound iron uptake and transferrin-mediated iron transport. *Chem. Biol.*, **11**, 407–416.

Bruns, C.M., Nowalk, A.J., Arvai, A.S., *et al.* (1997) Structure of *Haemophilus influenzae* Fe³⁺-binding protein reveals convergent evolution within a superfamily. *Nature Struct. Biol.*, **4**, 919–923.

Byrne, S.L., Chasteen, N.D., Steere, A.N. and Mason, A.B. (2010a) The unique kinetics of iron release from transferrin: the role of receptor, lobe-lobe interactions, and salt at endosomal pH. *J. Mol. Biol.*, **396**, 130–140.

Byrne, S.L., Steere, A.N., Chasteen, N.D. and Mason, A.B. (2010b) Identification of a kinetically significant anion binding (KISAB) site in the N-lobe of human serum transferrin. *Biochemistry*, **49**, 4200–4207.

Camaschella, C., Roetto, A., Cali, A., *et al.* (2000) The gene TFR2 is mutated in a new type of haemochromatosis mapping to 7q22. *Nat. Genet.*, **25**, 14–15.

Casey, J.D. and Chasteen, N.D. (1980) Vanadyl(IV) conalbumin. II. mixed metal and anion binding studies. *J. Inorg. Biochem.*, **13**, 127–136.

Chasteen, N.D. (1977) Human serotransferrin: structure and function. *Coord. Chem. Rev.*, **22**, 1–36.

Chasteen, N.D., Lord, E.M., Thompson, H.J. and Grady, J.K. (1986) Vanadium complexes of transferrin and ferritin in the rat. *Biochim. Biophys. Acta*, **884**, 84–92.

Chen, H., Attieh, Z.K., Syed, B.A., *et al.* (2012) Identification of zyklopen, a new member of the vertebrate multicopper ferroxidase family, and characterization in rodents and human cells. *J. Nutr.*, **140**, 1728–1735.

Chen, T.T., Li, L., Chung, D.H., *et al.* (2005) TIM-2 is expressed on B cells and in liver and kidney and is a receptor for H-ferritin endocytosis. *J. Exp. Med.*, **202**, 955–965.

Cheng, Y., Mason, A.B. and Woodworth, R.C. (1995) pH dependence of specific divalent anion binding to the N-lobe of recombinant human transferrin. *Biochemistry*, **34**, 14879–14884.

Cheng, Y., Zak, O., Aisen, P. *et al.* (2004) Structure of the human transferrin receptor-transferrin complex. *Cell*, **116**, 565–576.

Chevrier, B., d'Orchymont, H., Schalk, C., *et al.* (1996) The transmembrane segment of the human transferrin receptor functions as a signal peptide. *Eur. J. Biochem.*, **237**, 393–398.

Chua, A.C., Olynyk, J.K., Leedman, P.J. and Trinder, D. (2004) Nontransferrin-bound iron uptake by hepatocytes is increased in the Hfe knockout mouse model of hereditary hemochromatosis. *Blood*, **104**, 1519–1525.

Ciuraszkiewicz, J., Olczak, M. and Watorek, W. (2006) Isolation, cloning and sequencing of transferrins from red-eared turtle, African ostrich, and turkey. *Comp. Biochem. Physiol. B*, **144**, 301–310.

Dautry-Varsat, A., Ciechanover, A. and Lodish, H.F. (1983) pH and the recycling of transferrin during receptor-mediated endocytosis. *Proc. Natl Acad. Sci. USA*, **80**, 2258–2262.

de Jong, J.L. and Zon, L.I. (2005) Use of the zebrafish system to study primitive and definitive hematopoiesis. *Annu. Rev. Genet.*, **39**, 481–501.

Demeule, M., Bertrand, Y., Michaud-Levesque, J., *et al.* (2003) Regulation of plasminogen activation: a role for melanotransferrin (p97) in cell migration. *Blood*, **102**, 1723–1731.

Devireddy, L.R., Gazin, C., Zhu, X. and Green, M.R. (2005) A cell-surface receptor for lipocalin 24p3 selectively mediates apoptosis and iron uptake. *Cell*, **123**, 1293–1305.

Di Bona, K.R., Love, S., Rhodes, N.R., *et al.* (2011) Chromium is not an essential trace element for mammals: effects of a 'low-chromium' diet. *J. Biol. Inorg. Chem.*, **16**, 381–390.

Donovan, A., Brownlie, A., Zhou, Y., *et al.* (2000) Positional cloning of zebrafish ferroportin1 identifies a conserved vertebrate iron exporter. *Nature*, **403**, 776–781.

Donovan, A., Lima, C.A., Pinkus, J.L., *et al.* (2005) The iron exporter ferroportin/Slc40a1 is essential for iron homeostasis. *Cell Metab.*, **1**, 191–200.

Dubach, J., Gaffney, B.J., More, K., Eaton, G.R. and Eaton, S.S. (1991) Effect of the synergistic anion on electron paramagnetic resonance spectra of iron-transferrin anion complexes is consistent with bidentate binding of the anion. *Biophys. J.*, **59**, 1091–1100.

Dubljevic, V., Sali, A. and Goding, J.W. (1999) A conserved RGD (Arg-Gly-Asp) motif in the transferrin receptor is required for binding to transferrin. *Biochem. J.*, **341**, 11–14.

Dunkov, B. and Georgieva, T. (2006) Insect iron binding proteins: insights from the genomes. *Insect Biochem. Mol. Biol.*, **36**, 300–309.

Eckenroth, B.E., Mason, A.B., McDevitt, M.E., Lambert, L.A. and Everse, S.J. (2010) The structure and evolution of the murine inhibitor of carbonic anhydrase: a member of the transferrin superfamily. *Protein Sci.*, **19**, 1616–1626.

Eckenroth, B.E., Steere, A.N., Chasteen, N.D., Everse, S.J. and Mason, A.B. (2011) How the binding of human transferrin primes the transferrin receptor potentiating iron release at endosomal pH. *Proc. Natl Acad. Sci. USA*, **108**, 13089–13094.

Egan, T.J., Ross, D.C., Purves, L.R. and Adams, P.A. (1992) Mechanism of iron release from human serum C-terminal monoferric transferrin to pyrophosphate: Kinetic discrimination between alternative mechanisms. *Inorg. Chem.*, **31**, 1994–1998.

Eid, C., Hémadi, M., Ha-Duong, N.T. and El Hage Chahine, J.M. (2014) Iron uptake and transfer from ceruloplasmin to transferrin. *Biochim. Biophys. Acta*, **1840**, 1771–1781.

Escalante, R., Houdebine, L.-M. and Pamblanco, M. (1993) Transferrin gene expression in the mammary gland of the rat. The enhancing effect of 17β-oestradiol on the level of RNA is tissue-specific. *J. Mol. Endocrinol.*, **11**, 151–159.

Evans, R.W., Kong, X. and Hider, R.C. (2012) Iron mobilization from transferrin by therapeutic iron chelating agents. *Biochim. Biophys. Acta*, **1820**, 282–290.

Fantus, I.G., Deragon, G., Lai, R. and Tang, S. (1995) Modulation of insulin action by vanadate: evidence for a role for phosphotyrosine phosphatase activity to alter cellular signaling. *Mol. Cell. Biochem.*, **153**, 103–112.

Fisher, M., Gokhman, I., Pick, U. and Zamir, A. (1997) A structurally novel transferrin-like protein accumulates in the plasma membrane of the unicellular green alga *Dunaliella salina* grown in high salinities. *J. Biol. Chem.*, **272**, 1565–1570.

Fisher, M., Zamir, A. and Pick, U. (1998) Iron uptake by the halotolerant alga *Dunaliella* is mediated by a plasma membrane transferrin. *J. Biol. Chem.*, **273**, 17553–17558.

Fleming, R.F., Migas, M.C., Holden, C.C., *et al.* (2000) Transferrin receptor 2: continued expression in mouse liver in the face of iron overload and in hereditary hemochromatosis. *Proc. Natl Acad. Sci. USA*, **97**, 2214–2219.

Fleming, R.F., Ahmann, J.R., Migas, M.C., *et al.* (2002) Targeted mutagenesis of the murine transferrin receptor-2 gene produces hemochromatosis. *Proc. Natl Acad. Sci. USA*, **99**, 10653–10658.

Foley, A.A. and Bates, G.W. (1988) The influence of inorganic anions on the formation and stability of Fe^{3+}–transferrin–anion complexes. *Biochim. Biophys. Acta*, **965**, 154–162.

Food, M.R., Sekyere, E.O. and Richardson, D.R. (2002) The soluble form of the membrane-bound transferrin homologue, melanotransferrin, inefficiently donates iron to cells via nonspecific internalization and degradation of the protein. *Eur. J. Biochem.*, **269**, 4435–4445.

Forejtnikova, H., Vieillevoye, M., Zermati, Y., *et al.* (2010) Transferrin receptor 2 is a component of the erythropoietin receptor complex and is required for efficient erythropoiesis. *Blood*, **116**, 5357–5367.

Fox, P.L. (2003) The copper-iron chronicles: the story of an intimate relationship. *Biometals*, **16**, 9–40.

Fraenkel, P.G., Traver, D., Donovan, A., Zahrieh, D. and Zon, L.I. (2005) Ferroportin1 is required for normal iron cycling in zebrafish. *J. Clin. Invest.*, **115**, 1532–1541.

Frieden, E. and Hsieh, H.S. (1976) Ceruloplasmin: the copper transport protein with essential oxidase activity. *Adv. Enzymol.*, **44**, 187–236.

Fuchs, H., Lücken, U., Tauber, R., *et al.* (1998) Structural model of phospholipid-reconstituted human transferrin receptor derived by electron microscopy. *Structure*, **6**, 1235–1243.

Fujiwara, A., Unuma, T., Ohno, K. and Yamano, K. (2009) Molecular characterization of the major yolk protein of the Japanese common sea cucumber (*Apostichopus japonicus*) and its expression profile during ovarian development. *Comp. Biochem. Physiol. A*, **155**, 34–40.

Gaasch, J.A., Geldenhuys, W.J., Lockman, P.R., Allen, D.D. and Van der Schyf, C.J. (2007) Voltage-gated calcium channels provide an alternate route for iron uptake in neuronal cell cultures. *Neurochem. Res.*, **32**, 1686–1693.

Ganz, T. and Nemeth, E. (2006) Regulation of iron acquisition and iron distribution in mammals. *Biochim. Biophys. Acta*, **1763**, 690–699.

Garby, L. and Noyes, W.D. (1959) Studies on hemoglobin metabolism. II. Pathways of hemoglobin iron metabolism in normal man. *J. Clin. Invest.*, **38**, 1484–1486.

Geiser, D.L. and Winzerling, J.J. (2012) Insect transferrins: multifunctional proteins. *Biochim. Biophys. Acta*, **1820**, 437–451.

Gerstein, M., Anderson, B.F., Norris, G.E., *et al.* (1993) Domain closure in lactoferrin: two hinges produce a see-saw motion between alternative close-packed interfaces. *J. Mol. Biol.*, **234**, 357–372.

Giannetti, A.M., Snow, P.M., Zak, O. and Björkman, P.J. (2003) Mechanism for multiple ligand recognition by the human transferrin receptor. *PloS Biol.*, **1**, 341–350.

Giannetti, A.M., Halbrooks, P.J., Mason, A.B., *et al.* (2005) The molecular mechanism for receptor-stimulated iron release from the plasma iron transport protein transferrin. *Structure*, **13**, 1613–1623.

Grossmann, J.G., Neu, M., Pantos, E., *et al.* (1992) X-ray solution scattering reveals conformational changes upon iron uptake in lactoferrin, serum and ovo-transferrins. *J. Mol. Biol.*, **225**, 811–819.

Grossmann, J.G., Neu, M., Evans, R.W., *et al.* (1993) Metal-induced conformational changes in transferrins. *J. Mol. Biol.*, **229**, 585–590.

Groves, M.L. (1960) The isolation of a red protein from milk. *J. Am. Chem. Soc.*, **82**, 3345–3350.

Gruenberg, J. and Stenmark, H. (2004) The biogenesis of multivesicular endosomes. *Nat. Rev. Mol. Cell Biol.*, **5**, 317–323.

Gubler, C.J., Lahety, M.E., Cartwright, G.E. and Wintrobe, M.M. (1952) Studies on copper metabolism. X. Factors influencing the plasma copper level of the albino rat. *Am. J. Physiol.*, **171**, 652–658.

Gumerov, D.R. and Kaltashov, I.A. (2001) Dynamics of iron release from transferrin N-lobe studied by electrospray ionization mass spectrometry. *Anal. Chem.*, **73**, 2565–2570.

Gunshin, H., McKenzie, B., Berger, U.V., *et al.* (1997) Cloning and characterization of a mammalian proton-coupled metal-ion transporter. *Nature*, **388**, 482–488.

Gunshin, H., Fujiwara, Y., Custodio, A.O., *et al.* (2005) Slc11a2 is required for intestinal iron absorption and erythropoiesis but dispensable in placenta and liver. *J. Clin. Invest.*, **115**, 1258–1266.

Ha-Duong, N.T., Eid, C., Hémadi, M. and El Hage Chahine, J.M. (2010) In vitro interaction between ceruloplasmin and human serum transferrin. *Biochemistry*, **49**, 10261–10263.

Halbrooks, P.J., Mason, A.B., Adams, T.E., Briggs, S.K. and Everse, S.J. (2004) The oxalate effect on release of iron from human serum transferrin explained. *J. Mol. Biol.*, **339**, 217–226.

Halbrooks, P.J., He, Q.Y., Briggs, S.K., *et al.* (2005) Investigation of the mechanism of iron release from the C-lobe of human serum transferrin: mutational analysis of the role of a pH sensitive triad. *Biochemistry*, **42**, 3701–3707.

Han, J., Seaman, W.E., Di, X., *et al.* (2011) Iron uptake mediated by binding of H-ferritin to the TIM-2 receptor in mouse cells. *PLoS One*, **6**, e23800.

Haridas, M., Anderson, B.F. and Baker, E.N. (1995) Structure of human diferric lactoferrin refined at 2.2 Å resolution. *Acta Crystallogr. D Biol. Crystallogr.*, **51**, 629–646.

Harris, W.R. (1985) Thermodynamics of anion binding to human serum transferrin. *Biochemistry*, **24**, 7412–7418.

Harris, W.R. (1986) Estimation of the ferrous-transferrin binding constants based on thermodynamic studies of nickel(II)-transferrin. *J. Inorg. Biochem.*, **27**, 41–52.

Harris, W.R. (2012) Anion binding properties of the transferrins. Implications for function. *Biochim. Biophys. Acta*, **1820**, 348–361.

Harris, W.R. and Carrano, C.J. (1984) Binding of vanadate to human serum transferrin. *J. Inorg. Biochem.*, **22**, 201–218.

Harris, W.R. and Bali, P.K. (1988) Effects of anions on the removal of iron from transferrin by phosphonic acids and pyrophosphate. *Inorg. Chem.*, **27**, 2687–2691.

Harris, W.R., Friedman, S.B. and Silberman, D. (1984) Behavior of vanadate and vanadyl ion in canine blood. *J. Inorg. Biochem.*, **20**, 157–169.

Harris, W.R., Nesset-Tollefson, D., Stenback, J.Z. and Mohamed-Hani, N. (1990) Site selectivity in the binding of inorganic anions to serum transferrin. *J. Inorg. Biochem.*, **38**, 175–183.

Hartinger, C.A., Jakupec, M.A., Zorbas-Seifried, S., *et al.* (2008) KP1019, a new redox-active anticancer agent – preclinical development and results of a clinical phase I study in tumor patients. *Chem. Biodivers.*, **5**, 2140–2154.

He, Q.Y., Mason, A.B., Woodworth, R.C., *et al.* (1998) Mutations at nonliganding residues Tyr-85 and Glu-83 in the N-lobe of human serum transferrin. Functional second shell effects. *J. Biol. Chem.*, **273**, 17018–17024.

Hershko, C., Graham, G., Bates, G.W. and Rachmilewitz, E.A. (1978) Non-specific serum iron in thalassaemia: an abnormal serum iron fraction of potential toxicity. *Br. J. Haematol.*, **40**, 255–263.

Holmberg, C.G. and Laurell, C.B. (1947) Investigations in serum copper I. Nature of serum copper and its relation to the iron-binding protein in human serum. *Acta Chem. Scand.*, **1**, 944–950.

Hrkal, Z., Vodrazka, Z. and Kalousek, I. (1974) Transfer of heme from ferrihemoglobin and ferrihemoglobin isolated chains to hemopexin. *Eur. J. Biochem.*, **43**, 73–78.

Jakusch, T., Hollender, D., Enyedy, E.A., *et al.* (2009) Biospeciation of various antidiabetic $V^{IV}O$ compounds in serum. *Dalton Trans.*, **2428–2437**.

James, N.G., Byrne, S.L., Steere, A.N., *et al.* (2009) Inequivalent contribution of the five tryptophan residues in the C-lobe of human serum transferrin to the fluorescence increase when iron is released. *Biochemistry*, **48**, 2858–2867.

Jandl, J.M. and Katz, J.H. (1963) The plasma-to-cell cycle of transferrin. *J. Clin. Invest.*, **42**, 314–326.

Jandl, J.M., Inman, J.K., Simmons, R.L. and Allen, D.W. (1959) Transfer of iron from serum iron-binding protein to human reticulocytes. *J. Clin. Invest.*, **38**, 161–185.

Jeffrey, P.D., Bewley, M.C., MacGillivray, R.T., *et al.* (1998) Ligand-induced conformational change in transferrins: crystal structure of the open form of the N-terminal half-molecule of human transferrin. *Biochemistry*, **37**, 13978–13986.

Jeltsch, J.M. and Chambon, P. (1982) The complete nucleotide sequence of the chicken ovotransferrin mRNA. *Eur. J. Biochem.*, **122**, 291–295.

Jing, S. and Trowbridge, I.S. (1987) Identification of the intermolecular disulfide bonds of the human transferrin receptor and its lipid-attachment site. *EMBO J.*, **6**, 327–331.

Johansson, B. (1960) Isolation of an iron-containing red protein from human milk. *Acta Chem. Scand.*, **14**, 510–512.

Kaplan, J. (2002) Strategy and tactics in the evolution of iron acquisition. *Semin. Hematol.*, **39**, 219–226.

Kaplan, J. and Ward, D.M. (2012) Ferroportin-mediated iron transport: expression and regulation. *Biochim. Biophys. Acta*, **1823**, 1426–1433.

Katz, J.H. (1961) Iron and protein kinetic studies by means of doubly labelled human crystalline transferrin. *J. Clin. Invest.*, **40**, 2143–2152.

Kawabata, H., Yang, R., Hirama, T., *et al.* (1999) Molecular cloning of transferrin receptor 2. A new member of the transferrin receptor-like family. *J. Biol. Chem.*, **274**, 20826–20832.

Kawabata, H., Germain, R.S., Vuong, P.T., *et al.* (2000) Transferrin receptor 2-alpha supports cell growth both in iron-chelated cultured cells and in vivo. *J. Biol. Chem.*, **275**, 16618–16625.

Kawabata, H., Germain, R.S., Ikezoe, T., *et al.* (2004a) Regulation of expression of murine transferrin receptor 2. *Blood*, **98**, 1949–1954.

Kawabata, H., Tong, X., Kawanami, T., *et al.* (2004b) Analyses for binding of the transferrin family of proteins to the transferrin receptor 2. *Br. J. Haematol.*, **127**, 464–473.

Keel, S.B., Doty, R.T., Yang, Z., *et al.* (2008) A heme export protein is required for red blood cell differentiation and iron homeostasis. *Science*, **319**, 825–828.

Khan, J.A., Kumar, P., Paramasivam, M., *et al.* (2001) Camel lactoferrin, a transferrin-cum-lactoferrin: crystal structure of camel apolactoferrin at 2.6 Å resolution and structural basis of its dual role. *J. Mol. Biol.*, **309**, 751–761.

Kiss, T., Jakusch, T., Hollander, D., Enyedy, E.A. and Horvath, L. (2009) Comparative studies on the biospeciation of antidiabetic VO(IV) and Zn(II) complexes. *J. Inorg. Biochem.*, **103**, 527–535.

Kratz, F., Keppler, B.K., Hartmann, M., Messori, L. and Berger, M.R. (1996) Comparison of the antiproliferative activity of two antitumor ruthenium(III) complexes with their apotransferrin and transferrin-bound forms in a human colon cancer cell line. *Met.-Based Drugs*, **3**, 15–23.

Kretchmar, S.A. and Raymond, K.N. (1988) Effects of ionic strength on iron removal from the monoferric transferrins. *Inorg. Chem.*, **27**, 1436–1441.

Kristansen, M., Graversen, J.H., Jacobsen, C., *et al.* (2001) Identification of the haemoglobin scavenger receptor. *Nature*, **409**, 198–201.

Kumar, P., Yadav, S. and Singhet, T.P. (2002) Crystallization and structure determination of goat lactoferrin at 4.0 Å resolution: A new form of packing in lactoferrins with a high solvent content in crystals. *Indian J. Biochem. Biophys.*, **39**, 16–21.

Kumar, S., Sharma, A.K. and Singh, T.P. (2000) Metal substitution in lactoferrins: the crystal structure of manganese lactoferrin at 3.4Å resolution. *Ind. J. Phys.*, **74**, 143–146.

Kurokawa, H., Mikami, B. and Hirose, M. (1995) Crystal structure of diferric hen ovotransferrin at 2.4 Å resolution. *J. Mol. Biol.*, **254**, 196–207.

Kurokawa, H., Dewan, J.C., Mikami, B., Sacchettini, J.C. and Hirose, M. (1999) Crystal structure of hen apo-ovotransferrin. Both lobes adopt an open conformation upon loss of iron. *J. Biol. Chem.*, **274**, 28445–28452.

Lakadamyali, M., Rust, M.J. and Zhuang, X. (2006) Ligands for clathrin-mediated endocytosis are differentially sorted into distinct populations of early endosomes. *Cell*, **124**, 997–1009.

Lambert, L.A. (2012) Molecular evolution of the transferrin family and associated receptors. *Biochim. Biophys. Acta*, **1820**, 244–255.

Lambert, L.A. and Mitchell, S.L. (2007) Molecular evolution of the transferrin receptor/glutamate carboxypeptidase II family. *J. Mol. Evol.*, **64**, 113–128.

Lambert, L.A., Perri, H. and Meehan, T.J. (2005) Evolution of duplications in the transferrin family of proteins. *Comp. Biochem. Physiol. B Biochem. Mol. Biol.*, **140**, 11–25.

Laurell, C.B. and Ingelman, B. (1947) The iron-binding proteins of swine serum. *Acta Chem. Scand.*, **1**, 770–776.

Lawrence, C.M., Ray, S., Babyonyshev, M., *et al.* (1999) Crystal structure of the ectodomain of human transferrin receptor. *Science*, **286**, 779–782.

Lee, E.-H., Barcellos-Hoff, M.H., Chen, L.-H., *et al.* (1987) Transferrin is a major mouse milk protein and is synthesized by mammary epithelial cells. *In Vitro Cell. Dev. Biol.*, **23**, 221–226.

Le Gac, G., Ka, C., Joubrel, R., *et al.* (2013) Structure–function analysis of the human ferroportin iron exporter (SLC40A1): effect of hemochromatosis type 4 disease mutations and identification of critical residues. *Hum. Mutat.*, **34**, 1371–1380.

Leonard, D., Hayakawa, A., Lawe, D., *et al.* (2008) Sorting of EGF and transferrin at the plasma membrane and by cargo-specific signaling to EEA1-enriched endosomes. *Nat. Rev. Mol. Cell Biol.*, **5**, 317–323.

Leverence, R., Mason, A.B. and Kaltashov, I.A. (2013) Noncanonical interactions between serum transferrin and transferrin receptor evaluated with electrospray ionization mass spectrometry. *Proc. Natl Acad. Sci. USA*, **107**, 8123–8128.

Leveugle, B., Spik, G., Perl, D.P., *et al.* (1994) The iron-binding protein lactotransferrin is present in pathologic lesions in a variety of neurodegenerative disorders: a comparative immunohistochemical analysis. *Brain Res.*, **650**, 20–31.

Levina, A. Mitra, A. and Lay, P.A. (2009) Recent developments in ruthenium anticancer drugs. *Metallomics*, **1**, 458–470.

Li, J.Y., Paragas N., Ned, R.M., *et al.* (2009) Scara5 is a ferritin receptor mediating non-transferrin iron delivery. *Dev. Cell.*, **16**, 35–46.

Li, L., Fang, C.J., Ryan, J.C., *et al.* (2010) Binding and uptake of H-ferritin are mediated by human transferrin receptor-1. *Proc. Natl Acad. Sci. USA*, **107**, 3505–3510.

Li, Y., Llewellyn, L. and Moczydlowski, E. (1993) Biochemical and immunochemical comparison of saxiphilin and transferrin, two structurally related plasma proteins from *Rana catesbeiana. Mol. Pharmacol.*, **44**, 742–748.

Liang, Z., Sottrup-Jensen, L., Aspán, A., Hall, M. and Söderhäll, K. (1997) Pacifastin, a novel 155-kDa heterodimeric proteinase inhibitor containing a unique transferrin chain. *Proc. Natl Acad. Sci. USA*, **94**, 6682–6687.

Liboiron, B.D., Thompson, K.H., Hanson, G.R., *et al.* (2006) New insights into the interactions of serum proteins with bis(maltolato)oxovanadium(IV): transport and biotransformation of insulin-enhancing vanadium pharmaceuticals. *J. Am. Chem. Soc.*, **127**, 5104–5115.

Lindley, P.F. (1996) Iron in biology: a structural viewpoint. *Rep. Prog. Phys.*, **59**, 867–933.

Lindley, P.F., Card, G., Zaitseva, I., *et al.* (1997) An X-ray structural study of human ceruloplasmin in relation to ferroxidase activity. *J. Biol. Inorg. Chem.*, **2**, 454–463.

Liu, X.B., Yang, F. and Haile, D.J. (2005) Functional consequences of ferroportin 1 mutations. *Blood Cells Mol. Dis.*, **35**, 33–46.

Liuzzi, J.P., Aydemir, F., Nam, H., Knutson, M.D. and Cousins, R.J. (2006) Zip14 (Slc39a14) mediates non-transferrin-bound iron uptake into cells. *Proc. Natl Acad. Sci. USA*, **103**, 13612–13617.

Llewellyn, L.E., Bell, P.M. and Moczydlowski, E.G. (1997) Phylogenetic survey of soluble saxitoxin-binding activity in pursuit of the function and molecular evolution of saxiphilin, a relative of transferrin. *Proc. R. Soc. Lond. B.*, **264**, 891–902.

Ludwiczek, S., Theurl, I., Muckenthaler, M.U., *et al.* (2007) Ca^{2+} channel blockers reverse iron overload by a new mechanism via divalent metal transporter-1. *Nat. Med.*, **13**, 448–454.

Luecke, H. and Quiocho, F.A. (1990) High specificity of a phosphate transport protein determined by hydrogen bonds. *Nature*, **347**, 402–406.

MacGillivray, R.T.A. and Mason, A.B. (2002) Transferrins, in Cell and Molecular Biology of Iron Transport (ed. D.M. Templeton), Marcel Dekker, Inc., New York, pp. 41–69.

MacGillivray, R.T., Moore, S.A., Chen, J., *et al.* (1998) Two high-resolution crystal structures of the recombinant N-lobe of human transferrin reveal a structural change implicated in iron release. *Biochemistry*, **37**, 7919–7928.

Martin, A.W., Huebers, E., Huebers, H., Webb, J. and Finch, C.A. (1984) A mono-sited transferrin from a representative deuterostome: the ascidian *Pyura stolonifera* (subphylum Urochordata). *Blood*, **64**, 1047–1052.

Mason, A.B., Byrne, S.L., Everse, S.J., *et al.* (2009) A loop in the N-lobe of human serum transferrin is critical for binding to the transferrin receptor as revealed by mutagenesis, isothermal titration calorimetry, and epitope mapping. *J. Mol. Recognit.*, **22**, 521–529.

Mayle, L.M., Le, A.M. and Kamei, D.T. (2012) The intracellular trafficking pathway of transferrin. *Biochim. Biophys. Acta*, **1820**, 264–281.

McDermott, J.A., Huber, C.T., Osaki, S. and Frieden, E. (1968) Role of iron in the oxidase activity of ceruloplasmin. *Biochim. Biophys. Acta*, **151**, 541–557.

McKie, A.T., Marciano, P., Rolfs, A., *et al.* (2000) A novel duodenal iron-regulated transporter, IREG1, implicated in the basolateral transfer of iron to the circulation. *Mol. Cell*, **5**, 299–309.

Mecklenburg, S.L., Donohoe, R.J. and Olah, G.A. (1997) Tertiary structural changes and iron release from human serum transferrin. *J. Mol. Biol.*, **270**, 739–750.

Mizutani, K., Mikami, B. and Hirose, M. (2001) Domain closure mechanism in transferrins: new viewpoints about the hinge structure and motion as deduced from high resolution crystal structures of ovotransferrin N-lobe. *J. Mol. Biol.*, **309**, 937–947.

Mizutani, K., Mikami, B., Aibara, S. and Hirose, M. (2005) Structure of aluminium-bound ovotransferrin at 2.15 Angstroms resolution. *Acta Crystallogr. D*, **61**, 1636–1642.

Mizutani, K., Toyoda, M. and Mikami, B. (2012) X-ray structures of transferrins and related proteins. *Biochim. Biophys. Acta*, **1820**, 203–211.

Montreuil, J., Tonnelat, J. and Mullet, S. (1960) Preparation and properties of lactosiderophilin (lactotransferrin) of human milk. *Biochim. Biophys. Acta*, **45**, 413–421.

Morgan, W.T. and Smith, A. (1984) Domain structure of rabbit hemopexin. Isolation and characterization of a heme-binding glycopeptides. *J. Biol. Chem.*, **259**, 12001–12006.

Murayama, E., Takagi, Y., Ohira, T., *et al.* (2000) Fish otolith contains a unique structural protein, otolin-1. *Eur. J. Biochem.*, **269**, 688–696.

Nemeth, E. and Ganz, T. (2006) Regulation of iron metabolism by hepcidin. *Annu. Rev. Nutr.*, **26**, 323–342.

Nilsson, M.R. and Dobson, C.M. (2003) In vitro characterization of lactoferrin aggregation and amyloid formation. *Biochemistry*, **42**, 375–382.

Noll, H., Alcedo, J., Daube, M., *et al.* (2007) The toposome, essential for sea urchin cell adhesion and development, is a modified iron-less calcium-binding transferrin. *Dev. Biol.*, **310**, 54–70.

Nowalk, A.J., Tencza, S.B. and Mietzner, T.A. (1994) Coordination of iron by the ferric iron-binding protein of pathogenic *Neisseria* is homologous to the transferrins. *Biochemistry*, **33**, 12769–12775.

Ohgami, R.S., Campagna, D.R., Greer, E.L., *et al.* (2005) Identification of a ferrireductase required for efficient transferrin-dependent iron uptake in erythroid cells. *Nat. Genet.*, **37**, 1264–1269.

Osaki, S., Johnson, D.A. and Frieden, E. (1971) The mobilization of iron from the perfused mammalian liver by a serum copper enzyme, ferroxidase I. *J. Biol. Chem.*, **246**, 3018–3023.

Osborne, T.B. and Campbell, G.F. (1900) The protein constituents of egg white. *J. Am. Chem. Soc.*, **22**, 422–426.

Ota, K., Mikelj, M., Papler, T., *et al.* (2013) Ostreopexin: a hemopexin fold protein from the oyster mushroom, *Pleurotus ostreatus*. *Biochim. Biophys. Acta*, **1834**, 1468–1473.

Oudit, G.Y., Sun, H., Trivieri, M.G., *et al.* (2003) L-type Ca^{2+} channels provide a major pathway for iron entry into cardiomyocytes in iron-overload cardiomyopathy. *Nat. Med.*, **9**, 1187–1194.

Pakdaman, R., Petitjean, M. and El Hage Chahine, J.-M. (1998) A mechanism for iron uptake by lactoferrin. *Eur. J. Biochem.*, **254**, 144–153.

Paoli, M., Anderson, B.F., Baker, H.M., *et al.* (1999) Crystal structure of hemopexin reveals a novel high-affinity heme site formed between two beta-propeller domains. *Nat. Struct. Biol.*, **6**, 926–931.

Park, I., Schaeffer, E., Sidoli, A., *et al.* (1985) Organization of the human transferrin gene: direct evidence that it originated by gene duplication. *Proc. Natl Acad. Sci. USA*, **82**, 3149–3153.

Paz, Y., Katz, A. and Pick, U. (2007) A multicopper ferroxidase involved in iron binding to transferrins in *Dunaliella salina* plasma membranes. *J. Biol. Chem.*, **282**, 8658–8666.

Pflugrath, J.W. and Quiocho, F.A. (1988) The 2 Å resolution structure of the sulfate-binding protein involved in active transport in *Salmonella typhimurium*. *J. Mol. Biol.*, **200**, 163–180.

Polec-Pawlak, K., Abramski, J.K., Semenova, O., *et al.* (2006) Platinum group metallodrug-protein binding studies by capillary electrophoresis–inductively coupled plasma-mass spectrometry: a further insight into the reactivity of a novel antitumor ruthenium(III) complex toward human serum proteins. *Electrophoresis*, **27**, 1128–1135.

Quintanar, L., Stoj, C., Taylor, A.B., *et al.* (2007) Shall we dance? How a multicopper oxidase chooses its electron transfer partner. *Acc. Chem. Res.*, **40**, 445–452.

Rabin, M., McLelland, A., Kühn, L.C. and Ruddle, F.H. (1985) Regional localization of the human transferrin receptor gene to 3q26.2–qter. *Am. J. Hum. Genet.*, **37**, 1112–1116.

Ramírez-Gómez, F., Ortíz-Pineda, P.A., Rojas-Cartagena, C., Suárez-Castillo, E.C. and García-Arrarás, J.E. (2008) Immune-related genes associated with intestinal tissue in the sea cucumber *Holothuria glaberrima*. *Immunogenetics*, **60**, 57–71.

Ren, J., Wen, L., Gao, X., *et al.* (2009) DOG 1.0: illustrator of protein domain structures. *Cell Res.*, **19**, 271–273.

Roberts, R.M. (1989) Serendipity: Accidental Discoveries in Science, John Wiley & Sons Ltd, Chichester, pp. 270.

Rolland, Y., Demeule, M., Fenart, L. and Béliveau, R. (2009) Inhibition of melanoma brain metastasis by targeting melanotransferrin at the cell surface. *Pigment Cell Melanoma Res.*, **22**, 86–98.

Rose, T.M., Plowman, G.D., Teplow, D.B., *et al.* (1986) Primary structure of the human melanoma-associated antigen p97 (melanotransferrin) deduced from the mRNA sequence. *Proc. Natl Acad. Sci. USA*, **83**, 1261–1265.

Sabbioni, E. and Marafante, E. (1991) Relationship between iron and vanadium metabolism: *in vivo* incorporation of vanadium into iron proteins of the rat. *J. Toxicol. Environ. Health*, **8**, 419–429.

Sabbioni, E., Marafante, E., Amantini, L., Ubertalli, L. and Birattari, C. (1978) Similarity in metabolic patterns of different chemical species of vanadium in the rat. *Bioinorg. Chem.*, **8**, 503–515.

Sabbioni, E., Rade, J. and Bertolero, E. (1980) Relationship between iron and vanadium metabolism: the exchange of vanadium between transferrin and ferritin. *J. Inorg. Biochem.*, **12**, 307–315.

Sadrzadeh, S.M., Graf, E., Panter, S.S., Hallaway, P.E. and Eaton, J.W. (1984) Hemoglobin. A biologic Fenton reagent. *J. Biol. Chem.*, **259**, 14354–14356.

Sanna, D., Garribba, E. and Micera, G. (2009a) Interaction of VO^{2+} ion with human serum transferrin and albumin. *J. Inorg. Biochem.*, **103**, 648–655.

Sanna, D., Micera, G. and Garribba, E. (2009b) On the transport of vanadium in blood serum. *Inorg. Chem.*, **48**, 5747–5757.

Sanna, D., Micera, G. and Garribba, E. (2010a) New developments in the comprehension of the biotransformation and transport of insulin-enhancing vanadium compounds in the blood serum. *Inorg. Chem.*, **49**, 174–187.

Sanna, D., Buglyo, P., Micera, G. and Garribba, E. (2010b) A quantitative study of the biotransformation of insulin-enhancing VO^{2+} compounds. *J. Biol. Inorg. Chem.*, **15**, 825–839.

Sarkar, J., Seshadri, V., Tripoulas, N.A., Ketterer, M.E. and Fox, P.L. (2003) Role of ceruloplasmin in macrophage iron efflux during hypoxia. *J. Biol. Chem.*, **278**, 44018–44024.

Schade, A.L. and Caroline, L. (1944a) The preparation of a polyvalent dysentery bacteriophage in a dry and stable form: II. Factors affecting the stabilization of dysentery bacteriophage during lyophilization. *J. Bacteriol.*, **48**, 179–190.

Schade, A.L. and Caroline, L. (1944b) Raw hen egg-white and the role of iron in growth inhibition of *Shigella dysenteriae*, *Staphylococcus aureus*, *Escherichia coli* and *Saccharomyces cerevisiae*. *Science*, **100**, 14–15.

Schade, A.L. and Caroline, L. (1946) An iron-binding component in human blood plasma. *Science*, **104**, 340–341.

Schade, A.L., Reinhart, R.W. and Levy, H. (1949) Carbon dioxide and oxygen in complex formation with iron and siderophilin, the iron-binding component of human plasma. *Arch. Biochem. Biophys.*, **20**, 170–172.

Schlabach, M.R. and Bates, G.W. (1975) The synergistic binding of anions and Fe(III) by transferrin. *J. Biol. Chem.*, **250**, 2182–2188.

Schwarz, M., Sal-Man, N., Zamir, A. and Pick, U. (2003) A transferrin-like protein that does not bind iron is induced by iron deficiency in the alga *Dunaliella salina*. *Biochim. Biophys. Acta*, **1649**, 190–200.

Sharma, A.K., Rajashankar, K.R., Yadav, M.P. and Singh, T.P. (1999) Structure of mare apolactoferrin: the N and C lobes are in the closed form. *Acta Crystallogr. D Biol. Crystallogr.*, **55**, 1152–1157.

Shim, B.S., Lee, T.H. and Kang, Y.S. (1965) Immunological and biochemical investigations of human serum haptoglobin: composition of haptoglobin-haemoglobin intermediate, haemoglobin-binding sites and presence of additional alleles for beta-chain. *Nature*, **207**, 1264–1267.

Shindo, M., Torimoto, Y., Saito, H., *et al.* (2006) Functional role of DMT1 in transferrin-independent iron uptake by human hepatocyte and hepatocellular carcinoma cell, HLF. *Hepatol. Res.*, **35**, 152–162.

Sipe, D.M. and Murphy, R.F. (1991) Binding to cellular receptors results in increased iron release from transferrin at mildly acidic pH. *J. Biol. Chem.*, **266**, 8002–8007.

Smith, A. and Morgan, W.T. (1979) Haem transport to the liver by haemopexin. Receptor-mediated uptake with recycling of the protein. *Biochem. J.*, **182**, 47–54.

Smith, A. and Morgan, W.T. (1981) Haemopexin-mediated transport of heme into isolated rat hepatocytes. *J. Biol. Chem.*, **256**, 10902–10909.

Smith, A. and Hunt, R.C. (1990) Hemopexin joins transferrin as representative members of a distinct class of receptor-mediated endocytic transport systems. *Eur. J. Cell Biol.*, **53**, 234–245.

Smith, A. and Neuschatz, T. (1983) Haematoporphyrin, and O,O′-diacetyl-haematoporphyrin binding by serum and cellular proteins. Implications for the clearance of these photochemotherapeutic agents by cells. *Biochem. J.*, **214**, 503–509.

Smith, C.A., Anderson, B.F., Baker, H.M. and Baker, E.N. (1992) Metal substitution in the transferrins: the crystal structure of human copper-lactoferrin at 2.1Å resolution. *Biochemistry*, **31**, 4527–4533.

Smith, C.A., Ainscough, E.W., Baker, H.M., Brodie, A.M. and Baker, E.N. (1994) Specific binding of cerium by human lactoferrin stimulates the oxidation of Ce^{3+} to Ce^{4+}. *J. Am. Chem. Soc.*, **116**, 7889–7890.

Steere, A.N., Miller, B.F., Roberts, S.E., *et al.* (2011) Ionic residues of human serum transferrin affect binding to the transferrin receptor and iron release. *Biochemistry*, **51**, 686–694.

Steere, A.N., Byrne, S.L., Chasteen, N.D., *et al.* (2012) Kinetics of iron release from transferrin bound to the transferrin receptor at endosomal pH. *Biochim. Biophys. Acta*, **1820**, 326–339.

Sun, H., Li, H., Weir, R.A. and Sadler, P.J. (1998) The first specific Ti^{IV}–protein complex: potential relevance to anticancer activity of titanocenes. *Angew. Chem. Int. Ed. Engl.*, **37**, 1577–1579.

Surgenor, D.M., Koechlin, B.A. and Strong, L.E. (1949) Chemical, clinical and immunological studies on the products of human plasma fractionation. XXXVII. The metal-combining globulin of human plasma. *J. Clin. Invest.*, **28**, 73–96.

Suryo Rahmanto, Y., Dunn, L.L. and Richardson, D.R. (2007) The melanoma tumor antigen, melanotransferrin (p97): a 25-year hallmark – from iron metabolism to tumorigenesis. *Oncogene*, **26**, 6113–6124

Suryo Rahmanto, Y., Bal, S., Loh, K.H., Yu, Y. and Richardson, D.R. (2012) Melanotransferrin: search for a function. *Biochim. Biophys. Acta*, **1820**, 237–243.

Takahashi, N., Takahashi, Y. and Putnam, F.W. (1985) Periodicity of leucine and tandem repetition of a 24-amino acid segment in the primary structure of leucine-rich alpha 2-glycoprotein of human serum. *Proc. Natl Acad. Sci. USA*, **82**, 73–77.

Tang, S., Lu, B. and Fantus, I.G. (1998) Stimulation of ^{125}I-transferrin binding and ^{59}Fe uptake in rat adipocytes by vanadate: treatment time determines apparent tissue sensitivity. *Metabolism*, **47**, 630–636.

Taylor, A.B., Stoj, C.S., Ziegler, L., *et al.* (2005) The copper-iron connection in biology: Structure of the metallo-oxidase Fet3p. *Proc. Natl Acad. Sci. USA*, **102**, 15459–15464.

Teng, C.T. (2010) Lactoferrin: the path from protein to gene. *Biometals*, **23**, 359–364.

Thibodeau, S.N., Lee, D.C. and Palmiter, R.D. (1978) Identical precursors for serum transferrin and egg white conalbumin. *J. Biol. Chem.*, **253**, 3771–3774.

Tinoco, A.D., Peterson, C.W., Lucchese, B., Doyle, R.P. and Valentine, A.M. (2008) On the evolutionary significance and metal-binding characteristics of a monolobal transferrin from *Ciona intestinalis*. *Proc. Natl Acad. Sci. USA*, **105**, 3268–3273.

Turkewitz, A.P., Amatruda, J.F., Borhani, D., *et al.* (1988) A high yield purification of the human transferrin receptor and properties of its major extracellular fragment. *J. Biol. Chem.*, **263**, 8318–8325.

Unama, T., Okamoto, H., Konishi, K., Ohta, H. and Mori, K. (2001) Cloning of cDNA encoding vitellogenin and its expression in red sea urchin, *Pseudocentrotus depressus*. *Zool. Sci.*, **18**, 559–565.

Unuma, T., Yamamoto, T., Akiyama, T., Shiraishi, M. and Ohta, H. (2003) Quantitative changes in yolk protein and other components in the ovary and testis of the sea urchin Pseudocentrotus depressus. *J. Exp. Biol.* **206**, 365-72.

Unuma, T., Nakamura, A., Yamano, K. and Yokota, Y. (2010) The sea urchin major yolk protein is synthesized mainly in the gut inner epithelium and the gonadal nutritive phagocytes before and during gametogenesis. *Mol. Reprod. Dev.*, **77**, 59–68.

Uppal, R., Lakshmi, K.V. and Valentine, A.M. (2008) Isolation and characterization of the iron-binding properties of a primitive monolobal transferrin from *Ciona intestinalis*. *J. Biol. Inorg. Chem.*, **13**, 873–885.

Vachette, P., Dainese, E., Vasyliev, V.B., *et al.* (2002) A key structural role for active site type 3 copper ions in human ceruloplasmin. *J. Biol. Chem.*, **277**, 40823–40831

Vashchenko, G. and MacGillivray, R.T. (2013) Multi-copper oxidases and human iron metabolism. *Nutrients*, **5**, 2289–2313.

Vincent, J.B. (2014) Is chromium pharmacologically relevant? *J. Trace Elem. Med. Biol.*, **28**, 397–405.

Vincent, J.B. and Love, S. (2012) The binding and transport of alternative metals by transferrin. *Biochim. Biophys. Acta*, **1820**, 362–378.

Vulpe, C.D., Kuo, Y.M., Murphy, T.L., *et al.* (1999) Hephaestin, a ceruloplasmin homologue implicated in intestinal iron transport, is defective in the sla mouse. *Nat. Genet.*, **21**, 195–199.

Wallace, D.F., Summerville, L., Lusby, P.E. and Subramanian, V.N. (2005) First phenotypic description of transferrin receptor 2 knockout mouse, and the role of hepcidin. *Gut*, **54**, 980–986.

Wallace, D.F., Harris, J.M. and Subramaniam, V.N. (2010) Functional analysis and theoretical modeling of ferroportin reveals clustering of mutations according to phenotype. *Am. J. Physiol. Cell. Physiol.*, **298**, C75–C84.

Wally, J., Halbrooks, P.J., Vonrhein, C., *et al.* (2006) The crystal structure of iron-free human serum transferrin provides insight into inter-lobe communication and receptor binding. *J. Biol. Chem.*, **281**, 24934–24944.

Ward, D.M. and Kaplan, J. (2012) Ferroportin-mediated iron transport: expression and regulation. *Biochim. Biophys. Acta*, **1823**, 1426–1433.

Ward, P.P., Mendoza-Meneses, M., Cunningham, G.A. and Conneely, O.M. (2003) Iron status in mice carrying a targeted disruption of lactoferrin. *Mol. Cell Biol.*, **23**, 178–185.

West, A.P., Jr, Bennett, M.J., Sellers, V.M., *et al.* (2000) Comparison of the interactions of transferrin receptor and transferrin receptor 2 with transferrin and the hereditary hemochromatosis protein HFE. *J. Biol. Chem.*, **275**, 38135–38138.

Wheby, M.S. and Jones, L.G. (1963) Role of transferrin in iron absorption. *J. Clin. Invest.*, **42**, 1007–1016.

White, K.N., Conesa, C., Sanchez, L., *et al.* (2012) The transfer of iron between ceruloplasmin and transferrins. *Biochim. Biophys. Acta*, **1820**, 411–416.

Williams J. (1982) The evolution of transferrin. *Trends Biochem. Sci.*, **7**, 394–397.

Willsky, G.R., Goldfine, A.B., Kostyniak, P.J., *et al.* (2001) Effect of vanadium(IV) compounds in the treatment of diabetes: *in vivo* and *in vitro* studies with vanadyl sulfate and bis(maltolato)oxovanadium(IV). *J. Inorg. Biochem.*, **85**, 33–42.

Wuebbens, M.W., Roush, E.D., Decastro, C.M. and Fierke, C.A. (1997) Cloning, sequencing, and recombinant expression of the porcine inhibitor of carbonic anhydrase: a novel member of the transferrin family. *Biochemistry*, **36**, 4327–4336.

Young, S.P., Bomford, A. and Williams, R. (1984) The effect of the iron saturation of transferrin on its binding and uptake by rabbit reticulocytes. *J. Biol. Chem.*, **219**, 505–510.

Zak, O. and Aisen, P. (2003) Iron release from transferrin, its C-lobe, and their complexes with transferrin receptor: presence of N-lobe accelerates release from C-lobe at endosomal pH. *Biochemistry*, **42**, 12330–12334.

Zerial, M., Melancon, P., Schneider, C. and Garoff, H. (1986) The transmembrane segment of the human transferrin receptor functions as a signal peptide. *EMBO J.*, **5**, 1543–1550.

Zhang, Z., Zhang, F., An, P., *et al.* (2011) Ferroportin1 deficiency in mouse macrophages impairs iron homeostasis and inflammatory responses. *Blood*, **118**, 1912–1922.

Zhao, N., Gao, J., Enns, C.A. and Knutson, M.D. (2010) ZRT/IRT-like protein 14 (ZIP14) promotes the cellular assimilation of iron from transferrin. *J. Biol. Chem.*, **285**, 32141–32150.

Zohn, I.E., De Domenico, I., Pollock, A., *et al.* (2007) The flatiron mutation in mouse ferroportin acts as a dominant negative to cause ferroportin disease. *Blood*, **109**, 4174–4180.

7

Mammalian Iron Metabolism and Dietary Iron Absorption

7.1 An Overview of Mammalian Iron Metabolism

7.1.1 Introduction

In adult humans the total body iron content is normally 3–5 g (this corresponds to 40–50 mg Fe kg^{-1} body weight), with typically higher values in men than in women (50 mg kg^{-1} in men compared to 40 mg kg^{-1} in women). Body iron is unevenly distributed between three pools, the two larger of which – *functional* and *storage* – are connected by the much smaller *transport* pool (Figure 7.1). Circulating erythrocytes contain most of the *functional iron* bound in the haem prosthetic group of the oxygen transport protein haemoglobin (about 30 mg Fe kg^{-1}). A further 4 mg Fe kg^{-1} is found in the muscles in the form of the oxygen storage protein myoglobin, and about 2 mg Fe kg^{-1} in various tissues in the form of other haemoproteins, iron–sulphur proteins and non-haem, non iron–sulphur proteins, the complexity of which have been reviewed in Chapter 2. Most of the remaining iron (10–12 mg Fe kg^{-1} in men and around 5 mg Fe kg^{-1} in women) is in the *storage pool*, essentially in the liver, spleen, bone marrow and muscle, as ferritin and haemosiderin (see Chapter 9). Hepatocytes are the main location of iron stores, with considerable capacity to take up iron from the circulation, not only from transferrin, but also from non-transferrin-bound iron (NTBI), thereby protecting against toxic oxygen radicals. More importantly, as we will see in later chapters, the hepatocytes play a key role in maintaining the level of serum iron and in the global regulation of iron homeostasis (Ganz, 2011). The macrophages of the reticuloendothelial system are the second most important store, playing an important dual function. First, they are the main players in recycling iron from senescent erythrocytes to erythroid precursors, which accounts for most of the daily iron turnover under physiological conditions. Second, macrophages can immobilise iron in the storage form in the event of inflammation, representing the first line of iron storage, whereas storage in the

Iron Metabolism – From Molecular Mechanisms to Clinical Consequences, Fourth Edition. Robert Crichton.
© 2016 John Wiley & Sons, Ltd. Published 2016 by John Wiley & Sons, Ltd.

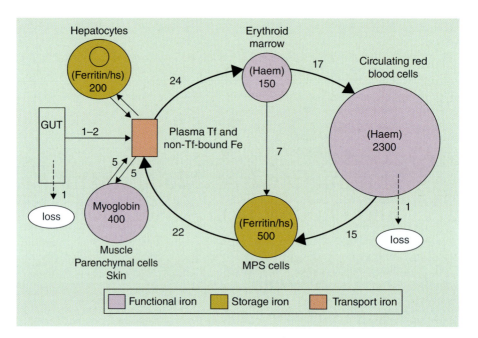

Figure 7.1 *Body iron stores and daily iron exchange. The figure shows a schematic representation of the routes of iron movement in normal adult male subjects. The plasma iron pool is about 4 mg (transferrin-bound iron and non-transferrin-bound iron), although the daily turnover is over 30 mg. The iron in parenchymal tissues is largely haem (in muscle) and ferritin/haemosiderin (in hepatic parenchymal cells). Dotted arrows represent iron loss through loss of epithelial cells in the gut or through blood loss. Numbers are in mg per day. Tf, transferrin; hs, haemosiderin; MPS, mononuclear phagocytic system, including macrophages in spleen and Kupffer cells in liver. Reproduced with permission from UNI-MED, Bremen from Crichton, R., Danielson B.G. and Geisser, P. (2008)* Iron Therapy With Special Emphasis on Intravenous Administration, *4th edition*

liver and other organs occurs only after the storage capacity of the macrophages has been saturated. Only a tiny fraction of total body iron, around 3 mg, circulates in the plasma and other extracellular fluids bound to the iron transport protein, transferrin (Bothwell *et al.*, 1979). This transport compartment plays a central role in iron metabolism and, despite its size, it is by far the most dynamic iron compartment in the body since, as we have seen earlier (Chapter 6), its iron normally is turned over at least ten times every day. It receives dietary iron from the duodenum and recycled iron from the breakdown of effete red blood cells; storage reserves (mostly liver hepatocytes) can also supply iron to the circulation, and are the main source of iron for haemoglobin synthesis in erythroid cell precursors. However, it also supplies iron to most other cells of the body, and is the source of maternal iron supplying the enormous requirements of the developing foetus during pregnancy.

The major pathways of internal iron exchange between different body compartments are well established in humans (Figure 7.1). As outlined below, iron absorption and excretion are mutually adjusted, and in the normal subject represent about 1 mg per day in each direction, such that iron homeostasis is tightly conserved. Transferrin in plasma and extracellular fluids transports iron between the different cellular compartments. About four-fifths of this exchange (under normal conditions, about 22 mg per day) cycles through the erythron and the mononuclear phagocytic system (MPS), which phagocytose senescent erythrocytes. Transferrin-bound iron in plasma and extracellular fluid cycles to the bone marrow, where it is incorporated into haem to supply the haemoglobin in newly formed red cell precursors. The erythrocytes circulate in the peripheral blood stream for about 120 days, and thereafter the old red blood cells are taken up by the reticuloendothelial MPS, consisting of the macrophages in the spleen and, to a lesser extent, the Kupffer cells in the liver. After lysis of the erythrocytes within the macrophages, the globin chains are digested within lyosomes, the haem is broken down via haem oxygenase (see Chapter 8), and its iron released to plasma transferrin.

During the course of each cycle a small amount of iron is transferred to storage sites where it is incorporated into ferritin and subsequently into haemosiderin. Some of the storage iron is released to the plasma, and a small proportion of the newly formed erythrocytes (ca. 10%) are destroyed within the bone marrow and their iron is released, thus escaping from the major circulatory part of the cycle: this is referred to as ineffective erythropoiesis. The numbers alongside the arrows in Figure 7.1 indicate the amount of iron (mg) that enters and leaves each of these compartments in normal healthy adults every day. Storage iron is usually present in roughly equal amounts in the macrophages of the reticuloendothelial system, in hepatic parenchymal cells, and in skeletal muscle. The overall extent of iron exchange by hepatocytes is much less (about one-fifth) than that by reticuloendothelial cells.

7.1.2   The Way Different Cells Handle Iron

Cellular iron transport involves both the *import* of iron from the external environment and its *export*, releasing iron from cells for its re-use somewhere else, with different mammalian cell types having distinctly different ways of handling iron (Figure 7.2). Some cells, like the precursors of red blood cells, are net *importers* of iron, taking up iron from circulating diferric transferrin and using it for haem synthesis. In contrast, polarised cells, like the enterocytes of the intestinal tract, *import* iron at one pole, transport it across the apical membrane, and *export* it at the opposite pole of the enterocyte through the basolateral membrane (Figure 7.2A). These cells move iron across the epithelial barrier between the gut and the circulation; in a similar manner, the syncytiotrophoblasts of the maternal placenta transport iron from the mother to the foetus. The transport of iron through the enterocytes from the gut to the plasma is discussed later in this chapter.

The precursors of red blood cells are unique in that they are net iron *importers*, with little evidence of any capacity for iron export (Figure 7.2B). These erythroid cells of the bone marrow, together with mature red blood cells, contain two-thirds of the total body iron in normal subjects. A single erythrocyte contains more than one billion iron atoms in the form of haem (Knutson and Wessling-Resnick, 2003), and during the course of their maturation they take up all of their iron via transferrin receptors (TfRs), using the transferrin-to-cell cycle described above. This distinguishes erythroid precursors from most other cells, which can also use nonTfR mechanisms to assimilate iron. The disruption of TfRs in mice results in embryonic lethality due to severe anaemia, although most tissues which are not involved in the production of red blood cells appear normal. Likewise, a deficiency of transferrin also results in severe anaemia, whereas nonhaematopietic cells develop massive iron overload, underlining both the importance of the transferrin–TfR cycle for erythroid cells and the fact that most other cells can assimilate iron without it.

Adult humans have about 25 trillion red blood cells (RBCs), and each second about five million of these are recycled by erythrophagocytosis (EP) in the macrophages of the reticuloendothelial system (White *et al.*, 2013). Tissue macrophages are responsible for the elimination of foreign particles, microorganisms, apoptotic cells, intracellular pathogens and senescent red blood cells. As such, they play a crucial role in active and passive immunity, tissue remodelling, defence

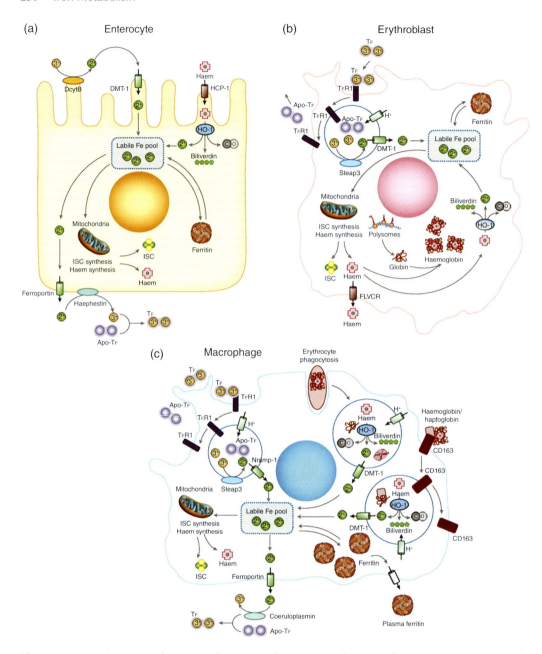

Figure 7.2 *Iron import, utilisation and export pathways according to cell type. (a) Enterocytes take up dietary iron at the apical pole and export it to transferrin at the basolateral poll, as described in detail later in the chapter. (b) Erythroblasts, the major iron-consuming cells in the organism, mainly take up transferrin-bound iron via transferrin receptor 1 (TfR1), and almost all is used for mitochondrial haem production and haemoglobin synthesis. (c) Macrophages exert a crucial role in iron recycling, phagocytosing senescent erythrocytes and releasing accumulated iron back into the circulation in a regulated manner, thus enabling iron recycling. More details can be found in Chapter 8. Reproduced with permission from BMJ Publishing Group, Ltd from Evstatiev, R. and Gasche, C. (2012) Iron sensing and signalling.* Gut, **61**, 933–952

against infection, and iron metabolism. In addition to their contribution to iron homeostasis, they are the principal source of iron for erythropoiesis, recycling the haem iron of senescent erythrocytes (Figure 7.2C). The first step in the process of erythrophagocytosis and the recycling of haem iron involves the specific recognition and internalisation by tissue macrophages of aged red blood cells. During the course of its life span the cell membrane of the red blood cell undergoes a number of biochemical modifications which constitute the signals that allow its elimination from the circulation by tissue macrophages. Following erythrophagocytosis and internalisation of the red blood cell in a phagosome, its cellular components are degraded (as described later). Macrophages, like the enterocytes of the gut, are both *importers* and *exporters* of iron, and the export in both cases is handled by ferroportin which, as we saw in Chapter 6, is expressed in specific cells that play critical roles in mammalian iron metabolism, including placental syncytiotrophoblasts, duodenal enterocytes, hepatocytes and reticuloendothelial macrophages.

Dietary iron absorption by the mature enterocytes at the villus tips of the duodenum (which will be discussed in detail later) is of the order of 1–2 mg per day, which is just enough normally to compensate for the loss of body iron, mostly by desquamatisation of epithelial cells. In contrast, the recycling of haem iron following the phagocytosis and catabolism of senescent red blood cells accounts for between 25–30 mg per day, corresponding to the billion iron atoms required for the daily production of haemoglobin in new erythrocytes. At the end of their natural lifespan (around 120 days in humans), senescent red cells are phagocytosed by tissue macrophages, mostly in the spleen, the bone marrow and the liver (Kupffer cells). The splenic pulp seems to be the most active site in the degradation of red blood cells. However, following splenectomy, the half-life of erythrocytes does not change, which suggests that the liver and bone marrow macrophages can rapidly compensate for the loss of spleen macrophages. The iron liberated by haem catabolism is then exported into the bloodstream to meet the demand for iron by the immature erythroid cells in the bone marrow. Thus, the bulk of the body iron is engaged in a perpetual exchange between these two cell types – the erythrocytes and their precursors on the one hand, and the macrophages on the other hand. Macrophages also take up iron from the haemoglobin–haptoglobin complex, as described in Chapter 6.

Other cells also exist, such as the hepatocytes of the liver which serve to store iron when it is abundant or in excess, but which can also release iron when it is required. These cells take up iron not only from transferrin but also from other sources, such as the haem–haemopexin complex when increased red cell haemolysis overwhelms the haemoglobin–haptoglobin pathway of haem clearance via macrophages and, when the iron-binding capacity of transferrin is saturated (as in iron-loading diseases) from non-transferrin-bound iron.

7.2 Mammalian Iron Absorption

7.2.1 Introduction

All mammals need to obtain iron from their food – they are more or less at the top of the global food chain, obtaining nutrients from a vast range of other animals, as well as from mineral and vegetable sources. However, in contrast to most other mammals, humans have considerable problems in regulating their iron requirements. There are no active excretory mechanisms for iron in humans, although small amounts are lost by exfoliation of skin and gastrointestinal cells, as well as in the bile and urine. The capacity of the human body to excrete iron is therefore severely limited – iron loss in human beings (per kg body weight) is only one-tenth that of other mammals (Finch *et al.*,

1978), and human dietary intake is only one-fiftieth to one-hundredth that of other mammals. It follows, as was originally suggested by McCance and Widdowson (1937), that iron balance in humans is primarily determined by iron absorption. As a consequence, body iron levels are principally controlled by regulating iron absorption from the jejunum and proximal duodenum, so that it precisely matches body iron losses.

The physiological regulation of iron absorption, as we will see later, is determined by the size of the iron storage pool and the demands of erythropoiesis. In subjects with normal erythropoiesis the levels of body iron are the main determinant of iron absorption, while serum ferritin levels are a good quantitative measure of iron stores (Cook *et al.*, 1974; Walters *et al.*, 1975).

7.2.2 The Intestinal Mucosa

Iron absorption is most active in the proximal small intestine near its junction with the stomach, essentially in the duodenum, but also to a lesser extent in the proximal jejunum. The future absorptive duodenal cells (enterocytes) originate by cell division within the crypts of Lieberkühn: at this stage, these crypt cells require iron for both cell division and development, but they lack absorptive capacity and must therefore obtain their iron from the plasma (Figure 7.3a). In contrast, as they differentiate while migrating to the villus tips, within the space of approximately 48 h, the enterocytes will progressively absorb iron from the lumen of the intestinal tract. These absorptive enterocytes (Figure 7.3b) are often called 'brush-border' cells, because of the brush-like mass of microvilli on their apical surface, which serves to increase the area of apical membrane actively involved in the transport of nutrients, including iron, from the intestinal tract into the cells.

The small intestine has a huge surface area (around 200 m^3) due to folds of the mucosa, their villi, or finger-like projections, and the microvillar structure of the brush-border membrane, which makes up the surface layer of the villi. These adaptations result in a 600-fold increase in the surface area of the small intestine compared to a cylinder of the same diameter. The enterocytes are polarised cells with the apical microvillus brush-border separated from the basolateral cell membrane (which is in contact with the circulation), while the enterocytes are connected to each other by tight junctions and by desmosomes (Figure 7.3b), forming a mechanical seal such that there is no mixing of the interstitial fluid with the contents of the lumen. Since, under normal conditions, there is little paracellular transport[1] of iron, this implies that iron must cross both the apical and the basolateral membranes in order to gain access to the circulation. It is, therefore, logical to assume that there will be specific transporter proteins at each of these membranes to ensure transmembrane transport, as well as oxidoreductases to change the oxidation state of iron.

Already in 1963, William Crosby advanced the hypothesis of a regulation of iron balance by the intestinal mucosa (Crosby, 1963) based on the observation that, subsequent to alterations in body iron levels, a delay of two to three days is required before any change in iron absorption occurs – a delay which corresponds approximately to the life span of the enterocyte. The idea was that, within the crypts of Leiberkühn, as the future enterocytes are formed they are programmed with 'messenger iron' which is a direct reflection of body iron stores (Conrad and Crosby, 1963). As they differentiate into enterocytes and migrate into the absorptive zone of the villus, this messenger iron regulates iron absorption, possibly by interaction with iron carriers, potentially at both the apical and the basolateral membrane.

At the villus tips, the enterocytes are sloughed off (together with their intracellular content) to be phagocytosed in the intestinal tract, and those nutritive elements such as iron which have been

---

[1] Paracellular transport involves passage between cells rather than through the polarised absorptive cells.

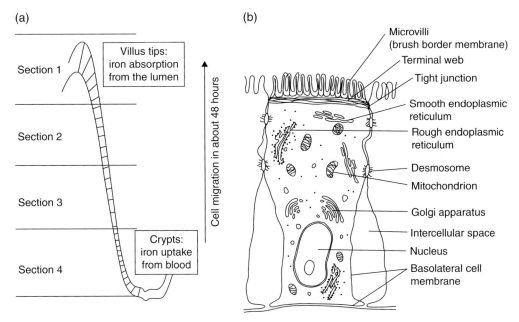

Figure 7.3 *(a) Rat duodenal cells divide in the crypts of Lieberkühn and differentiate while migrating to the villus tips within approximately 48 h. The crypt cells take up iron from the blood and are thereby able to sense the body's state of iron repletion. They migrate to the villus tips, where this information determines their iron-absorption capacity from the intestinal lumen. Reproduced with permission from John Wiley & Sons from Schumann, K., Moret, R., Kunzle, H. and Kühn, L.C. (1999) Iron regulatory protein as an endogenous sensor of iron in rat intestinal mucosa. Possible implications for the regulation of iron absorption. Eur. J. Biochem., **260**, 362–372. (b) Ultrastructure of a small intestinal epithelial cell (enterocyte)*

taken up during the villal phase of their cycle, but have not been transferred across the cells to the bloodstream at the basolateral surface, are lost.

7.2.3 Sources of Dietary Iron

As indicated above, the principal site of iron absorption is the upper part of the gastrointestinal tract (the duodenum). Both, the amount and bioavailability of dietary iron, together with the pH and motility of the gut lumen and other factors, influence iron absorption. These different factors do not, however, regulate iron absorption: this is thought to be carried out by the intestinal mucosa, which under normal circumstances adjusts the amount of dietary iron absorbed, so that it just compensates the iron which is lost by excretion. Since the human body lacks an effective means of iron excretion, this means that only very small amounts of dietary iron are absorbed (see Section 7.2.4, Iron losses).

Iron absorption from the diet depends not only on the iron content but also on its composition. Typical Western diets contain about 5–6 mg of iron per 1000 kcal, of which about 1 mg iron per 1000 kcal will be absorbed. There is very little variation from meal to meal in food iron, which therefore corresponds to a total daily intake of 12–18 mg for most subjects. There are two major pools of dietary iron: haem iron and non-haem iron. The primary sources of haem iron are haemoglobin and myoglobin from the consumption of meat, poultry and fish, while non-haem iron is obtained from cereals, pulses, legumes, fruits and vegetables. Non-haem iron, which essentially is inorganic iron, is by far the most predominant form of iron in dietary components of plant origin, and accounts for 80–90% of the iron in a standard diet (Hallberg, 1981; Carpenter and Mahoney, 1992); the remainder is accounted for by haem iron.

Haem iron is highly bioavailable and well absorbed (typically 15–35%), and dietary factors or physiological variables have little effect on its absorption (FAO/WHO, 2001). In contrast, non-haem iron is less well absorbed (2–20%), with absorption being strongly influenced by other food components (Hurrell and Egli, 2010). Thus, despite its relative paucity in the diet, haem iron is absorbed much more efficiently than non-haem iron and may contribute up to 50% of the total iron absorbed by the body (Hallberg, 1981; Bezwoda *et al.*, 1983; Carpenter and Mahoney, 1992). The haem iron in meat, essentially in the form of haemoglobin and myoglobin, when exposed to the low pH of the stomach, coupled with the action of proteolytic enzymes in both stomach and small intestine, is released as an intact metalloporphyrin. Haem itself is poorly absorbed, due to the formation of dimers and higher polymers in aqueous solution (Conrad *et al.*, 1966). In contrast, haem given as haemoglobin is well absorbed as it is maintained in its monomeric state by the primary amines released during the proteolysis of globin. Haem bioavailability can be substantially reduced by baking or prolonged frying. Despite its limited solubility, haem forms soluble complexes with a number of dietary components in the gut lumen. Haem uptake from the gut appears to involve specific, high-affinity mucosal brush-border haem-binding sites, which may represent a receptor-mediated process.

Despite its lower bioavailability, since the quantity of non-haem iron is so much greater than haem iron in most diets, non-haem iron generally contributes more to iron nutrition (FAO/WHO, 2001). Non-haem iron in food enters an exchangeable pool where it is subject to the interplay of luminal factors which both promote and inhibit its absorption (Abbaspour *et al.*, 2014; Hurrell and Egli, 2010). The major enhancers of non-haem iron absorption are meat and organic acids, of which ascorbate and citrate are the most important, acting as weak chelators to solubilise iron in the duodenum. Ascorbate can, in addition, reduce poorly soluble ferric Fe(III) iron to the more soluble ferrous Fe(II) state (Conrad and Umbreit, 1993; Sharp, 2010). Cooking, industrial processing and storage lead to the destruction of ascorbic acid and have a deleterious effect on the bioavailability of iron (Teucher *et al.*, 2004) – so don't cook the life out of green vegetables! A number of other organic acids (malic, lactic and tartaric acids) also enhance non-haem iron bioavailability. Ascorbic acid is the only enhancer of iron absorption in vegetarian diets, and therefore iron absorption from vegetarian and vegan meals can be best optimised by the inclusion of ascorbate-containing vegetables (Lynch and Cook, 1980). The enhancing effect of meat, fish or poultry on iron absorption from vegetarian meals has been clearly established (Lynch *et al.*, 1989a), but increases reported vary from two- to threefold (Bjorn-Rasmussen and Hallberg, 1979) to a modest 35–50% increase (Reddy *et al.*, 2006; Bach-Kristensen *et al.*, 2005).

In plant-based diets, phytates (myo-inositol hexakisphosphate), which constitute 1–2% by weight of many cereals, nuts and legumes, are the main inhibitor of non-haem iron absorption (Hurrell and Egli, 2010); their effects are dose-dependent, and start at very low concentrations (2–10 mg per meal) (Siegenberg *et al.*, 1991; Hurrell *et al.*, 1992). Polyphenols and tannins, found in vegetables, fruits, some cereals and legumes, tea, coffee and wine also decrease the absorption of non-haem iron. Other inhibitors of non-haem iron absorption are thought to be wheat bran and other components of dietary fibre complexes, calcium and phosphorus acting together, perhaps due to the formation of poorly available calcium–phosphate–iron complexes and dietary protein, particularly from soy beans, nuts and lupines (Abbaspour *et al.*, 2014).

Ascorbic acid will overcome the negative effect of all inhibitors of iron absorption, which include phytate, polyphenols, the calcium and proteins in milk products, and also increases the absorption of fortification iron (Hallberg *et al.*, 1989; Siegenberg *et al.*, 1991, Steckel *et al.*, 1986), although the enhancing effect of ascorbic acid in fruit and vegetables is often cancelled out by the inhibitory effect of polyphenols (Ballot *et al.*, 1987).

Diets rich in enhancers such as meat and/or ascorbate have high iron bioavailability (about 3 mg absorbed per day), whereas diets with inhibitors such as polyphenols and phytates are poor sources of iron (less than 1 mg per day) (Bothwell *et al.*, 1989). Clearly, the human body is genetically adapted to haem iron absorption, a throwback to the days when man was a hunter. The progressive change in dietary habits, which began with the introduction of the cultivation of grain about 10 000 years ago, has led to the replacement of well-absorbed haem iron by less-well absorbed non-haem iron from a cereal diet. The poor availability of dietary iron, particularly amongst the economically underprivileged, explains in large part the estimated more than 500 million persons throughout the world suffering from anaemia due to dietary iron deficiency (see Chapter 11). With the current tendency in Western society to adopt a vegetarian regime – particularly among young women – a significant increase in anaemia can be expected, exacerbated by the progressive decrease in caloric intake (which of course correlates with dietary iron). As noted in Chapter 11, an appropriately planned and well-balanced vegetarian diet is nonetheless compatible with adequate iron status. (Craig, 2009; Saunders *et al.*, 2013). And, at the opposite extreme, an only slightly enhanced excessive mucosal iron absorption can lead to parenchymal iron overload sufficient to cause tissue damage, a condition unique to humans; indeed, genetic haemochromatosis is probably the most frequently inherited disease in humans (see Chapter 11).

The absorption of haem iron is only modestly influenced by iron status (Lynch *et al.*, 1989b; Roughead and Hunt, 2000), whereas the absorption of non-haem iron is tightly regulated by iron stores (Bothwell *et al.*, 1979). Non-haem iron absorption can also be decreased by the chronic use of proton pump inhibitors for gastric acid reflux, *Helicobacter pylori* infection, and inflammatory conditions (e.g. celiac disease) (Collins and Anderson, 2012).

7.2.4   Iron Loss and Effects on Uptake

In the basal state, iron is lost passively in cells that are shed from the skin surface or the epithelial lining of internal organs. Small amounts of red blood cells are also lost via the gastrointestinal tract. The normal amount of iron lost in men is of the order of 14 µg kg^{-1} per day; these losses are distributed between the gastrointestinal tract, the skin and the urinary tract in a ratio of 6:3:1. In a 70-kg man, this basal loss would average 0.98 mg per day, whereas for a 55-kg woman this would be 0.77 mg per day. Menstruation increases the amount of iron loss, and to maintain balance in 95% of women the absorption of 2.84 mg per day of iron is required. In iron deficiency these losses may be reduced by 50%, whereas in iron overload they are slightly increased (Crichton *et al.*, 2008; Crichton, 2013).

The other physiological cause of increased iron loss is *pregnancy*. Although a pregnant woman should be in positive iron balance during the course of the pregnancy, it is not unusual for the pregnancy and parturition to result in a net loss of iron from the mother's body. The iron requirements specific to pregnancy over the nine-month gestational period, for a 55-kg woman, are calculated to be 320 mg for basal losses, 360 mg for the products of conception (foetus, 270 mg; placenta and umbilical cord, 90 mg), and approximately 150 mg as peripartum blood loss. An additional 450 mg of iron is required for expanded maternal red cell mass; however, this iron will not be lost with parturition but will be returned to the mother during postpartum contraction of the red cell mass. The greatest increases in total requirements (up to 6 mg Fe per day) are for foetal growth and erythroid expansion during the second and third trimesters, which are only slightly offset by the diminished iron loss as a result of the amenorrhea of pregnancy. Lactation results in a further iron loss of 0.3–0.6 mg per day postpartum in the milk, but this additional loss is largely balanced by the accompanying amenorrhea.

Growth markedly increases iron requirements for the formation of both erythroid and non-erythroid tissues. Because of more efficient oxygen delivery to tissues, the newborn infant initially experiences a decrease in haemoglobin concentration, with a shift of iron into stores. Growth and erythropoiesis exhaust this supply of iron within six months, so that in the first year of life the infant must absorb 0.3 mg Fe per day to maintain iron homeostasis. In the second year of life, growth causes this figure to rise to 0.4 mg per day. Slow growth from this time until puberty results in a gradual increase in requirements to 0.5 to 0.8 mg per day. Puberty and adolescent growth spurts increase iron requirements to 1.6 mg per day in young men and to 2.4 mg per day in young women. The higher requirement in young women reflects concomitant menarche.

Basal iron losses and physiologically enhanced losses as in menstruation, pregnancy and lactation are normal iron losses. Iron loss may be increased in situations of pathological and nonpathological blood loss. Pathological losses occur in such situations as bleeding from the urinary, genital and gastrointestinal tracts. The gastrointestinal tract is the most common site of pathological bleeding, secondary to conditions such as oesophagitis, gastritis, varices, peptic ulcers, neoplasms, diverticulosis, angiodysplasia and inflammatory bowel disease. In developing regions of the world, infection with parasites such as hookworm may increase iron loss. Heavy infestation may cause bleeding of sufficient magnitude to increase requirements of iron by as much as 3–5 mg per day. Nonpathological increases in blood loss may be secondary to the effects of aspirin or nonsteroidal anti-inflammatory drugs, which may cause gastric bleeding, or to voluntary blood donation.

Stimulation of erythropoiesis by administered erythropoietin, which is used to treat various disease states (e.g. renal failure), or by endogenous erythropoietin, which is elevated in haemolytic states related to abnormalities in haemoglobin formation (e.g. thalassemia or sickle cell disease), further increases iron requirements. Endogenous erythropoietin production by the kidney is stimulated when oxygen delivery to the kidney is reduced, as in anaemia.

7.3 Molecular Mechanisms of Mucosal Iron Absorption

7.3.1 Iron Uptake at the Apical Pole

The absorption of dietary iron by the intestinal mucosal cells occurs in three distinct steps: (i) the *uptake* of iron from the lumen of the gut, across the brush-border at the apical pole of the intestinal mucosal cell; (ii) the *transport* of iron across the mucosal cell, associated with its eventual sequestration into an intramucosal ferritin pool which can potentially be lost when the mucosal cell reaches the end of its short life cycle; and (iii) the *release* of iron at the basolateral pole of the mucosal cell and its incorporation into the plasma transport protein, transferrin. These steps will now be discussed in turn, and are outlined in Figure 7.2A.

Mucosal cells can take up dietary iron from the lumen across their brush-border membranes by at least two separate pathways, one specific for non-haem iron and the other for haem iron. Non-haem dietary iron seems most likely to be taken across the brush-border membrane by reduction of Fe^{3+} and subsequent transport of the Fe^{2+} by a divalent metal ion transporter protein.

Dietary non-haem iron can be reduced to Fe^{2+} by ascorbate in the intestinal tract and by brush-border ferrireductases. This not only increases its solubility but also supplies the requisite substrate, for the divalent metal transporter. The first candidate ferrireductase to be identified, Dcytb, was isolated using a subtractive cloning strategy from the iron-deficient rat (McKie *et al.*, 2001). Dcytb (duodenal cytochrome *b*) is similar to the ascorbate-reducible cytochrome *b*561 of the adrenal chromaffin granule (Figure 7.4), though with some differences in midpoint potentials of the haems (Oakhill *et al.*, 2008). Cytochromes *b*561 (Cyts-*b*561) are ascorbate-reducible, *trans*-membrane, di-haem proteins identified in a great variety of organisms, including invertebrates, vertebrates and plants (Tsubaki *et al.*, 2005). All Cyts-*b*561 are predicted to consist of six *trans*-membrane helices, with four highly conserved His residues involved in the haem coordination. They use ascorbate as an electron donor, functioning as monodehydroascorbate reductases, regenerating ascorbate, and in the opposite direction as, Fe^{3+}-reductases, providing reduced iron for *trans*-membrane transport. Their physiological functions include stress defence, cell wall modifications, iron metabolism, tumour suppression, and various neurological processes, including memory retention (for recent reviews, see Asard *et al.*, 2013; Lüthje *et al.*, 2013). Dcytb is highly expressed in the brush-border membrane of duodenal enterocytes and induces ferric reductase activity when expressed in *Xenopus* oocytes and cultured cells. Duodenal expression levels of Dcytb in the rat are regulated by physiological modulators of iron absorption; they are increased in iron deficiency (McKie *et al.*, 2001; Collins *et al.*, 2005; Latunde-Dada *et al.*, 2002) and hypoxia (McKie *et al.*, 2001; Latunde-Dada *et al.*, 2011) and decreased in response to an oral bolus of iron (Frazer *et al.*, 2003), indicating that Dcytb plays an important role in the regulation of the iron absorption pathway. Increased levels of Dcytb mRNA were also found in iron-loaded, HFE-deficient mice (Herrmann *et al.*, 2004; Ludwiczek *et al.*, 2005). It was shown that Dcytb is not required for iron absorption in mice

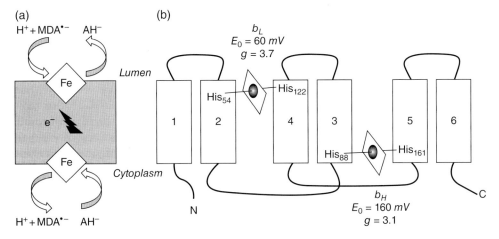

Figure 7.4 *Electron transport via AdCytb (a) and the topological arrangement of AdCytb in the membrane of chromaffin granules (b). (a) According to the current paradigm, cytoplasmic ascorbate (AH⁻) is oxidised by AdCytb to monodehydroascorbate (MDA•⁻). The resulting electrons are transferred to the lumen (matrix) of chromaffin granules to replenish ascorbate consumed in the process of norepinephrine synthesis by reducing intragranular MDA. (b) The transmembrane helices of AdCytb numbered 1–6 are connected by the extramembrane segments. Two haems are bound to the apoprotein by histidine residues 122 and 54 and histidine residues 161 and 88. The crosslinked binding of haems to the four central helices constitutes a 'core domain' (note that the order of helices 3 and 4 is inverted for the sake of clarity). Reprinted with permission from da Silva, G.F., Shinkarev, V.P., Kamensky, Y.A. and Palmer, G. (2012) Spectroscopic evidence of the role of an axial ligand histidinate in the mechanism of adrenal cytochrome b561. Biochemistry, **51**, 8730–8742; © 2012, American Chemical Society*

(Gunshin *et al.*, 2005a), although more recent studies with knockout mice have shown that DcytB is the primary iron-regulated duodenal ferric reductase in the gut and that Dcytb is necessary for optimal iron metabolism (Choi *et al.*, 2012). Members of the STEAP (six transmembrane epithelial antigen of prostate proteins), which can also reduce Fe^{3+} to Fe^{2+}, are also present in the brush border of the duodenum (Ohgami *et al.*, 2006).

Subsequent to its reduction, Fe^{2+} is transported across the brush-border membrane of enterocytes via the divalent metal transporter 1, DMT1, encoded by the *SLC11A2* gene (Mackenzie and Garrick, 2005). DMT1 was encountered previously in the transferrin-to-cell cycle, transporting Fe^{2+} across the endosomal membrane and into the cytoplasm (see Chapter 6). DMT1, also known as solute carrier family 11, member 2 (SLC11A2), Nramp2 and DCT1, is a member of the natural resistance-associated macrophage (Nramp) family of 12 transmembrane segment proteins, and has been implicated in the rapid uptake of dietary Fe(II) from the intestinal mucosa (Fleming *et al.*, 1997; Gunshin *et al.*, 1997, 2005b). Members of the SLC11 (NRAMP) family of membrane proteins are present in all kingdoms of life with a high degree of sequence conservation. DMT1 is a proton symporter, using the acid microclimate at the brush-border to provide the H^+ electrochemical gradient to drive transport of Fe^{2+} into the enterocyte. However, DMT1 is not specific for Fe^{2+} and transports other divalent metal ions such as Mn^{2+} and Cd^{2+}, whereas Zn^{2+} is a poor substrate (Mackenzie *et al.*, 2006; Illing *et al.*, 2012). It does not transport the alkaline earth metal ions Ca^{2+} and Mg^{2+} (Shawki and Mackenzie, 2010), and this is important because their high concentration in the duodenum would interfere with the absorption of Fe^{2+}. The crystal structure of *Staphylococcus capitis* DMT (ScaDMT), a close prokaryotic homologue of the family, has been recently determined (Ehrnstorfer *et al.*, 2014), and it has been shown that the substrate-binding site located in the centre of the transporter, is composed of conserved residues, which coordinate Mn^{2+}, Fe^{2+} and Cd^{2+} but not Ca^{2+}. DMT1 is dramatically upregulated in the intestine by restriction of dietary iron and by increased demand for iron. There are two splice variants of DMT1 mRNA in the intestine, the predominant form of which has an IRE in its 3′-untranslated region. Binding of IRP to this IRE when intracellular iron is low would protect the mRNA from degradation, and explain the upregulation, as discussed in detail in Chapter 10.

The essential role of DMT1 for both intestinal iron absorption and erythropoiesis is underlined by the severe iron-deficiency anaemia that results from deletion (Gunshin *et al.*, 2005b) or mutation (Fleming *et al.*, 1997, 1998) of the gene in rodents. Global and selective inactivation of the murine gene that encodes DMT1 showed that foetal DMT1 is not needed for materno-foetal iron transfer, but that its activity is essential for intestinal non-haem iron absorption after birth. It is also required for normal haemoglobin production during the development of erythroid precursors. However, hepatocytes, brain and most other cells seem to have an alternative, as yet unknown, iron-uptake mechanism (Gunshin *et al.*, 2005b). The high expression of DMT1 in specific brain regions (Gunshin *et al.*, 1997) underlines its likely important role there, reinforced by the observation that the expression of DMT1 in primary hippocampal cultures after *N*-methyl-D-aspartate (NMDA) receptor stimulation or spatial memory training increased (Haeger *et al.*, 2010). Mutations in human DMT1 have been found in patients with congenital anaemia (Beaumont *et al.*, 2006; Iolascon *et al.*, 2006; Iolascon and De Falco, 2009; Mims *et al.*, 2005). Unlike the situation in rodents, these patients develop hepatic iron overload. This may simply reflect increased gut iron absorption from the preferred human iron source, haem, to compensate for the defective delivery of iron to erythroid cells, reflected by the anaemic condition of the patients.

Haem iron is also taken up by mucosal cells, and it seemed reasonable to suppose that haem would be taken up by a receptor-mediated uptake pathway. A novel transporter, designated haem carrier protein 1 (HCP1), also designated SLC46A1, was proposed to mediate haem transport in mice enterocytes (Shayeghi *et al.*, 2005), but it was subsequently reported that SLC46A1 is in fact a transporter of the vitamin folic acid (K_m 0.8 µM compared to 125 µM for haem) rather than haem (Qui *et al.*, 2006), and the name proton-coupled folate transporter (PCFT) was proposed. A loss-of-function mutation in SLC46A1 was also identified in a family with hereditary folate malabsorption: the affected children required high doses of supplemental folate, but appeared to have no defect in iron metabolism. Subsequent studies have indicated that while PCFT is undoubtedly a primary folate transporter, it may still play a physiological role in iron metabolism as a low-affinity haem transporter (Laftah *et al.*, 2009; Le Blanc *et al.*, 2012). From studies in the worm *Caenorhabditis elegans* which, like related helminthes, is a natural haem auxotroph acquiring environmental haem for incorporation into haemoproteins, another candidate, haem-responsive gene 1, *HRG-1*, has been identified (Rajagopal *et al.*, 2008).

7.3.2   Iron Transit Through and Storage in Enterocytes

Once within the cytosol of the enterocyte, Fe^{2+} enters the labile iron pool (see Figure 7.2A), the communal 'melting pot' through which all the cellular iron fluxes of the cell pass (more of this in Chapter 8). Current opinion is that both haem and non-haem iron arrive within the enterocyte as Fe^{2+}, the former after its release from haem by haem oxygenase, which is also discussed in Chapter 8.

The *transport* step involves the passage of iron that has been taken up at the apical, brush-border membrane across the mucosal epithelial cell to the basolateral membrane, where it will be transferred into the circulation. When body iron demand is high this step will be rapid. However, when demand is low, not all of the iron taken up from the lumen into the cell is transferred, and it can be used for intracellular purposes in mitochondria, for example, or stored in ferritin within the cytoplasm of the enterocyte. When iron is sequestered in ferritin, it will eventually be discarded into the gastrointestinal tract when the cell exfoliates. The administration of a large bolus of oral iron to anaemic animals blocked the absorption of subsequent smaller doses of ^{59}Fe (Hahn *et al.*, 1943), and this 'mucosal block' lasted for several days after the administration of the blocking dose and correlated with the expression of intestinal ferritin (Granick, 1946). Hahn *et al.* (1943) suggested that iron absorbed from the gut in excess of body requirements might be incorporated into mucosal cell ferritin, where it would somehow function as a 'mucosal block' against unnecessary assimilation of dietary iron. The mucosal cell would thus function as a gate-keeper, preventing the onward transfer of unwanted dietary iron. This notion will be discussed in greater detail in Chapter 10, when the regulation of systemic iron homeostasis is considered. However, it clearly implies that some kind of signal couples the amount of iron entering the mucosa from the lumen, and the proportion which is subsequently transferred into the plasma, to the body's iron requirements.

7.3.3   Iron Efflux across the Basolateral Membrane

Basolateral transfer of iron from duodenal enterocytes into the circulation involves a transporter of Fe^{2+}, ferroportin, a protein originally called IREG1 (iron-regulated gene 1), while a new member of the pantheon of classical Greek mythology, called hephaestin, is also involved in iron egress from the intestine (Figure 7.2A).

The iron transporter of the basolateral membrane of the enterocyte responsible for the exportation of iron from the enterocytes into the portal vein circulation, was discovered almost simultaneously by three groups (McKie *et al.*, 2001; Donovan *et al.*, 2000; Abboud and Haile, 2000). The first of these, IREG1, was isolated and characterised as a novel cDNA from duodenal mucosa of homozygous atransferrinaemic mice which exhibit abnormally high rates of iron absorption (McKie *et al.*, 2001). Ferrroportin (Donovan *et al.*, 2000) was cloned as the gene responsible for the hypochromic anaemia of the zebrafish mutant with the delightful oenological appellation 'chardonnay' (vintage unspecified), while MTP1 (Metal Transporter Protein 1) was found expressed in tissues involved in body iron homeostasis, including the reticuloendothelial system, the duodenum and the pregnant uterus (Abboud and Haile, 2000). IREG1, ferroportin1 (FPN1) and MTP1 are identical, and constitute the unique member of the *SLC40A* family (McKie and Barlow, 2004; Montalbetti *et al.*, 2013); FPN1 has a 10–12 predicted transmembrane secondary structure, has no obvious homology to DMT1. As we discussed in Chapter 6, a model of the three-dimensional (3D) structure of ferroportin has been proposed recently based on homology to the crystal structure of a Major Facilitator Superfamily member (EmrD) (Le Gac *et al.*, 2013). It has an apparent IRE in the 5′-untranslated region of its mRNA. The importance of IREG1 in iron absorption and iron homeostasis is underlined by its targeted disruption in mice (Donovan *et al.*, 2005), which results in defects in materno-embryonic iron transport, in basolateral iron transport out of enterocytes and, as seen in Chapter 8, in the export of iron from tissue macrophages. *SLC40A1* gene mutations in humans are rare, but constitute an important subset of iron-loading disorders, which are discussed in Chapter 11.

FPN1 transports Fe^{2+} across the basolateral membrane into the circulation, and it is thought that the Fe^{2+} must be oxidised to Fe^{3+} in order to ensure its incorporation into apotransferrin. This implies a ferroxidase activity either in the basolateral membrane itself, or in the blood with which it is in contact. One potential candidate for such ferroxidase activity is ceruloplasmin (Cp), the major copper-binding protein of blood plasma, whose ferroxidase activity in iron incorporation into apotransferrin has been discussed in Chapter 6. However, no evidence was found in support of a role for ceruloplasmin as an intestinal ferroxidase (Hellman and Gitlin, 2002), and *Cp*-knockout mice do not show a noticeable disruption in iron absorption (Harris *et al.*, 1999; Yamamoto *et al.*, 2002). In contrast, a potential role for Cp in iron absorption accompanying stimulated erythropoiesis was observed in severely bled *Cp-/-* mice (Cherukuri *et al.*, 2005).

This intestinal ferroxidase activity was finally discovered during the course of genome sequencing projects in the mouse (Vulpe *et al.*, 1999) and human (Syed *et al.*, 2002) X chromosome. The predicted polypeptide had 50% sequence identity with ceruloplasmin, including conservation of the cysteinyl residues involved in ceruloplasmin disulphide binding and the histidine, cysteinyl and methionine residues involved in copper coordination. The candidate gene in mice was designated *Heph* – for hephaestin.[2] Hephaestin (HEPH) is a multicopper ferroxidase inserted into the basolateral membrane by a GPI (Glyco-Phospho-Inositol) anchor, which appears to be necessary for iron egress from intestinal enterocytes into the circulation, and which represents a major link between iron and copper metabolism in mammals (see Chapter 14). The colocalisation of FPN1 and HEPH has been observed both *in vivo* and *in vitro* (Han and Kim, 2007; Yeh *et al.*, 2009, 2011). Ferroxidase activity has been observed in the cytosolic fraction of isolated rodent enterocytes (Ranganathan *et al.*, 2012a) which does not seem to be associated with hephaestin, since the activity remained present in enterocytes isolated from *Heph* KO mice (Ranganathan *et al.*, 2012b).

The way in which these different partners may be involved in iron uptake across the intestine is summarised in Figure 7.2A. The reduction of ferric complexes to the Fe^{2+} form is achieved by the action of the brush-border ferric reductase. The Fe^{2+} is transported across the brush-border membrane by the proton-coupled divalent cation transporter (DCT1), where it enters an unknown

---

[2] Hephaestus (Vulcan) was the Greek god of fire and husband of Aphrodite (Venus). See Chapter 14 for more on the relationship of Vulcan, Venus (copper) and Mars (iron).

compartment in the cytosol. Fe^{2+} is then transported across the basolateral membrane by IREG1, where the membrane-bound copper oxidase hephaestin (Hp) promotes release and binding of Fe^{3+} to circulating apotransferrin.

7.3.4 Regulation of Iron Uptake by the Enterocyte

When we consider the situation of the crypt cell at the beginning of its differentiation into an enterocyte, before it has begun its climb towards the tip of the villus, it is reasonable to assume that at this stage in its development it has no absorptive capacity and that it will only take up the iron necessary for its future differentiation and growth from circulating diferritransferrin (Fe_2Tf) via the transferrin receptors in its basolateral membrane. This level of intracellular iron, in the form of the labile iron pool (LIP), would then programme the crypt cell's potential for iron uptake when it reaches the developmental stage of an absorptive enterocyte, thereby determining not only the amount of iron taken up by the enterocyte but also the amount of iron that would be retained within the enterocyte as ferritin, and lost when the cell is sloughed at the end of its short life span. The way in which this could be achieved at both the cellular and the systemic level is described in Chapter 10. The regulation of the expression of proteins involved in iron uptake, storage and egress at the level of transcription employs the IRP/IRE system, while the regulation of systemic iron balance is controlled by the levels of expression of the circulating peptide hormone hepcidin, which can act on basolateral iron transport by interacting with ferroportin and also affect the enterocyte LIP.

References

Abbaspour, R., Hurrell, R. and Kelishadi, R. (2014) Review on iron and its importance for human health. *J. Res. Med. Sci.*, **19**, 164–174.

Abboud, S. and Haile, D.J. (2000) A novel mammalian iron-regulated protein involved in intracellular iron metabolism. *J. Biol. Chem.*, **275**, 19906–19912.

Asard, H., Barbaro, R., Trost, P. and Bérczi, A. (2013) Cytochromes b561: ascorbate mediated transmembrane electron transport. *Antioxid. Redox Signal.*, **19**, 1026–1035.

Bach-Kristensen, M., Hels, O., Morberg, C., *et al.* (2005) Pork meat increases iron absorption from a 5-day fully controlled diet when compared to a vegetarian diet with similar vitamin C and phytic acid content. *Br. J. Nutr.*, **94**, 78–83.

Ballot, D., Baynes, R.D., Bothwell, T.H., *et al.* (1987) The effects of fruit juices and fruits on the absorption of iron from a rice meal. *Br. J. Nutr.*, **57**, 331–343.

Beaumont, C., Delaunay, J., Hetet, G., *et al.* (2006) Two new human DMT1 gene mutations in a patient with microcytic anemia, low ferritinemia, and liver iron overload. *Blood*, **107**, 4168–4170.

Bezwoda, W.R., Bothwell, T.H., Charlton, R.W., *et al.* (1983) The relative dietary importance of haem and non-haem iron. *S. Afr. Med. J.*, **64**, 552–556.

Bjorn-Rasmussen, E. and Hallberg, L. (1979) Effect of animal proteins on the absorption of food iron in man. *Nutr. Metab.*, **23**, 192–202.

Bothwell, T.H., Charlton, R.W., Cook, J.D. and Finch, C.A. (1979) *Iron metabolism in man*, 1st edn. Blackwell Scientific Publications, Oxford, pp. 576.

Bothwell, T.H., Baynes, R.D., MacFarlane, B.J. and MacPhail, A.P. (1989) Nutritional iron requirements and food iron absorption. *J. Intern. Med.*, **226**, 357–365.

Carpenter, C.E. and Mahoney, A.W. (1992) Contributions of heme and nonheme iron to human nutrition. *Crit. Rev. Food Sci. Nutr.*, **31**, 333–367.

Cherukuri, S., Potla, R., Sarkar, J., *et al.* (2005) Unexpected role of ceruloplasmin in intestinal iron absorption. *Cell. Metab.*, **2**, 309–319.

Choi, J., Masaratana, P., Latunde-Dada, G.O., *et al.* (2012) Duodenal reductase activity and spleen iron stores are reduced and erythropoiesis is abnormal in Dcytb knockout mice exposed to hypoxic conditions. *J. Nutr.*, **142**, 1929–1934.

Collins, J.F. and Anderson, G.J. (2012) Molecular mechanisms of intestinal iron transport, in *Physiology of the Gastrointestinal Tract*, 5th edition, Elsevier, New York.

Collins, J.F., Franck, C.A., Kowdley, K.V. and Ghishan, F.K. (2005) Identification of differentially expressed genes in response to dietary iron deprivation in rat duodenum. *Am. J. Physiol. Gastrointest. Liver Physiol.*, **288**, G964–G971.

Conrad, M.E. and Crosby, W.H. (1963) Intestinal mucosal mechanisms controlling iron absorption. *Blood*, **22**, 406–415.

Conrad, M.E. and Umbreit, J.N. (2002) Pathways of iron absorption. *Blood Cells Mol. Dis.*, **29**, 336–355.

Conrad, M.E., Cortell, S., Williams, H.L. and Foy, A.L. (1966) Polymerization and intraluminal factors in the absorption of hemoglobin-iron. *J. Lab. Clin. Med.*, **68**, 659–668.

Cook, J.D., Marsaglia, G., Eschbach, J.W., Funk, D.D. and Finch, C.A. (1970) Ferrokinetics: a biologic model for plasma iron exchange in man. *J. Clin. Invest.*, **49**, 197–205.

Cook, J.D., Lipschitz, D.A., Miles, L.E. and Finch, C.A. (1974) Serum ferritin as a measure of iron stores in normal subjects. *Am. J. Clin. Nutr.*, **27**, 681–687.

Craig, W.J. (2009) Health effects of vegan diets. *Am. J. Clin. Nutr.*, **89**, 1627S–1633S.

Crichton, R.R. (2013) Iron, in *Biochemical, Physiological, Molecular Aspects of Human Nutrition*, 2nd edition (eds M.H. Stipanuk and M.A. Caudill), Saunders-Elsevier, St Louis, pp. 801–827.

Crichton, R.R., Danielson, B. and Geisser, P. (2008) *Iron Therapy with Special Emphasis on Intravenous Administration*, 4th edition, UNI-MED Verlag, AG, Bremen, pp. 128.

Crosby, W.H. (1963) The control of iron balance by the intestinal mucosa. *Blood*, **22**, 441–449.

da Silva, G.F., Shinkarev, V.P., Kamensky, Y.A. and Palmer, G. (2012) Spectroscopic evidence of the role of an axial ligand histidinate in the mechanism of adrenal cytochrome b561. *Biochemistry*, **51**, 8730–8742.

Donovan, A., Brownlie, A., Zhou, Y., *et al.* (2000) Positional cloning of zebrafish ferroportin1 identifies a conserved vertebrate iron exporter. *Nature*, **403**, 776–781.

Donovan, A., Lima, C.A., Pinkus, J.L., *et al.* (2005) The iron exporter ferroportin/Slc40a1 is essential for iron homeostasis. *Cell Metab.*, **1**, 191–200.

Ehrnstorfer, I.A., Geertsma, E.R., Pardon, E., Steyaert, J. and Dutzler, R. (2014) Crystal structure of a SLC11 (NRAMP) transporter reveals the basis for transition-metal ion transport. *Nat. Struct. Mol. Biol.*, **21**, 990–996.

Evstatiev, R. and Gasche, C. (2012) Iron sensing and signalling. *Gut*, **61**, 933–952.

FAO/WHO (Food and Agriculture Organization/World Health Organization) (2001) Food-based approaches to meeting vitamin and mineral requirements, Human vitamin and mineral requirements. Rome, pp. 7–25.

Finch, C.A., Ragan, H.A., Dyer, I.A. and Cook, J.D. (1978) Body iron loss in animals. *Proc. Soc. Exp. Biol. Med.*, **159**, 335–338.

Fleming, M.D., Trenor, C.C., Su, M.A., *et al.* (1997) Microcytic anaemia mice have a mutation in *Nramp2*, a candidate iron transporter gene. *Nat. Genet.*, **16**, 383–386.

Fleming, M.D., Romano, M.A., Su, M.A., *et al.* (1998) *Nramp2* is mutated in the anemic Belgrade (b) rat: evidence of a role for Nramp2 in endosomal iron transport. *Proc. Natl Acad. Sci. USA*, **95**, 1148–1153.

Frazer, D.M., Wilkins, S.J., Becker, E.M., *et al.* (2003) A rapid increase in the expression of DMT1 and Dcytb but not Ireg1 or hephaestin explains the mucosal block phenomenon of iron absorption. *Gut*, **52**, 340–346.

Ganz, T. (2011) Hepcidin and iron regulation, 10 years later. *Blood*, **117**, 4425–4433.

Granick, S. (1946) Ferritin; increase of the protein apoferritin in the gastrointestinal mucosa as a direct response to iron feeding; the function of ferritin in the regulation of iron absorption. *J. Biol. Chem.*, **164**, 737–746.

Gunshin, H., McKenzie, B., Berger, U.V., *et al.* (1997) Cloning and characterization of a mammalian proton-coupled metal-ion transporter. *Nature*, **388**, 482–488.

Gunshin, H., Starr, C.N., Direnzo, C., *et al.* (2005a) Cybrd1 (duodenal cytochrome b) is not necessary for dietary iron absorption in mice. *Blood*, **106**, 2879–2883.

Gunshin, H., Fujiwara, Y., Custodio, A.O., *et al.* (2005b) Slc11a2 is required for intestinal iron absorption and erythropoiesis but dispensable in placenta and liver. *J. Clin. Invest.*, **115**, 1258–1266.

Haeger, P., Alvarez, A., Leal, N., *et al.* (2010) Increased hippocampal expression of the divalent metal transporter 1 (DMT1) mRNA variants 1B and +IRE and DMT1 protein after NMDA-receptor stimulation or spatial memory training. *Neurotox. Res.*, **17**, 238–247.

Hahn, P.F., Bale, W.F., Ross, J.F., *et al.* (1943) Radioactive iron absorption by gastrointestinal tract: influence of anemia, anoxia and antecedent feeding distribution in growing dogs. *J. Exp. Med.*, **78**, 169–188.

Hallberg, L. (1981) Bioavailability of dietary iron in man. *Annu. Rev. Nutr.*, **1**, 123–147.

Hallberg, L., Brune, M. and Rossander, L. (1989) Iron absorption in man: ascorbic acid and dose-dependent inhibition by phytate. *Am. J. Clin. Nutr.*, **49**, 140–144.

Han, O. and Kim, E.Y. (2007) Colocalization of ferroportin-1 with hephaestin on the basolateral membrane of human intestinal absorptive cells. *J. Cell. Biochem.*, **101**, 1000–1010.

Harris, Z.L., Durley, A.P., Man, T.K. and Gitlin, J.D. (1999) Targeted gene disruption reveals an essential role for ceruloplasmin in cellular iron efflux. *Proc. Natl Acad. Sci. USA*, **96**, 10812–10817.

Hellman, N.E. and Gitlin, J.D. (2002) Ceruloplasmin metabolism and function. *Annu. Rev. Nutr.*, **22**, 430–458.

Herrmann, T., Muckenthaler, M., van der Hoeven, F., *et al.* (2004) Iron overload in adult Hfe-deficient mice independent of changes in the steady-state expression of the duodenal iron transporters DMT1 and Ireg1/ferroportin. *J. Mol. Med.*, **82**, 39–48.

Hurrell, R. and Egli, I. (2010) Iron bioavailability and dietary reference values. *Am. J. Clin. Nutr.*, **91**, 1461S–1467S.

Hurrell, R.F., Juillerat M.A., Reddy, M.B., *et al.* (1992) Soy protein, phytate, and iron absorption in humans. *Am. J. Clin. Nutr.*, **56**, 573–578.

Illing, A.C., Shawki, A., Cunningham, C.L. and Mackenzie, B. (2012) Substrate profile and metal-ion selectivity of human divalent metal-ion transporter-1. *J. Biol. Chem.*, **287**, 30485–30496.

Iolascon, A. and De Falco, L. (2009) Mutations in the gene encoding DMT1: clinical presentation and treatment. *Semin. Hematol.*, **46**, 358–370.

Iolascon, A., d'Apolito, M., Servedio, V., *et al.* (2006) Microcytic anemia and hepatic iron overload in a child with compound heterozygous mutations in DMT1 (SCL11A2). *Blood*, **107**, 349–354.

Knutson, M. and Wessling-Resnick, M. (2003) Iron metabolism in the reticuloendothelial system. *Crit. Rev. Biochem. Mol. Biol.*, **38**, 61–88.

Laftah, A.H., Latunde-Dada, G.O., Fakih, S., *et al.* (2009) Haem and folate transport by proton-coupled folate transporter/haem carrier protein 1 (SLC46A1). *Br. J. Nutr.*, **101**, 1150–1156.

Latunde-Dada, G.O., Van der Westhuizen, J., Vulpe, C.D., *et al.* (2002) Molecular and functional roles of duodenal cytochrome B (Dcytb) in iron metabolism. *Blood Cells Mol. Dis.*, **29**, 356–360.

Latunde-Dada, G.O., Xiang, L., Simpson, R.J. and McKie, A.T. (2011) Duodenal cytochrome b (Cybrd 1) and HIF-2α expression during acute hypoxic exposure in mice. *Eur. J. Nutr.*, **50**, 699–704.

Le Blanc, S., Garrick, M.D. and Arredondo, M. (2012) Heme carrier protein 1 transports heme and is involved in heme-Fe metabolism. *Am. J. Physiol. Cell Physiol.*, **302**, C1780–C1785.

Le Gac, G., Ka, C., Joubrel. R., *et al.* (2013) Structure–function analysis of the human ferroportin iron exporter (SLC40A1): effect of hemochromatosis type 4 disease mutations and identification of critical residues. *Hum. Mutat.*, **34**, 1371–1380.

Ludwiczek, S., Theurl, I., Bahram, S., *et al.* (2005) Regulatory networks for the control of body iron homeostasis and their dysregulation in HFE mediated hemochromatosis. *J. Cell. Physiol.*, **204**, 489–499.

Lüthje, S., Möller, B., Perrineau, F.C. and Wöltje, K. (2013) Plasma membrane electron pathways and oxidative stress. *Antioxid. Redox Signal.*, **18**, 2163–2183.

Lynch, S.R. and Cook, J.D. (1980) Interaction of vitamin C and iron. *Ann. N. Y. Acad. Sci.*, **355**, 32–44.

Lynch, S.R., Hurrell, R.F., Dassenko, S.A. and Cook, J.D. (1989a) The effect of dietary proteins on iron bioavailability in man. *Adv. Exp. Med. Biol.*, **249**, 117–132.

Lynch, S.R., Skikne, B.S. and Cook, J.D. (1989b) Food iron absorption in idiopathic hemochromatosis. *Blood*, **74**, 2187–2193.

Mackenzie, B. and Garrick, M.D. (2005) Iron imports. II. *Iron uptake at the apical membrane in the intestine*. *Am. J. Physiol. Gastrointest. Liver Physiol.*, **289**, G981–G986.

Mackenzie, B., Ujwal, M.L., Chang, M.H., Romero, M.F. and Hediger, M.A. (2006) Divalent metal-ion transporter DMT1 mediates both H$^+$-coupled Fe^{2+} transport and uncoupled fluxes. *Pflugers Arch.*, **451**, 544–558.

McCance, R.A. and Widdowson, E.M. (1937) Absorption and excretion of iron. *Lancet*, **ii**, 680–684.

McKie, A.T. and Barlow, D. (2004) The SLC40 basolateral iron transporter family (IREG1/ferroportin/MTP1). *Pflugers Arch.*, **447**, 9801–9806.

McKie, A.T., Barrow, D., Latunde-Dada, G.O., *et al.* (2001) An iron-regulated ferric reductase associated with the absorption of dietary iron. *Science*, **291**, 1755–1759.

Mims, M.P., Guan, Y., Pospisilova, D., *et al.* (2005) Identification of a human mutation of DMT1 in a patient with microcytic anemia and iron overload. *Blood*, **105**, 1337–1342.

Montalbetti, N., Simonin, A., Kovacs, G. and Hediger, M.A. (2013) Mammalian iron transporters: families SLC11 and SLC40. *Mol. Aspects Med.*, **34**, 270–287.

Oakhill, J.S., Marritt, S.J., Gareta, E.G., Cammack, R. and McKie, A.T. (2008) Functional characterization of human duodenal cytochrome b (Cybrd1): Redox properties in relation to iron and ascorbate metabolism. *Biochim. Biophys. Acta*, **1777**, 260–268.

Ohgami, R.S., Campagna, D.R., McDonald, A. and Fleming, M.D. (2006) The Steap proteins are metalloreductases. *Blood*, **108**, 1388–1394.

Qiu, A., Jansen, M., Sakaris, A., *et al.* (2006) Identification of an intestinal folate transporter and the molecular basis for hereditary folate malabsorption. *Cell*, **127**, 917–928.

Rajagopal, A., Rao, A.U., Amigo, J., *et al.* (2008) Haem homeostasis is regulated by the conserved and concerted functions of HRG-1 proteins. *Nature*, **453**, 1127–1131.

Ranganathan, P.N., Lu, Y., Fuqua, B.K. and Collins, J.F. (2012a) Discovery of a cytosolic/soluble ferroxidase in rodent enterocytes. *Proc. Natl Acad. Sci. USA*, **109**, 3564–3569.

Ranganathan, P.N., Lu, Y., Fuqua, B.K. and Collins, J.F. (2012b) Immunoreactive hephaestin and ferroxidase activity are present in the cytosolic fraction of rat enterocytes. *Biometals*, **25**, 687–695.

Reddy, M.B., Hurrell, R.F. and Cook, J.D. (2006) Meat consumption in a varied diet marginally influences nonheme iron absorption in normal individuals. *J. Nutr.*, **136**, 576–581.

Roughead, Z.K. and Hunt, J.R. (2000) Adaptation in iron absorption: iron supplementation reduces nonheme-iron but not heme-iron absorption from food. *Am. J. Clin. Nutr.*, **72**, 982–989.

Saunders, A.V., Craig, W.J., Baines, S.K. and Posen, J.S. (2013) Iron and vegetarian diets. *Med. J. Aust.*, **199**, S11–S16.

Schumann, K., Moret, R., Kunzle, H. and Kühn, L.C. (1999) Iron regulatory protein as an endogenous sensor of iron in rat intestinal mucosa. Possible implications for the regulation of iron absorption. *Eur. J. Biochem.*, **260**, 362–372.

Sharp, P.A. (2010) Intestinal iron absorption: regulation by dietary and systemic factors. *Int. J. Vitam. Nutr. Res.*, **80**, 231–242.

Shawki, A. and Mackenzie, B. (2010) Interaction of calcium with the human divalent metal-ion transporter-1. *Biochem. Biophys. Res. Commun.*, **393**, 471–475.

Shayeghi, M., Latunde-Dada, G.O., Oakhill, J.S., *et al.* (2005) Identification of an intestinal heme transporter. *Cell*, **122**, 789–801.

Siegenberg, D., Baynes, R.D., Bothwell, T.H., *et al.* (1991) Ascorbic acid prevents the dose-dependent inhibitory effects of polyphenols and phytates on nonheme-iron absorption. *Am. J. Clin. Nutr.*, **53**, 537–541.

Stekel, A., Olivares, M., Pizarro, F., *et al.* (1986) Absorption of fortification iron from milk formulas in infants. *Am. J. Clin. Nutr.*, **43**, 917–922.

Syed, B.A., Beaumont, N.J., Patel, A., *et al.* (2002) Analysis of the human hephaestin gene and protein: comparative modelling of the N-terminus ectodomain based upon ceruloplasmin. *Protein Eng.*, **15**, 205–214.

Teucher, B., Olivares, M. and Cori, H. (2004) Enhancers of iron absorption: Ascorbic acid and other organic acids. *Int. J. Vitam. Nutr. Res.*, **74**, 403–419.

Tsubaki, M., Takeuchi, F. and Nakanishi, N. (2005) Cytochrome *b*561 protein family: expanding roles and versatile transmembrane electron transfer abilities as predicted by a new classification system and protein sequence motif analyses. *Biochim. Biophys. Acta*, **1763**, 174–200.

Vulpe, C.D., Kuo, Y.M., Murphy, T.L., *et al.* (1999) Hephaestin, a ceruloplasmin homologue implicated in intestinal iron transport, is defective in the *sla* mouse. *Nat. Genet.*, **21**, 195–199.

Walters, G.O., Jacobs, A., Worwood, M., Trevett, D. and Thomson W. (1975) Iron absorption in normal subjects and patients with idiopathic haemochromatosis: relationship with serum ferritin concentration. *Gut*, **16**, 188–192.

White, C., Yuan, X., Schmidt, P.J., *et al.* (2013) HRG1 is essential for heme transport from the phagolysosome of macrophages during erythrophagocytosis. *Cell Metab.*, **17**, 261–270.

Yamamoto, K., Yoshida, K., Miyagoe, Y., *et al.* (2002) Quantitative evaluation of expression of iron-metabolism genes in ceruloplasmin-deficient mice. *Biochim. Biophys. Acta*, **1588**, 195–202.

Yeh, K.Y., Yeh, M., Mims, L. and Glass, J. (2009) Iron feeding induces ferroportin 1 and hephaestin migration and interaction in rat duodenal epithelium. *Am. J. Physiol. Gastrointest. Liver Physiol.*, **296**, G55–G65.

Yeh, K.Y., Yeh, M. and Glass, J. (2011) Interactions between ferroportin and hephaestin in rat enterocytes are reduced after iron ingestion. *Gastroenterology*, **141**, 292–299.

8

Intracellular Iron Utilisation

8.1 Intracellular Iron Pools

8.1.1 Introduction

As pointed out earlier, while nearly all forms of life require iron, the element has undesirable chemical properties in aqueous solution around neutral pH: the readily available Fe^{3+} hydrolyses and polymerises, leading to the formation of insoluble ferric-hydroxide polymers, while the more reactive Fe^{2+} generates toxic free radicals. After considering how iron is transported between cells, we now consider the different pools of iron within cells, which sequester the metal in a nontoxic, soluble and bioavailable form. This excludes the storage pool, which is discussed in Chapter 9.

Cells contain many different iron-containing proteins (see Chapter 2), which can be classified based on their metal coordination chemistry into three broad types: (i) haemoproteins, notably O_2 carriers, O_2 activators or electron transfer proteins; (ii) iron–sulphur cluster-containing proteins, many of which are involved in electron transfer, but also catalytic iron–sulphur clusters; and (iii) non-haem, non-iron–sulphur, iron-containing proteins which include enzymes, and also proteins of iron storage and transport. Since iron-containing proteins are located in essentially every subcellular compartment, this implies that iron, either as pre-formed haem or Fe–S cofactors, or as 'free' iron must travel to every compartment in the cell. These cofactors must then be distributed to nascent proteins in the mitochondria, in the cytosol, and in membrane-bound organelles. Recent evidence suggests that iron cofactors are distributed within the cell by specific systems, which include membrane transporters, protein chaperones, specialised carriers, and small molecules (Philpott and Ryu, 2014).

Iron Metabolism – From Molecular Mechanisms to Clinical Consequences, Fourth Edition. Robert Crichton.
© 2016 John Wiley & Sons, Ltd. Published 2016 by John Wiley & Sons, Ltd.

8.1.2 The Cytosolic Labile Iron Pool (LIP)

The idea of a 'labile iron pool' (LIP) in erythroid cells is not new (Greenberg and Wintrobe, 1946; Ross, 1946), and during the 1960s and 1970s evidence began to appear for the existence of non-haem intermediates, clearly distinct from ferritin and transferrin not only in erythroid cells but also in other cell types (reviewed in Jacobs, 1977). It also became clear that this pool of iron could be removed from cells by the iron chelator desferrioxamine, whether it was iron involved in erythro-poiesis (Lipschitz *et al.*, 1971) or iron flow induced by haemolysis (Cumming *et al.*, 1967).

The importance of this intracellular iron pool can be seen from its numerous known reactions, which include equilibrating iron between transport and storage pools, iron supply to haem, non-haem and other iron-containing compounds, access to chelation and potential toxicity, and have not changed significantly since this 'intracellular iron pool' was proposed by Allan Jacobs in 1977 (Jacobs, 1977). As Jacobs presciently pointed out then, "It is the focal point of intracellular iron metabolism and its interaction with extracellular transferrin and thus similar transit pools in other tissues, provides a pool of exchangeable iron which allows an equilibrium to be estab-lished not only between various metabolic processes in the cell but also between different organs of the body".

In nonpathological conditions, plasma iron is tightly bound in a nonlabile form to transferrin, and the physiological process of receptor-mediated endocytosis of transferrin-bound iron serves in all mammalian cells as the key route for regulated iron uptake. Within the cytoplasm and the intra-cellular compartments of the cell (e.g. mitochondria, endoplasmic reticulum and Golgi apparatus, lysosomes) the vast majority (>95%) of iron is protein-bound, either directly to amino acid resi-dues or via prosthetic groups such as haem or Fe–S clusters in iron-containing proteins. The remainder constitutes the LIP as defined above (Jacobs, 1977; Crichton, 2009) and, as pointed out in a recent excellent review by Ioav Cabantchik, it also denotes the combined redox properties of iron and its amenability to exchange between ligands, including chelators (Cabantchik, 2014).

Most of the iron taken up by the cell initially enters this kinetically labile, exchangeable pool in the cytosol (Shvartsman and Ioav Cabantchik, 2012; Cabantchik, 2014), and the majority of iron in the LIP is delivered to the mitochondria (Shvartsman and Ioav Cabantchik, 2012), where it is incorporated into haem and iron–sulphur clusters, as well as into non-haem, non-iron–sulphur iron proteins. Haem and some of the Fe–S cluster assembly machinery are also exported from the mito-chondria for utilisation in the cytosol and nucleus. It has been proposed that in haemoglobin-synthesizing reticulocytes, iron derived from transferrin-bound iron by receptor-mediated endocytosis is transferred directly from endosomes to the mitochondria (Zheng *et al.*, 2005; Sheftel *et al.*, 2007), via the 'kiss and run' mechanism, familiar to many utilisers of public transport. In this proposed pathway, vesicle–mitochondria interactions were proposed to provide bridges or channels for the transvesicular transfer of Fe^{2+} directly from transferrin-containing endosomes to mitochondria for haem biosynthesis, thereby bypassing the oxygen-rich cytosol.

That the LIP functions under normal physiological conditions is manifested by the capacity of permeating iron chelators to inhibit both iron-dependent cell functions and the reactive oxygen species (ROS) formation attributed to it in basal and peroxide-stimulated conditions (Glickstein *et al.*, 2005). Conceptually, the LIP must be both kinetically labile and metabolically accessible to allow iron to be distributed to the sites of utilisation, transport or storage as required (Jacobs, 1977; Crichton, 2009; Hider and Kong, 2013; Cabantchik, 2014). The LIP is made up of chelatable com-plexes of both Fe^{2+} and Fe^{3+} associated with a diverse population of mostly low-molecular-weight ligands, which can potentially participate in the generation of ROS and can be scavenged by chela-tors that permeate the cells. Earlier attempts to measure the LIP required disruption of the cells, which could lead to both redistribution of the metal among putative ligands and changes in the relative amounts of Fe^{2+} and Fe^{3+} due to exposure to O_2. To circumvent this problem, *in-vivo* approaches have been developed, based on the assumption that the LIP is made up of relatively low-affinity iron complexes, in which the iron is in dynamic equilibrium and amenable to chelation (Epsztjn *et al.*, 1997; Petrat *et al.*, 2002). Using this approach with fluorescent chelators (Esposito *et al.*, 2002), cytosolic LIP has been measured with calcein and found to be in the range 0.3 to 1.6 μM with different cell types. The principles of labile iron detection with fluorescent metal sensors using fluorescence microscopy imaging are outlined in Figure 8.1. Methodological aspects

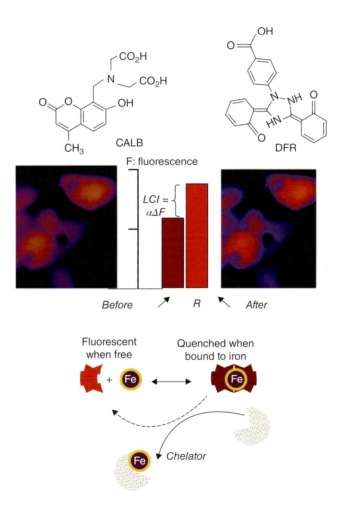

Figure 8.1 *Principle of labile iron detection with fluorescent metal sensors (FMS) using fluorescence microscopy imaging. Calcein blue (CALB) as FMS paradigm. The blue fluorescent umbelliferyl iminodiacetic acid binds Fe(III) with a 2:1 or 3:1 stoichiometry and undergoes fluorescence (F) quenching which can be reversed by the addition of excess amounts of the chelator deferasirox (DFR). Reproduced from Cabantchik, Z.I. (2014) Labile iron in cells and body fluids: physiology, pathology, and pharmacology.* Front. Pharmacol., **5**, *45. This is an open-access article distributed under the terms of the Creative Commons Attribution License (CC BY)*

related to the analysis of labile cytosolic iron (LCI) and its counterpart in plasma, labile plasma iron (LPI), are the subject of a number of reviews (Esposito *et al.*, 2002; Kakhlon and Cabantchik, 2002; Petrat *et al.*, 2002; Kruszewski, 2003; Breuer *et al.*, 2007; Brissot *et al.*, 2012).

On the presumption that the cytosolic LIP is predominantly Fe^{2+}, which seems less than certain, the ligands of LIP should be good Fe(II) chelators, and on this basis it has been proposed that *in vitro* reduced glutathione (GSH) could be the major cytosolic ligand for Fe(II) (Hider and Kong, 2011). Support for this comes from genetic studies in yeast (Sipos *et al.*, 2002; Kumar *et al.*, 2011). As we will see later, additional studies suggest that Fe–GSH, in conjunction with monothiol glutaredoxins, has a direct role in the formation and transfer of cytosolic Fe–S clusters (Rodriguez-Manzaneque *et al.*, 2002; Wingert *et al.*, 2005; Ye *et al.*, 2010). Glutaredoxins may have a broader role in cytosolic iron homeostasis (reviewed in Rouhier *et al.*, 2010; Philpott and Ryu, 2014).

However, despite numerous efforts to characterise the molecular composition of LIP, the nature of this 'Holy Grail' of intracellular iron metabolism still remains undefined, "…somewhat like the Loch Ness monster, only to disappear from view before its presence, or indeed its nature, can be confirmed" (Crichton, 1984). As Ioav Cabantchik has recently pointed out, while various Fe^{3+} complexes have been proposed as potential LCI candidates (Weaver and Pollack, 1989; Hider and Kong, 2011) "…those implications should be interpreted with caution as changes in environments (including pH and redox potential) that result from cell de-compartmentalisation are likely to result in metal redistribution among potential metal binders" (Cabantchik, 2014).

8.1.3 Distribution of Iron in the Cytosol

Once iron has entered the cytosolic LIP it will be redistributed, not only to the mitochondria, to where most of it will be delivered (*vide infra*) but also to other partners within the cytosol (Figure 8.2) (Philpott and Ryu, 2012). In Figure 8.2 iron is shown entering the cell as Fe(II) from DMT1, which was encountered in Chapter 6 as the mediator of iron egress from transferrin-bound iron taken up by receptor-mediated endocytosis, but which can also take up iron from other sources (Shawki *et al.*, 2012). Once within the LIP, which is schematically represented as Fe(II)–GSH complexes, the iron can be utilised by a number of other pathways which are enumerated below.

Metallochaperones–proteins that specifically deliver metal ions to target enzymes or transporters via metal-mediated protein–protein interactions–are extensively involved in copper metabolism (see Chapter 14). The family of poly C-binding proteins (PCBPs) has been shown to have iron chaperone activity for ferritin (Shi *et al.*, 2008), and this is discussed in greater detail in Chapter 9. Recently, two enzymes of the family of iron and α-ketoglutarate-dependent dioxygenases (see Chapter 2), prolyl hydroxylase (PHD) and asparaginyl hydroxylase (FIH1), which modify hypoxia-inducible factor α (HIFα), have been identified as targets of PCBP1 (Nandal *et al.*, 2011). HIFs are heterodimeric transcription factors which mediate the cellular adaptation to hypoxia, and are discussed further in Chapter 10. The dinuclear non-haem family of enzymes (Chapter 2) contain an iron-binding site that is structurally related to the ferroxidase site of ferritin which, as noted above, is a known target for PCBPs. Very recently it was shown that deoxyhypusine hydroxylase (DOHH) is a target for PCBPs (Frey *et al.*, 2014). The unusual basic amino acid, hypusine [*N*(epsilon)-(4-amino-2-hydroxybutyl)-lysine], is a lysine residue which has been modified by the addition of a 4-aminobutyl moiety derived from the polyamine spermidine. Hypusine is the product of a unique posttranslational modification that occurs in only one cellular protein, eukaryotic translation initiation factor 5A (eIF5A; Park *et al.*, 2010). Hypusine is synthesised exclusively in eIF5A by two sequential enzymatic steps involving deoxyhypusine synthase (DHS) and deoxyhypusine hydroxylase (DOHH). The conversion of the conserved Lys to hypusine in eIF5A is essential in all

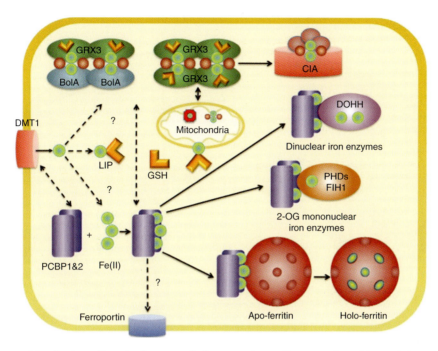

Figure 8.2 *Distribution of iron in the cytosol of mammalian cells. Reproduced from Philpott, C.C. and Ryu, M.-S. (2014) Special delivery: distributing iron in the cytosol of mammalian cells.* Front. Pharmacol., **5**, *173. This is an open-access article distributed under the terms of the Creative Commons Attribution License (CC BY)*

eukaryotes, since it enables the translation of peptides and proteins containing polyproline sequences (Gutierrez *et al.*, 2013).

It has been proposed that PCBPs can regulate the cellular distribution of labile iron by either depositing it in the cellular iron reservoir ferritin and/or by directing it to sites of utilisation as an inorganic cofactor for cytosolic non-haem iron enzymes (Philpott and Ryu, 2014). Very recently, Yanatori *et al.* (2014) have demonstrated that PCBP2 physically interacts directly with both DMT1, the major iron importer, and also with FPN1 (ferroportin 1), the only iron exporter. These new data suggest that PCBP2 may be a component of an as-yet-to-be-described Fe-transport metabolon that engages in Fe channelling to and from Fe transporters and intracellular sites (Lane and Richardson, 2014).

As discussed below, homodimers of Grx3 or heterooligomers of Grx3 and BolA2 coordinate [2Fe–2S] clusters with the help of GSH (Figure 8.3), which may be used for the metallation of cytosolic Fe–S enzymes (via the cytosolic iron–sulphur cluster assembly machinery; CIA) and may have a role in mitochondrial iron delivery in erythroid tissues.

8.1.4 Other Intracellular Iron Pools

Historically, the first pool of iron to be observed within mammalian cells was haemosiderin, originally identified histologically as iron-rich granules in tissues, which gave an intense Prussian blue reaction with potassium ferrocyanide (Perls, 1867). Haemosiderin was first isolated by Cook (1929) and described as consisting of 'organic granules impregnated with some form of ferric

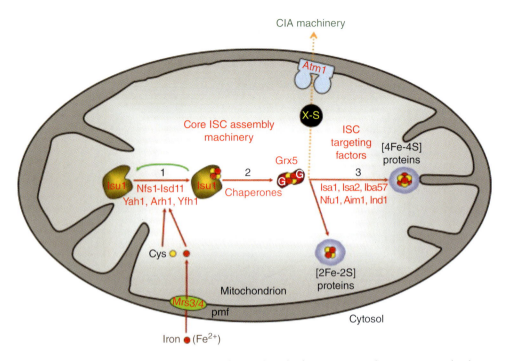

Figure 8.3 *An overview of the three steps of mitochondrial Fe–S protein biogenesis. In the first step, a [2Fe–2S] cluster is assembled on the Isu1 scaffold protein. This process requires ferrous iron, which is imported into mitochondria via the mitochondrial carriers Mrs3/4 and possibly other carriers, a mechanism driven by the proton motive force (pmf), cysteine desulfurase complex Nfs1–Isd11, the [2Fe–2S] ferredoxin Yah1, the ferredoxin reductase Arh1, and frataxin. In the second step, the Fe–S cluster is released from Isu1, involving a dedicated chaperone system and the glutaredoxin Grx5 which, together with glutathione (G), binds a [2Fe–2S] cluster. The ISC components of steps 1 and 2 constitute the core ISC assembly machinery and are sufficient for the assembly of mitochondrial [2Fe–2S] proteins. Moreover, these components are involved in the biogenesis of extra mitochondrial Fe–S proteins via the ISC export machinery. Its central component is the ABC transporter Atm1 which exports an unknown sulphur-containing moiety (X–S) towards the cytosolic Fe–S protein assembly (CIA) machinery for the maturation of cytosolic and nuclear Fe/S proteins (dotted arrow). In the third step, dedicated ISC targeting factors, including Isa1–Isa2 and Iba57, allow for the formation of [4Fe–4S] clusters and their target-specific insertion into mitochondrial apoproteins. Reproduced from Stehling, O., Wilbrecht, C. and Lill, R. (2014) Mitochondrial iron-sulfur protein biogenesis and human disease. Biochimie,* **100***, 61–77; © 2014, Elsevier*

oxide'. It is insoluble, visible by light microscopy as golden yellow intracellular granules, and in iron-loaded animals is localised in membranous structures termed siderosomes (Richter, 1978), which appear to be derived from lysosomes. It has a variable but higher iron content than ferritin, and represents the vast majority of the excess iron stored in clinical iron-overloading disorders. This constitutes the lysosomal iron pool in iron-loaded subjects or animals.

There is also a pool of iron within the mitochondria, which is the site of haem and Fe–S cluster biosynthesis, some of it associated with mitochondrial ferritin, as we will see shortly. A protein which possibly functions as a mitochondrial iron chaperone, frataxin, is thought to deliver iron for the scaffold protein involved in Fe–S cluster biosynthesis, and may also be the iron donor for haem synthesis. A deficiency of frataxin leads to mitochondrial iron accumulation in the neurodegenerative disease Friedreich's ataxia (which is described in detail in Chapter 15).

8.2 Mitochondrial Iron Metabolism

8.2.1 Mitochondrial Iron Uptake and Storage

In eukaryotic cells, the mitochondria are organelles which are often described as the 'powerhouse of the cell' on account of their important role in cellular energy supply. However, they also play a role in a multitude of other important metabolic processes, including cell signalling, cell differentiation, and apoptotic cell death. They are the cell's major consumers of iron, and play an important role in iron metabolism, since they are the unique site of iron insertion into protoporphyrin IX, the final step of haem biosynthesis, and the major site of [Fe–S] cluster biogenesis. In yeast, iron is imported into the mitochondria in a membrane potential-dependent manner via the Mrs3/4 mitochondrial solute carriers (Lange *et al.*, 1999; Foury and Roganti, 2002; Mühlenhoff *et al.*, 2003a). In vertebrates, homologues of Mrs3 and Mrs4 and of the zebrafish protein frascati, mitoferrins 1 and 2, are implicated in delivering iron to the mitochondria (Figure 8.3). Their expression is tissue-specific; mitoferrin 2 is expressed ubiquitously whereas mitoferrin 1 is essential for mitochondrial iron import in developing erythroid cells (Shaw *et al.*, 2006; Paradkar *et al.*, 2009).

Some mammalian tissues express a homopolymeric mitochondrial-specific ferritin with a high level of sequence identity, and similar capacity to oxidise and store iron to H-ferritin (Arosio and Levi, 2010). Whereas the highest expression of is observed in the testis (spermatozoa), it appears to be completely absent from typical iron-storage tissues such as liver and spleen (Santambrogio *et al.*, 2007). High levels of mitochondrial ferritin are also expressed in sideroblasts (erythroblasts with iron granules) of patients with sideroblastic anaemia (Santambrogio *et al.*, 2007; Cazzola *et al.*, 2003).

8.2.2 Mitochondrial Fe–S Protein Biogenesis

Fe–S proteins were first identified as redox cofactors involved in electron transfer in bacterial and mitochondrial respiratory complexes I–III, photosystem I of photosynthetic organisms, ferredoxins and hydrogenases. However, some Fe–S proteins like aconitase are required for enzymatic catalysis, whereas others play a role in the regulation of gene expression. For example, in the absence of its Fe–S cofactor, human iron regulatory protein 1 (IRP1) is active as an mRNA-binding protein, modulating the biosynthesis of proteins involved in iron metabolism (Volz, 2008). Other proteins such as the bacterial FNR (fumarate and nitrate reduction) regulatory proteins or the IscR protein have oxygen-sensitive Fe–S clusters which function as O_2 sensors (Kiley and Beinert, 1999; Giel *et al.*, 2012; Zhang *et al.*, 2012). Recently, proteins involved in DNA replication and repair, including the eukaryotic replicative DNA polymerases (Pol α, Pol ε, Pol δ and Pol ζ) and the DNA helicases involved in DNA damage repair such as XPD and FancJ, have been shown to have Fe–S clusters which stabilise their structure (Rudolf *et al.*, 2006; Netz *et al.*, 2012). In eukaryotes, Fe–S proteins are found in the mitochondria, cytosol, nucleus and plastids. However, the mitochondria are the primary site for the biosynthesis of Fe–S clusters. Recent reviews on mitochondrial Fe–S protein biogenesis can be found in Stehling *et al.* (2014), Rouault (2015), Miao and Rouault (2014), Stehling and Lill (2013), and Lill *et al.* (2012).

Most Fe–S clusters in eukaryotes are either the rhomboid [2Fe–2S] or the cubane [4Fe–4S] clusters, although, as we saw in Chapter 2, more complex forms – which can also involve metal ions other than iron–have been characterised, predominantly in bacterial species. Fe–S clusters are typically bound to cysteine residues of the polypeptide chain, but other amino acid residues including histidine, arginine, and serine are also used; for example, the [2Fe–2S] Rieske cluster of respiratory complex III in which one of the two Fe ions is coordinated by two histidine residues.

The Fe–S cluster (ISC) assembly machinery was inherited from bacteria in an endosymbiotic event (Muller and Martin, 1999), and in recent years its function has been elucidated in particular detail using the model eukaryote *Saccharomyces cerevisiae* (Lill, 2009; Lill and Mühlenhoff, 2008; Lill *et al.*, 2012; Stehling and Lill, 2013; Stehling *et al.*, 2014). The core ISC assembly factors involved in *de novo* Fe–S cluster synthesis (yeast name/human name) are the scaffold proteins Isu1, Isu2/ISCU, the sulphur donor Nfs1/NFS1, Isd11/ISD11, Yfh1/frataxin (FXN), and the electron transport proteins Yah1/ferredoxin2 (FDX2) and Arh1/ferredoxin reductase (FDXR). In this section, the yeast nomenclature is used. The mitochondrial assembly of Fe–S proteins falls into three major steps (Figure 8.4). In the first step, a [2Fe–2S] cluster is assembled *de novo* in a transient fashion on the heterodimeric scaffold protein Isu1 (and in yeast its paralogue Isu2). In the second step, the Fe–S cluster is released from the scaffold by a dedicated chaperone system, and the [2Fe–2S] cluster then transiently binds to the monothiol glutaredoxin Grx5 from which it can be directly inserted into [2Fe–2S] target proteins. In the third step, the Isa and Iba57 proteins help to convert the [2Fe–2S] cluster into [4Fe–4S] clusters, which are then inserted into apoproteins by various ISC targeting factors, such as Nfu1 and Ind1.

Six components are known to contribute to the *de-novo* formation of a transiently bound [2Fe–2S] cluster on the scaffold protein Isu1 (Figure 8.4) (Kispal *et al.*, 1999; Garland *et al.*, 1999; Mühlenhoff *et al.*, 2003b). The Fe^{2+} required is imported into the mitochondria by the

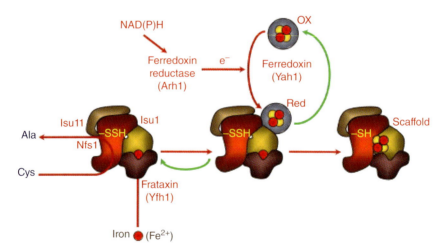

Figure 8.4 De-novo [2Fe–2S] cluster formation on the scaffold protein Isu1. The desulfurase complex Nfs1–Isd11 converts cysteine to alanine and releases sulphur, which is transiently bound in form of a persulphide group on a conserved cysteine residue on Nfs1. After putative transfer to a cysteine residue on the scaffold protein Isu1, the sulphane sulphur is reduced to sulphide to allow for Fe–S cluster formation. Sulphur reduction is presumably mediated by the electron transport chain comprised of NAD(P)H, Arh1, and Yah1. Yah1 binds to Isu1 only in its reduced (red) but not in its oxidised (ox) state. The delivery of iron to Isu1 might involve frataxin (Yfh1) which is needed for maximal desulphurase activity of Nfs1. Reproduced from Stehling, O., Wilbrecht, C. and Lill, R. (2014) Mitochondrial iron-sulfur protein biogenesis and human disease. Biochimie, **100**, 61–77; © 2014, Elsevier

mitochondrial carriers Mrs3/4 and possibly by other carriers, driven by the proton motive force (pmf). The cysteine desulfurase Nfs1 together with Isd11 in the complex Nfs1–Isd11 converts cysteine to alanine. During this reaction sulphur is released from cysteine and transiently bound as a persulphide group to a conserved cysteine residue on the desulfurase (Zheng *et al.*, 1994; Kaiser *et al.*, 2000). The function of Nfs1 *in vivo* depends on the eukaryote-specific, LYRM family protein Isd11 (Angerer, 2013), forming a hetero-oligomer with Nfs1 (Adam *et al.*, 2006; Wiedemann *et al.*, 2006; Terali *et al.*, 2013). Isd11 seems to be a stabilizing partner of Nfs1 and may not directly participate in the desulphurase reaction, as it is not essential for desulphurase activity but for Fe–S cluster synthesis (Stehling *et al.*, 2014). The persulphide sulphur may then be transferred from Nfs1 to Isu1, likely involving the formation of a persulphide group on one of the three cysteine residues of the scaffold. For subsequent cluster assembly the sulphur needs to be reduced from sulphane sulphur (S°) to sulphide (S^{2-}). The electrons required for the reduction process are probably provided by an electron transport chain including NAD(P)H, the ferredoxin reductase Arh1, and the ferredoxin Yah1 (Lange *et al.*, 2000; Mühlenhoff *et al.*, 2003b; Li *et al.*, 2001). The [2Fe–2S] cluster synthesis on Isu has been recently reconstituted in a reaction depending on Nfs1, Isd11, frataxin, Yah1, Arh1 and NADPH (Webert *et al.*, 2014). In marked contrast to the bacterial system, frataxin is an essential part of Fe/S cluster biosynthesis and is required simultaneously and stoichiometrically to Yah1. Reduced but not oxidised Yah1 tightly interacts with apoIsu1, and nuclear magnetic resonance (NMR) structural studies have identified the YAh1–Isu1 interaction surface and suggested a pathway for electron flow from reduced ferredoxin to Isu1. Taken together, this study defines the molecular function of the ferredoxin Yah1 and its human orthologue FDX2 in mitochondrial Fe–S cluster synthesis.

The way in which the imported iron obtains access to the scaffold complex is still under debate, although Yfh1 (frataxin in humans) is presumed to play a role in iron delivery. It might act directly as an iron-donor for the scaffold protein Isu1, which is consistent with the finding that Yfh1 tightly interacts with the Nfs1–Isd11–Isu1 complex (Gerber *et al.*, 2003; Schmucker *et al.*, 2011). Recently, Yfh1 was shown to significantly stimulate the desulfurase activity of Nfs1, which raises the alternative possibility that Yfh1 acts as an allosteric activator of the cysteine desulfurase (Tsai and Barondeau, 2010; Colin *et al.*, 2013). Both models are not mutually exclusive.

The [2Fe–2S] cluster on Isu1 has to be released from the scaffold and transferred for insertion into target proteins in the second step, involving the mtHsp70 chaperone system and also the monothiol glutaredoxin Grx5 (Mühlenhoff *et al.*, 2003b). Most eukaryotes, including humans, rely on the action of a single, multifunctional mitochondrial Hsp70 protein which performs protein import, folding, and Fe–S cluster insertion (Pukszta *et al.*, 2010. However, a subset of fungi, which includes *S. cerevisiae*, contain a dedicated chaperone mtHsp70 involved in iron–sulphur (Fe–S) cluster biogenesis, Ssq1. In yeast, dissociation of the Fe–S cluster from Isu1 requires a chaperone system comprising Ssq1, the co-chaperone Jac1, and the nucleotide exchange factor Mge1 (Dutkiewicz *et al.*, 2006) (Figure 8.5). The process of release of the transient [2Fe–2S] cluster is initiated by the binding of Jac1 to the scaffold, which allows the scaffold to interact via its conserved LPPVK loop with Ssq1 in its ATP-bound form (Hoff *et al.*, 2003; Dutkiewicz *et al.*, 2004). This triggers the ATPase activity of Ssq1 which causes a conformational change resulting in stronger binding to Isu1 (Dutkiewicz *et al.*, 2003; Vickery and Cupp-Vickery, 2007). ATP hydrolysis is believed to induce a conformational change on Isu1, which weakens [2Fe–2S] cluster binding to Isu1, accompanied by the dissociation of Jac1 from the complex (Chandramouli and Johnson, 2006; Shakamuri *et al.*, 2012). The monothiol glutaredoxin Grx5 now intervenes in the process, binding to Ssq1 at a site which is in close proximity to, but not overlapping with, the peptide-binding region of Ssq1 where Isu1 is attached to the chaperone (Uzarska *et al.*, 2013). Dimerisation

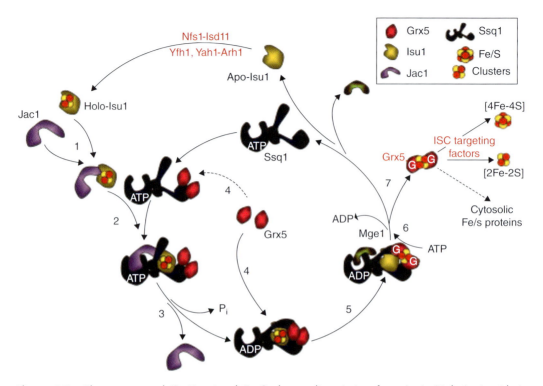

Figure 8.5 *Chaperone- and Grx5-assisted Fe–S cluster dissociation from Isu1. Holo-Isu1 with its transient [2Fe–2S] cluster is recruited by the co-chaperone Jac1 and guided to the ATP-bound form of the Hsp70 chaperone Ssq1 (step 1). Ssq1 binds to the conserved LPPVK loop of Isu1 (step 2), thus triggering the ATPase activity of Ssq1 which in turn leads to a tight binding of Isu1 and the release of Jac1 (step 3). ATP hydrolysis is believed to induce a conformational change on Isu1 to weaken Fe–S cluster binding to Isu1. The monothiol glutaredoxin Grx5 binds to Ssq1 in close vicinity to Isu1 (step 4), thereby enabling Fe–S cluster transfer from the scaffold to Grx5 (step 5). Next, ADP is exchanged for ATP by the exchange factor Mge1, triggering a conformational change of the peptide-binding domain of Ssq1 from the closed to an open state. Subsequently, the Ssq1–Isu1 complex disassembles, allowing the components to resume with a new cycle (steps 6 and 7). The Fe–S cluster on holo-Grx5 is required for the maturation of all cellular Fe/S proteins, comprising the mitochondrial [4Fe–4S] and [2Fe–2S] proteins and the cytosolic-nuclear Fe–S proteins. Reproduced from Stehling, O., Wilbrecht, C. and Lill, R. (2014) Mitochondrial iron-sulfur protein biogenesis and human disease. Biochimie, **100**, 61–77; © 2014, Elsevier*

of Grx5 allows coordination of the bridging [2Fe–2S] cluster via the active-site cysteine residue and non-covalently bound GSH (Bandyopadhyay *et al.*, 2008; Johansson *et al.*, 2011; Picciocchi *et al.*, 2007). At the end of the chaperone cycle the nucleotide exchange factor Mge1 binds to Ssq1 and drives the exchange of ADP for ATP (Dutkiewicz *et al.*, 2003). This results in the release of all components from Ssq1 including the [2Fe–2S]-bound Grx5 which supports maturation of all cellular Fe–S proteins, either directly or via the participation of additional ISC and CIA factors (Uzarska *et al.*, 2013). Apo-Isu1 and the chaperones are then ready for another cycle.

In the third phase of mitochondrial Fe–S protein biogenesis the [2Fe–2S] clusters can be converted to a [4Fe–4S] cluster by the A-type ISC proteins Isa1 and Isa2, and the folate-binding protein

Iba57 (Gelling *et al.*, 2008; Mühlenhoff *et al.*, 2011; Sheftel *et al.*, 2012), which physically interact by forming a complex (Gelling *et al.*, 2008). Both, Isa1 and Isa2 interact with Grx5 supporting a role of this glutaredoxin in linking the early and late phases of mitochondrial Fe–S protein assembly (Rodriguez-Manzaneque *et al.*, 2002; Kim *et al.*, 2010). How the Isa proteins and Iba57 use iron or the rhombic [2Fe–2S] cluster to assist the assembly of a cubic [4Fe–4S] cluster remains to be determined.

There are a number of more specialised targeting factors which assist in the maturation of dedicated subsets of [4Fe–4S] proteins. Nfu1, which like Isu1 can transiently coordinate a [4Fe–4S] cluster (Tong *et al.*, 2003), is specifically required for the assembly of a subset of [4Fe–4S] clusters, including subunits of the respiratory chain complexes I and II, as well as lipoic acid synthase (Cameron *et al.*, 2011; Navarro-Sastre *et al.*, 2011), as is Aim1 (Cameron *et al.*, 2011). Lipoic acid is essential for the key metabolic enzymes pyruvate dehydrogenase (PDH), α-ketoglutarate dehydrogenase (α-KGDH), branched-chain ketoacid dehydrogenase (BCKDH), as well as the H protein of the glycine cleavage system. Even more specific is Ind1, which is involved in the maturation of [4Fe–4S] clusters of respiratory chain complex I (Bych *et al.*, 2008; Sheftel *et al.*, 2009). Ind1 is not present in *S. cerevisiae*, which does not have respiratory complex I. Neither [2Fe–2S] proteins nor the mitochondrial [4Fe–4S] aconitase are dependent on Nfu1.

8.2.3 Maturation of Cytosolic and Nuclear Fe–S Proteins

There are numerous cytosolic and nuclear Fe–S proteins which perform key functions in metabolic catalysis, iron regulation, protein translation, tRNA base modification, DNA synthesis and repair, and telomere length regulation. An inventory of cytosolic and nuclear Fe–S proteins in eukaryotes is shown in Table 8.1. Eukaryotes contain the iron–sulfur cluster (ISC) assembly machinery in mitochondria, the CIA (cytosolic iron–sulphur protein assembly) machinery in the cytosol, and the SUF (mobilisation of sulphur) machinery in the chloroplasts (Lill and Mühlenhoff, 2006) The ISC and SUF proteins were inherited during the course of evolution from similar components of the bacterial ancestors of mitochondria and plastids, respectively (Ayala-Castro *et al.*, 2008; Py and Barras, 2010; Roche *et al.*, 2013).

The biogenesis of cytosolic and nuclear Fe–S proteins depends strictly on the core ISC assembly machinery (Kispal *et al.*, 1999; Gerber *et al.*, 2004; Biederbick *et al.*, 2006; Fosset *et al.*, 2006; Lill *et al.*, 2014), which is why this point is discussed here. The process depends on the interplay between the mitochondrial core ISC assembly machinery, the ISC export machinery and the CIA machinery. Table 8.2 lists the protein components required for the maturation of human and yeast cytosolic and nuclear Fe–S proteins, while Figure 8.6 presents the domain structure and functional modules of each of the components of the yeast CIA. For reviews of the CIA machinery, see Lill and Mühlenhoff (2008), Netz *et al.* (2014), and Paul and Lill (2015). The process can be dissected into two major steps, which depend on mitochondrial function, the CIA machinery and a glutaredoxin.

A working model for the maturation of cytosolic and nuclear Fe–S is presented in Figure 8.7. The core ISC machinery of the mitochondria generates a sulphur-containing compound (designated X-S in Figure 8.7), which is delivered to the cytosol by the ISC export machinery to allow the formation of extramitochondrial Fe–S cofactors. The export of X-S is mediated by the ABC transporter ABCB7 (Atm1 in yeast) of the mitochondrial inner membrane, and the export reaction further requires the function of the intermembrane space sulfhydryl oxidase ALR (Erv1 in

Table 8.1 *Inventory of cytosolic and nuclear Fe–S proteins in eukaryotes[a]*

Fe–S protein (human)	Yeast homolog	Fe–S cluster type	Proposed main function
DNA maintenance			
PRIM2	Pri2	[4Fe–4S]	Primase, synthesis of RNA primers for DNA replication
POLA	Pol1	[4Fe–4S]	Catalytic subunit of polymerase α, DNA replication
POLE1	Pol2	[4Fe–4S]	Catalytic subunit of polymerase ε, DNA replication
POLD1	Pol3	[4Fe–4S]	Catalytic subunit of polymerase δ, DNA replication
REV3L	Rev3	[4Fe–4S]	Catalytic subunit of polymerase ζ, DNA repair
FANCJ	absent	[4Fe–4S]	Helicase, DNA repair
NTHL1	Ntg2	[4Fe–4S]	DNA glycosylase, DNA repair
XPD	Rad3	[4Fe–4S]	Helicase, nucleotide excision repair
MUTYH	absent	[4Fe–4S]	DNA glycosylase, DNA repair
RTEL1	absent	[4Fe–4S]	Helicase, telomere stability, anti-recombinase
CHLR1	Chl1	[4Fe–4S]	Helicase, chromosome segregation
DNA2	Dna2	[4Fe–4S]	Helicase/nuclease, DNA repair Okazaki fragment processing,
Amino acid and nucleotide metabolism			
Absent	Leu1	[4Fe–4S]	Isopropylmalate isomerase (leucine biosynthesis)
Absent	Ecm17	[4Fe–4S]	Sulphite reductase, required for biosynthesis of methionine
Absent	Glt1	[4Fe–4S]	Glutamate synthase
AOX1	Absent	2× [2Fe–2S]	Aldehyde oxidase (catabolism of xenobiotics)
DPYD	Absent	4× [4Fe–4S]	Dihydropyrimidine dehydrogenase (pyrimidine catabolism)
GPAT	Absent	[4Fe–4S]	Phosphoribosyl pyrophosphate amidotransferase (purine biosynthesis)
XDH	Absent	2× [2Fe–2S]	Xanthine dehydrogenase/oxidase
Ribosome function and tRNA modification			
ABCE1	Rli1	2× [4Fe–4S]	Ribosome biogenesis, translation initiation and termination
ELP3	Elp3	2× [4Fe–4S]	Elongator protein 3 (tRNA wobble base modification), SAM
TYW1	Tyw1	2× [4Fe–4S]	tRNA wybutosine biosynthesis, SAM
CDKAL1	Absent	[4Fe–4S]	tRNA modification
CDKRAP1	Absent	[4Fe–4S]	tRNA modification
Other processes			
GRX3 (PICOT)	Grx3–Grx4	[2Fe–2S]	Intracellular iron homeostasis
IRP1	Absent	[4Fe–4S]	Intracellular iron regulation
RSAD1 (Viperin)	Absent	[4Fe–4S]	Antiviral activity, SAM
mitoNEET (CISD1)	Absent	[2Fe–2S]	Insulin sensitivity, unknown (located in mitochondrial outer membrane facing cytosol)
MINER1 (NAF1, CISD2)	Absent	[2Fe–2S]	Ca²⁺ metabolism, unknown
MINER2	Absent	[2Fe–2S]	Ca²⁺ metabolism, unknown

[a] Known Fe/S proteins of the cytosol and nucleus are provided for human and yeast cells. Alternative names are provided in parentheses. Note that four additional Fe–S proteins are members of the CIA machinery (see Table 8.2). SAM, *S*-adenosyl-methionine as an additional cofactor.

Reprinted with permission from Elsevier from Netz, D.J., Mascarenhas, J., Stehling, O., Pierik, A.J. and Lill, R. (2014) Maturation of cytosolic and nuclear iron-sulfur proteins. *Trends Cell Biol.*, **24**, 303–312.

Table 8.2 *Components of the CIA machinery* [a]

Human CIA proteins	Yeast CIA proteins	Important functional groups	Proposed main function
CFD1 (NUBP2)	**Cfd1**	Bridging [4Fe–4S] cluster with Nbp35	Scaffold complex, assembly, and transient binding of [4Fe–4S] cluster
NBP35 (NUBP1)	**Nbp35**	Bridging [4Fe–4S] cluster with Cfd1; N-terminal [4Fe–4S] cluster	Scaffold complex, assembly, and transient binding of [4Fe–4S] cluster
CIAPIN1 (Anamorsin)	**Dre2**	[2Fe–2S] and [4Fe–4S] clusters	Electron acceptor from NADPH–Tah18
NDOR1	**Tah18**	FAD, FMN	Electron transfer from NADPH to Dre2
IOP1 (NARFL)	**Nar1**	2× [4Fe–4S] clusters	CIA adaptor protein, mediates contact between early and late parts of CIA machinery
CIA1 (CIAO1)	**Cia1**	–	Docking site of the CIA targeting complex
CIA2B (FAM96B, MIP18)	**Cia2**	Hyper-reactive Cys	Insertion of Fe–S clusters into target apoproteins
CIA2A (FAM96A)	–	Hyper-reactive Cys?	Insertion of Fe–S clusters into IRP1
MMS19	**Mms19** (Met18)	–	Insertion of Fe–S clusters into target apoproteins

[a] Known yeast and human CIA proteins are listed. Note that in this review the yeast nomenclature (bold face) is mainly used. Alternative names are provided in parentheses.

Reprinted with permission from Elsevier from Netz, D.J., Mascarenhas, J., Stehling, O., Pierik, A.J. and Lill, R. (2014) Maturation of cytosolic and nuclear iron-sulfur proteins. *Trends Cell Biol.*, **24**, 303–312.

yeast) and GSH (Kispal *et al.*, 1999; Lange *et al.*, 2001; Sipos *et al.*, 2002; Lill and Muhlenhoff, 2006; Cavadini *et al.*, 2007; Miao *et al.*, 2009). GSH may be part of the exported X-S molecule, since the very recent determination of the crystal structures of the yeast Atm1 and its bacterial homologue (Lee *et al.*, 2014; Srinivasan *et al.*, 2014) both contain GSH bound in a positively charged pocket. For recent reviews on the export machinery and the nature of X-S, see Qi *et al.* (2013), Lill *et al.* (2014), and Schaedler *et al.* (2014). The precise role of the FAD-dependent sulphydryl oxidase ERV1 is not clear, but its function in the introduction of disulphide bridges in mitochondrial pre-proteins during their MIA40-dependent import into the intermembrane space seems clear (Mesecke *et al.*, 2005). Once the X-S molecule has been exported into the cytosol, the nine known components of the CIA machinery carry out the assembly of Fe–S clusters and their insertion into extra-mitochondrial target proteins (Sharma *et al.*, 2010; Basu *et al.*, 2014; Netz *et al.*, 2014).

The first step of cytosolic Fe–S protein biogenesis involves the assembly and transient binding of a [4Fe–4S] cluster (Figure 8.7) on the cytosolic scaffold complex formed by the two P-loop NTPases CFD1 and NBP35 (Roy *et al.*, 2003; Hausmann *et al.*, 2005; Netz *et al.*, 2007; Stehling *et al.*, 2008). CFD1 and NBP35 form a heterotetrameric scaffold which coordinates two different kinds of [4Fe–4S] cluster (Netz *et al.*, 2012): a loosely bound [4Fe–4S] cluster bound to a conserved CX_2C motif found in the C terminus of both proteins, which bridges the two subunits, and a second [4Fe–4S] cluster which binds at the N terminus of NBP35 where it is tightly associated to a ferredoxin-like $CX_{13}CX_2CX_5C$ motif and essential for NBP35 function (Netz *et al.*, 2007, 2012; Pallesen *et al.*, 2013). The differential lability of the two clusters was underlined by a

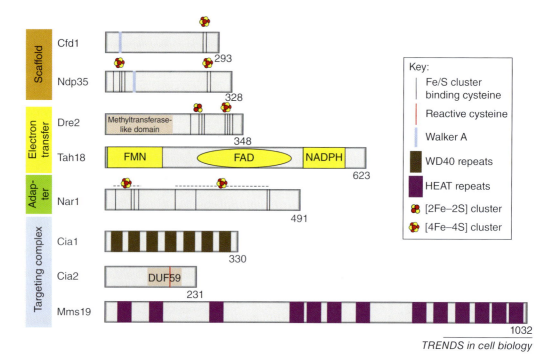

Figure 8.6 *The domain structure and functional modules of each of the components of the yeast CIA. The numbers indicate the length of each CIA protein. The functional units and features are described in the box. Reproduced with permission from Elsevier from Netz, D.J., Mascarenhas, J., Stehling, O., Pierik, A.J. and Lill, R. (2014) Maturation of cytosolic and nuclear iron-sulfur proteins.* Trends Cell Biol., **24**, *303–312*

pulse-chase experiment (Pallesen *et al.*, 2013), and the loose binding of the C-terminal [4Fe–4S] cluster may be an important determinant for its transfer and incorporation into dedicated target proteins in the second step of biogenesis. Electrons are required for the assembly reaction, just as in the case of ferredoxin and its reductase in the mitochondrial ISC machinery which generates the [2Fe–2S] cluster (Webert *et al.*, 2014). The electron transfer chain of the CIA system is composed of NADPH, the diflavin protein NDOR1, and the Fe–S protein CIAPIN1 (Banci *et al.*, 2013; Netz *et al.*, 2010). The domain structure of Dre2, the yeast homologue of CIAPIN1, incorporates an N-terminal *S*-adenosylmethionine (SAM) methyltransferase-like domain which is not known to bind SAM, connected by a flexible linker to a C-terminal Fe–S domain (Banci *et al.*, 2011; Soler *et al.*, 2012). This domain has two pairs of four conserved cysteine residues which were suggested to coordinate one [2Fe–2S] and one [4Fe–4S] cluster (Zhang *et al.*, 2008a,b; Netz *et al.*, 2010, 2014). Dre2 and CIAPIN1 physically interact with Tah18, the yeast homologue of NDOR1 (Vernis *et al.*, 2009). Electron paramagnetic resonance (EPR) studies using the yeast counterparts unravelled the fact that electrons are transferred from NADPH via the FAD and FMN centres of Tah18 to the [2Fe–2S] cluster of Dre2. Cytosolic and nuclear Fe–S protein biogenesis additionally depends on the multidomain glutaredoxin GLRX3, although its exact function and site of action is unknown to date (Muhlenhoff *et al.*, 2010; Haunhorst *et al.*, 2013).

In the second step of Fe–S protein biogenesis, the Fe–S clusters are released from Cfd1–Nbp35 and transferred to apoproteins (Apo) in a reaction mediated in yeast by the Fe–S protein Nar1

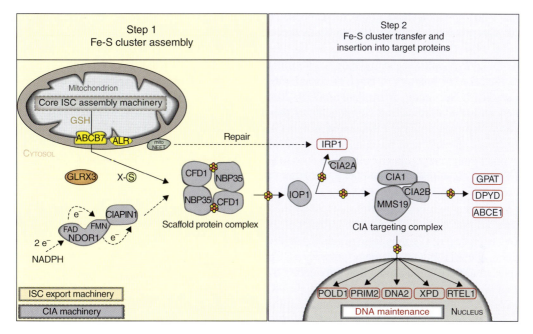

Figure 8.7 *A working model for the maturation of cytosolic and nuclear Fe–S proteins. The process can be dissected into two major steps. In Step 1, a bridging [4Fe–4S] cluster is assembled and loosely bound to the scaffold complex consisting of CFD1 and the Fe–S protein NBP35. In Step 2, the newly assembled Fe–S cluster is transferred from the scaffold protein complex onto apoproteins. This transfer is performed by the CIA targeting complex consisting of CIA1, CIA2B and MMS19, which mediate direct interactions with dedicated apoproteins. For details, see the text. Cytosolic target Fe–S proteins matured by these machineries execute diverse cellular functions, including nucleotide metabolism (GPAT, DPYD) or translation initiation and termination (ABCE1). Nuclear Fe–S proteins conduct functions in DNA replication (POLD1, PRIM2, DNA2) as well as in DNA repair processes (XPD) or the regulation of telomere length (RTEL1), thus contributing to the maintenance of genome integrity. Reproduced with permission from Elsevier from Paul, V.D. and Lill, R. (2015) Biogenesis of cytosolic and nuclear iron-sulfur proteins and their role in genome stability.* Biochim. Biophys. Acta, **1853**, *1528–1539*

(Balk *et al.*, 2004) and the CIA targeting complex Cia1–Cia2–Mms19 (Balk *et al.*, 2005; Weerapana *et al.*, 2010; Gari *et al.*, 2012; Stehling *et al.*, 2012; Stehling and Lill, 2013). The WD40-repeat protein Cia1 crystal structure shows a β-propeller structure, with seven pseudo-symmetrically oriented blades around a central axis (Srinivasan *et al.*, 2007). Cia2 is a small acidic protein with a C-terminal domain of unknown function, while MMS19 is a very large, 1032-residue protein with a number of HEAT repeats, which are enriched at its C terminus, forming a predicted armadillo structure. In humans, this reaction requires the coordinated function of IOP1 (iron-only hydrogenase-like protein) and the CIA targeting complex composed of CIA1, CIA2B (one of the two human homologues of yeast Cia2), and MMS19. CIA1, CIA2B and MMS19 form binary and ternary complexes in yeast and mammalian cells, and undergo direct interactions with numerous cytosolic and nuclear Fe–S target proteins (Srinivasan *et al.*, 2007; Weerapana *et al.*, 2010; Gari *et al.*, 2012; Stehling *et al.*, 2012; Stehling and Lill, 2013; van Wietmarschen *et al.*, 2012; Seki *et al.*, 2013). IOP1, while exhibiting sequence homology to bacterial [FeFe] hydrogenases (Mulder *et al.*, 2011; Nicolet and Fontecilla-Camps, 2012), lacks the active site of the hydrogenases, although it coordinates two [4Fe–4S] cofactors that are similar to those in the hydrogenases (Balk *et al.*, 2004; Urzica *et al.*, 2009). Studies on the yeast homologue Nar1 showed that these clusters are bound to N- and C-terminal motifs with four conserved cysteine residues each. Both motifs are required for the function of Nar1. A considerable body of evidence (extensively reviewed in Lill *et al.*, 2014; Netz *et al.*, 2014; Paul and Lill, 2015) has led to the assumption that IOP1–Nar1 connects early- and late-acting components of the CIA machinery by an as yet unknown mode of action (Figure 8.7). The WD40-repeat protein CIA1 represents the putative docking site of the CIA targeting complex, with the conserved, surface-exposed residue R127 as a potential docking site for other components of cytosolic Fe–S protein assembly. However, so far it is not fully understood how CIA1 recognises its complex partners and thus mediates the formation of the CIA targeting complex by interacting with CIA2B and MMS19.

Cytosolic target Fe–S proteins matured by these machineries (Figure 8.7) execute diverse cellular functions, such as: (i) in nucleotide metabolism – glutamine phosphoribosyl-pyrophosphate amidotransferase (GPAT), dihydropyrimidine dehydrogenase (DPYD) or translation initiation and termination, the ATP-binding cassette protein (ABCE1). Nuclear Fe–S proteins are involved in DNA replication, the catalytic subunit of polymerase δ, POLD1, the subunit of DNA primase, involved in DNA synthesis and double-strand break repair PRIM2, and the helicase/nuclease, DNA2, involved in DNA repair, Okazaki fragment maturation and telomere maintenance; and (ii) in DNA repair processes – the helicase, XPD involved in nucleotide excision repair or and the helicase, RTEL1, involved in the regulation of telomere length, thus contributing to the maintenance of genome integrity.

In marked contrast to yeast, human cells express two Cia2-like proteins, CIA2A and CIA2B (Stehling *et al.*, 2012), and the components of the human CIA targeting complex components show a high degree of specificity for reactions involving the maturation of dedicated Fe–S proteins (Stehling *et al.*, 2012; Stehling and Lill, 2013; Gari *et al.*, 2012). Thus, whereas CIA2B, like the yeast Cia2, acts in general Fe-S protein maturation, CIA2A has a much more restricted clientele, and exerts a huge influence on the cellular iron status of human cells. The target-specific maturation of Fe–S apoproteins involving late-acting human CIA proteins is illustrated in Figure 8.8.

As mentioned above, the differential and highly specialised requirement of the three CIA targeting complex components for the maturation of the individual target Fe–S apoproteins in human cells was rapidly established (Stehling *et al.*, 2012; Stehling and Lill, 2013; Gari *et al.*, 2012), and, together with the observation that CIA1, CIA2B, and MMS19 form various binary and ternary subcomplexes, it therefore seems reasonable to assume that the three components interact dynamically (Figure 8.7). Thus, it appeared that different types of subcomplex might receive the [4Fe–4S] clusters assembled on CFD1–NBP35 and deliver them in a target-specific fashion to dedicated cytosolic Fe–S proteins, such as glutamine phosphoribosyl-pyrophosphate amidotransferase (GPAT), dihydropyrimidine dehydrogenase (DPYD) and the ATP-binding cassette protein ABCE1 or nuclear Fe–S proteins such as XPD and POLD1 (Figure 8.8). The ternary CIA targeting complex appears to have the broadest substrate spectrum mediating the maturation of numerous Fe–S proteins such as DPYD, ABCE1 and XPD. MMS19 plays only a minor role in the maturation of GPAT, while CIA2B is not crucially required for DNA polymerase δ (POLD1) assembly (Stehling and Lill, 2013). This functional data was corroborated by proteomic studies which unravelled the selective binding of one, two or three components of the CIA targeting complex to different target Fe–S proteins established (Stehling *et al.*, 2012; Stehling and Lill, 2013; Gari *et al.*, 2012; van Wietmarschen *et al.*, 2012; Seki *et al.*, 2013). The list of CIA1, CIA2B, and MMS19 interaction partners established by proteomic studies may potentially contain additional cytosolic or nuclear Fe–S proteins and new CIA factors.

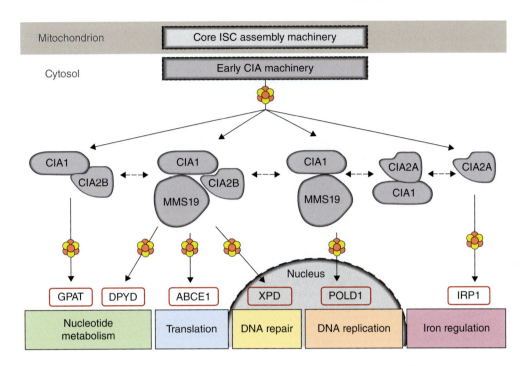

Figure 8.8 *Different late-acting human CIA proteins mediate the target-specific maturation of Fe–S apoproteins. The figure presents the current view of the target specificity of the late-acting CIA components. The [4Fe–4S] clusters are delivered from the early step of cytosolic Fe–S cluster assembly (cf. Figure 8.7) to dedicated cytosolic–nuclear target Fe–S proteins with the help of the late-acting CIA components CIA1, CIA2B, and MMS19. These CIA proteins form several subcomplexes. The majority of the Fe–S proteins (e.g., DPYD, ABCE1, XPD) are matured with the help of the trimeric targeting complex consisting of CIA1, CIA2B (functional orthologue of yeast Cia2) and MMS19. In contrast, maturation of GPAT and POLD1 was hardly affected by the absence of MMS19 or CIA2B, respectively. The human CIA system possesses a second Cia2 isoform termed CIA2A that is not found in yeast. This CIA component is specifically required for the maturation of IRP1, thus contributing to the regulation of iron homeostasis in human cells. No dedicated function has been assigned to a CIA2A–CIA1 subcomplex. The respective cellular functions of the individual Fe–S target proteins are depicted at the bottom to indicate the importance of Fe–S protein biogenesis for many aspects of cell homeostasis and viability. Reproduced with permission from Elsevier from Paul, V.D. and Lill, R. (2015) Biogenesis of cytosolic and nuclear iron-sulfur proteins and their role in genome stability.* Biochim. Biophys. Acta, **1853**, *1528–1539*

The impact of the human CIA system on cellular iron homeostasis is twofold and mainly connected to CIA2A (Figures 8.8 and 8.9). CIA2A functions as a dedicated Fe–S cluster maturation factor for IRP1 and is also a stabiliser for IRP2, thus integrating the functions of the two IRPs in intracellular iron homeostasis in human cells. First, CIA2A is specifically required for the maturation of cytosolic aconitase, the [4Fe–4S] holoform of IRP1 (Figure 8.9) which, with IRP2, is a key regulator of cellular iron homeostasis in mammals (Stehling and Lill, 2013). Both, IRP1 and IRP2 exert their regulatory functions via complex post-transcriptional mechanisms (as discussed in detail in Chapter 10), which modulate the expression of proteins involved in intracellular iron trafficking, storage and utilisation. Under iron-replete conditions the equilibrium between apo- and holo-IRP1 is shifted towards the Fe–S cluster form, whose assembly strictly depends on the

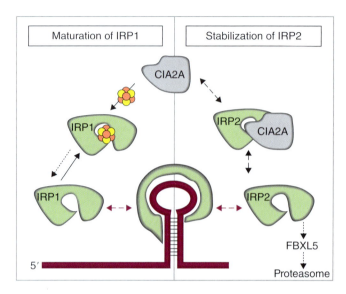

Figure 8.9 *CIA2A performs a dual role in human iron homeostasis. In mammalian cells the iron-regulatory proteins IRP1 and IRP2 are key components of regulating the intracellular iron supply and distribution. IRP1 is a cytosolic aconitase whose activity depends on the coordination of a [4Fe–4S] cluster. Maturation of this Fe–S protein depends on the mitochondrial ISC assembly and export systems, and further involves the early-acting CIA components and the late-acting CIA factor CIA2A, while the CIA targeting complex is dispensable. Upon iron starvation or during oxidative stress, IRP1 loses its cluster. The resulting apoform, after undergoing a major conformational change, can bind to iron-responsive elements (IREs; magenta line) of mRNAs which encode proteins involved in iron trafficking, storage and utilisation. IRP–IRE binding can alter the translation efficiency or stability of the mRNA. IRP2 does not contain a Fe–S cluster but is regulated by iron- and oxygen-dependent proteasomal degradation mediated by the E3 ubiquitin ligase FBXL5. Under iron-replete conditions, IRP2 is poly-ubiquitinated and degraded, whereas it is stable under low iron conditions. IRP2 can additionally be stabilised by binding to CIA2A, demonstrating the dual role of CIA2A in iron homeostasis. Reproduced with permission from Elsevier from Paul, V.D. and Lill, R. (2015) Biogenesis of cytosolic and nuclear iron-sulfur proteins and their role in genome stability.* Biochim. Biophys. Acta, **1853**, 1528–1539

early-acting CIA components and CIA2A, but not on CIA2B or MMS19 (Stehling and Lill, 2013). MitoNEET is a small mitochondrial protein located at the mitochondrial outer membrane which binds a unique three-Cys- and one-His-ligated [2Fe–2S] cluster. The holo-form of mitoNEET is resistant to NO and H_2O_2, and is capable of repairing oxidatively damaged [4Fe–4S] clusters of iron regulatory protein 1 (IRP1) (Ferecatu *et al.*, 2014).

Second, CIA2A binds to and stabilises IRP2, the other important regulatory factor for intracellular iron supply and distribution (Figure 8.10). IRP2 does not contain a Fe–S cluster but its protein level is regulated in an iron- and oxygen-dependent fashion. Under iron-replete conditions IRP2 is polyubiquitinated by the E3 ubiquitin ligase FBXL5, which responds to increased iron and oxygen levels resulting in proteasomal degradation of IRP2, whereas under low-iron or low-oxygen conditions FBXL5 is destabilised and degraded, leading to increased levels of IRP2. CIA2A can tightly bind to and stabilise IRP2 and prevent it from FBXL5-mediated proteasomal degradation. CIA1 also interacts with the CIA2A–IRP2 complex, yet depletion of CIA1 had no major effect on the cellular iron metabolism (Stehling and Lill, 2013).

8.2.4   Haem Biosynthesis

Haem biosynthesis occurs in all cells, although in haemopoietic erythroid cells it is tightly coupled to iron acquisition and globin gene expression. The two major sites of haem biosynthesis are developing red blood cells in the bone marrow, which synthesise around 85% of the body's haem groups, and the liver, which synthesises most of the remainder for haem-containing enzymes. A major function of haem in the liver is as the prosthetic group of cytochrome P450 (as discussed in Chapter 2). The P450 family of enzymes, which reside in the endoplasmic reticulum (ER) of the mammalian liver, function together with their redox partners cytochrome P450 reductase (CPR) and cytochrome b_5 (b_5) in the oxidative metabolism and elimination of numerous endo- and xenobiotics.

The liver cell must continue to synthesise cytochrome P450 throughout its lifetime in quantities that vary according to the environmental conditions. This is in marked contrast to the developing erythroid cell, which only engages in haem synthesis upon differentiation, embarking on a once-in-a-lifetime orgy of haem and globin synthesis, which ceases upon red cell maturation, thereby ensuring the haemoglobin content which will last for the lifetime of the erythrocyte. As a consequence, haem synthesis in liver and erythroid cells are regulated in quite different ways.

The haem biosynthetic pathway (Figure 8.10) begins in the mitochondrion, with the reaction catalysed by ALA synthase (ALAS); this involves the condensation of succinyl CoA derived from the citric acid cycle with glycine to form δ-aminolaevulinic acid (ALA), which is exported into the cytoplasm. There are two isoforms of ALAS, which are encoded by separate genes. ALAS1 is ubiquitously expressed and plays a housekeeping role, providing haem for non-erythroid tissues, whereas ALAS2 is expressed exclusively in erythroid cells, where it is essential for the terminal maturation of red blood cells (Harigae *et al.*, 1998). During the course of erythroid differentiation, pro-erythroblasts increase their iron uptake through the upregulation of TfR1. At the same time, the activity of ALAS2 also increases to provide the large amounts of haem required for haemoglobin production. Soon after its synthesis, haem activates the transcription and translation of globin chains, thus allowing haemoglobin synthesis. The increased expression of *Alas*2 is a prerequisite for the full induction of the other genes of the haem biosynthetic pathway (Sadlon *et al.*, 1999). Erythroid-specific transcription factors such as GATA1 regulate the expression of *Alas*2, while the post-transcriptional regulation of ALAS2 expression is regulated by iron, linking haem biosynthesis to iron availability. The presence of an IRE in the 5′-untranslated region (UTR) of the *Alas*2 mRNA (see Chapter 10) means that when iron is in short supply, IRPs bind to the mRNA to prevent its translation; in contrast, when intracellular iron levels are increased the inhibitory binding no longer occurs, allowing the translation of ALAS2 mRNA.

Once it has been synthesised, ALA must be exported to the cytoplasm where the next steps in the haem biosynthetic pathway take place. Two proteins have been proposed to export ALA, namely SLC25A38 (solute carrier family 25, member 38) and ABCB10. SLC25A38 is a member of the inner mitochondrial membrane (IMM) transporters, which promote the exchange of one metabolite for another across the IMM (Palmieri, 2013). The gene is expressed in large amounts exclusively in erythroid cells. Because mutations in *SLC25A38* cause congenital sideroblastic anaemia, which is most likely due to defective haem biosynthesis, it has been proposed that SLC25A38 either imports glycine into the mitochondria or exchanges cytosolic glycine for mitochondrial ALA across the mitochondrial membrane (Guernsey *et al.*, 2009); that is, it would transport one or two substrates required in the first steps of haem biosynthesis. ABCB10 has been proposed to facilitate mitochondrial ALA synthesis or its export from mitochondria (Bayeva *et al.*, 2013).

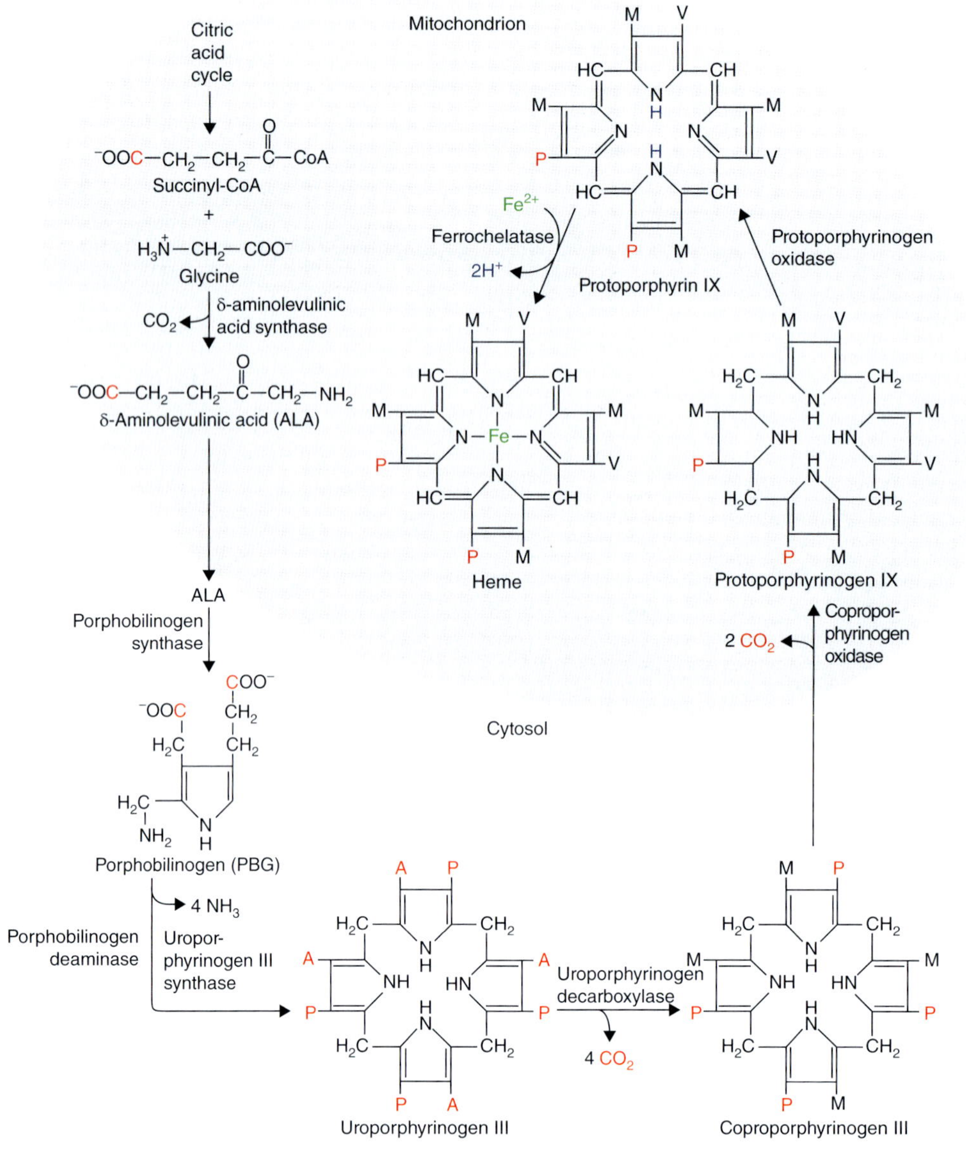

Figure 8.10 *The overall pathway of haem biosynthesis. δ-aminolaevulinic acid (ALA) is synthesised in the mitochondrion and transferred to the cytosol, where it is converted to porphobilinogen, four molecules of which condense to form a porphyrin ring. The next three steps involve oxidation of the pyrrole ring substituents to give protoporphyrinogen IX, whose formation is accompanied by its transport back into the mitochondrion. After oxidation to protoporphyrin IX, ferrochelatase inserts Fe^{2+} to yield haem. A, P, M and V represent, respectively, acetyl, propionyl, methyl and vinyl ($-CH_2=CH_2$) groups. Illustration © 2011, John Wiley & Sons Ltd*

Once ALA is in the cytoplasm, synthesis of the tetrapyrrole porphyrin nucleus continues apace, until the step at which uroporphyrinogen decarboxylase converts uroporphyrinogen II to coproporphyrinogen III. Coproporphyrinogen III is then imported into the mitochondrial intermembrane space, and it is proposed that the transfer from the cytosol involves ABCB6 (Krishnamurthy *et al.*, 2006), although this remains controversial. Coproporphyrinogen III then undergoes oxidative decarboxylation to protoporphyrinogen IX. The penultimate step is the oxidation of protoporphyrinogen IX to protoporphyrin IX, catalysed by protoporphyrinogen oxidase, which requires three molecules of molecular oxygen and generates three molecules of hydrogen peroxide. The terminal step of haem synthesis is the insertion of ferrous iron into the protoporphyrin macrocycle to yield the final product, haem, catalysed by ferrochelatase (FECH). All of the genes involved in haem biosynthesis have been cloned, and the crystal structures of the enzymes have been determined (Hamza and Dailey, 2012). For reviews of haem biosynthesis, see Ajioka *et al.* (2006), Dailey and Meissner (2013), and Chiabrando *et al.* (2014).

The specific insertion of a number of different metal ions (Fe, Mg, Co or Ni) into tetrapyrroles resulting in the formation of haem, chlorophyll, cobalamin and coenzyme F_{430}, respectively, is carried out by a class of enzymes called chelatases. The most extensively studied enzyme within the chelatase class is ferrochelatase, which catalyses the insertion of ferrous iron into PPIX to form haem. This reaction unites the biochemically synchronised pathways of porphyrin synthesis and iron transport in nearly all living organisms (Hunter *et al.*, 2011). The ferrochelatases are an evolutionarily diverse family of enzymes, and sequence data is available for a large number of prokaryotic and eukaryotic ferrochelatases, although the enzymes from *Bacillus subtilis* and mammalian ferrochelatases, particularly human, have been studied most extensively. They represent the greatest diversity between ferrochelatases examined at present, with <10% sequence identity. Most of the conserved residues are located in the active-site pocket. The *B. subtilis* enzyme is a water-soluble, monomeric protein with no cofactors (Al-Karadaghi *et al.*, 1997), whereas the human enzyme is a mitochondrial inner membrane-associated homodimer with a [2Fe–2S] cluster in each subunit (Burden *et al.*, 1999). The redox state of the enzyme is not important for function, and while the iron–sulphur cluster may be required for structural reasons it is not involved in the reaction. Despite the low degree of sequence homology, the two enzymes – for which some 40 X-ray structures have been deposited at the RCSB Protein Data Bank – have close structural similarity (Al-Karadaghi *et al.*, 1997; Wu *et al.*, 2001). When the three-dimensional structure of ferrochelatase is compared to other known protein structures, it emerges that its overall fold is most similar to that of bacterial periplasmic binding proteins (see Chapter 3), with the polypeptide folded into two similar domains each with a four-stranded parallel β-sheet flanked by α-helices (Figure 8.11).

Distortion of the porphyrin macrocycle has long been recognised to be a critical step in porphyrin metallation (Hambright and Chock, 1974; Lavallee, 1988). Porphyrin distortion facilitates metal chelation by endowing the porphyrin with an appropriate configuration for metal ion complexation. In this configuration, the lone pair orbitals of the pyrrole nitrogen atoms are exposed to the incoming metal ion (Hambright and Chock, 1974). The crystal structure of ferrochelatase complexed with *N*-methylmesoporphyrin (*N*-MeMP), a potent inhibitor of ferrochelatase which mimics a strained substrate, is shown in Figure 8.11 (Al-Karaghi *et al.*, 2006). This has served as the basis for a mechanistic model of ferrochelatases (Al-Karadaghi *et al.*, 2006), which involves as the first step a distortion of the tetrapyrrole porphyrin upon binding to the enzyme to give a saddled structure (Figure 8.12a). In this structure, two opposite pyrrole rings are slightly tilted upwards, while the other two pyrrole rings are tilted slightly downwards, giving a distortion of the porphyrin ring of about 36° (Lecerof *et al.*, 2000). The two unprotonated nitrogen atoms of the pyrrole rings

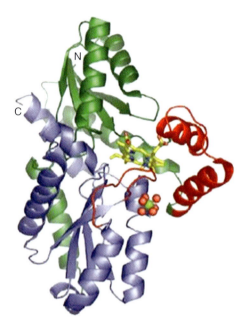

Figure 8.11 *Structure of* B. subtilis *ferrochelatase in complex with the transition state inhibitor N-methylmesoporphyrin (N-MeMP). The structure is composed of two Rossmann-type domains (green and blue), in which a central four-stranded β-sheet is flanked by α-helices. A cleft defined by structural elements (red) from both domains accommodates the porphyrin- and metal-binding sites. The inhibitor N-MeMP is shown in the cleft (carbon atoms, yellow; oxygen, red; nitrogen, blue). Reprinted with permission from Elsevier from Al-Karadaghi, S., Franco, R., Hansson, M., Shelnutt, J.A., et al. (2006) Chelatases: distort to select?* Trends Biochem. Sci., *31, 135–142*

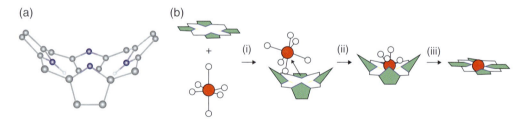

Figure 8.12 *(a) Out-of-plane saddle structure in which two pyrrole rings with unprotonated nitrogens (blue spheres) point upwards, while the other two, protonated (blue and white spheres) point downwards. (b) Steps in the mechanism for incorporation of the metal ion (red) into the porphyrin (pyrrole rings in green), as described in the text. Reprinted with permission from Elsevier from Al-Karadaghi, S., Franco, R., Hansson, M., Shelnutt, J.A., et al. (2006) Chelatases: distort to select?* Trends Biochem. Sci., *31, 135–142*

point upwards, while the two protonated nitrogens point downwards. Following distortion of the porphyrin ring, the first metal–porphyrin bond is formed (Figure 8.12b), followed by other ligand-exchange steps leading to the formation of a complex in which the iron atom is sitting on top of the porphyrin, with two of its nitrogen atoms coordinated to the metal while the other two are still protonated. This is followed by a sequential deprotonation of the two pyrrole nitrogen atoms, coupled with formation of the metallated porphyrin. Although close to 50 ferrochelatase structures are available, the exact mechanism for iron insertion into porphyrin is still a matter for debate.

Since *in vivo* both of the substrates of ferrochelatase, Fe^{2+} iron and PPIX, are potentially toxic to the cell they must be delivered directly to FECH. A reasonable solution to delivering protoporphyrin IX would be the proposed transient protein–protein complex formed between protoporphyrinogen oxidase and FECH (Ferreira *et al.*, 1988; Proulx *et al.*, 1993; Koch *et al.*, 2004). Indeed, a ternary complex has been modelled involving the three terminal enzymes of the pathway CPOCX, PPOX and FECH (Koch *et al.*, 2004). It has been proposed that FECH is part of a complex in the IMM with the iron import protein mitoferrin1 (MFRN1) and the ABCB10 transporter (Chen *et al.*, 2009, 2010). The interaction between FECH and MFRN1 would couple iron import into the mitochondria with its incorporation into the porphyrin ring, while the role of ABCB10 may be to stabilise MFRN1 expression.

If, as proposed above, Fe^{2+} is delivered by MFRN1 also forming a complex with FECH, the role of the channels (Medlock *et al.*, 2012), which enables both substrates and products to enter and leave FECH, may prove as important for ultimately understanding the mechanism of this intriguing enzyme as the conformational dynamics induced by substrate binding (Asuru *et al.*, 2012), and the distortion of the porphyrin macrocycle in the mechanism proposed by Al-Karadaghi *et al.* (2006).

Ferrochelatase expression increases during erythroid differentiation, controlled by transcription factors Sp1, NF-E2 and GATA elements (Tugores *et al.*, 1994). Since human FECH is an iron–sulphur cluster protein, its expression is controlled at the post-transcriptional level by the availability of newly formed iron–sulphur clusters whose biogenesis is dependent on iron as well as on functional iron–sulphur cluster assembly machinery (Crooks *et al.*, 2010). The downregulation of *FECH* was observed during iron-deficient erythropoiesis in *IRP2^{-/-}* mice, in iron-limited erythroid differentiation of MEL cells, and under conditions of impaired iron–sulphur cluster biogenesis (Crooks *et al.*, 2010). It has recently been shown that TMEM14C, an IMM protein that is enriched in vertebrate haematopoietic tissues, is essential for erythropoiesis and haem synthesis *in vivo*, and appears to facilitate the import of protoporphyrinogen IX into the mitochondrial matrix for haem synthesis and subsequent haemoglobin production (Yien *et al.*, 2014).

8.3 Haem Oxygenase

8.3.1 Structure and Catalytic Cycle

The recycling of iron from effete red blood cells represents the most important source of daily iron requirements. The degradation of haem is catalysed by the haem oxygenase (HO) system, which oxidatively cleaves haem (Fe-protoporphyrin IX) to produce CO, biliverdin and free iron (Figure 8.13). There are two isoforms of HO, encoded by two distinct genes: (i) a constitutive form (HO-2), which is highly expressed in neuronal and vascular tissues; and (ii) an inducible form (HO-1), which is a major stress-inducible protein in mammalian cells.

Mammalian haem oxygenases catalyse the conversion of haem to biliverdin IXα, with the release of CO and Fe^{2+} (Matsui *et al.*, 2010; Ortiz de Montellano, 2000), and were originally considered to be 'housekeeping' enzymes, their principal role being to recycle iron. They are now recognised as playing an important role in antioxidant defence and cellular signaling, and as we saw in Chapter 4, pathogenic bacteria utilise HOs to acquire iron from their hosts. The HO-dependent conversion of haem to biliverdin consumes three molecules of dioxygen in three

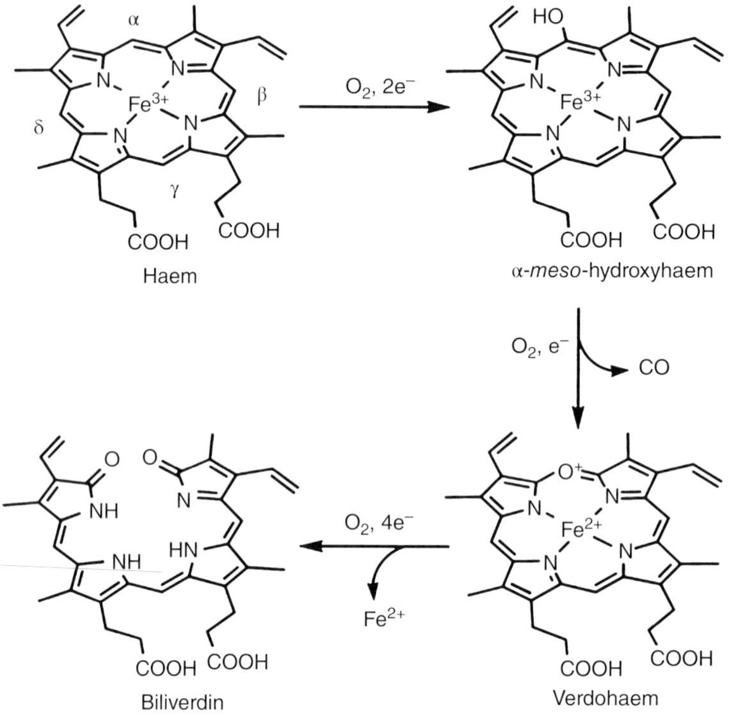

Figure 8.13 *Haem degradation scheme catalysed by HO. Reprinted with permission from Matsui, T., Iwasaki, M., Sugiyama, R., Unno, M. and Ikeda-Saito, M. (2010) Dioxygen activation for the self-degradation of heme: reaction mechanism and regulation of heme oxygenase.* Inorg. Chem., ***49,*** *3602–3609 ; © 2010, American Chemical Society*

successive steps of O_2 activation involving the uptake of seven electrons (Figure 8.13) which, in mammals, are supplied by NADPH-cytochrome P-450. The biliverdin is converted to bilirubin by the action of biliverdin reductase, whereas in plants, algae and cyanobacteria, a ferredoxin-dependent HO generates biliverdin as a precursor for the synthesis of light-harvesting bilins (Montgomery and Lagarias, 2002; Dammeyer and Frankenberg-Dinkel, 2008): no physiological electron donors have been identified for the classical (canonical) bacterial HOs (Ratliff *et al.*, 2001). A number of bacterial IsdG/1-like HOs (non-canonical), convert haem to oxo-bilirubins (staphylobilins) or else catalyse oxidative ring cleavage with retention of the α-mesocarbon as formaldehyde (Figure 8.14).

  O_2 activation by haem enzymes (peroxidase, catalase, and cytochrome P450; see Chapter 2) has been extensively studied, and involves a common reactive species compound I, a ferryl ($O{=}Fe^{IV}$) haem paired with a porphyrin cation radical. Haem degradation through the action of HO is unusual in that it utilises haem both as a substrate and as a cofactor for its own degradation. HO catalysis is unique in that all of the O_2 activations are performed by the substrate itself, as shown by the absence of any other cofactor (Yoshida and Kikuchi, 1978; Ortiz de Montellano, 1998). The conventional haem enzymes, such as peroxidase, catalase and cytochrome P450, strictly avoid such self-oxidation of the prosthetic group, which would result in enzyme inactivation. Thus, the HO enzyme must have a protein architecture that enables the unique O_2 activation for haem self-degradation. The initial O_2 activation of HO is similar to cytochrome P450, involving reduction of the ferric haem iron to the ferrous state, which binds O_2 (Figure 8.15), followed by one-electron

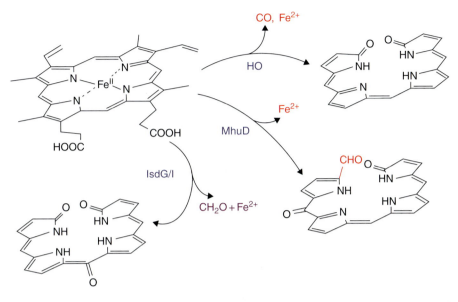

Figure 8.14   *Reaction products of the canonical haem oxygenase (HO) and non-canonical IsdG/I-like HOs. Reprinted with permission from Elsevier from Wilks, A. and Heinzl, G. (2014) Heme oxygenation and the widening paradigm of heme degradation. Arch. Biochem. Biophys., **15** (544), 87–95*

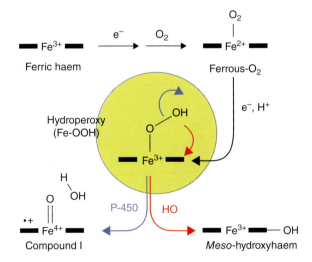

Figure 8.15   *Comparison of O_2 activation by HO and cytochrome P450. Reprinted with permission from Matsui, T., Iwasaki, M., Sugiyama, R., Unno, M. and Ikeda-Saito, M. (2010) Dioxygen activation for the self-degradation of heme: reaction mechanism and regulation of heme oxygenase. Inorg. Chem., **49**, 3602–3609; © 2010, American Chemical Society*

reduction and protonation of the ferrous-O_2 haem to give a ferric hydroperoxy species (FeOOH). In cytochrome P450, as well as peroxidase and catalase, the terminal oxygen of FeOOH is thought to be liberated as water to give compound I or its equivalent as an active species. The crystal structures of HO show that the haem pocket is not designed for enhancing O–O bond heterolysis (Figure 8.16). Indeed, even when HO compound I is generated artificially it has been shown not to be responsible for haem hydroxylation (Matsui *et al.*, 2006). HO was proposed to utilise the FeOOH species, but not conventional ferryl haems, as a reactive intermediate for self-hydroxylation, and low-temperature, mutational and crystallographic studies have revealed that the protonation of FeOOH by a distal water molecule is critical in promoting the unique self-hydroxylation (Matsui *et al.*, 2010). The second oxygenation is a rapid, spontaneous autooxidation of the reactive alpha-*meso*-hydroxyhaem in which the HO enzyme does not play a critical role, while further O_2 activation by verdohaem cleaves its porphyrin macrocycle to form biliverdin and free ferrous iron. This third step is considered to be a major rate-determining step of HO catalysis to regulate enzyme activity (Matsui *et al.*, 2010). Biliverdin can then be converted to bilirubin by the cytosolic enzyme biliverdin reductase.

Both, bilirubin and CO have cytoprotective activity, whereas the Fe^{2+} released from the activity of HO can generate ROS, notably the highly reactive hydroxyl radical via the Fenton reaction, with deleterious cellular consequences (these will be discussed in Chapter 13). Both, biliverdin and bilirubin produced from HO activity potentially contribute to cellular antioxidant balance prior to their excretion. CO is also associated with cytoprotection and cellular homeostasis in several distinct cell types and tissues, mainly targeting mitochondria (Almeida *et al.*, 2015). Eukaryotic organisms use endogenous CO as a neurotransmitter and a signal molecule. CO sensors act as signal transducers by coupling a 'regulatory' haem-binding domain to a 'functional' signal transmitter. Although high CO concentrations generally inhibit haem protein action, low CO levels can influence several signalling pathways, including those regulated by soluble guanylate cyclase and/or mitogen-activated protein kinases (Gullotta *et al.*, 2012). Direct exposure to CO may protect cells or organs from various disease insults, and it has been suggested that this may have protective effects and therapeutic potential in liver diseases and liver transplantation (Bosch and Tsui, 2012), and also during and after cardiopulmonary bypass (Loop *et al.*, 2012).

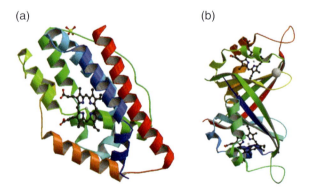

(a) (b)

Figure 8.16 *Overall fold of the canonical HemO of P. aeruginosa and IsdI of S. aureus. (a) HemO shown with haem in red and active site hydrogen bond contributing residues shown in stick form. (b) IsdG shown with haem in red and active site residues in stick form. Protein Data Bank (PDB) codes 1SK7 (HemO) and 3LGM (IsdI)*

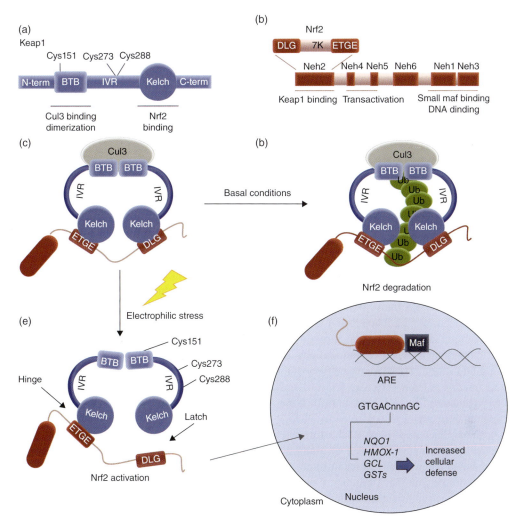

Figure 8.17 *Proposed mechanism for activation of the Keap1–Nrf2–ARE-pathway. (a, b) Domain structures of Keap1 and Nrf2. Keap1 have the following domains: N-terminal domain, BTB domain, IVR, Kelch domain, and C-terminal domain. Nrf2 consists of six Neh domains. Two different motifs of Neh2 domain, DLG and ETGE motifs, bind the Keap1 Kelch domain, resulting in an Nrf2–Keap1 complex of 1:2 stoichiometry (c). Under basal conditions, Keap1 functions as an adaptor protein in the Cul3-based E3 ligase complex, resulting in rapid ubiquitination of the lysine residues located between the ETGE and the DLG motifs, and subsequent degradation of Nrf2 (d). On activation, electrophiles can directly bind Keap1 cysteines such as Cys151, Cys273, and Cys288, resulting in a conformational change in Keap1 leading to detachment of the weaker binding DLG motif (Latch) and disturbed ubiquitination of Nrf2 (e). In this setting, the Keap1-ETGE binding remains (Hinge), but Nrf2 escapes the degradation pathway, translocates to the nucleus, binds to the ARE, and promotes the transcription of antioxidant genes such as NQO1, HMOX1, GCL, and GSTs (f). Reproduced with permission from Elsevier from Kansanen, E., Jyrkkänen, H.-K. and Levonen A.-L. (2012) Activation of stress signaling pathways by electrophilic oxidized and nitrated lipids.* Free Radical Biol. Med., **52**, *973–982*

8.3.2 Activation of Haem Oxygenase 1 (HO-1)

The induction of the gene *HO-1* occurs as a general response to cellular stress. In addition to the substrate haem, a broad spectrum of stimuli can induce *HO-1* expression, including nitric oxide (NO), cytokines, heavy metals, hormones, growth factors, thiol-reactive substances, oxidants, extreme oxygen environments, ischaemia/reperfusion injury, and ultraviolet-A radiation (Ryter *et al.*, 2006). Since many of these inducing conditions are associated with the stimulation of pro-oxidant states, HO-1 is considered an inducible defence mechanism against oxidative cellular stress. *HO-1* gene expression is tightly regulated at the transcriptional level (Paine *et al.*, 2010), and its induction is controlled by a number of redox-dependent transcriptional activators such as NF-E2-related factor 2 (Nrf2), NF-κB and AP-1 along with the transcription repressor BTB and CNC homologue 1 (Bach1) (reviewed in Naito *et al.*, 2014). The Keap1–Nrf2 pathway is the major regulator of cytoprotective responses to endogenous and exogenous stresses caused by ROS and electrophiles (Kansanen *et al.*, 2012). The key signalling proteins within the pathway are the transcription factor Nrf2 (nuclear factor erythroid 2-related factor 2) which, together with small Maf proteins, binds to the antioxidant response element (ARE) in the regulatory regions of target genes, and Keap1 (Kelch ECH-associating protein). Keap1 is a very cysteine-rich protein, and three Cys residues, C151, C273 and C288, have been shown to play a functional role by altering the conformation of Keap1 (Taguchi *et al.*, 2011). In basal conditions, Keap1 functions as an adaptor protein in the Cul3-based E3 ligase complex, resulting in a rapid ubiquitination of the lysine residues located between the ETGE and the DLG motifs, and proteasomal degradation of Nrf2 (Figure 8.17). On activation, electrophiles can directly bind Keap1 cysteines such as Cys151, Cys273 and Cys288, resulting in a conformational change in Keap1 and leading to detachment of the weaker binding DLG motif (Latch) and disturbed ubiquitination of Nrf2 (E). In this setting, the Keap1-ETGE binding remains (Hinge), but Nrf2 escapes the degradation pathway, translocates to the nucleus, binds to the ARE, and promotes the transcription of antioxidant genes, including HO1 (Kansanen *et al.*, 2012).

Under baseline conditions, Bach1 forms a heterodimer with small Maf proteins which repress transcription of the *HMOX1* gene by binding upstream of the site to which Nrf2 binds. In contrast, an increase in haem results in haem-binding to Bach1, displacing Bach1 from the *HMOX1* gene, which in turn permits Nrf2 binding. Consequently, intracellular haem ultimately regulates HO-1 transcription via modification of the status of Bach1 and Nrf2.

References

Adam, A.C., Bornhövd, C., Prokisch, H., Neupert, W. and Hell K. (2006) The Nfs1 interacting protein Isd11 has an essential role in Fe/S cluster biogenesis in mitochondria. *EMBO J.*, **25**, 174–183.

Ajioka, R.S., Phillips, J.D. and Kushner, J.P. (2006) Biosynthesis of heme in mammals. *Biochim. Biophys. Acta*, **1763**, 723–736.

Al-Karadaghi, S., Hansson, M., Nikonov, S., *et al.* (1997) Crystal structure of ferrochelatase: the terminal enzyme in heme biosynthesis. *Structure*, **5**, 1501–1510.

Al-Karadaghi, S., Franco, R., Hansson, M., *et al.* (2006) Chelatases: distort to select? *Trends Biochem. Sci.*, **31**, 135–142.

Almeida, A.S., Figueiredo-Pereira, C. and Vieira, H.L. (2015) Carbon monoxide and mitochondria-modulation of cell metabolism, redox response and cell death. *Front. Physiol.*, **6**, 33.

Angerer, H. (2013) The superfamily of mitochondrial Complex1_LYR motif-containing (LYRM) proteins. *Biochem. Soc. Trans.*, **41**, 1335–1341.

Arosio, P. and Levi, S. (2010) Cytosolic and mitochondrial ferritins in the regulation of cellular iron homeostasis and oxidative damage. *Biochim. Biophys. Acta*, **1800**, 783–792.

Asuru, B.P., An, M. and Busenlehner, L.S. (2012) Dissection of porphyrin-induced conformational dynamics in the heme biosynthesis enzyme ferrochelatase. *Biochemistry*, **51**, 7116–7127.

Ayala-Castro, C., Saini, A. and Outten, F.W. (2008) Fe-S cluster assembly pathways in bacteria. *Microbiol. Mol. Biol. Rev.*, **72**, 110–125.

Balk, J., Pierik, A.J., Netz, D.J., Mühlenhoff, U. and Lill, R. (2004) The hydrogenase-like Nar1p is essential for maturation of cytosolic and nuclear iron-sulphur proteins. *EMBO J.*, **23**, 2105–2115.

Balk, J., Pierik, A.J., Aguilar Netz, D.J., Mühlenhoff, U. and Lill, R. (2005) Nar1p, a conserved eukaryotic protein with similarity to Fe-only hydrogenases, functions in cytosolic iron-sulphur protein biogenesis. *Biochem. Soc. Trans.*, **33**, 86–89.

Banci, L., Bertini, I., Ciofi-Baffioni, S., *et al.* (2011) Anamorsin is a [2Fe–2S] cluster-containing substrate of the Mia40-dependent mitochondrial protein trapping machinery. *Chem. Biol.*, **18**, 794–804.

Banci, L., Bertini, I., Calderone, V., *et al.* (2013) Molecular view of an electron transfer process essential for iron–sulfur protein biogenesis. *Proc. Natl Acad. Sci. USA*, **110** 7136–7141.

Bandyopadhyay, S., Gama, F., Molina-Navarro, M.M., *et al.* (2008) Chloroplast monothiol glutaredoxins as scaffold proteins for the assembly and delivery of [2Fe-2S] clusters. *EMBO J.*, **27**, 1122–1133.

Basu, S., Netz, D.J., Haindrich, A.C., *et al.* (2014) Cytosolic iron–sulphur protein assembly is functionally conserved and essential in procyclic and bloodstream *Trypanosoma brucei*. *Mol. Microbiol.*, **93**, 897–910.

Bayeva, M., Khechaduri, A., Wu, R., *et al.* (2013) ATP-binding cassette B10 regulates early steps of heme synthesis. *Circ. Res.*, **113**, 279–287.

Biederbick, A., Stehling, O., Rosser, R., *et al.* (2006) Role of human mitochondrial Nfs1 in cytosolic iron–sulfur protein biogenesis and iron regulation. *Mol. Cell. Biol.*, **26**, 5675–5687.

Bosch, F. and Tsui, T.Y. (2012) Carbon monoxide, a two-face for the protection of the liver. *Curr. Pharm. Biotechnol.*, **13** (6), 803–812.

Breuer, W., Shvartsman, M. and Cabantchik, Z.I. (2007) Intracellular labile iron. A review. *Int. J. Biochem. Cell Biol.*, **40**, 350–354.

Brissot, P., Ropert, M., Le Lan, C. and Loreal, O. (2012) Non-transferrin bound iron: a key role in iron overload and iron toxicity. *Biochim. Biophys. Acta*, **1820**, 403–410.

Burden, A.E., Wu, C., Dailey, T.A., *et al.* (1999) Human ferrochelatase: crystallization, characterization of the [2Fe–2S] cluster and determination that the enzyme is a homodimer. *Biochem. Biophys. Acta*, **1435**, 191–197.

Bych, K., Kerscher, S., Netz, D.J., *et al.* (2008) The iron-sulphur protein Ind1 is required for effective complex I assembly. *EMBO J.*, **27**, 1736–1746.

Cabantchik, Z.I. (2014) Labile iron in cells and body fluids: physiology, pathology, and pharmacology. *Front. Pharmacol.*, **5**, 45.

Cameron, J.M., Janer, A., Levandovskiy, V., *et al.* (2011) Mutations in iron-sulfur cluster scaffold genes NFU1 and BOLA3 cause a fatal deficiency of multiple respiratory chain and 2-oxoacid dehydrogenase enzymes. *Am. J. Hum. Genet.*, **89**, 486–495.

Cavadini, P., Biasiotto, G., Poli, M., *et al.* (2007) RNA silencing of the mitochondrial ABCB7 transporter in HeLa cells causes an iron-deficient phenotype with mitochondrial iron overload. *Blood*, **109**, 3552–3559.

Cazzola, M., Invernizzi, R., Bergamaschi, G., *et al.* (2003) Mitochondrial ferritin expression in erythroid cells from patients with sideroblastic anemia. *Blood*, **101**, 1996–2000.

Chandramouli, K. and Johnson, M.K. (2006) HscA and HscB stimulate [2Fe-2S] cluster transfer from IscU to apoferredoxin in an ATP-dependent reaction. *Biochemistry*, **45**, 11087–11095.

Chen, W., Paradkar, P.N., Li, L., *et al.* (2009) Abcb10 physically interacts with mitoferrin-1 (Slc25a37) to enhance its stability and function in the erythroid mitochondria. *Proc. Natl Acad. Sci. USA*, **106**, 16263–16268.

Chen, W., Dailey, H.A. and Paw, B.H. (2010) Ferrochelatase forms an oligomeric complex with mitoferrin-1 and Abcb10 for erythroid heme biosynthesis. *Blood*, **116**, 628–630.

Chiabrando, D., Mercurio, S. and Tolosano, E. (2014) Heme and erythropoiesis: more than a structural role. *Haematologica*, **99**, 973–983.

Colin, F., Martelli, A., Clémancey, M., *et al.* (2013) Mammalian frataxin controls sulfur production and iron entry during de novo Fe4S4 cluster assembly. *J. Am. Chem. Soc.*, **135**, 733–740.

Cook, S.F. (1929) The structure and composition of hemosiderin. *J. Biol. Chem.*, **82**, 595–609.

Crichton, R.R. (1984) Iron uptake and utilization by mammalian cells II. Intracellular iron utilization. *Trends Biochem. Sci.*, **9**, 283–286.

Crichton, R.R. (2009) *Inorganic Biochemistry of Iron Metabolism from Molecular Mechanisms to Clinical Consequences*, 3rd edition, John Wiley & Sons, Chichester, pp. 183–222.

Crooks, D.R., Ghosh, M.C., Haller, R.G., Tong, W.H. and Rouault, T.A. (2010) Posttranslational stability of the heme biosynthetic enzyme ferrochelatase is dependent on iron availability and intact iron-sulfur cluster assembly machinery. *Blood*, **115**, 860–869.

Cumming, R.L., Goldberg, A., Morrow, J. and Smith, J.A. (1967) Effect of phenylhydrazine-induced haemolysis on the urinary excretion of iron after desferrioxamine. *Lancet*, **1**, 71–74.

Dailey, H.A. and Meissner, P.N. (2013) Erythroid heme biosynthesis and its disorders. *Cold Spring Harb. Perspect. Med.*, **3**, a011676.

Dammeyer, T. and Frankenberg-Dinkel, N. (2008) Function and distribution of bilin biosynthesis enzymes in photosynthetic organisms. *Photochem. Photobiol. Sci.*, **7**, 1121–1130.

Dutkiewicz, R., Schilke, B., Knieszner, H., *et al.* (2003) Ssq1, a mitochondrial Hsp70 involved in iron-sulfur (Fe/S) center biogenesis. Similarities to and differences from its bacterial counterpart. *J. Biol. Chem.*, **278**, 29719–29727.

Dutkiewicz, R., Schilke, B., Cheng, S., *et al.* (2004) Sequence-specific interaction between mitochondrial Fe-S scaffold protein Isu and Hsp70 Ssq1 is essential for their in vivo function. *J. Biol. Chem.*, **279**, 29167–29174.

Dutkiewicz, R., Marszalek, J., Schilke, B., *et al.* (2006) The Hsp70 chaperone Ssq1p is dispensable for iron-sulfur cluster formation on the scaffold protein Isu1p. *J. Biol. Chem.*, **281**, 7801–7808.

Epsztejn, S., Kakhlon, O., Glickstein, H., *et al.* (1997) Fluorescence analysis of the labile iron pool of mammalian cells. *Anal. Biochem.*, **248**, 31–40.

Esposito, B.P., Epsztejn, S., Breuer, W., and Cabantchik, Z.I. (2002). A review of fluorescence methods for assessing labile iron in cells and biological fluids. *Anal. Biochem.*, **304**, 1–18.

Ferecatu, I., Goncalves, S., Golinelli-Cohen, M.P., *et al.* (2014) The diabetes drug target MitoNEET governs a novel trafficking pathway to rebuild an Fe–S cluster into cytosolic aconitase/iron regulatory protein 1. *J. Biol. Chem.*, **289**, 28070–28086.

Ferreira, G.C., Andrew, T.L., Karr, S.W. and Dailey, H.A. (1988) Organization of the terminal two enzymes of the heme biosynthetic pathway. *Orientation of protoporphyrinogen oxidase and evidence for a membrane complex. J. Biol. Chem.*, **263**, 3835–3839.

Foury, F. and Roganti, T. (2002) Deletion of the mitochondrial carrier genes *MRS3* and *MRS4* suppresses mitochondrial iron accumulation in a yeast frataxin-deficient strain. *J. Biol. Chem.*, **277**, 24475–24483.

Fosset, C., Chauveau, M.J., Guillon, B., *et al.* (2006) RNA silencing of mitochondrial m-Nfs1 reduces Fe–S enzyme activity both in mitochondria and cytosol of mammalian cells. *J. Biol. Chem.*, **28**, 25398–25406.

Frey, A.G., Nandal, A., Park, J.H. and Smith, P.M. (2014). The iron chaperones PCBP1 and PCBP2 mediate the metallation of the dinuclear iron enzyme deoxyhypusine hydroxylase. *Proc. Natl Acad. Sci. USA*, **111** 8031–8036.

Gari, K., León Ortiz, A.M., Borel, V., *et al.* (2012) MMS19 links cytoplasmic iron-sulfur cluster assembly to DNA metabolism. *Science*, **337**, 243–245.

Garland, S.A., Hoff, K., Vickery, L.E. and Culotta, V.C. (1999) *Saccharomyces cerevisiae* ISU1 and ISU2: members of a well-conserved gene family for iron-sulfur cluster assembly. *J. Mol. Biol.*, **294**, 897–907.

Gelling, C., Dawes, I.W., Richhardt, N., Lill, R. and Mühlenhoff, U. (2008) Mitochondrial Iba57p is required for Fe/S cluster formation on aconitase and activation of radical SAM enzymes. *Mol. Cell. Biol.*, **28**, 1851–1861.

Gerber, J., Mühlenhoff, U. and Lill, R. (2003) An interaction between frataxin and Isu1/Nfs1 that is crucial for Fe/S cluster synthesis on Isu1. *EMBO Rep.*, **4**, 906–911.

Gerber, J., Neumann, K., Prohl, C., Muhlenhoff, U. and Lill, R. (2004) The yeast scaffold proteins Isu1p and Isu2p are required inside mitochondria for maturation of cytosolic Fe/S proteins. *Mol. Cell. Biol.*, **24**, 4848–4857.

Giel, J.L., Nesbit, E.L., Mettert, A.S., *et al.* (2012) Regulation of iron-sulphur cluster homeostasis through transcriptional control of the Isc pathway by [2Fe-2S]-IscR in *Escherichia coli. Mol. Microbiol.*, **87**, 478–492.

Glickstein, H., Ben El, R., Shvartsman, M. and Cabantchik, Z.I. (2005) Intracellular labile iron pools as direct targets of iron chelators: a fluorescence study of chelator action in living cells. *Blood*, **106**, 3242–3450.

Greenberg, G.R. and Wintrobe, M.M. (1946) A labile iron pool. *J. Biol. Chem.*, **165**, 397.

Guernsey, D.L., Jiang, H., Campagna, D.R., *et al.*, (2009) Mutations in mitochondrial carrier family gene SLC25A38 cause nonsyndromic autosomal recessive congenital sideroblastic anemia. *Nat. Genet.*, **41**, 651–653.

Gullotta, F., di Masi, A., Coletta, M. and Ascenzi, P. (2012) CO metabolism, sensing, and signaling. *Biofactors*, **38**, 1–13.

Gutierrez, E., Shin, B.S., Woolstenhulme, C.J., *et al.* (2013). eIF5A promotes translation of polyproline motifs. *Mol. Cell*, **51**, 35–45.

Hambright, P. and Chock, P.B. (1974) Metal–porphyrin interactions. III. A dissociative-interchange mechanism for metal ion incorporation into porphyrin molecules. *J. Am. Chem. Soc.*, **96**, 3123–3131.

Hamza, I. and Dailey, H.A. (2012) One ring to rule them all: trafficking of heme and heme synthesis intermediates in the metazoans. *Biochim. Biophys. Acta*, **1823**, 1617–1632.

Harigae, H., Suwabe, N., Weinstock, P.H., *et al.* (1998) Deficient heme and globin synthesis in embryonic stem cells lacking the erythroid-specific delta-aminolevulinate synthase gene. *Blood*, **91**, 798–805.

Haunhorst, P., Hanschmann, E.M., Bräutigam, L., *et al.* (2013) Crucial function of vertebrate glutaredoxin 3 (PICOT) in iron homeostasis and hemoglobin maturation. *Mol. Biol. Cell*, **24**, 1895–1903

Hausmann, A., Aguilar Netz, D.J., Balk, J., *et al.* (2005) The eukaryotic P loop NTPase Nbp35: an essential component of the cytosolic and nuclear iron-sulfur protein assembly machinery. *Proc. Natl Acad. Sci. USA*, **102**, 3266–3271.

Hider, R.C. and Kong, X. (2013). Iron speciation in the cytosol: an overview. *Dalton Trans.*, **42**, 3220–3229.

Hoff, K.G., Cupp-Vickery, J.R. and Vickery, L.E. (2003) Contributions of the LPPVK motif of the iron–sulfur template protein IscU to interactions with the Hsc66-Hsc20 chaperone system. *J. Biol. Chem.*, **278**, 37582–37589.

Hunter, G.A., Al-Karadaghi, S. and Ferreira, G.C. (2011) Ferrochelatase: the convergence of the porphyrin biosynthesis and iron transport pathways. *J. Porphyr. Phthalocyanines*, **15**, 350–356.

Jacobs, A. (1977) Low-molecular-weight intracellular iron transport compounds. *Blood*, **50**, 433–439.

Johansson, C., Roos, A.K., Montano, S.J., *et al.* (2011) The crystal structure of human GLRX5: iron-sulfur cluster co-ordination, tetrameric assembly and monomer activity. *Biochem. J.*, **433**, 303–311.

Kaiser, J.T., Clausen, T., Bourenkow, G.P., *et al.* (2000) Crystal structure of a NifS-like protein from *Thermotoga maritima*: implications for iron sulphur cluster assembly. *J. Mol. Biol.*, **297**, 451–464.

Kakhlon, O. and Cabantchik, Z.I. (2002) The labile iron pool: characterization, measurement, and participation in cellular processes. *Free Radic. Biol. Med.*, **33**, 1037–1046.

Kansanen, E., Jyrkkänen, H.-K. and Levonen, A.-L. (2012) Activation of stress signaling pathways by electrophilic oxidized and nitrated lipids. *Free Radical Biol. Med.*. **52**, 973–982.

Kiley, P.J. and Beinert, H. (1999) Oxygen sensing by the global regulator, *FNR: the role of the iron-sulfur cluster. FEMS Microbiol. Rev.*, **22**, 341–352.

Kim, K.D., Chung, W.H., Kim, H.J., Lee, K.C. and Roe, J.H. (2010) Monothiol glutaredoxin Grx5 interacts with Fe-S scaffold proteins Isa1 and Isa2 and supports Fe-S assembly and DNA integrity in mitochondria of fission yeast. *Biochem. Biophys. Res. Commun.*, **392**, 467–472.

Kispal, G., Csere, P., Prohl, C. and Lill, R. (1999) The mitochondrial proteins Atm1p and Nfs1p are essential for biogenesis of cytosolic Fe/S proteins. *EMBO J.*, **18**, 3981–3989.

Koch, M., Breithaupt, C., Kiefersauer, R., *et al.* (2004) Crystal structure of protoporphyrinogen IX oxidase: a key enzyme in haem and chlorophyll biosynthesis. *EMBO J.*, **23**, 1720–1728.

Krishnamurthy, P.C., Du, G., Fukuda, Y., *et al.* (2006) Identification of a mammalian mitochondrial porphyrin transporter. *Nature*, **443**, 586–589.

Kruszewski, M. (2003) Labile iron pool: the main determinant of cellular response to oxidative stress. *Mutat. Res.*, **29**, 81–92.

Kumar, C., Igbaria, A., D'autreaux, B., Planson, A.G., Junot, C., Godat, E., *et al.* (2011) Glutathione revisited: a vital function in iron metabolism and ancillary role in thiol-redox control. *EMBO J.*, **30**, 2044–2056.

Lane, D.J.R. and Richardson, D.R. (2014) Chaperone turns gatekeeper: PCBP2 and DMT1 form an iron-transport pipeline. *Biochem. J.*, **462**, e1–e3.

Lange, H., Kispal, G. and Lill, R. (1999) Mechanism of iron transport to the site of heme synthesis inside yeast mitochondria. *J. Biol. Chem.*, **274**, 18989–18996.

Lange, H., Kaut, A., Kispal, G. and Lill, R. (2000) A mitochondrial ferredoxin is essential for biogenesis of cellular iron-sulfur proteins. *Proc. Natl Acad. Sci. USA*, **97**, 1050–1055.

Lange, H., Lisowsky, T., Gerber, J., *et al.* (2001) An essential function of the mitochondrial sulfhydryl oxidase Erv1p/ALR in the maturation of cytosolic Fe/S proteins. *EMBO Rep.*, **2**, 715–720.

Lavallee, D.C. (1988) Porphyrin metallation reactions in biochemistry. *Mol. Struct. Energ.*, **9**, 279–314.

Lecerof, D., Fodje, M., Hansson, A., Hansson, M. and Al-Karadaghi, S. (2000) Structural and mechanistic basis of porphyrin metallation by ferrochelatase. *J. Mol. Biol.*, **297**, 221–232.

Lee, J.Y., Yang, J.G., Zhitnitsky, D., Lewinson, O. and Rees, D.C. (2014) Structural basis for heavy metal detoxification by an Atm1-type ABC exporter. *Science*, **343**, 1133–1136.

Li, J., Saxena, S., Pain, D. and Dancis, A. (2001) Adrenodoxin reductase homolog (Arh1p) of yeast mitochondria required for iron homeostasis. *J. Biol. Chem.*, **276**, 1503–1509.

Lill, R. (2009) Function and biogenesis of iron-sulphur proteins. *Nature*, **460**, 831–838.

Lill, R. and Mühlenhoff, U. (2006) Iron-sulfur protein biogenesis in eukaryotes: components and mechanisms. *Annu. Rev. Cell. Dev. Biol.*, **22**, 457–486.

Lill, R. and Mühlenhoff, U. (2008) Maturation of iron-sulfur proteins in eukaryotes: mechanisms, connected processes, and diseases. *Annu. Rev. Biochem.*, **77**, 669–700.

Lill, R., Hoffmann, B., Molik, S., *et al.* (2012) The role of mitochondria in cellular iron-sulfur protein biogenesis and iron metabolism. *Biochim. Biophys. Acta*, **1823**, 1491–1508.

Lill, R., Srinivasan, V. and Mühlenhoff, U. (2014) The role of mitochondria in cytosolic-nuclear iron–sulfur protein biogenesis and in cellular iron regulation. *Curr. Opin. Microbiol.*, **22C**, 111–119.

Lipschitz, D.A., Dugard, J., Simon, M.O., Bothwell, T.H. and Charlton, R.W. (1971) The site of action of desferrioxamine. *Br. J. Haematol.*, **20**, 395–404.

Loop, T., Schlensak, C. and Goebel, U. (2012) Cytoprotection by inhaled carbon monoxide before cardiopulmonary bypass in preclinical models. *Curr. Pharm. Biotechnol.*, **13**, 797–802.

Matsui, T., Kim, S.H., Jin, H., *et al.* (2006) Compound I of heme oxygenase cannot hydroxylate its heme meso-carbon. *J. Am. Chem. Soc.*, **128**, 1090–1091.

Matsui, T., Iwasaki, M., Sugiyama, R., Unno, M. and Ikeda-Saito, M. (2010) Dioxygen activation for the self-degradation of heme: reaction mechanism and regulation of heme oxygenase. *Inorg. Chem.*, **49**, 3602–3609.

Medlock, A.E., Najahi-Missaoui, W., Ross, T.A., *et al.* (2012) Identification and characterization of solvent-filled channels in human ferrochelatase. *Biochemistry*, **51**, 5422–5433.

Mesecke, N., Terziyska, N., Kozany, C., *et al.* (2005) A disulfide relay system in the intermembrane space of mitochondria that mediates protein import. *Cell*, **121**, 1059–1069.

Miao, N. and Rouault, T.A. (2014) Iron-sulfur cluster biogenesis in mammalian cells: New insights into the molecular mechanisms of cluster delivery. *Biochim. Biophys. Acta*, **1853**, 1493–1512.

Miao, R., Kim, H., Koppolu, U.M., *et al.* (2009) Biophysical characterization of the iron in mitochondria from Atm1p-depleted *Saccharomyces cerevisiae*. *Biochemistry*, **48**, 9556–9568.

Montgomery, B.L. and Lagarias, J.C. (2002) Phytochrome ancestry: sensors of bilins and light. *Trends Plant Sci.*, **7**, 357–366.

Mühlenhoff, U., Stadler, J., Richhardt, N. *et al.* (2003a) A specific role of the yeast mitochondrial carriers Mrs3/4p in mitochondrial iron acquisition under iron-limiting conditions. *J. Biol. Chem.*, **278**, 40612–40620.

Mühlenhoff, U., Gerber, J., Richhardt, N. and Lill, R. (2003b) Components involved in assembly and dislocation of iron-sulfur clusters on the scaffold protein Isu1p. *EMBO J.*, **22**, 4815–4825.

Mühlenhoff, U., Molik, S., Godoy, J.R., *et al.* (2010) Cytosolic monothiol glutaredoxins function in intracellular iron sensing and trafficking via their bound iron-sulfur cluster. *Cell Metab.*, **12**, 373–385.

Mühlenhoff, U., Richter, N., Pines, O., Pierik, A.J. and Lill, R. (2011) Specialized function of yeast Isa1 and Isa2 proteins in the maturation of mitochondrial [4Fe-4S] proteins. *J. Biol. Chem.*, **286**, 41205–41216.

Mulder, D.W., Shepard, E.M., Meuser, J.E., *et al.* (2011) Insights into [FeFe]-hydrogenase structure, mechanism, and maturation. *Structure*, **19**, 1038–1052.

Müller, M. and Martin, W. (1999) The genome of *Rickettsia prowazekii* and some thoughts on the origin of mitochondria and hydrogenosomes. *BioEssays*, **21**, 377–381.

Naito, Y., Takagi, T. and Higashimura, Y. (2014) Heme oxygenase-1 and anti-inflammatory M2 macrophages. *Arch. Biochem. Biophys.*, **564**, 83–88.

Nandal, A., Ruiz, J.C., Subramanian, P., *et al.* (2011) Activation of the HIF prolyl hydroxylase by the iron chaperones PCBP1 and PCBP2. *Cell Metab.*, **14**, 647–657.

Navarro-Sastre, A., Tort, F., Stehling, O., *et al.* (2011) A fatal mitochondrial disease is associated with defective NFU1 function in the maturation of a subset of mitochondrial Fe-S proteins. *Am. J. Hum. Genet.*, **89**, 656–667.

Netz, D.J., Pierik, A.J., Stümpfig, M., Mühlenhoff, U. and Lill, R. (2007) The Cfd1-Nbp35 complex acts as a scaffold for iron-sulfur protein assembly in the yeast cytosol. *Nat. Chem. Biol.*, **3**, 278–286.

Netz, D.J., Stümpfig, M., Dove, C., *et al.* (2010) Tah18 transfers electrons to Dre2 in cytosolic iron–sulfur protein biogenesis. *Nat. Chem. Biol.*, **6**, 758–765.

Netz, D.J., Stith, C.M., Stümpfig, M., *et al.* (2012) Eukaryotic DNA polymerases require an iron-sulfur cluster for the formation of active complexes. *Nat. Chem. Biol.*, **8**, 125–132.

Netz, D.J., Mascarenhas, J., Stehling, O., Pierik, A.J. and Lill, R. (2014) Maturation of cytosolic and nuclear iron-sulfur proteins. *Trends Cell Biol.*, **24**, 303–312.

Nicolet, Y. and Fontecilla-Camps, J.C. (2012) Structure–function relationships in [FeFe]-hydrogenase active site maturation. *J. Biol. Chem.*, **287**, 13532–13540.

Ortiz de Montellano, J.R. (1998) Heme oxygenase mechanism: evidence for an electrophilic, ferric peroxide species. *Acc. Chem. Res.*, **31**, 543–549.

Ortiz de Montellano, J.R. (2000) The mechanism of heme oxygenase. *Curr. Opin. Chem. Biol.*, **4**, 221–227.

Paine, A., Eiz-Vesper, B., Blasczyk, R. and Immenschuh, S. (2010) Signaling to heme oxygenase-1 and its anti-inflammatory therapeutic potential. *Biochem. Pharmacol.*, **80**, 1895–1903.

Pallesen, L.J., Solodovnikova, N., Sharma, A.K. and Walden, W.E. (2013) Interaction with Cfd1 increases the kinetic lability of FeS on the Nbp35 scaffold. *J. Biol. Chem.*, **288**, 23358–23367.

Palmieri, F. (2013) The mitochondrial transporter family SLC25: identification, properties and physiopathology. *Mol. Aspects Med.*, **34**, 465–484.

Paradkar, P.N., Zumbrennen, K.B., Paw, B.H., Ward, D.M. and Kaplan, J. (2009) Regulation of mitochondrial iron import through differential turnover of mitoferrin 1 and mitoferrin 2. *Mol. Cell. Biol.*, **29**, 1007–1016.

Park, M.H., Nishimura, K., Zanelli, C.F. and Valentini, S.R. (2010) Functional significance of eIF5A and its hypusine modification in eukaryotes. *Amino Acids*, **38**, 491–500.

Paul, V.D. and Lill, R. (2015) Biogenesis of cytosolic and nuclear iron-sulfur proteins and their role in genome stability. *Biochim Biophys Acta*, **1853**, 1528–1539.

Perls, M. (1867) Nachweis von Eisenoxyd in gewissen Pigmenten. *Virchows Arch. A*, **39**, 42–48.

Petrat, F., De Groot, H., Sustmann, R. and Rauen, U. (2002) The chelatable iron pool in living cells: a methodically defined quantity. *Biol. Chem.*, **383**, 489–502.

Philpott, C.C. and Ryu, M-S. (2014) Special delivery: distributing iron in the cytosol of mammalian cells. *Front. Pharmacol.*, **5**, 173.

Picciocchi, A., Saguez, C., Boussac, A., Cassier-Chauvat, C. and Chauvat, F. (2007) CGFS type monothiol glutaredoxins from the cyanobacterium *Synechocystis* PCC6803 and other evolutionary distant model organisms possess a glutathione-ligated [2Fe-2S] cluster. *Biochemistry*, **46**, 15018–15026.

Proulx, K.L., Woodard, S.I. and Dailey, H.A. (1993) In situ conversion of coproporphyrinogen to heme by murine mitochondria: terminal steps of the heme biosynthetic pathway. *Protein Sci.*, **2**, 1092–1098.

Pukszta, S., Schilke, B., Dutkiewicz, R., *et al.* (2010) Co-evolution-driven switch of J protein specificity towards an Hsp70 partner. *EMBO Rep.*, **11**, 360–365.

Py, B. and Barras, F. (2010) Building Fe-S proteins: bacterial strategies. *Nat. Rev. Microbiol.*, **8**, 436–446.

Qi, W., Li, J., Chain, C.Y., *et al.* (2013) Glutathione-complexed iron–sulfur clusters. Reaction intermediates and evidence for a template effect promoting assembly and stability. *Chem. Commun.*, **4**, 6313–6315.

Ratliff, M., Zhu, W., Deshmukh, R., Wilks, A. and Stojiljkovic, I. (2001) Homologues of neisserial heme oxygenase in gram-negative bacteria: degradation of heme by the product of the pigA gene of *Pseudomonas aeruginosa*. *J. Bacteriol.*, **183**, 6394–6403.

Richter, G.W. (1978) The iron-loaded cell-the cytopathology of iron storage. *A review. Am. J. Pathol.*, **91**, 363–397.

Roche, B., Aussel, L., Ezraty, B., *et al.* (2013) Iron/sulfur proteins biogenesis in prokaryotes: formation, regulation and diversity. *Biochim. Biophys. Acta*, 1827, 455–469.

Rodriguez-Manzaneque, M.T., Tamarit, J., Belli, G., Ros, J. and Herrero E. (2002). Grx5 is a mitochondrial glutaredoxin required for the activity of iron/sulfur enzymes. *Mol. Biol. Cell*, **13**, 1109–1121.

Ross, J.F. (1946) The metabolism of inorganic and haemoglobin iron. *J. Clin. Invest.*, **25**, 933.

Rouault, T.A. (2015) Mammalian iron-sulphur proteins: novel insights into biogenesis and function. *Nat. Rev. Mol. Cell Biol.*, **16**, 45–55.

Rouhier, N., Couturier, J., Johnson, M.K. and Jacquot J. P. (2010). Glutaredoxins: roles in iron homeostasis. *Trends Biochem. Sci.*, **35**, 43–52.

Roy, A., Solodovnikova, N., Nicholson, T., Antholine, W. and Walden, W.E. (2003) A novel eukaryotic factor for cytosolic Fe-S cluster assembly. *EMBO J.*, **22**, 4826–4835.

Rudolf, J., Makrantoni, V., Ingledew, W.J., Stark, M.J. and White, M.F. (2006) The DNA repair helicases XPD and FancJ have essential iron-sulfur domains. *Mol. Cell*, **23**, 801–808.

Ryter, S.W., Alam, J. and Choi, A.M.K. (2006) Heme oxygenase-1/carbon monoxide: from basic science to therapeutic applications. *Physiol Rev.*, **86**, 583–650.

Sadlon, T.J., Dell'Oso, T., Surinya, K.H. and May, B.K. (1999) Regulation of erythroid 5-aminolevulinate synthase expression during erythropoiesis. *Int. J. Biochem. Cell Biol.*, **31**, 1153–1167.

Santambrogio, P., Biasiotto, G., Sanvito, F., *et al.* (2007) Mitochondrial ferritin expression in adult mouse tissues. *J. Histochem. Cytochem.*, **55**, 1129–1137.

Schaedler, T.A., Thornton, J.D., Kruse, I., *et al.* (2014) A conserved mitochondrial ATP-binding cassette transporter exports glutathione polysulfide for cytosolic metal cofactor assembly. *J. Biol. Chem.*, **289**, 23264–23274.

Schmucker, S., Martelli, A., Colin, F., *et al.* (2011) Mammalian frataxin: an essential function for cellular viability through an interaction with a preformed ISCU/NFS1/ISD11 iron-sulfur assembly complex. *PLoS One*, **6**, e16199.

Seki, M., Takeda, Y., Iwai, K. and Tanaka, K. (2013) IOP1 protein is an external component of the human cytosolic iron–sulfur cluster assembly (CIA) machinery and functions in the MMS19 protein-dependent CIA pathway. *J. Biol. Chem.*, **288**, 16680–16689.

Shakamuri, P., Zhang, B. and Johnson, M.K. (2012) Monothiol glutaredoxins function in storing and transporting [Fe2S2] clusters assembled on IscU scaffold proteins. *J. Am. Chem. Soc.*, **134**, 15213–15216.

Sharma, A.K., Pallesen, L.J., Spang, R.J. and Walden, W.E. (2010) Cytosolic iron–sulfur cluster assembly (CIA) system: factors, mechanism, and relevance to cellular iron regulation. *J. Biol. Chem.*, **285**, 26745–26751.

Shaw, G.C., Cope, J.J., Li, L., *et al.* (2006) Mitoferrin is essential for erythroid iron assimilation. *Nature*, **440**, 96–100.

Shawki, A., Knight, P.B., Maliken, B.D., Niespodzany, E.J. and Mackenzie, B. (2012) H(+)-coupled divalent metal-ion transporter-1: functional properties, physiological roles and therapeutics. *Curr. Top. Membr.*, **70**, 169–214.

Sheftel, A.D., Zhang, A.S., Brown, C., Shirihai, O.S. and Ponka, P. (2007) Direct interorganellar transfer of iron from endosome to mitochondrion. *Blood*, **110**, 125–132.

Sheftel, A.D., Stehling, O., Pierik, A.J., *et al.* (2009) Human ind1, an iron–sulfur cluster assembly factor for respiratory complex I. *Mol. Cell. Biol.*, **29**, 6059–6073.

Sheftel, A.D., Wilbrecht, C., Stehling, O., *et al.* (2012) The human mitochondrial ISCA1, ISCA2, and IBA57 proteins are required for [4Fe-4S] protein maturation. *Mol. Biol. Cell*, **23**, 1157–1166.

Shi, H., Bencze, K.Z., Stemmler, T.L. and Philpott C.C. (2008). A cytosolic iron chaperone that delivers iron to ferritin. *Science*, **320**, 1207–1210.

Shvartsman, M. and Ioav Cabantchik, Z. (2012) Intracellular iron trafficking: role of cytosolic ligands. *Biometals*, **25**, 711–723.

Sipos, K., Lange, H., Fekete, Z., *et al.* (2002). Maturation of cytosolic iron-sulfur proteins requires glutathione. *J. Biol. Chem.*, **277**, 26944–26949.

Soler, N., Craescu, C.T., Gallay, J., *et al.* (2012) A *S*-adenosylmethionine methyltransferase-like domain within the essential, Fe–S-containing yeast protein Dre2. *FEBS J.*, **279**, 2108–2119.

Srinivasan, V., Netz, D.J., Webert, H., *et al.* (2007) Structure of the yeast WD40 domain protein Cia1, a component acting late in iron–sulfur protein biogenesis. *Structure*, **15**, 1246–1257.

Srinivasan, V., Pierik, A.J. and Lill, R. (2014) Crystal structures of nucleotide-free and glutathione-bound mitochondrial ABC transporter Atm1. *Science*, **343**, 1137–1140.

Stehling, O. and Lill, R. (2013) The role of mitochondria in cellular iron–sulfur protein biogenesis: mechanisms, connected processes, and diseases. *Cold Spring Harb. Perspect. Med.*, **3**, 1–17.

Stehling, O., Netz, D.J., Niggemeyer, B., *et al.* (2008) Human Nbp35 is essential for both cytosolic iron–sulfur protein assembly and iron homeostasis. *Mol. Cell. Biol.*, **28**, 5517–5528.

Stehling, O., Mascarenhas, J., Vashisht, A.A., *et al.* (2012) Human CIA2A-FAM96A and CIA2B-FAM96B integrate iron homeostasis and maturation of different subsets of cytosolic-nuclear iron-sulfur proteins. *Cell Metab.*, **18**, 187–198.

Stehling, O., Wilbrecht, C. and Lill, R. (2014) Mitochondrial iron-sulfur protein biogenesis and human disease. *Biochimie*, **100**, 61–77.

Taguchi, K., Motohashi, H. and Yamamoto, M. (2011) Molecular mechanisms of the Keap1–Nrf2 pathway in stress response and cancer evolution. *Genes Cells*, **16**, 123–140.

Terali, K., Beavil, R.L., Pickersgill, R.W. and van der Giezen, M. (2013) The effect of the adaptor protein Isd11 on the quaternary structure of the eukaryotic cysteine desulphurase Nfs1. *Biochem. Biophys. Res. Commun.*, **440**, 235–240.

Tong, W.H., Jameson, G.N., Huynh, B.H. and Rouault, T.A. (2003) Subcellular compartmentalization of human Nfu, an iron-sulfur cluster scaffold protein, and its ability to assemble a [4Fe-4S] cluster. *Proc. Natl Acad. Sci. USA*, **100**, 9762–9767.

Tsai, C.L. and Barondeau, D.P. (2010) Human frataxin is an allosteric switch that activates the Fe-S cluster biosynthetic complex. *Biochemistry*, **49**, 9132–9139.

Tugores, A., Magness, S.T. and Brenner, D.A. (1994) A single promoter directs both housekeeping and erythroid preferential expression of the human ferrochelatase gene. *J. Biol. Chem.*, **269**, 30789–30797.

Urzica, E., Pierik, A.J., Muhlenhoff, U. and Lill, R. (2009) Crucial role of conserved cysteine residues in the assembly of two iron–sulfur clusters on the CIA protein Nar1. *Biochemistry*, **48**, 4946–4958.

Uzarska, M.A., Dutkiewicz, R., Freibert, S.A., Lill, R. and Mühlenhoff, U. (2013) The mitochondrial Hsp70 chaperone Ssq1 facilitates Fe/S cluster transfer from Isu1 to Grx5 by complex formation. *Mol. Biol. Cell*, **24**, 1830–1841.

van Wietmarschen, N., Moradian, A., Morin, G.B., *et al.* (2012) The mammalian proteins MMS19, MIP18, and ANT2 are involved in cytoplasmic iron–sulfur cluster protein assembly. *J. Biol. Chem.*, **287**, 43351–43358.

Vernis, L., Facca, C., Delagoutte, E., *et al.* (2009) A newly identified essential complex, Dre2–Tah18, controls mitochondria integrity and cell death after oxidative stress in yeast. *PLoS ONE*, **4**, e4376.

Vickery, L.E. and Cupp-Vickery, J.R. (2007) Molecular chaperones HscA/Ssq1 and HscB/Jac1 and their roles in iron-sulfur protein maturation. *Crit. Rev. Biochem. Mol. Biol.*, **42**, 95–111.

Volz, K. (2008) The functional duality of iron regulatory protein 1. *Curr. Opin. Struct. Biol.*, **18**, 106–111.

Weaver, J. and Pollack, S. (1989) Low-Mr iron isolated from guinea pig reticulocytes as AMP-Fe and ATP-Fe complexes. *Biochem. J.*, **261**, 787–792.

Webert, H., Freibert, S.A., Gallo, A., *et al.*, (2014) Functional reconstitution of mitochondrial Fe/S cluster synthesis on Isu1 reveals the involvement of ferredoxin. *Nat. Commun.*, **5**, 5013.

Weerapana, E., Wang, C., Simon, G.M., *et al.* (2010) Quantitative reactivity profiling predicts functional cysteines in proteomes. *Nature*, **468**, 790–795.

Wiedemann, N., Urzica, E., Guiard, B., *et al.* (2006) Essential role of Isd11 in mitochondrial iron-sulfur cluster synthesis on Isu scaffold proteins. *EMBO J.*, **25**, 184–195.

Wilks, A. and Heinzl, G. (2014) Heme oxygenation and the widening paradigm of heme degradation. *Arch. Biochem. Biophys.*, **15** (544), 87–95.

Wingert, R.A., Galloway, J.L., Barut, B., *et al.* (2005) Deficiency of glutaredoxin 5 reveals Fe-S clusters are required for vertebrate haem synthesis. *Nature*, **436** 1035–1039.

Wu, C.K., Dailey, H.A., Rose, J.P., *et al.* (2001) The 2.0 Å structure of human ferrochelatase, the terminal enzyme of heme biosynthesis. *Nat. Struct. Biol.*, **8**, 156–160.

Yanatori, I., Yasui, Y., Tabuchi, M. and Kishi, F. (2014) Chaperone protein involved in transmembrane transport of iron. *Biochem. J.*, **462**, 25–37.

Ye, H., Jeong, S.Y., Ghosh, M.C., *et al.* (2010). Glutaredoxin 5 deficiency causes sideroblastic anemia by specifically impairing heme biosynthesis and depleting cytosolic iron in human erythroblasts. *J. Clin. Invest.*, **120**, 1749–1761.

Yien, Y.Y., Robledo, R.F., Schultz, I.J., *et al.* (2014) TMEM14C is required for erythroid mitochondrial heme metabolism. *J. Clin. Invest.*, **124**, 4294–4304.

Yoshida, T. and Kikuchi, G. (1978) Features of the reaction of heme degradation catalyzed by the reconstituted microsomal heme oxygenase system. *J. Biol. Chem.*, **253**, 4230–4236.

Zhang, B., Crack, J.C., Subramanian, S., *et al.* (2012) Reversible cycling between cysteine persulfide-ligated [2Fe-2S] and cysteine-ligated [4Fe-4S] clusters in the FNR regulatory protein. *Proc. Natl Acad. Sci. USA*, **109**, 15734–15739.

Zhang, Y., Li, H., Zhang, C., *et al.* (2008a) Conserved electron donor complex Dre2 Tah18 is required for ribonucleotide reductase metallocofactor assembly and DNA synthesis. *Proc. Natl Acad. Sci. USA*, **111**, E1695–E1704.

Zhang, Y., Lyver, E.R., E. Nakamaru-Ogiso, E., *et al.* (2008b) Dre2, a conserved eukaryotic Fe/S cluster protein, functions in cytosolic Fe/S protein biogenesis. *Mol. Cell. Biol.* **28**, 5569–5582.

Zheng, L., White, R.H., Cash, V.L. and Dean, D.R. (1994) Mechanism for the desulfurization of L-cysteine catalyzed by the nifS gene product. *Biochemistry*, **33**, 4714–4720.

9

Iron Storage Proteins

9.1 Introduction

The ubiquitous labile iron pool (LIP) together with the panoply of reactions involving iron in the biosynthesis of Fe–S proteins and in the biosynthesis and degradation of haem has been reviewed in Chapter 8. There is, however, one aspect of intracellular iron metabolism which has not been addressed, which is the pool of storage iron deposited within ferritin and haemosiderin in mammals, and in the Dps proteins in many microbial species. The importance of storage as a necessary complement to transport was pithily summarised by Gideon Bauer at a meeting on Transport by Proteins (Crichton, 1978), when he pointed out that "…transport firms all over the world usually keep big warehouses for storage". Clearly, in the case of iron, these iron storage proteins represent not only a way to maintain iron in a soluble, non-toxic and bioavailable form, but they also constitute a reserve which the organism can draw on when iron availability becomes a problem. In this chapter, the ferritin superfamily of iron storage proteins is discussed before attention is turned to the mineral core deposited within the protein shell and the product of ferritin aggregation and degradation, haemosiderin, which is found in iron overload. The mechanisms involved in iron uptake into ferritin are then addressed, followed by a brief overview of how storage iron might be mobilised from the storage proteins. Finally, a brief review is provided of some ways in which the apoferritin protein shell can be used as a 'nanoreactor' for the formation of a variety of non-native, unusual, mineralised nanoparticles.

Iron Metabolism – From Molecular Mechanisms to Clinical Consequences, Fourth Edition. Robert Crichton.
© 2016 John Wiley & Sons, Ltd. Published 2016 by John Wiley & Sons, Ltd.

9.2 The Ferritin Superfamily and Haemosiderins

9.2.1 The Ferritin Superfamily

Historically, the first pool of iron to be observed within mammalian cells was haemosiderin, originally identified histologically as iron-rich granules in tissues, which gave an intense Prussian blue reaction with potassium ferrocyanide (Perls, 1867). Haemosiderin was first isolated by Cook (1929) and was described as consisting of 'organic granules impregnated with some form of ferric oxide'. It is insoluble, visible by light microscopy as golden yellow intracellular granules, and in iron-loaded animals is localised in membranous structures termed siderosomes (Richter, 1978), which appear to be derived from lysosomes. Haemosiderin has a variable, but higher iron content than ferritin, and represents the vast majority of the excess iron stored in clinical iron-overloading disorders. This constitutes the lysosomal iron pool in iron-loaded subjects or animals.

Haemosiderin is derived from the soluble storage form, ferritin, which was first crystallised from horse spleen by the Czech physiologist Vilem Laufberger[1] as an 'iron-rich protein', which he correctly speculated served as a depot for iron in the body (Laufberger, 1937). The name was adapted from the iron-rich protein that Naunyn Schmiedeberg had isolated from pig liver in 1894 and had called 'ferratin'. Both, ferritin and haemosiderin consist of a central inorganic ferric oxyhydroxide core, which in ferritin is surrounded by a well-organised apoferritin protein shell. The protein component of haemosiderin is poorly characterised, but seems to contain some apoferritin, or degradation products of apoferritin. Haemosiderin is thought to be derived from the intralysosomal aggregation and degradation of ferritin.

In normal human subjects some 25% of total body iron (800–1000 mg) is present in the storage forms, mostly as ferritin. Whereas it is likely that all mammalian cell types contain some ferritin, haemosiderin in normal subjects is essentially restricted to cells of the reticuloendothelial system. Ferritin turns out to be almost universal in its distribution: ferritin and ferritin-like proteins have been found in all organisms except for yeasts and one or two archaebacteria. In contrast, haemosiderin has not been found to any extent outside of iron-loaded animals, except for a brief report of a phytosiderin in pea seeds (Laulhere *et al.*, 1989).

Classically, ferritins can be defined as oligomeric proteins of 24 identical or similar subunits, forming a hollow protein shell, capable of storing iron (in mammalian ferritins up to 4500 atoms) in a water-soluble, non-toxic, bioavailable form, often as ferric hydroxyphosphate micelles (Crichton, 2009). This definition does not encompass other members of the ferritin superfamily, like the 24-subunit artemins of the brine shrimp, which do not retain iron (Chen *et al.*, 2007), and the bacterial Dps proteins which, unlike classical ferritins, contain only 12 subunits (Su *et al.*, 2005), but still sequester iron inside a hollow protein shell. In this section, the members of the evolutionary dynasty represented by the *ferritin superfamily*, are discussed, all of which have diverse functions but all are thought to share a common structural motif, namely a four-helical bundle (or part thereof) (Finn *et al.*, 2010; Lundin *et al.*, 2012). The ferritins are ancient proteins, common in all three domains of life, which have travelled a considerable evolutionary journey, derived from the far more simplistic rubrerythrin-like molecules which play roles in defence against toxic oxygen species.

---

[1] Laufberger had tried to obtain the protein from horse liver, but it did not crystallise and, as he pointed out to me when I met him in Prague some years ago, in the 1930s crystallization was *the* criterion of purity. Although James Sumner had crystallised jack bean urease in 1926, his preparations were somewhat impure, and it was only in the mid-1930s, when John Northrop and Moses Kunitz showed that there is a direct correlation between the enzymatic activities of crystalline pepsin, trypsin and chymotrypsin that the protein nature of enzymes was generally accepted.

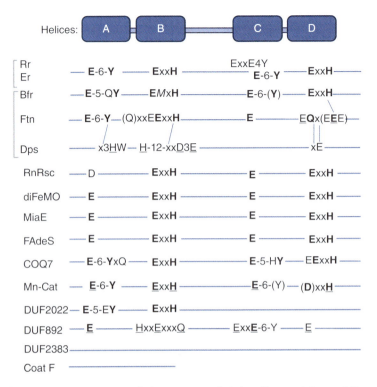

Figure 9.1 *Schematic representation of the conserved defined/potential metal ligands within the ferritin-like superfamily. Approximate positions of key conserved residues within the four long helices of the helical bundle are indicated schematically. Residues in bold are those associated with the central dinuclear iron site and are widely conserved across the superfamily with structurally equivalent locations. Those residues in brackets are partially conserved. Reprinted with permission from Elsevier from Andrews, S.C. (2010) The ferritin-like superfamily: Evolution of the biological iron storeman from a rubrerythrin-like ancestor.* Biochim. Biophys. Acta, ***1800****, 691–705*

The ferritin 'superfamily' consists of some 11 500 members within the *Pfamseq* database (Finn *et al.*, 2010), distributed between at least 12 'subfamilies' (Figure 9.1), of which the ferritins are the most abundant (34%) (Andrews, 2010). Within the superfamily, there are three distinct types of iron-storing (or iron-detoxifying) protein: (i) the classical 24-meric ferritins; (ii) the haem-containing 24-meric bacterioferritins of prokaryotes; and (iii) the prokaryotic 12-meric Dps proteins, which bind to and protect DNA. These three ferritin types are similar, but also possess unique properties that distinguish them and enable them to achieve their specific physiological purposes. The 24-meric ferritins utilise very similar intrasubunit ferroxidase centres to catalyse iron oxidation, whereas the 12-meric Dps proteins employ an intersubunit ferroxidase centre (Andrews, 2010). Figure 9.1 presents the conserved or potential metal ligands within the ferritin superfamily. Several of the better-known members of the other 'subfamilies' are briefly described here. Class 1 ribonucleotide reductases (RnRsc) are common in bacteria and eukaryotes, but are rare in the archaea, and the smaller of their two polypeptide chains is a ferritin-like protein (see Chapter 2), which contains both the active site Tyr radical and the di-iron site responsible for its formation. The six di-iron ligands, one Asp, two His and three Glu residues, closely match the di-iron binding motif of the ferritin-like superfamily and are located at structurally similar positions within the ferritin-like four-helical bundle (Nordlund *et al.*, 1990). The rubrerythrins/erythrins (Rr, Er) found in many microaerophilic and anaerobic bacteria and archae, particularly sulphate-reducing bacteria, have an N-terminal ferritin-like four-helix bundle which contains a similar di-iron cluster together with a C-terminal rubredoxin-like domain containing an Fe–Cys$_4$ cluster (deMaré *et al.*, 1996; Sieker *et al.*, 2000). They act as a defence against toxic oxygen species (Kurtz, 2006), and appear to be the precursors of the ferritin superfamily (Andrews, 2010). Hydrocarbon oxidation in multicomponent monooxygenases, such as methane monooxygenase (diFeMO), which catalyse the hydroxylation of a variety of hydrocarbon substrates, including alkanes, alkenes and aromatics, has also evolved from a common ancestral di-iron containing, ferritin-like protein (Leahy *et al.*, 2003; Sazinsky and Lippard, 2006), while the bacterial and plant type 2 fatty acid desaturases (Fades), which catalyse the formation of a double bond in fatty acids (Shanklin *et al.*, 2009), the MiaE bacterial tRNA hydroxylases (Mathevon *et al.*, 2007) and the Mn-catalases (Mn-Cat) (Barynin *et al.*, 2001), constitute other subfamilies.

The ferritins are an unusual example of a family of proteins that possess an overall three-dimensional (3D) shape which is entirely critical for their function (Crichton and Declercq, 2010). Many proteins are built around a substrate-binding site, a ligand-binding site, a transport channel, and so on, which specifies the role of the protein, whilst the rest of the protein surrounding the critical functional part acts as little more than a relatively inert scaffold, holding the reactive site in place. But for ferritins, the 3D shape is all important and essentially defines their function. The ferritins are polymers of identical (or highly similar) subunits which act as building blocks for the assembly of a large, hollow protein which is roughly spherical in shape (Crichton and Declercq, 2010). The subunits consist of a characteristic four-helical bundle (helices A–D) (Figure 9.2), which can itself be divided into two homologous pairs of anti-parallel helices with helix B linked to helix C via a long loop that traverses the full length of the helical bundle (Figure 9.2): helices A–B are evolutionarily related to helices C–D (Kurtz and Prickril, 1991; deMaré *et al.*, 1995). The striking similarity of the global subunit fold in ferritins and Dps proteins, particularly the central four-helix bundle is illustrated in Figure 9.3. This presents ribbon diagrams of the subunit structure of recombinant human H and horse L chain ferritins (HuHF and HoLF), non-haem-containing bacterioferritin (FTN) from *Escherichia coli*, haem-containing bacterioferritin (BFR) from *Desulfovibrio desulfuricans*, and one of the DPS proteins from *Deinococcus radiodurans*.

The first ever apoferritin sequences, horse spleen L-chain (Heusterspreute and Crichton, 1981) and human L-chain (Wustefeld and Crichton, 1982), were determined by what are now considered to be almost prehistoric, so-called 'direct' methods. Subsequently, innumerable ferritin sequences, obtained either by DNA sequencing,[2] as in the case of human H ferritin, or by genome sequencing, have been reported. Ferritins are found in a wide range of species, including animals, plants, fungi, eubacteria and archaebacteria, but are notably absent from many fungal species (e.g. *Saccharomyces cerevisiae*) as well as the eubacteria *Mycoplasma genitalium*, *Streptococcus pyogenes* and two archaebacterial *Pyrococcus* genomes (*P. horikoshii* and *P. abyssi*). Some ferritins have N-terminal extensions which lie on the outside of the assembled shell and target the ferritin to a specific destination such as plastids in plants and yolk sac in snails (Andrews *et al.*, 1992; Lobréaux *et al.*, 1992). For example, pea ferritin is synthesised with an N-terminal extension of 75 residues, which is missing from the mature protein. The first part of this extension is a chloroplast-targeting sequence of 47 residues, which is lost on entry into the plastid. The second part, an extension

---

[2]When the human spleen apoferritin was published, we included, together with the main sequence, the sequences of some 70 residues which did not fit into the principal sequence, pointing out that it was probably that of the H-subunit. The complete H-sequence, based on cDNA sequencing, was published a short time later (Costanzo *et al.*, 1984; Boyd *et al.*, 1985).

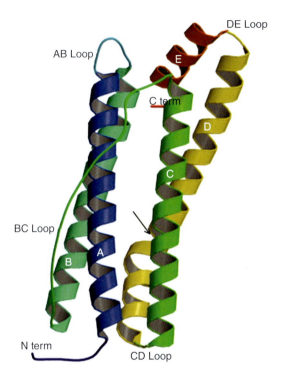

Figure 9.2 *Ribbon diagram of recombinant horse L apoferritin, PDB 2v2i, showing the relationship of the secondary structure elements to the inner and outer surface of the 24-mer. The outer surface (front) consists of helices A and C and the loop BC, while the inner surface (behind) is made up of helices B and D. Helix E is inclined at ~60° to the four-helix bundle. The subunit is coloured progressively from blue at the N terminus to red at the C terminus. The kink in the D helix is indicated by the arrow. Produced with MOLSCRIPT (Kraulis, 1991). Reprinted with permission from Elsevier from Crichton, R.R. and Declercq, J.P. (2010) X-ray structures of ferritins and related proteins. Biochim. Biophys. Acta, **1800**, 706–718*

peptide, is lost prior to assembly of the 24-subunit oligomer, and its loss is a prerequisite for assembly (Proudhon *et al.*, 1989). The ferritin-like protein, artemin, has C-terminal extensions which fill the cavity within the shell, and prevent iron storage (Chen *et al.*, 2007), while (as will be seen in Chapter 15) in the human neurodegenerative disease neuroferrinopathy the patients have pathogenic mutations in the light chain of ferritin which are all predicted to alter the carboxy-terminal sequence of the protein, preventing iron incorporation (Keogh *et al.*, 2012). For a detailed review of the ferritins and other members of the ferritin superfamily, and their evolution from far more simplistic rubrerythrin-like molecules which play roles in defence against toxic oxygen species, see Andrews (2010).

9.2.2 Structure of Vertebrate and Invertebrate Ferritins

Ferritins are tetracosameric protein shells (24-mers) made up of identical or similar subunits, which form a hollow protein shell within which a non-toxic, water-soluble, yet bioavailable, iron core is stored. Mammalian ferritins are typically heteropolymers, made up of two subunits with distinct amino acid sequences, known as H (predominant in heart, designated heavy) and L (predominant in liver, designated light). The H chain ferritins are characterised by a di-iron,

(a)   (b)   (c)

(d)   (e)

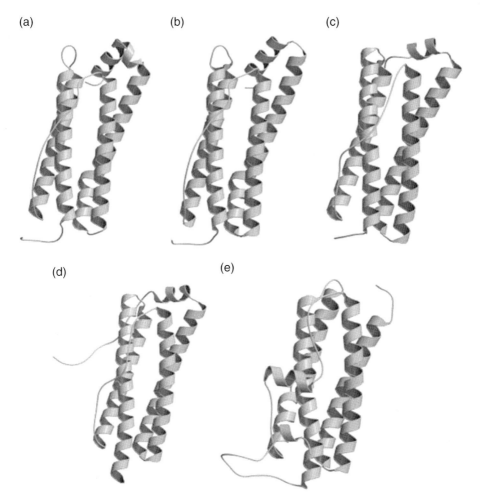

Figure 9.3 *Ribbon diagram of the subunit structure of mammalian H- and L-subunits, bacterioferritin (FTN) haem-containing bacterioferritin (BFR) and Dps protein. (a) human H-chain ferritin, PDB 2fha; (b) horse L-chain ferritin, PDB 2v2i; (c) E. coli bacterioferritin (FTN), PDB 2htn; (d) haem-containing D. desulfuricans bacterioferritin (BFR), PDB 1nfv; and (e) D. radiodurans DPS protein, PDB 2c2u. Produced with MOLSCRIPT (Kraulis, 1991). Reprinted with permission from Elsevier from Crichton, R.R. and Declercq, J.P. (2010) X-ray structures of ferritins and related proteins. Biochim. Biophys. Acta, 1800, 706–718*

ferroxidase centre, involved in the oxidation of Fe^{2+} to Fe^{3+}, whereas the L chains are thought to be involved in the nucleation of the iron core of ferritin (*vide infra*). The H chain is typically longer than L, at both the N and the C terminus (in the rest of this chapter, numbering is based on the H subunit). Whereas the H and L sequences show only about 54% identity, about 90% of H chain residues are identical between species, while 85% of L chain residues are identical. However, when only residues which are responsible for interactions between subunits are considered, the conservation of primary structure between H and L chains rises to 79% (Chasteen and Harrison, 1999). Variations in the amount of the two subunits between different human tissues mean that, for example, in liver and spleen – which play an important role in iron storage – the population of ferritin molecules has a much greater content of the L subunit, whereas in human heart and brain – which play a more important role in iron detoxification – heteropolymers rich in H subunits are predominant, As will be seen later, the effective storage of iron in mammalian ferritins requires contributions from both types of subunit. This seems to explain why heteropolymers rather than homopolymers are normally found. Homopolymers are only found in pathological situations such as the Hereditary Hyperferritinaemia Cataract Syndrome (HHCS), where L chain homopolymers, devoid of iron, are present (Levi *et al.*, 1998).

Some species have a third, intermediate chain, designated M, such as tadpole (Dickey *et al.*, 1987), the Antarctic teleost *Trematomus bernacchii*, and the Atlantic salmon *Salmo salar* (Andersen *et al.*, 1995; Mignogna *et al.*, 2002); these M chain sequences are much more similar to the mammalian H chain than to the L chain.

The subunit structure consists of a closed, four-helical bundle with a left-handed twist with one crossover connection between helix B and helix C. This is illustrated as a ribbon diagram for recombinant horse L apoferritin subunit in Figure 9.2. Nearly three-quarters of the 174 residues of the subunit are disposed within five α helices designated A, B,C, D, and E, corresponding approximately to residues 14–40, 49–76, 96–123, 127–161, and 163–173 (H chain numbering). Helices A–D constitute a characteristic long central bundle of four parallel and anti-parallel helices, with the fifth short helix, E, butting on to one end of the α-helical bundle. The relationship of the secondary structure elements to the inner and outer surface of the 24-mer is such that the outer surface consists of helices A and C and the loop BC (in the front), while the inner surface (behind) is made up of helices B and D.

The first 3D structure of a ferritin to be determined, at a final resolution of 2.6 Å (Rice *et al.*, 1983; Ford *et al.*, 1984) (although unfortunately, the coordinates were never deposited), was that of horse spleen apoferritin, with an average composition of about $L_{21}H_3$ (the crystallisation step may have selected a population with an even higher content of L subunits). Since, in the cubic space group F432 all subunits are statistically equivalent, the electron density contours can be interpreted solely in terms of the predominant L subunit. It has generally proved very difficult to crystallise heteropolymers, and the best results in crystallographic terms have therefore been obtained with recombinant homopolymers. However, while the study of homopolymers of mammalian ferritins represents a great convenience, it constitutes a physiological simplification since, as pointed out above and discussed in greater detail later, mammalian ferritins usually have both subunit types present within the 24-mer, and both subunit types appear to play important roles in the iron-storage function of the molecule.

The compact, symmetrical and extremely stable apoferritin shell is the outcome of the assembly of 24 subunits with octahedral 432 symmetry. The shell has the approximate geometry of a rhombic dodecahedron (Figure 9.4), the faces of which consist of two subunits related by a twofold symmetry axis at its centre (e.g., I and II or III and VI), with each subunit I interacting with five other subunits (III–VII). A characteristic structural feature of ferritins, and indeed Dps proteins, is their propensity to form dimers. Even if the overall pathway, or pathways, of oligomerisation remain unclear there is a general consensus that the subunit dimer is almost certainly the first intermediate to be formed (Stefanini *et al.*, 1987; Gerl and Jaenicke, 1987a,b). The interface between the two participating subunits I and II along this long (22 Å) interface involves the helices A and B, as well as the BC loops, the N terminus and the AB turn. There is extensive contact, which can be divided into two equivalent, symmetry-related halves involving many hydrophobic residues, with several hydrophilic interactions clustered at the ends of the interface. In L chain apoferritins, towards the centre of the interface, a cluster of four glutamate side chains from the B helix (Glu57, 60, 61, 64) extend into the cavity in a diamond-shaped array and are thought to participate in iron micelle formation (see later).

(a)

(b)

(c)

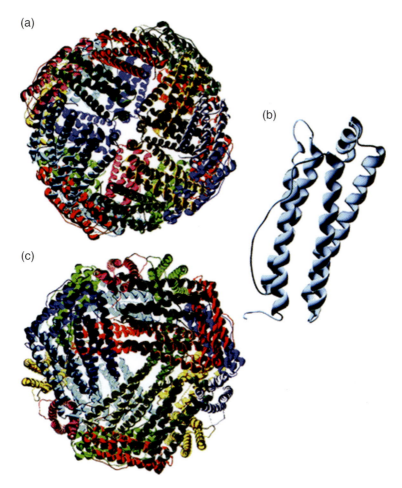

Figure 9.4   *(a) Schematic diagram indicating labelling used for symmetry-related subunits. Reproduced with permission from Hempstead, P.D., Yewdall, S.J., Fernie, A.R. et al. (1997) Comparison of the three-dimensional structures of recombinant human H and horse L ferritins at high resolution. J. Mol. Biol.,* ***268****, 424–448; © 1997, Elsevier. (b) 24-meric human H-chain ferritin molecule viewed down the fourfold symmetry axis. (c) 24-meric human H-chain ferritin molecule viewed down the threefold symmetry axis. Reproduced with permission of The Royal Society of Chemistry from Lewin, A., Moore, G.R. and Le Brun, N.E. (2005) Formation of protein-coated iron minerals. Dalton Trans., 3597–3610*

The other long side of subunit I interacts with the ends of subunits III and VI, while the two ends of subunit I also interact with subunits IV and VII (Figure 9.4). Most of the intersubunit interactions involving both hydrophobic and hydrophilic interactions lie within these interfaces, between the threefold and fourfold axes. The threefold axis-related interactions I–III and IV–I are identical, as are those around the fourfold axis (I–VI and VII–I), while there are only limited contacts across the fourfold axis (I–V).

The subunit arrangement viewed down the four- and threefold axes of symmetry is shown in Figure 9.4, and there are two clearly discernible channels leading from the outside to the inside of the protein shell along the fourfold and threefold axes of symmetry, with the six fourfold channels essentially hydrophobic, whereas the eight threefold axes are extremely hydrophilic with three

Glu134 residues, towards the outer surface of the protein shell, and three Asp 131 residues, towards the inner surface, which are conserved in both H and L subunits. These channels allow iron (and other small molecules) to enter and exit the protein, as will be seen later. The hollow cavity enclosed within the confines of the apoferritin protein shell is a crucial part of the design since it allows ferritins to function as 'molecular cages' for the storage of large amounts of iron.

In insects, ferritins are secreted proteins and are thought to play a major role in both iron storage and transport (Strickler-Dinglasan *et al.*, 2006; Wang *et al.*, 2009; Kim *et al.*, 2009). The crystal structure of insect ferritin also shows a tetrahedral symmetry consisting of 12 heavy chain and 12 light chain subunits, in contrast to that of mammalian ferritin. Insect ferritins are often glycosylated and are synthesised with a signal peptide which targets them to the vacuolar system where they serve as iron transporters – quite the opposite of mammalian ferritins, which are mainly cytoplasmic and serve as iron-storage proteins (Pham and Winzerling, 2010). Both, H and L subunits have secretion signals that direct them to the endoplasmic reticulum (ER) during translation and, as a result, their ferritin is confined to the secretory pathway (ER, Golgi complexes, and secretory vesicles) and is abundant in the haemolymph but not in the cytosol (Nichol *et al.*, 2002; Pham and Winzerling, 2010). In non-blood-feeding insects such as fruit flies and moths, secreted ferritin consists of equal numbers of H and L subunits (Hamburger *et al.*, 2005; Missirlis *et al.*, 2007). The crystal structure of the secreted ferritin from the lepidopteran *Trichoplusia ni* (cabbage looper) has been determined (Hamburger *et al.*, 2005), and is presented in Figure 9.5. The 12 H- and 12 L-chain subunits are arranged with tetrahedral (32) symmetry, which creates two distinct types of threefold axis pores. Structural analysis indicates that Cys residues present on each of the subunits allow the formation of such a tetrahedral structure with intra-subunit disulfide bridges involving Cys21 and Cys130 in the H-chain and Cys4 and Cys24 in the L-chain, together with an inter-subunit disulphide bond between Cys3 of the H chain and Cys12 of the L chain. Some of the Cys residues required for this configuration are not conserved in the mosquito ferritins (Pham and Winzerling, 2010). Another notable difference from mammalian ferritins is an N-terminal extension in both H- and L-subunits, unique to secreted insect ferritins, which form extended loops that bridge adjacent subunits on the outside of the ferritin shell.

9.2.3 Plant and Bacterial Ferritins

As mentioned in Chapter 5, plant ferritins have some unique structural features, notably the presence of two plant-specific N-terminal amino acid sequences, the transit peptide (TP) and the extension peptide (EP). This characteristic is found not only in ferritins from land plants, such as monocots and dicots, but also in algal ferritins. Whereas ferritins from cyanobacteria and diatoms have sequences which are rather similar to bacterioferritins (Laulhère *et al.*, 1992; Keren *et al.*, 2004; Marchetti *et al.*, 2009), green algae have plant ferritin-like molecules (Long *et al.*, 2008; Wu *et al.*, 2009). The TP is responsible for targeting plant ferritin to plastids, and is removed from the N terminus after entering the plastid (Lescure *et al.*, 1991). The EP, downstream from the TP, constitutes the N-terminal region of the mature plant ferritin, and has been reported to be cleaved from the core region in the germination process in legume seeds (Ragland *et al.*, 1990) to generate the 22 kDa form, which readily associates to form insoluble phytosiderin, thereby destabilizing the protein shell (Van Wuytswinkel *et al.*, 1995). The crystal structure of soybean ferritin 4 has been determined, revealing that it has high structural similarity to vertebrate ferritin, except for the N-terminal EP region, the short C-terminal E-helix, and the end of the BC loop (Masuda *et al.*, 2010a). The EP forms a helix which lies along the outer surface of the protein shell. In further studies, the crystalline structure of plant ferritin from the green algea *Ulva pertusa* (sea lettuce)

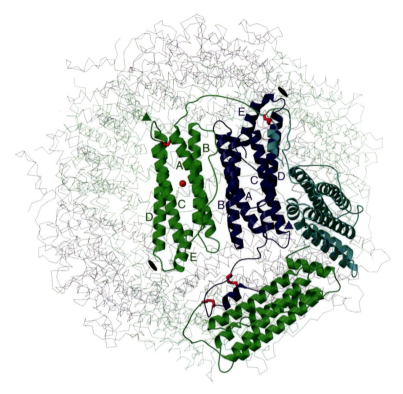

Figure 9.5 *Structures of* T. ni *ferritin H- and L-chains. Ribbon diagrams of the H- (green) and L- (blue and light blue) subunits. The Fe^{3+} at the ferroxidase site is shown in red. Also shown are the approximate locations of the threefold axes (blue and green triangles) and the pseudo fourfold axes (black ovals). Disulphide-bonded cysteine residues are shown in magenta in ball-and-stick representation. The N-terminal region of each subunit extends on the outside of the ferritin shell and forms a disulphide bond with a non-adjacent subunit of the opposite type. Helices A–E are labelled in green for the H-chain and in blue for the L-chain. Reprinted with permission from Elsevier from Hamburger, A.E., West, A.P. Jr, Hamburger, Z.A., et al. (2005) Crystal structure of a secreted insect ferritin reveals a symmetrical arrangement of heavy and light chains.* J. Mol. Biol., **349**, *558–569*

(Masuda *et al.*, 2012) has been established (Figure 9.6), showing that EP interacts with the neighbouring threefold symmetry-related subunit, contributing to both shell stability and surface hydrophobicity.

There are two types of ferritin in bacteria, the archetypal ferritins of the H type similar to those found in eukaryotes (usually designated Ftn), and the haem-containing bacterioferritins (designated Bfrs). Ftn homologues have also been identified and characterised in archaeon species. There has been some confusion in the literature, since some Ftns have been cited as Bfrs, despite the fact that they do not have bound haem; examples include BfrB from *Mycobacterium tuberculosis* (Khare *et al.*, 2011) and BfrA from *Pseudomonas aeruginosa* (Yao *et al.*, 2011). The high-resolution structure of one of the two non-haem-containing ferritins of *E. coli*, EcFTNA (Stillman *et al.*, 2001), shows considerable structural similarity to human H chain ferritin (rms deviation of main chain atoms 0.066 nm), despite the low sequence identity (only 22%). While little conservation of residues involved in intersubunit interactions is found,

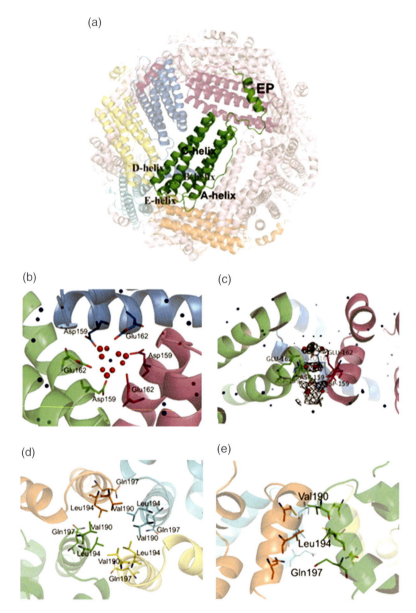

Figure 9.6 *(a) Overall structure of UpFER. A single subunit is highlighted in green. (b and c) The metal entry channel around a threefold symmetry axis. This image is viewed down a threefold symmetry axis from outside of the shell (b) and viewed perpendicular to the axes (c). Calcium ions are shown as red balls. Water molecules (oxygen) are shown as blue balls. Asp159 and Glu162 of UpFER correspond to Asp131 and Glu134 of human H-chain ferritin. (d and e) The structure of UpFER around the fourfold symmetry axis. The fourfold channels are represented by two different orientations: (d) aligned on the fourfold axis and (b) perpendicular to the axis. Val190 and Leu194 of UpFER correspond to Leu165 and Leu169 of human H-chain ferritin, respectively. Reproduced with permission from John Wiley & Sons from Masuda, T., Morimoto, S., Mikami, B. and Toyohara, H. (2012) The extension peptide of plant ferritin from sea lettuce contributes to shell stability and surface hydrophobicity.* Protein Sci., **21**, 786–796

many of the conserved residues are clustered in the centre of the four-helix bundle. All seven residues of the ferroxidase centre of HuHF are found in EcFTN, although one of the Glu ligands (Glu61 in HuHF) is derived from a different part of the polypeptide chain in EcFTN (Glu130).

Among the FTN structures deposited at the PDB are those from *E. coli* (PDB code 1eum[3]; Stillman *et al.*, 2001), *Campylobacter jejuni* (PDB code: 1krq; unpublished work), *Archaeoglobus fulgidus* (PDB code: 1s3q; Johnson *et al.*, 2005), *Pyrococcus furiosus* (PDB code: 2jd6; Tatur *et al.*, 2007), *Helicobacter pylori* (PDB code: 3egm; Cho *et al.*, 2009), *Thermotoga maritima* (PDB code:1vlg; unpublished work), *Pseudomonas aeruginosa* (PDB code: 3r2k; Yao *et al.*, 2011) and *Mycobacterium tuberculosis* (PDB code: 3qd8; Khare *et al.*, 2011; 3oj5, 3uno: unpublished work). Three of these are illustrated in Figure 9.7 (upper). Although the structure of the ferritin monomer from the hyperthermophilic Archaeon *Archaeoglobus fulgidus* has a high degree of structural similarity with ferritins from *E. coli* and humans, its quaternary structure is novel, since the 24 subunits assemble into a shell with tetrahedral (2–3) rather than the canonical octahedral (4–3–2) symmetry of archetypal ferritins (Johnson *et al.*, 2005). The difference in assembly opens four large (~45 Å) pores in the *A. fulgidus* ferritin shell (Figure 9.7, top left), when compared with other Ftns and Bfrs.

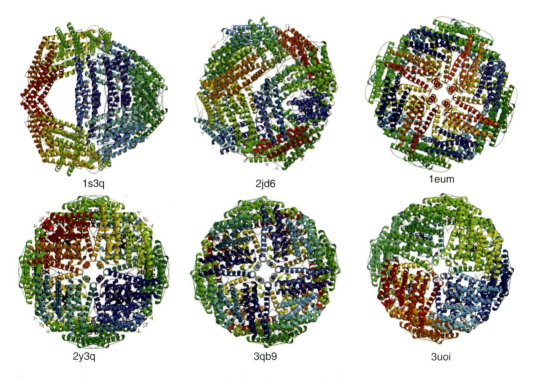

1s3q 2jd6 1eum

2y3q 3qb9 3uoi

Figure 9.7 *The quaternary structures of selected Ftns and Bfns. Ftn structures (top, left to right)* Archaeoglobus fulgidus *(PDB code: 1s3q);* Pyrococcus furiosus *(PDB code: 2jd6);* Escherichia coli *(PDB code 1eum). Bfn structures (lower, left to right)* Escherichia coli *(PDB code: 2y3q);* Mycobacterium tuberculosis *(PDB code: 3qb9);* Mycobacterium tuberculosis *(PDB code: 3uoi)*

---

[3] Where possible for protein structures the PDB reference as well as the relevant publication are cited – however some structures deposited at the PDB are unpublished, and only the PDB number is given.

The second class of ferritins in bacteria, BFRs, contain haem and were first unequivocally iden-tified by Steifel and Watt (1979), since when they have been isolated from many bacteria and identified in the gene sequences of many others. They are homopolymers of H chain-type subunits and they all contain an iron-protoporphyrin as an integral part of the protein, which is usually protoporphyrin IX (Fe(II)-protoporphyrin IX is haem), although in the case of *Desulphovibrio desulfuricans*, Fe-coproporphyrin III is the haem cofactor, the first example of such a haem in a biological system (Romao *et al.*, 2000). A number of Bfr structures are known, including those from *E. coli* (PDB code: 1bcf; Frolow *et al.*, 1994; PDB code: 1bfr; Dautant *et al.*, 1998; Frolow and Kalb, 2001; PDB code: 2htn; van Eerde *et al.*, 2006; PDB code: 2vxi; Willies *et al.*, 2009; PDB code: 3eil; Crow *et al.*, 2009; PDB code: 2y3q; Antonyuk and Hough, 2011), *Rhodobacter capsulatus* (PDB code: 1jgc; Cobessi *et al.*, 2002), *Desulphovibrio desulfuricans* (PDB code: 1nf6; Macedo *et al.*, 2003), *Azotobacter vinelandii* (PDB code: 1sof; Liu *et al.*, 2004; PDB code: 2fkz; Swartz *et al.*, 2006), *Mycobacterium tuberculosis* (PDB code: 2wtl; Gupta *et al.*, 2009: PDB code: 3uoi: unpublished work), *Pseudomonas aeruginosa* (PDB code:3isf; Weeratunga *et al.*, 2010), *Brucella melitensis* (PDB code: 3fvb: unpublished work), *Campylobacter jejuni* (PDB code: 3kwo: unpublished work).

The structures of three Bfrs are illustrated in Figure 9.7 (lower). The EcBfr subunit has a hydro-philic region at the centre of its four-helical bundle with hydrophobic regions at each extremity, which contains, in common with HuHF and EcFTN, five of the residues of the ferroxidase site which is described below. The long, mostly hydrophobic I:II intersubunit contact supplies a relatively uncrowded central pocket in the dimer interface in which haem is bound (Figure 9.8), usually with

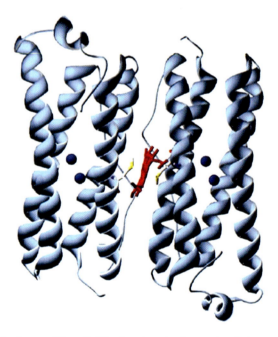

Figure 9.8 *The subunit dimer of* E. coli *Bfr showing the intersubunit haem-binding site. The haem group (in red) is ligated by Met52 and Met52 (shown in grey/yellow) from the two subunits, respectively. The position of the intrasubunit ferroxidase centres of each subunit is shown (blue spheres) Reproduced with permission from the Royal Society of Chemistry from Lewin, A., Moore, G.R. and Le Brun, N.E. (2005) Formation of protein-coated iron minerals.* Dalton Trans., *3597–3610*

two symmetry-related Met residues as axial ligands to the metal centre. The haem-binding pocket in all of the bacterioferritins is symmetrical – it is found at a perfect twofold rotation axis between two equivalent monomers. However, given the nonsymmetrical structure of the *b*-type haem and of Fe-coproporphyrin III, this is impossible, and it is therefore not surprising that in the structures of several bacterioferritins, the haem has been proposed to adopt several conformations (e.g. Cobessi *et al.*, 2002; Macedo *et al.*, 2003; Swartz *et al.*, 2006).

In studies on mammalian apoferritins, haem binding results in the cleavage and demetallation of haem, generating an alkyl protoporphyrin (Précigoux *et al.*, 1994; Michaux *et al.*, 1996; Crichton *et al.*, 1997; Carette *et al.*, 2006; de Val *et al.*, 2012). In the Bfr from *Mycobacterium tuberculosis* the incorporation of selenomethionine is also observed to result in cleavage and demetallation of haem (Gupta *et al.*, 2009).

In BFRs, the threefold channels are hydrophilic in character, as in mammalian ferritins, whereas the fourfold channels of most BFRs are hydrophilic, in contrast to their hydrophobic character in mammalian ferritins. In the structures of both *D. desulfuricans* Bfr and *A. vinelandii* Bfr, a pore distinct from the three- and fourfold symmetry pores was observed associated with a concentrated negative charge (Macedo *et al.*, 2003; Swartz *et al.*, 2006), While the exact role of this pore is uncertain, it is clear that this pore is sufficiently large to accommodate an iron atom.

9.2.4 Dps Proteins and Rubrerythrins

The first member of the Dps protein family, isolated from starved *E. coli* cells, was found to bind to DNA without apparent sequence specificity, and was therefore called 'DNA-binding protein from starved cells' (Almiron *et al.*, 1992). Dps is the most abundant protein in the bacterial cytoplasm during the stationary phase of *E. coli* growth with the DNA entrapped in DNA-Dps crystals, and it was concluded that the physical interaction with DNA was the basis of its DNA protection (Wolff *et al.*, 1999). However, this did not explain the key observation that Dps expression is associated with resistance to H_2O_2 and increases during the log phase of growth in conditions of oxidative stress (Altuvia *et al.*, 1994). The explanation came from the progressive recognition that the 'ferritin' from the Gram-positive bacterium *Listeria innocua* (Bozzi *et al.*, 1997) is indeed a Dps protein (Grant *et al.*, 1998; Ilari *et al.*, 2000; Su *et al.*, 2005), with the highly conserved ferroxidase centre (Ilari *et al.*, 2000) which confers a 'ferritin-like' activity to all Dps proteins. This represents the link to its biological activity in response to oxidative stress (Chiancone and Ceci, 2010a). Dps proteins are widely distributed in the bacterial kingdom, with most bacterial genomes encoding at least one Dps protein. A search of the PROSITE database using the *E. coli* protein as a probe identified over 300 Dps sequences (Chiancone and Ceci, 2010a).

The X-ray structure of the Dps monomer from *L. innocua* shown in Figure 9.9a consists of a central core composed of the four-helix bundle, similar to other ferritins, with greatest similarity to L-chain ferritin, together with N- and C-terminal regions of variable length containing a varying number of positive charges. The packing of the four helices (A–D) involves essentially hydrophobic interactions, with helices B and C connected by a long loop which, unlike ferritins, has a short helix in the middle. The other major difference is at the C terminus, where the smaller *Listeria* protein lacks the fifth E helix. Indeed, as was first shown for the *E. coli* Dps protein (Grant *et al.*, 1998), the quaternary structure of the Dps proteins, unlike classical ferritins, contains 12 rather than 24 subunits (Figure 9.9b and c), assembled into a spherical dodecamer with 23 symmetry. The central cavity has a diameter of ~40 Å, which corresponds to about one-eighth that of typical ferritin shells, in excellent agreement with their respective capacity to store iron (~500 Fe(III) atoms for Dps proteins versus 4500 Fe(III) atoms for ferritins). The 23 symmetry defines two types of

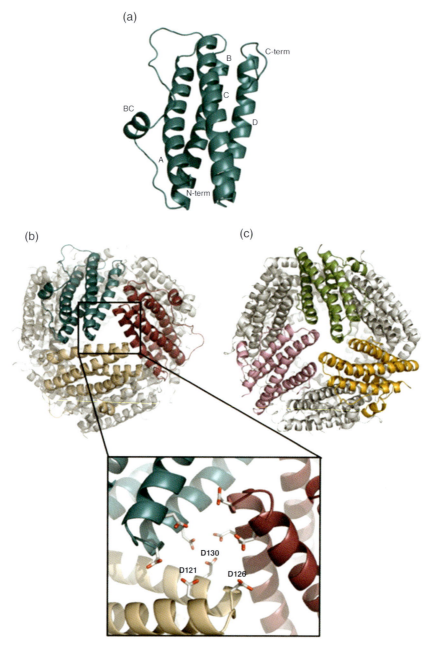

Figure 9.9 *Structural organisation of Dps proteins. Dps fold (a), 12-mer assembly: view along the ferritin-like (b) and Dps-type (c) pores formed respectively by the N- and C-terminal regions of the subunits. In (b) the blow-up shows the aspartate residues lining the ferritin-like pore in* L. innocua *Dps. Reprinted with permission from Elsevier from Chiancone, E. and Ceci, P. (2010a) The multifaceted capacity of Dps proteins to combat bacterial stress conditions: Detoxification of iron and hydrogen peroxide and DNA binding.* Biochim. Biophys. Acta, **1800**, *798–805*

environments at the threefold symmetry axes, such that there are two different types of channel (Figure 9.9b and c): (i) relatively large, negatively charged 'ferritin-like' channels, formed by the C-terminal ends of the subunits, which may provide the pathway for iron entry into the negatively charged internal cavity; and (ii) 'Dps-like' channels of unknown function, formed by the C-terminal ends of the subunits.

Dps protein sequences contain a highly conserved ferroxidase centre which represents the most distinctive structural signature of the Dps family. However, it is located at the interface of twofold symmetry-related subunits rather than within the four-helix bundle of a single subunit, as in all known ferroxidases (Figure 9.10) (Ilari *et al.*, 2000). This signature is not present in the Dps-like dodecameric proteins from two Archaea, *Pyrococcus furiosus* and *Sulfolobus solfataricus* (Ramsay *et al.*, 2006; Gauss *et al.*, 2006), which possess an intrasubunit ferroxidase centre resembling that of bacterioferritins and apparently belonging to a different branch of the ferritin superfamily. The mechanism of iron deposition in Dps proteins will be discussed later in the chapter. In addition to the localisation of the ferroxidase centre referred to earlier, another distinctive feature of Dps proteins is that they typically prefer H_2O_2 which is typically 100-fold more efficient than O_2 in iron oxidation (Tonello *et al.*, 1999; Zhao *et al.*, 2002; Franceschini *et al.*, 2006).

The DNA-binding ability displayed by the prototypic *E. coli* Dps (Almiron *et al.*, 1992; Wolf *et al.*, 1999) is not shared by all members of the family, since it requires specific structural elements within the Dps molecule in order to establish electrostatic interactions with the negatively charged DNA backbone. These most likely involve positively charged lysine or arginine residues, which protrude from the external surface of the Dps spherical assembly, in N- and C-terminal helices of variable length. Based on the X-ray crystal structure of *E. coli* Dps the highly mobile N-terminal region was recognised as the DNA-interacting element (Grant *et al.*, 1998). The N terminus reaches out from the surface of the molecule into solvent and contains three lysine residues which can

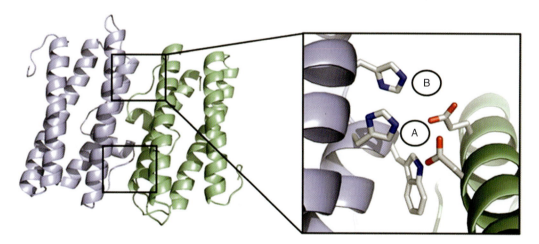

Figure 9.10 *Dimeric interface and ferroxidase centre of Dps proteins. Twofold symmetry interface (left) and blow-up of the intersubunit ferroxidase centre located at the interface (right). The positions of the high-affinity (A) and low-affinity (B) iron-binding sites are indicated along with those of the conserved metal ligands, namely two histidine residues, one aspartic acid and one glutamic acid. Reprinted with permission from Elsevier from Chiancone, E. and Ceci, P. (2010a) The multifaceted capacity of Dps proteins to combat bacterial stress conditions: Detoxification of iron and hydrogen peroxide and DNA binding. Biochim. Biophys. Acta,* **1800**, *798–805*

interact with the phosphate groups on DNA (Grant *et al.*, 1998; Ceci *et al.*, 2004). The importance of this N-terminal region for DNA binding is borne out by the fact that it has been shown to be directly involved in *M. smegmatis* and *D. radiodurans* Dps proteins (Roy *et al.*, 2008; Grove and Wilkinson, 2005; Bhartacharyya and Grove, 2007), and that some 20 Dps family members have N-terminal sequences resembling that of *E. coli* Dps (Chiancone and Ceci, 2010a). At physiological pH values, these three positively charged Lys form large complexes that enclose many Dps molecules and one or more DNA plasmids, the so-called 'DNA condensates'. When the pH increases, deprotonating the Lys residues, large complexes are no longer formed and simple DNA binding takes place. Not only are the Lys residues required for DNA binding (Chiancone and Ceci, 2010a), but flexibility of the N terminus is also required, as illustrated by studies on Dps proteins from *A. tumefaciens* and *Lactobacillus lactis* (Ceci *et al.*, 2003; Stillman *et al.*, 2005; Chiancone and Ceci, 2010b).

Two other DNA-binding signatures have been identified, respectively in the C terminus of *M. Smegmatis* Dps 1 protein, which has a truncated N terminus, but a highly mobile 26-residue C terminus (Gupta and Chatterji, 2003; Roy *et al.*, 2007; Ceci *et al.*, 2005), and in the *H. pylori* Dps (also known as HPNAP because of its neutrophil-activating properties), characterised by a positively charged protein surface which at physiological pH values can be used to bind to DNA (Ceci *et al.*, 2007). A similar mechanism may operate in the Dps protein from *Trichodesmium erythraeum*, which has no positively charged residues at the N terminus and a truncated C terminus, but nonetheless binds DNA at pH 8.0 without condensing it into large Dps–DNA complexes (Castruita *et al.*, 2006).

It has been suggested (Bozzi *et al.*, 1997; Grant *et al.*, 1998) that Dps and *L. Innocua* Dps proteins represent examples of a family of ancestral dodecameric protein which had a function to trap – but not to mineralise – metal ions, and that the ability to efficiently oxidise and mineralise iron and to form fourfold interactions came later. The hollow-cored dodecameric motif exemplified by Dps has clearly been adapted to a number of functions, since in addition to DNA binding and iron storage other family members include a novel pilin, a bromoperoxidase and several other proteins of unknown function (Grant *et al.*, 1998).

Rubrerythrin is the trivial name given to a family of homodimeric non-haem iron proteins found in a many air-sensitive bacteria and archaea. which contain a unique combination of a rubredoxin-like and a non-sulphur, oxo/dicarboxylato-bridged di-iron site. Each subunit (Figure 9.11a) contains an N-terminal 'ferritin-like' four-helix bundle domain which contains a di-iron site with a μ-oxo bridge and a C-terminal rubredoxin-like domain which contains a $[Fe(Cys)_4]$ centre (LeGall *et al.*, 1988; deMaré *et al.*, 1996; Sieker *et al.*, 2000). Some members of the family, such as sulerythrin (Wakagi, 2003; Fushinobo *et al.*, 2003), lack the C-terminal rubredoxin-like domain usually referred to as erythrins (Andrews, 2010), while other rubrerythrin-like proteins (e.g. from *Clostridium acetobutylicum*) have been found to have the domain orders reversed (Figure 9.11b) (May *et al.*, 2004). At the time of its initial isolation, since its function was unknown, the protein was given the trivial name rubrerythrin (Rbr), a contraction of rubredoxin and haemerythrin. The subsequent X-ray crystal structure of recombinant oxidised (all ferric) *D. vulgaris* Rbr (Rbr_{ox}) confirmed the initial spectroscopic identifications of these iron sites (deMaré *et al.*, 1996).

More than a dozen Rbr homologues or their genes have been identified from a variety of air-sensitive bacteria and archaea. Rbr has been implicated as one component of a novel oxidative stress protection system in these microorganisms, whereby Rbr can function as a hydrogen peroxide reductase (peroxidase). Kinetic results show that the two ferrous iron atoms at the di-iron site of Rbr are oxidised in a concerted manner by H_2O_2, which is rapidly reduced to water (Mishra and Imlay, 2012; Zhao *et al.*, 2007; Kawasaki *et al.*, 2007; Riebe *et al.*, 2009). The K_M for H_2O_2 is as low as 2

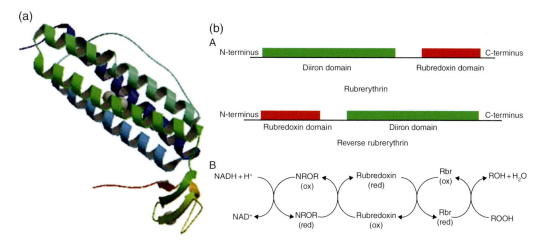

Figure 9.11 *(a) Ribbon diagram of D. vulgaris rubrerythrin (PDF code: 1LKO). (b) Domain organisation of rubrerythrins. (A, B) Scheme of electron delivery to recycle rubrerythrin (Rbr). NROR: NADH:rubredoxin oxidoreductase. Reprinted with permission from Elsevier from Mishra, M. and Imlay, J. (2012) Why do bacteria use so many enzymes to scavenge hydrogen peroxide?* Arch. Biochem. Biophys., **525**, *145–160*

µM, and *in-vitro* systems have achieved turnover numbers as high as 5000 min^{-1}. The reduced Rbr (Rbr$_{red}$) reacts with H$_2$O$_2$ on the millisecond time scale or faster, whereas its reaction with O$_2$ is orders of magnitude slower (several minutes). Completion of the catalytic cycle requires the movement of two consecutive electrons from the rubredoxin site to the di-ferric site. In turn, the oxidised rubredoxin site probably is then reduced *in vivo* by an authentic rubredoxin protein, as its structural gene is sometimes located in an operon together with that of the rubrerythrin. A complete peroxidase system has been reconstituted *in vivo* using NADH:rubredoxin oxidoreductase (NROR), rubredoxin, and rubrerythrin (Rbr) (Figure 9.11b) (Riebe *et al.*, 2009; Zhao *et al.*, 2007).

High-resolution structures of the best-characterised DvRbrs, rubrerythrin from *Desulfovibrio vulgaris* DvRbr, and a second Rbr homologue, called nigerythrin (DvNgr), which has significantly higher peroxidase activity than DvRbr, have been determined using X-ray crystallography (Jin *et al.*, 2002; Iyer *et al.*, 2005). As we will discuss later, the di-iron site of ferritins is characterised by a six-ligand motif pattern, whereas rubrerythrins are unusual in that they contain a seventh metal-ligating residue. This additional ligand is a glutamate that resides within a π-helical bulge of core helix C and reflects an insertion compared to other ferritin-like superfamily (FLSF) proteins (Cooley *et al.*, 2010). It gives rubrerythrins the unusual ability among FLSF proteins to preferentially react with H$_2$O$_2$ rather than with dioxygen (Coulter *et al.*, 2000). As a result, rubrerythrins are believed to act as peroxidases *in vivo* in order to mitigate toxicity from reactive oxygen species (ROS) (Zhao *et al.*, 2007; Mishra and Imlay, 2012), particularly in anaerobes where they are widely distributed (Gomes *et al.*, 2001).

Rubrerythrins have the most plastic metallocentre among FLSF proteins in that although seven residues are involved in metal ligation in the di-iron site, only six residues coordinate the metal-locentre at any one time. In the diferric state, the His from helix B is not a ligand; however, upon reduction to the diferrous state, Fe1 shifts by ~2.0 Å so that it breaks its bond with the additional glutamate from helix C and makes a new ligand bond with the His from helix B (Jin *et al.*, 2002; Iyer *et al.*, 2005). This redox-dependent toggling of Fe1 positions is thought to be part of rubrerythrin's catalytic cycle (Dillard *et al.*, 2011).

The metallocentre of symerythrin, a novel rubrerythrin variant from the oxygenic phototroph *Cyanophora paradoxa*, has a unique eighth ligating residue compared to rubrerythrin – an additional glutamate inserted into helix A of the four-helix bundle that resides on a π-helical segment (Cooley *et al.*, 2011). Symerythrin has high internal symmetry, which supports the notion that its four-helix bundle core was formed by the gene duplication and fusion of a two-helix peptide (Figure 9.12). The authors proposed that, contrary to previous assumptions, there have been multiple gene fusion events that have generated the single-chain FLSF fold.

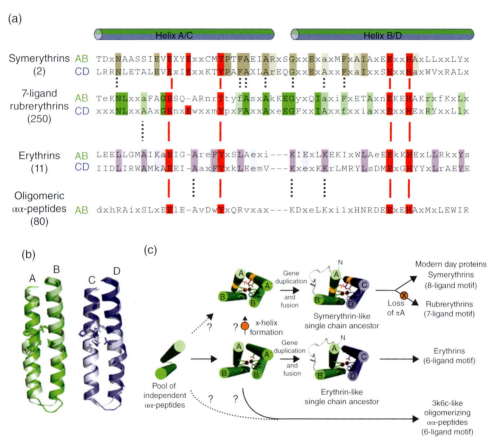

Figure 9.12 *Internal sequence similarities of three ferritin-like superfamily (FLSF) families and a model for their origins. (a) Internal alignment of consensus sequences from helix pairs A–B and C–D of symerythrins, of rubrerythrin family members with seven metal-ligating residues, of erythrins, and of an oligomerising αα-peptide family. In parentheses below the family name is the number of sequences used to generate the consensus sequences for that group. (b) Overlay of helix pairs A–B and C–D of symerythrin (dark green and dark blue, respectively) on the equivalent helices of erythrin (light green and light blue, respectively; PDB ID: 2fzf) showing the structural difference associated with the three-residue gap in erythrins compared to rubrerythrins. Side chains of metallocentre residues are shown as sticks. (c) Schematic for the origins of modern-day symerythrins, seven-ligand rubrerythrins, erythrins, and oligomerising αα-peptides. Continuous lines represent a simple direct pathway for the formation of each modern-day family, assuming that the dimerising two-helix peptides are homologous with each other. Reprinted with permission from Elsevier from Cooley, R.B., Arp, D.J. and Karplus, P.A. (2010) Symerythrin structures at atomic resolution and the origins of rubrerythrins and the ferritin-like superfamily. J. Mol. Biol., **413**, 177–194*

9.2.5 The Mineral Core

The 24-mer hollow-sphere architecture of ferritins has an outer diameter of 12 nm and an inner diameter of 8 nm, within which the hydrated ferric iron core is deposited. The amount of iron in the core is variable, and can range from zero to a maximum of approximately 4500 atoms (Fischbach and Anderegg, 1965), although the average iron content of animal ferritins is around 1000–3000 atoms per protein shell. In mammalian ferritins, which typically have a rather low phosphate content (about 1 P per 10 Fe atoms in horse spleen ferritin), the mineral cores are highly ordered, consisting essentially of the mineral phase ferrihydrite (see Chapter 1 for a more detailed review), with varying degrees of crystallinity as judged by X-ray or electron diffraction, electron microscopy, Mössbauer spectroscopy and EXAFS (Chasteen and Harrison, 1999; Ward *et al.* 2000; Uchida *et al.*, 2010). The ferritins often consist of a single well-defined nanoparticle crystallite encapsulated within the protein shell, clearly visible by transmission electron microscopy (Evans and Browning, 2013). In contrast, the iron cores of most bacterial ferritins are almost completely amorphous, show poor crystallinity, and consist essentially of hydrated ferric phosphate, reflecting their P:Fe ratios of 1:1 to 1:2.

The global process of storing iron within the nanocage of the apoferritin protein shell can be summarised as follows:

$$4Fe^{2+} + O_2 + 6H_2O \rightarrow 4Fe(O)OH + 8H^+$$

However, the reality of the process of iron oxidation and subsequent entrapment within the protein shell is considerably more complex, and quite a lot of the intermediate steps between initial binding of Fe^{2+} and core formation remain unresolved. The mineralisation of the iron core will be discussed in the next section of this chapter, followed by a brief review of potential applications of the ferritin protein nanocages in drug delivery, imaging, biocatalysis and the development of novel nanomaterials.

9.2.6 Haemosiderins

Haemosiderin was the first storage form of iron to be identified (Perls, 1867) and isolated (Cook, 1929). The name is perhaps misleading – while the original source of haemosiderin iron may well be haem, the iron cores of haemosiderin contain non-haem iron, which is derived from ferritin. Whereas haemosiderin is only found in conditions of iron overload, usually associated with toxic pathological states in humans, it is frequently found as a normal physiological response without any toxicity in many migratory birds and, seasonally, in certain animals (e.g. horses and reindeers; reviewed in Ward *et al.*, 2000). Electron micrographs of iron-loaded tissue and of haemosiderin from human and avian (Order Passeriformes[4]) spleen are presented in Figure 9.13. Haemosiderin, as isolated, is typically a water-insoluble protein of ill-defined nature with a much higher iron to protein ratio than ferritin, which is consistent with it being a lysosomal degradation product of ferritin (Richter, 1978; Ward *et al.*, 1992, 1994).

On the basis of a number of physico-chemical methods (Mössbauer spectroscopy, electron diffraction, EXAFS), the iron cores of naturally occurring haemosiderins isolated from various iron-loaded animals and human (horse, reindeer, birds and human old age) were consistently shown to have ferrihydrite-like iron cores similar to those of ferritin (Ward *et al.*, 1992, 1994, 2000).

---

[4] Better known as the common starling.

(a)

(b)

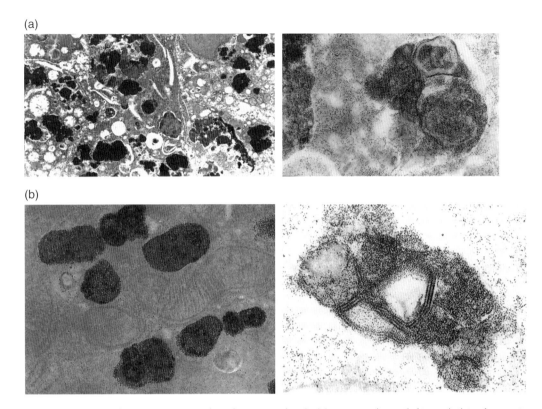

Figure 9.13 *(a) Electron micrographs of iron-overloaded human spleen (left) and (b) of an avian species (order Passeriformes) (left) showing clumps of densely stained material throughout the tissue, haemosiderin. Electron micrographs of siderosomes (right) (a) from human spleen and (b) from an avian species (order Passeriformes). Iron-rich particles can be seen within the membrane-bound structures. Reprinted with permission from Elsevier from Ward, R.J., Legssyer, R., Henry, C. and Crichton, R.R. (2000) Does the haemosiderin iron core determine its potential for chelation and the development of iron-induced tissue damage?* J. Inorg. Biochem., **79**, *311–317*

As we will see in later chapters, the use of the iron core of ferritin as a means of evaluating tissue iron by non-invasive techniques *in vivo*, typically relaxometry, magnetic field correlation imaging and phase-based contrast (Dusek *et al.*, 2013), has developed extensively in recent years. In particular, cerebral tissue iron concentrations are proving important in studying physiological age-related disorders, as well as pathological conditions in neurodegenerative, neuroinflammatory, and vascular diseases.

9.3 Iron Uptake and Release from Ferritin

9.3.1 Iron Uptake in Ferritins

Before entering into a detailed analysis of iron uptake into ferritins and Dps proteins, it is essential to remind the reader that whereas ferritins of plant and bacterial origin (e.g. Dps proteins) are homopolymers, mammalian ferritin are heteropolymers, composed of two or occasionally three classes of subunits, which have considerable structural identity, although they differ considerably in their amino acid sequence. In most mammalian ferritins the two subunits, H-chain (heavy) and L-chain (light), self-assemble to form hetero-24-mers with different ratios of each subunit, depending on the organ from which the ferritin is isolated. Indeed, with the exception of serum ferritin and mitochondrial ferritin (Chasteen and Harrison, 1999; Corsi *et al.*, 2002) and pathological conditions such as hereditary hyperferritinaemia cataract syndrome (HHCS) (see Chapter 9; Millonig *et al.*, 2010) and neuroferritinopathy (see Chapter 14; Keogh *et al.*, 2013), in which the L-chain is overexpressed, there are no situations in which a mammalian tissue would have ferritin homopolymers, and this should be taken into account when evaluating data obtained from studies on recombinant H- or L-chain homopolymers. As we will see below, the H-chain has a well-conserved ferroxidase site which catalyses the oxidation of Fe^{2+}, whereas the L-chain has clusters of acidic residues (Glu and Asp) on its interior surface which constitute potential sites for nucleation of the mineral core. For recent reviews on iron uptake and mineralisation in ferritins, see Honarmand Ebrahimi *et al.* (2014), Bradley *et al.* (2014), Lalli and Turano (2013) and Theil (2013).

The earliest studies (Bielig and Bayer, 1955) clearly established that apoferritin catalyses the oxidation of ferrous iron by dioxygen: the ferric iron then undergoes hydrolysis and is deposited within the protein shell in mammalian ferritins, as ferrihydrite. Globally, the process of iron uptake in mammalian ferritins is now assumed to involve the following steps which are described in greater detail below: (i) entry of Fe(II) into the protein shell through channels in the apoferritin protein shell; (ii) oxidation of ferrous iron by the dinuclear ferroxidase sites situated within the four-helix bundle of H-chain subunits by molecular O_2, producing H_2O_2; (iii) migration of Fe(III) from the ferroxidase sites to nucleation sites on the interior surface of the L-chain subunits of the protein shell, which facilitate mineralisation; and (iv) growth of the ferrihydrite mineral core via iron oxidation and mineralisation on the surface of the growing crystallite. These steps will be discussed separately for mammalian heteropolymeric ferritins.

9.3.1.1 Entry of Fe(II) into the Protein Shell

It is assumed that all substances involved in ferritin iron deposition or mobilisation – Fe^{2+}, Fe^{3+}, O_2, reductants, chelators, and so on – gain access to the interior of the apoferritin protein shell. Four possible pathways, described variously as channels or pores, have been identified by which they might penetrate into the interior cavity of the protein. These are: (i) the six channels along the fourfold axes; (ii) the eight channels along the threefold axes; (iii) the four so-called B pores located near each of the fourfold axes, at the intersection of three subunits, not aligned by any axis of symmetry in the structure, which are found in the protein shells of bacterial ferritins (Bfr and Ftn); and (iv) a 'one-fold' ferroxidase channel in each subunit. However, before considering which route is used, we need to ask first in what form is Fe^{2+} presented? As mentioned earlier, the family of poly C binding proteins (PCBPs) was proposed to have iron chaperone activity for mammalian ferritins (Shi *et al.*, 2008), and PCBP1 and -2 are reported to form a complex for iron delivery to ferritin. It is proposed that all four PCBPs may share iron chaperone activity (Leidgens *et al.*, 2013). While the evidence, obtained using heterologous expression of human PCBP and H and L ferritins in yeast (which does not have any ferritin, as we saw in Chapter 5) is convincing, further studies would seem to be required to confirm these important suggestions.

For mammalian ferritins it is generally agreed that the polar, hydrophilic channels along the threefold axes are the most likely port of access for metal ions. The eight threefold axes (Figure 9.14) are funnel-shaped with a wider entrance at the outside of the molecule and a narrower passage at the inside (0.34 nm wide and about 0.6 nm long). The amino acid residues

322 *Iron Metabolism*

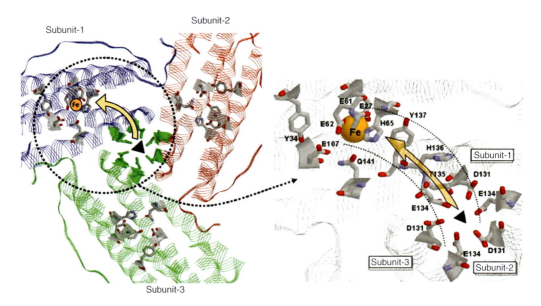

Figure 9.14 *Internal view of the threefold channel of ferritin (left panel). The right panel shows a putative Fe(II) pathway from the threefold channel to the ferroxidase centre of the protein. Reprinted with permission from Elsevier from Bou-Abdallah F. (2010) The iron redox and hydrolysis chemistry of the ferritins.* Biochim. Biophys. Acta, **1800**, *719–731*

that neighbour and line these channels include residues from the C terminus of helix C and the N terminus of helix D, which are highly conserved in both L- and H-subunits although there are a number of positions where H-chains differ from L-chains. Many of the H for L changes are found in or close to the wider end of the channel, whereas the narrow region is highly conserved in all ferritins. The channel is extremely hydrophilic in the narrow inner region, with three Glu134 residues, towards the outer surface of the protein shell, and three Asp131 residues, towards the inner surface (one from each of the three D helices), which are conserved in both H- and L-subunits, and predominantly hydrophilic in its wider entrance region. The funnel-shaped design of the channels could allow ions or molecules approaching the shell to find these channels more easily than if they were narrow throughout their length. The pathway to the ferroxidase centre through the threefold channels would involve passing through the 1.2 nm-long channel, and then traversing a further distance of about 0.8 nm along a hydrophilic pathway from the inside of the channel to the ferroxidase site. In the known crystal structures, one to three metal ions are seen in the threefold channels (Cd^{2+}, Zn^{2+}, Ca^{2+}, Mg^{2+}, Co^{2+}, Tb^{3+}), often binding to the six conserved carboxylates (Hempstead *et al.*, 1997; Toussaint *et al.*, 2007; Tosha *et al.*, 2010). [113]Cd NMR spectroscopy (Stefanini *et al.*, 1989), as well as electrostatic potential calculations (Douglas and Ripoll, 1998) and fluorescence quenching studies, also indicated that the threefold channels are the only avenues for rapid access of Fe^{2+} to the ferroxidase centre (Bou-Abdallah *et al.*, 2008). Translocation of iron from the entry channel to the ferroxidase site, has been proposed to involve a novel metal-binding 'transit site', observed in the crystal structures of both soybean ferritin and human H ferritin (Masuda *et al.*, 2010a,b), involving Glu140 of the human H- and L-chains. Almost all of the reported sequences of vertebrate ferritin have this glutamate residue. An exception is a Glu-Lys substitution in the sequence of the mouse L-chain, which may account for the low iron incorporation activity of the mouse L-chain compared with the human L-chain (Santambrogio *et al.*, 2000). A recent molecular dynamics simulation study confirms the threefold channel as the main entrance pathway, and also identifies an explicit pathway from the channel to the ferroxidase centre (Laghaei *et al.*, 2013). Diffusion of Fe^{2+} from the inner opening of the channel to the ferroxidase site located in the interior region of the protein coat is assisted by Thr135, His136 and Tyr137, with the Fe^{2+} binding preferentially to site A of the ferroxidase site. Figure 9.14 shows the threefold channel and the putative pathway from the threefold channel to the ferroxidase centre of the protein.

In prokaryote Ftns and Bfns, the pathway of Fe^{2+} from the outside of the protein shell is not well established (reviewed in Honarmand Ebrahimi *et al.*, 2014), although in *H. pylori* Ftn it has been suggested that the hydrophilic fourfold channels are involved (Cho *et al.*, 2009), while in *Pyrococus furiosus*, it has been suggested that the site C (*vide infra*) might be involved in the translocation of Fe^{2+}/Fe^{3+} into/out of the ferroxidase centre (Honarmand Ebrahimi *et al.*, 2012).

9.3.1.2   Oxidation of Fe^{2+} by Ferroxidase Sites

Mammalian H-chain ferritins catalyse Fe^{2+} oxidation much faster than L-chain ferritins (Levi *et al.*, 1988), and this is attributed to the presence of a di-iron 'ferroxidase centre' located in the middle of the four-helix bundle which constitutes the central core of each subunit. The four-helix bundle and di-iron site (as we saw earlier in Chapter 2) is characteristic of other members of the ferritin superfamily (Sazinsky and Lippard, 2006), and its absence from mammalian L-chain subunits implies that the L-subunit must contribute some other important function to the essential role of ferritin – storing iron in a soluble, non-toxic yet bioavailable form within cells. The role of the L-chain will be returned to shortly.

As we saw in Chapter 2, the di-iron centres of members of the ferritin superfamily are in many respects quite similar, with adjacent (~4 Å apart) sites which bind two metal ions in a coordination environment rich in carboxylate residues (most often four glutamates), with one histidine ligand per metal subsite. Each of the proteins function by reaction of their carboxylate-bridged di-iron cluster with dioxygen, and mechanistic studies have suggested that [μ-(hydro)peroxo]-Fe_2(III/III) intermediates, formed by the bridging, oxidative addition of O_2 to the Fe_2(II/II) cofactors, are common to most, if not all, of the reactions (Liu *et al.*, 1994; Tong *et al.*, 1996; Broadwater *et al.*, 1998; Pereira *et al.*, 1998; Yun *et al.*, 2007; Murray *et al.*, 2007).

A great many members of the ferritin superfamily use their di-iron centre for objectives rather than for iron storage, catalysing an ever-expanding repertoire of reactions, as illustrated in Figure 9.15 (Krebs *et al.*, 2011). However, at no time are the iron atoms released from these catalytic centres, which instead function as redox cofactors, oscillating between the Fe^{2+} and Fe^{3+} states. In contrast, in the ferritins, protonation and dissociation of the peroxide prevents either further oxidation of the iron ions or oxidation of a substrate (Jamieson *et al.*, 2002). The two ferrous ions are the 'substrate', generating an oxo/hydroxo diferric product which is released at the end of the oxidation cycle from the ferroxidase site and stored within the ferric mineral core (Schwartz *et al.*, 2008).

The metal coordination of the ferroxidase centre of rHuH ferritin is shown in Figure 9.16. In marked contrast to the catalytic cofactor sites described above, the ferroxidase site of mammalian ferritins has only one μ-1,3-carboxylate bridging ligand, Glu62. Three coordinating atoms from residues Glu27, His65 and Glu62 and one water molecule coordinate the zinc ion from site A, while the second oxygen atom of Glu62 and the two oxygen atoms of Glu107 coordinate the zinc ion from site B; Glu 107 in turn interacts with Gln141 and Tyr34, which are highly conserved among eukaryotic ferritins. The coordinating environment of the ferroxidase site is not only distinct

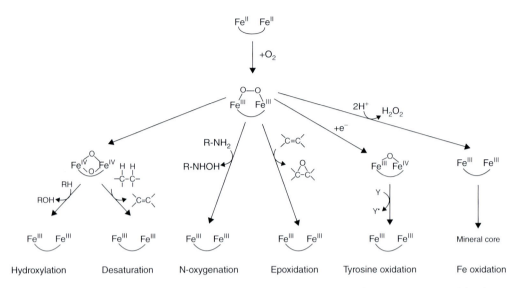

Figure 9.15 *Diverse reaction pathways of the peroxo-Fe$_2$(III/III) intermediates in reactions of the ferritin-like di-iron-carboxylate proteins. For simplicity, the peroxo-Fe$_2$(III/III) intermediate is depicted as having a μ-1,2 bridging mode, although many other binding modes have been discussed. Aromatic hydroxylation is believed to proceed by a mechanism similar to that labelled as 'epoxidation'. Reproduced from Krebs, C., Bollinger, J.M. Jr and Booker, S.J. (2011) Cyanobacterial alkane biosynthesis further expands the catalytic repertoire of the ferritin-like 'di-iron-carboxylate' proteins. Curr. Opin. Chem. Biol., **15**, 291–303*

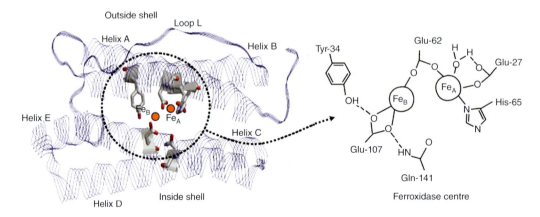

Figure 9.16 *Schematic view of the di-iron ferroxidase centre on the four-helix of the H-chain ferritin (left panel). Dinuclear ferroxidase centre diagram (right panel) showing residues from the Tb-derivative X-ray structure of ferritin. Reprinted with permission from Elsevier from Bou-Abdallah F. (2010) The iron redox and hydrolysis chemistry of the ferritins. Biochim. Biophys. Acta, **1800**, 719–731*

from that of the cofactor sites, the metal ions are also more weakly bound to the protein, allowing the diferric product to leave the active site for formation of the ferric mineral core. This difficulty is underlined by the paucity of structural information with Fe bound in the ferroxidase centre, although the structure of the ferroxidase centre of bullfrog M-chain ferritin, with the same coordination of sites A and B as human H-chain, has been determined in the Fe^{3+}-bound state (Bertini *et al.*, 2012).

In the Tb^{3+}-bound rHuH structure a third metal site is found (Lawson *et al.*, 1991) which may correspond to the C site described below for bacterial ferritins. NMR experiments have given indications that, upon leaving the ferroxidase centre, the Fe^{3+} follows a route along the long axis of the subunit, emerging at the fourfold axis where it enters the cavity (Turano *et al.*, 2010).

The ferroxidase centres of Ftn proteins are very similar to those of H-chain ferritin subunits, as illustrated in Figure 9.16 for *E. coli* Ftn (Hempstead *et al.*, 1994; Stillman *et al.*, 2001). The protein ligands to the A site are the same, involving the bridging Glu50, a His53 and a monodentate Glu17. However, as well as the bridging Glu50 and bidentate Glu94, the B site has an additional Glu130. This additional Glu130 is a bridging ligand to a third iron-binding site (site C), which has three further Glu ligands, Glu49, Glu126 and Glu129, and two water molecules. The Fe–Fe distance for Fe_A–Fe_B is 3.24 Å, implying the presence of a bridging oxo- or hydroxo species (Stillman, 2001), whereas the Fe_B–Fe_C distance is 5.8 Å. The occupancy of site B is low compared to sites A and B. Fe_C and ferroxidase centre ligands are highly conserved in other prokaryote Ftns (Tatur *et al.*, 2007) and in the archael Ftns from *Archaeoglobus fulgidis* and *Pyrococcus furiosus* (Johnson *et al.*, 2005; Tatur *et al.*, 2007). The Fe_A–Fe_B and Fe_B–Fe_C distances are also similar, and for the latter the C site is occupied at the expense of site B. The structure of the eukaryote ferritin from the pinnate diatom *Pseudo-nitzschia multiseries* which, like other diatoms, is composed of a single type of subunit (Marchetti *et al.*, 2009), reveals that it is an Ftn-type ferritin with a C site similar to, but distinct from, prokaryotic Ftn (Marchetti *et al.*, 2009; Pfaffen *et al.*, 2013). Glu130 appears to have flexible coordination between sites B, C and bridging between them (Pfaffen *et al.*, 2013). Two additional potential nucleation sites were observed on the inner surface.

The structures of haem-containing Bfrs from several bacteria have been determined with both Fe^{2+} and Fe^{3+} bound in the ferroxidase centre (Macedo *et al.*, 2003; Swartz *et al.*, 2006; Crow *et al.*, 2009; Weeratunga *et al.*, 2010). The coordination geometry of the di-iron site differs significantly from both H-chain and Ftn-type centres, and closely resembles that of class II dinuclear iron centres, including the R2 subunit of ribonucleotide reductase and the hydroxylase subunit of methane monooxygenase (Nordlund *et al.*, 1990; Rosenzweig *et al.*, 1993). Three distinct catalytic states of the ferroxidase centre have been revealed for *E. coli* Bfr (Figure 9.17) (Crow *et al.*, 2009). The apoprotein structure shows that the centre is preformed, with the side chains of the ferroxidase centre residues (Glu18, Glu51, His54, Glu94, Glu127, and His130) clearly in position to bind metal ions. In crystals soaked in Fe^{2+} for 2 minutes, the two irons are 3.71 Å apart, in the ferroxidase centre, which is roughly twofold rotationally symmetric, with each iron ligated by one histidine nitrogen and four carboxyl oxygens. Two of these oxygen ligands arise from a bidentate glutamate carboxyl (Glu18 in one site, and Glu94 in the second), and the others are supplied by Glu51 and Glu127 which bridge the two irons. An additional iron site has been observed, located directly below the ferroxidase centre on the inner face of each subunit, associated with Asp50 and His46 (Figure 9.17b), 9.2 Å from the nearest ferroxidase centre iron, and clearly protrudes into the central cavity. Asp50 in Bfr is equivalent to, but conformationally distinct from, the Fe_C ligand Glu49 in Ftn., and is almost universally conserved in Bfr sequences, whereas His46 is only conserved in γ-proteobacteria and cyanobacteria. As mentioned above, the Bfrs contain up to 12 haems per 24-mer, located at intersubunit sites (Frolow *et al.*, 1994; Andrews *et al.*, 1995).

9.3.1.3 *Mineralisation of the Iron Core*

Iron oxidation/mineralisation in human ferritin is thought to occur by at least three different phases (Yang *et al.*, 1998; Zhao *et al.*, 2003). In the first phase, once two Fe^{2+} ions have bound to the A and B ferroxidase sites of H-chain ferritin (Treffry *et al.*, 1997; Bou-Abdallah *et al.*,

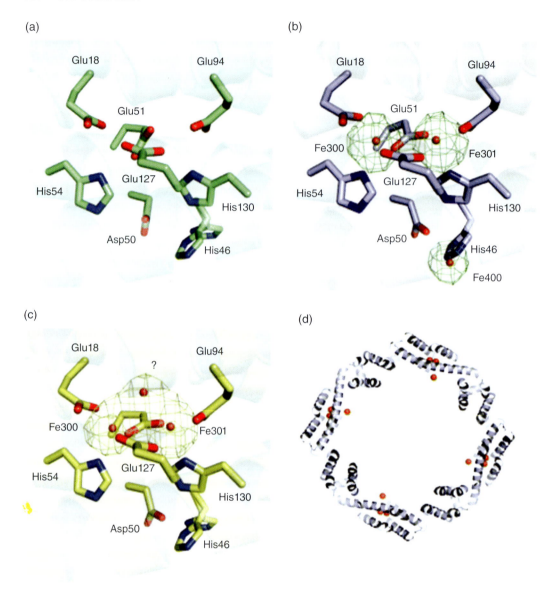

Figure 9.17 *Crystal structures of Bfr showing three distinct catalytic states of the ferroxidase centre. (a) Apo-ferroxidase centre obtained after soaking an apo-BFR crystal aerobically (at pH 7) in a cryoprotectant solution devoid of iron. (b) Structure of a di-Fe^{2+} ferroxidase centre intermediate with an additional iron site located on the inner face of each subunit obtained after a 2.5 min exposure to Fe^{2+}. The 12-fold NCS-averaged anomalous map constructed using diffraction data collected at the iron peak is shown as a green mesh (12 σ, 2.7 Å). (c) Structure of a probable μ-oxo-bridged diferric intermediate, obtained in a 65 min aerobic soak using an anaerobically prepared solution of Fe^{2+}. A 12-fold NCS-averaged omit map (12 σ) is shown as a yellow mesh, with a question mark and red sphere denoting the additional bridging electron density. (d) A cross-section of the biological unit (with metal ions shown as orange spheres) confirming that iron associated with Asp50 and His46 is located on the inside face of the BFR molecule and is associated with all 24 protein subunits. Reprinted with permission from Crow, A., Lawson, T.L., Lewin, A., Moore, G.R. and Le Brun, N.E. (2009) Structural basis for iron mineralization by bacterioferritin. J. Am. Chem. Soc., **131**, 6808–6813; © 2009, American Chemical Society*

2002a), dioxygen binds and, as was proposed many years ago (Crichton and Roman, 1978), a diferric peroxo intermediate is formed. The protein-catalyzed oxidation of Fe(II) generates H_2O_2 as the product of O_2 reduction (Xu and Chasteen, 1991; Waldo and Theil, 1993; Sun *et al.*, 1993; Zhao *et al.*, 2001), and a mineral core of Fe(III) is subsequently produced, written for simplicity as $Fe(O)OH_{(core)}$ (Eq. 9.1). Second, some of the H_2O_2 generated in Eq. 9.1 reacts with additional Fe(II) in the detoxification reaction (Eq. 9.2) to produce H_2O (Yang *et al.*, 1998). Once a mineral core of sufficient size has developed, in the third phase, Fe(II) autoxidation becomes significant and iron oxidation and hydrolysis occur primarily on the growing surface of the mineral through an autocatalytic process (Xu and Chasteen, 1991; Yang *et al.*, 1998; Zhao *et al.*, 2003) where O_2 is reduced completely to H_2O (Eq. 9.3):

$$2Fe^{2+} + O_2 + 4H_2O \rightarrow 2Fe(O)OH_{(core)} + H_2O_2 + 4H^+ \qquad (9.1)$$

$$2Fe^{2+} + H_2O_2 + 2H_2O \rightarrow 2Fe(O)OH_{(core)} + 4H^+ \qquad (9.2)$$

$$4Fe^{2+} + O_2 + 6H_2O \rightarrow 4Fe(O)OH_{(core)} + 8H^+ \qquad (9.3)$$

The two-electron ferroxidase reaction results in an $Fe:O_2$ ratio of 2:1 (Eq. 9.1) (Bou-Abdallah *et al.*, 2002b; Jamieson *et al.*, 2002; Zhao *et al.*, 2003), and can be followed directly via the formation and decay of a characteristic blue diferric peroxo intermediate (Treffry *et al.*, 1995: Pereira *et al.*, 1998; Moenne-Loccoz *et al.*, 1999; Bou-Abdallah *et al.*, 2002b, 2005; Zhao *et al.*, 2005), using its characteristic absorbance at 650 nm (Treffry *et al.*, 1995; Zhao *et al.*, 1997; Pereira *et al.*, 1998). While many of the Mössbauer and Raman spectroscopic parameters resemble those of peroxodiferric species (Bou-Abdallah *et al.*, 2002b; Pereira *et al.*, 1997, 1998), the precise nature of the blue intermediate remains uncertain, and a number of possible structures are presented in Figure 9.18. A tyrosyl radical on Tyr34, close to the ferroxidase centre, has been detected during the ferroxidase reaction (Chen-Barrett *et al.*, 1995), but its role in the process remains unclear.

What happens next has been the subject of intense discussion in two very recent review articles. Bradley *et al.* (2014) argue that there is no universal mechanism for ferritin iron mineralisation, whereas Honarmand Ebrahimi *et al.* (2014), in marked contrast, propose that there is a common mechanism for iron storage in all three classes of ferritins.

Bradley *et al.* (2014) propose different mechanisms for each of the three classes of ferritins. For H-chain-type ferritins (Figure 9.19a), the ferroxidase centre operates as a gated iron site (i.e. iron transfer can only occur following the oxidation of Fe^{2+} to Fe^{3+}), and since the μ-1,2-oxodiferric species is unstable, it undergoes hydrolysis, forming [2FeOOH], and regenerating the apo-form of the ferroxidase centre for further rounds of Fe^{2+} binding and oxidation. Once a mineral core has been established, the surface of the mineral competes with the ferroxidase centre as a catalytic site. Mineralisation in Ftn-type ferritins (Figure 9.19b) occurs by a mechanism related to that described for H-chain ferritin, but is complicated by the presence of the Fe_C site. Two pathways may operate: in one pathway the Fe_C site is involved in Fe^{2+} oxidation, while in the other it functions as a transit/ holding site for iron which has been oxidised at the ferroxidase centre. In Bfr-type ferritins (Figure 9.19c) the ferroxidase centre operates as a true cofactor, cycling its oxidation state as Fe^{2+} is oxidised in the cavity. Once a mineral core is established, the mineral itself conducts electrons toward the ferroxidase centre.

For mammalian ferritins, the μ-1,2-oxodiferric species is thought to be unstable and to undergo hydrolysis, releasing protons (Yang *et al.*, 1998), H_2O_2, and forming [2FeOOH] which becomes

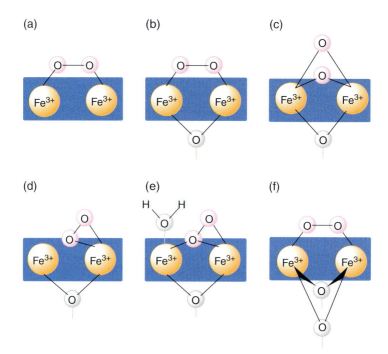

Figure 9.18 *Possible molecular structures of the blue intermediate in ferritin. Comparison of the spectroscopic properties of the diamagnetic Fe(III) intermediate in ferritin with those of different model compounds suggests several different possible molecular structures for the Fe(III) species with blue colour. (a) Structure is less likely because of the long Fe–Fe distance that is observed for similar structures with model compounds. Mössbauer and resonance Raman parameters of the blue intermediate in different ferritins can be compared with those of (μ-O)(μ-1,2-O$_2$) bonding in model compounds with Fe$_2$(O)(O$_2$) core structure (b), with those of η^2-O$_2$ bonding in model compounds with Fe$_2$(O$_2$) core structure (c), or with side-on (η^2-O$_2$) bonding mode in the Fe(O$_2$) core structure (d, e). (e) Structure has been proposed for the intermediate P with blue colour in soluble methane monooxygenase. (f) Structure has been suggested for BfMF because of an unusually short Fe–Fe distance of 2.54 Å for the blue intermediate. A short Fe(III)–Fe(III) distance (2.7 Å) has been reported for (μ-O)$_2$ bonding in a model compound. Reprinted with permission from Honarmand Ebrahimi, K.H., Hagedoorn, P.L. and Hagen, W.R. (2014) Unity in the Biochemistry of the Iron-Storage Proteins Ferritin and Bacterioferritin.* Chem. Rev., ***115**, 295–326; © 2014, American Chemical Society*

part of the nascent mineral core. The movement of the Fe(III)–O(H)–Fe(III) product out of the ferroxidase centres is accompanied by the formation of small iron clusters, as demonstrated using Mossbauer spectroscopy for human H-chain and bullfrog M-chain ferritins (Bauminger *et al.*, 1993; Pereira *et al.*, 1997; Bou-Abdallah *et al.*, 2002b). The regeneration of the apo-form of the H-chain ferroxidase centre for further Fe^{2+} oxidation (Waldo and Theil, 1993; Yang *et al.*, 1998; Bou-Abdallah *et al.*, 2005) suggests that the ferroxidase site is a 'gated' iron site. However, it is important to note that the rate of iron migration out of the ferroxidase centre is significantly enhanced by addition of further Fe^{2+}, suggestive of a displacement mechanism (Bou-Abdallah *et al.*, 2005; Honarmand Ebrahimi *et al.*, 2012).

In eukaryotic ferritins, the gateway ferroxidase centre was thought to function as a substrate site, catalysing the oxidation of two Fe(II) ions, followed by spontaneous release of the hydrolysis

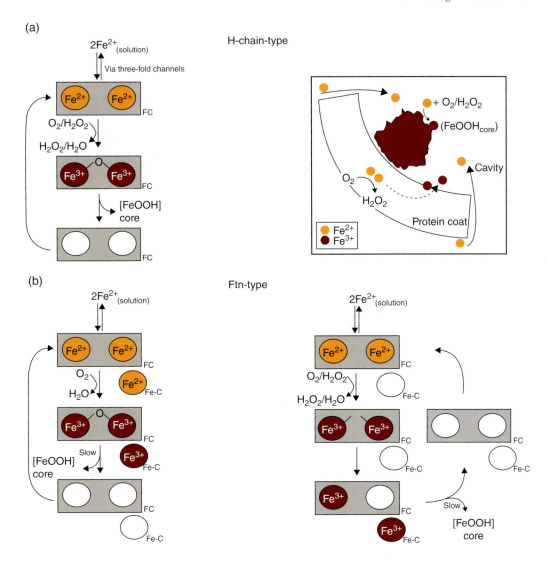

Figure 9.19 *Mechanisms of mineralisation in 24-mer ferritins. (a) Mechanism for H-chain-type ferritins describing how the ferroxidase centre operates as a gated iron site (left-hand side). When a mineral core is established, the surface of the mineral competes as a catalytic site. (b) Mechanistic schemes for Ftn-type ferritins. On the left, the Fe–C site is involved in Fe^{2+} oxidation, while on the right, it functions as a transit/holding site for iron oxidised at the ferroxidase centre. (c) Mechanism for E. coli BFR-type ferritins describing how the ferroxidase centre operates as a true cofactor, cycling its oxidation state as Fe^{2+} is oxidised in the cavity (left-hand side). When a mineral core is established, the mineral itself conducts electrons toward the ferroxidase centre. Reproduced with permission from Springer Verlag from Bradley, J.M., Moore, G.R. and Le Brun, N.E. (2014) Mechanisms of iron mineralization in ferritins: one size does not fit all. J. Biol. Inorg. Chem., **19**, 775–785*

(c)

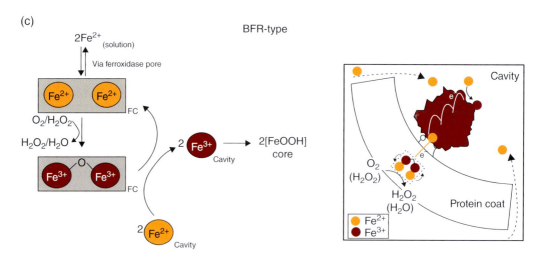

Figure 9.19 (*Continued*)

products of the μ-1,2-oxodiferric intermediate (Figure 9.19a). However, this conclusion has been cast into doubt by more recent studies which show that the Fe(III) resides in a metastable state in the ferroxidase centre until it is displaced by Fe(II), and is subsequently stored in the internal cavity via an as yet unknown pathway. After oxidation of Fe(II) in the ferroxidase centre of *P. furiosus* Ftn, reductive titration monitored using electron paramagnetic resonance (EPR) spectroscopy showed the formation of a mixed-valence [Fe(II)–Fe(III)] cluster in the ferroxidase centre (Tatur and Hagen, 2005). X-ray crystallography provided direct evidence that Fe(III) remains in the ferroxidase centre of *P. furiosus* Ftn and does not spontaneously leave this site (Tatur *et al.*, 2007). This observation has subsequently been confirmed by crystallographic studies on the bacterial Ftns of *Pseudomonas aeruginosa* (Yao *et al.*, 2011) and *Chlorobium tepidum* (Arenas-Salinas, *et al.*, 2014) and, most importantly, on the eukaryote bull-frog M-chain ferritin (Bertini *et al.*, 2012). This suggests that the Fe(III)-O(H)–Fe(III) product of the ferroxidase centre may act as a prosthetic group to catalyse the oxidation of subsequently added Fe(II), or alternatively be displaced from the centre by incoming Fe(II) (Honarmand Ebrahimi *et al.*, 2009). The outcome of a study of iron incorporation into recombinant human H-chain ferritin (thought to follow the eukaryotic mechanism) and *P. furiosus* ferritin (the bacterial mechanism) using a combination of binding experiments, isotopic labelling studies and spectroscopic analysis (Honarmand Ebrahimi *et al.*, 2012), satisfied neither mechanism, and the authors proposed a unifying mechanism in which the Fe(III)–O–Fe(III) unit resides in the ferroxidase centre until it is sequentially displaced by incoming Fe(II) (Figure 9.20). The model posits that Fe^{2+} is distributed between three sites – the A and B sites of the ferroxidase centre and a third site, C. This might not only be the third site described for Ftns and Bfrs, but also the nucleation centre(s) furnished by the L-subunit in most mammalian ferritins. Two possible pathways are envisaged, in the first of which two Fe^{2+} ions bind to the ferroxidase centre, and there is no Fe^{2+} present in site C of the ferroxidase centre gateway. In this case, two Fe^{2+} are oxidised simultaneously via a blue-coloured intermediate and molecular oxygen is reduced to hydrogen peroxide. In the second pathway, two Fe^{2+} ions bind to the ferroxidase centre, and an Fe^{2+} ion binds to site C in the ferroxidase centre gateway. In this situation the two Fe^{2+} in the ferroxidase centre are simultaneously oxidised to form a blue intermediate. The third Fe^{2+} either reacts with this intermediate or is oxidised by the peroxide that is released as

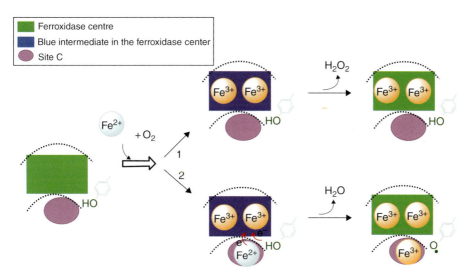

Figure 9.20 *Mechanism of Fe(II) oxidation by ferritin. Because of the distribution of Fe(II) among three binding sites, oxidation of Fe(II) occurs via at least two pathways. Pathway 1: Two Fe(II) ions bind to the ferroxidase centre, and there is no Fe(II) present in site C of the ferroxidase centre gateway. In this case, two Fe(II) are oxidised simultaneously via an intermediate with blue colour and molecular oxygen is reduced to hydrogen peroxide. Pathway 2: Two Fe(II) ions bind to the ferroxidase centre, and an Fe(II) ion binds to site C in the ferroxidase centre gateway. In this situation the two Fe(II) in the ferroxidase centre are simultaneously oxidised to form a blue intermediate. The third Fe(II) either reacts with this intermediate or it is oxidised by the peroxide that is released as the blue intermediate decays. The fourth electron for complete reduction of molecular oxygen to water is proposed to be provided by the conserved tyrosine in the vicinity of the ferroxidase centre. Reprinted with permission from Honarmand Ebrahimi, K.H., Hagedoorn, P.L. and Hagen, W.R. (2014) Unity in the biochemistry of the iron-storage proteins ferritin and bacterioferritin. Chem. Rev., **115**, 295–326; © 2014, American Chemical Society*

the blue intermediate decays. The fourth electron for complete reduction of molecular oxygen to water is proposed to be provided by the conserved tyrosine in the vicinity of the ferroxidase centre, which acts as a single-electron capacitor (Ebrahimi *et al.*, 2013; Honarmand Ebrahimi *et al.*, 2014). As we saw previously, in bacterial and archael ferritins site C has a higher affinity for Fe^{2+} than site C in eukaryotic ferritins, and therefore more Fe^{2+} would be oxidised at this site in bacterial and archael ferritins than in eukaryotic ferritins.

Models for the mechanism of iron storage by mammalian ferritins and bacterial Ftns are illustrated in Figure 9.21 (Honarmand Ebrahimi *et al.*, 2014). Of the two versions of the displacement model (Honarmand Ebrahimi *et al.*, 2012) which were described earlier, the evidence strongly favours sequential displacement of the two Fe(III) in the ferroxidase centre. In the light of the seeming perennity of iron at the ferroxidase centre after the initial round of oxidation, the substrate site model, despite the experimental data marshalled in its support (Bradley *et al.*, 2014), now appears fragile. However, at the very least it is consistent with the Fe(III)–Fe(II) displacement model, confirming the point that the opposing views can often be reconciled.

There remains the question of the haem-containing Bfrs. For three bacterioferritins, namely, *P. aeruginosa* bacterioferritin (PaBFR) (Weeratunga *et al.*, 2010), *A. vinelandii* bacterioferritin (AvBFR) (Swartz *et al.*, 2006) and *D. desulfuricans* bacterioferritin (DdBFR) (Macedo *et al.*, 2003),

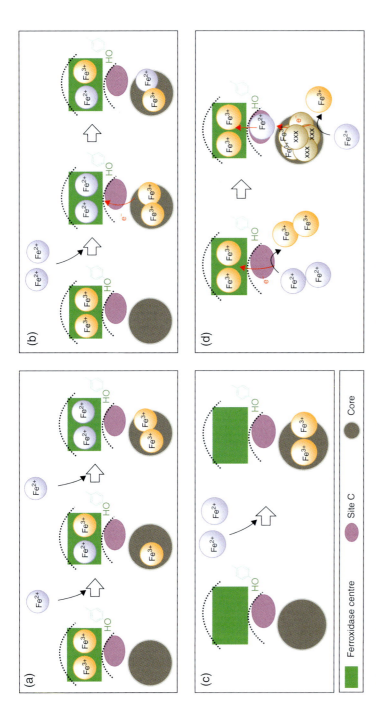

Figure 9.21 Models for the mechanism of iron storage by ferritin and bacterioferritin. (a, b) Fe(III) displacement model for ferritin. On the basis of this model, after oxidation of Fe(II) in the ferroxidase centre the Fe(III) stays metastably in the ferroxidase centre. Movement of Fe(III) from the ferroxidase centre requires the presence of Fe(II). (a) Fe(II) either sequentially displaces the two Fe(III) in the ferroxidase centre or (b) it displaces both Fe(III) simultaneously. (c) Substrate site model for ferritin. On the basis of this model two Fe(II) simultaneously bind to the ferroxidase centre and, after oxidation, Fe(III) spontaneously leave the centre to form the Fe(III) mineral core. As a result the ferroxidase centre is left empty. There is no direct experimental evidence to support this model, and all data on which this model was proposed are consistent with the Fe(III)–Fe(II) displacement model. (d) Complex cofactor site model proposed for EcBFR. In this model the Fe(III) in the ferroxidase centre acts as a cofactor. When there is no core present, Fe(II) ions bind to a third binding site and are oxidised at this site via an electron transfer mechanism to the Fe(III) in the ferroxidase centre, where molecular oxygen is reduced to hydrogen peroxide. When enough Fe(III)–mineral core is formed, the Fe(II) ions are oxidised on the surface of a core and the electrons are transferred to the Fe(III) in the ferroxidase centre via the proposed Fe(II) binding site. Subsequently, molecular oxygen is reduced in the ferroxidase centre to water. Experimental data on which this complex model was based can be interpreted in the frame of the simplified Fe(III)–Fe(II) displacement model. Reprinted with permission from Honarmand Ebrahimi, K.H., Hagedoorn, P.L. and Hagen, W.R. (2014) Unity in the Biochemistry of the Iron-Storage Proteins Ferritin and Bacterioferritin. Chem. Rev., *115*, 295–326; © 2014, American Chemical Society

structural data suggested that Fe(II) may reach the ferroxidase centre through a ferroxidase channel, and that the ferroxidase centre acts as a gateway from where the Fe(III) product of oxidation of Fe(II) somehow enters the protein cavity. Details of this mechanism remain to be explored, but it is possible that the Fe(III)–Fe(II) displacement model (Figure 9.21a/b) could apply (Honarmand Ebrahimi *et al.*, 2014). For *E. coli* BFR (EcBFR) a different model has been proposed (Bradley *et al.*, 2014; Crow *et al.*, 2009), namely that the ferroxidase centre functions as a true enzyme cofactor site (Figure 9.19c), continually cycling its redox state (Le Brun *et al.*, 1995; Yang *et al.*, 2000; Baaghil *et al.*, 2003; Crow *et al.*, 2009; Lawson *et al.*, 2009). The similarity between the BFR ferroxidase centre and the di-iron sites of other well-characterised di-iron enzymes (Le Brun *et al.*, 1995) was already pointed out earlier. Since there clearly is a third iron-binding site in EcBFR, it does not seem impossible that the displacement mechanism evoked above could also apply.

9.3.2 Iron Uptake in Dps Proteins

The ferroxidase centre of Dps proteins is highly conserved and has an unusual location, not within the four-helix bundle of one subunit but rather, in most cases, at the interface of twofold symmetry-related subunits (see Figure 9.9) (Ilari *et al.*, 2000). Two known exceptions are the Dps-like dodeca-meric proteins from the Archae *Pyrococcus furiosus* (Ramsay *et al.*, 2006) and *Sulfolobus solfataricus* (Gauss *et al.*, 2006), in which the ferroxidase centre resembles the bacterioferritins; they probably belong to a different branch of the ferritin superfamily. In Dps proteins, both subunits provide the iron ligands, usually two histidines from one subunit and two carboxylates from the other (Chiancone and Ceci, 2010a). The occupancy of the two iron-binding sites varies significantly in the known crystal structures, indicating that the amino acids in the second coordination sphere influence the affinity of the ferroxidase centre for iron (Chiancone and Ceci, 2010a). The ferroxi-dase centre of Dps proteins has another striking feature which distinguishes it from those of ferritins and bacterioferritins. Whereas ferritins in general use O_2 as oxidant, generating H_2O_2 (Zhao *et al.*, 2003), and bacterioferritins can use both O_2 and H_2O_2 (Bunker *et al.*, 2005), Dps proteins prefer H_2O_2, which usually catalyses the ferroxidation reaction between 100- and 1000-fold faster than O_2 (Tonello *et al.*, 1999; Zhao *et al.*, 2002; Su *et al.*, 2005; Franceschini, *et al.*, 2006). The only reported exception is Dps2 from *B. anthracis*, which reacts with Fe(II) and H_2O_2 only threefold faster than with O_2 (Liu *et al.*, 2006). After oxidation, Fe^{3+} moves to the internal Dps protein cavity, forming a microcrystalline core that can contain up to 400–500 iron atoms (Ilari *et al.*, 2002).

9.3.3 Iron Release from Ferritin

Storage iron, whether it be haemosiderin or ferritin, can be mobilised to meet body iron require-ments, particularly in conditions of iron demand. Yet, despite many efforts over a long period the molecular mechanisms that allow iron release *in vivo* are not understood. A great many *in-vitro* studies have been carried out which show that the incubation of mammalian ferritin or haemosid-erin with either chelators alone or with reducing agents in the presence of Fe(II) chelators can lead to iron release. The fastest rates were observed with dihydroflavins in conjunction with a suitable Fe(II) chelator (Sirivech *et al.*, 1974; Jones *et al.*, 1978; Funk *et al.*, 1985), and it was concluded that redox reactions involving the ferritin core can occur without direct interaction of the redox reagent at the mineral core surface (Funk *et al.*, 1985; Watt *et al.*, 1988). It has also been proposed *in vitro* that the channels along the threefold symmetry axes of ferritin control both Fe(II) entry and exit (Theil, 2011; Theil *et al.*, 2008; Tosha *et al.*, 2010). The manipulation of a specific group of conserved channel amino acids which eliminate conserved ionic or hydrophobic interactions between Arg72 and Asp122 and between Leu110 and Leu134 increases unfolding of the channel structure and selectively increases mineral dissolution and Fe^{2+} exit after the addition of reductants (Tosha *et al.*, 2012). It remains to be established whether the generation of Fe^{2+} ions within ferritin results from direct contact with external reductants, or from electron transfer through the protein. The recent suggestion that the iron in the ferroxidase centre of mammalian ferritins might be directly scavenged *in vivo* by transferrin (Honarmand Ebrahimi *et al.*, 2012, 2014) appears to be physiologically unrealistic. In the case of haem-containing Bfrs it has been proposed that iron release from Bfr was significantly increased in the presence of haem (Yasmin *et al.*, 2011).

Currently, there are two models for ferritin iron mobilisation based on *in-vivo* experimentation. The first model implies that cytosolic ferritin must gain access to lysosomes, and that ferritin degradation within the lysosome is responsible for iron release, based on studies in which iron demand was induced by desferrioxamine (DFO) treatment (Bridges, 1987; Kidane *et al.*, 2006), and has been recently reviewed (Linder, 2013). Figure 9.22 summarises the most plausible steps

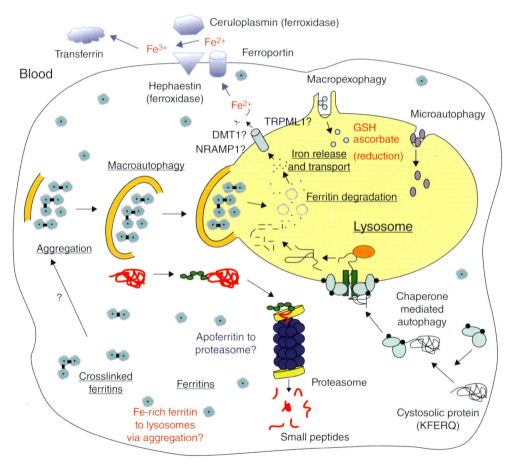

Figure 9.22 *Summary of the potential and most likely steps involved in mobilisation of iron stored in cytosolic ferritin when the need arises. A description of the steps is given in the text. Various forms of lysosomal autophagy, including those not involved in ferritin uptake, are also depicted. From Linder, M.C. (2013) Mobilization of stored iron in mammals: a review.* Nutrients, **5**, *4022–4050. This article is an open access article distributed under the terms and conditions of the Creative Commons Attribution license*

involved which may be summarised as follows (Linder, 2013). It is suggested that, in response to iron deprivation (resulting in a decreased content of the labile iron pool) and/or decreased oxygen tension, cytosolic ferritin is taken up by lysosomes via autophagy. The nuclear receptor coactivator 4 (NCOA4) was recently identified as the cargo-receptor protein mediating autophagy of ferritin heavy and light chains (Mancias *et al.*, 2014). The form of autophagy is unclear, but once in the lysosomes the ferritin shell is degraded by cathepsins, exposing the iron within the ferrihydrite core to reduction/chelation, and transport into the cytosol. There, it joins the labile iron pool either for redistribution within the cell or for export into the extracellular medium.

The second mechanism, based on studies using expression of the iron exporter ferroportin to deplete cytosolic iron, indicated that iron was released from ferritin in the cytosol and apoferritin degraded by the proteasome (De Domenico *et al.*, 2006). Subsequent studies indicated that cell-permeable chelators induce ferritin degradation via the proteosome, while confirming that the poorly permeable DFO induced ferritin degradation by lysosomes (De Domenico *et al.*, 2009). It is possible that the two hypotheses are complementary, in the sense that the lysosome may preferentially target iron-rich ferritin whereas apoferritin and iron-poor ferritin are degraded in the cytosol by the proteasome, in order to minimise the reincorporation of iron into ferritin (Linder, 2013).

It has been shown that the bis-Met-coordinated haems in *E. coli* BFR play an important role in iron release from the mineral core, with the electron transfer of electrons into the inner cavity being the rate-limiting step of the release reaction, whereas the ferroxidase centre is not involved in iron release (Yasmin *et al.*, 2011).

9.4 Biotechnological Applications of Ferritins

The potential to utilizing the apoferritin protein shell as a 'nanoreactor' for the formation of a variety of non-native, unusual, mineralised nanoparticles has been exploited for a considerable number of years. Early examples included the generation of magnetic cores of mixed-valence minerals, magnetite (Fe_3O_4) and/or maghaemite (γ-Fe_2O_3) (Meldrum *et al.*, 1992; Wong *et al.*, 1998), cores of amorphous iron sulphide (Douglas *et al.*, 1995), and of manganese oxyhydroxide (MnOOH) (Meldrum *et al.*, 1995). In both, mammalian ferritins (Douglas and Stark, 2000) and *L. innocua* Dps protein (Allen *et al.*, 2003), mineral cores of cobalt and oxygen can be generated by the protein-catalysed oxidation of Co^{2+} to Co^{3+}, and ferritin cores containing cadmium sulphide (Wong and Mann, 1996), iron and cobalt oxide and metallic nanoparticles (Hosein *et al.*, 2004), nickel and chromium nanoparticles (Okuda *et al.*, 2003). Cu and CuFe Prussian Blue derivative nanoparticles (Gálvez *et al.*, 2005) have also been prepared. The iron core of ferritins has also been used to photocatalyse the formation of Cu(0) colloids from aqueous Cu^{2+} within the protein cavity (Ensign *et al.*, 2004).

More recently, nanoparticle-based drugs have emerged as an important category of therapeutics, and a myriad array of nanoparticles, including metals, metal oxides, carbon nanotubes, liposomes and polymers, have been investigated as drug-delivery nanocarriers (Hughes, 2005; Peer *et al.*, 2007), although to date, few nanoparticle-based drugs have been approved for therapeutic use (Zhen *et al.*, 2014). With their large central cavity, which can be loaded with various transition metals or, indeed, with molecules such as drugs or photosensitisers with high efficiency (Zhen *et al.*, 2013; Sun *et al.*, 2011), and with a surface that can be easily modified chemically or genetically to introduce functionalities (Hainfeld, 1992; Lin *et al.*, 2011), apoferritins represent a powerful system with potential for use in both imaging and drug delivery. Recent progress on the use of ferritins as a platform to construct functional nanoparticles for applications in magnetic resonance imaging, optical imaging, cell tracking, and drug delivery are reviewed by Zhen *et al.* (2014).

The incorporation of drugs within the ferritin protein shell can, in principle, be used to vectorise the drug to key biological targets. As pointed out in Chapter 6, TfR1 has been found to bind human H-chain ferritin, and while the physiological implications are unclear the fact that Tfr1 is upregulated in cancer cells has led to strategies to target anticancer drugs to tumour cells using H-chain ferritin (Fan *et al.*, 2012, 2013), both for tumour detection and therapy. Examples are the use of ferritin to vehicle anticancer drugs, such as doxorubicin (Kilic *et al.*, 2012; Liang *et al.*, 2014) or photosensitisers (Yan *et al.*, 2008; Zhen *et al.*, 2013) to cancer cells.

The haem-containing bacterioferritins are an attractive protein scaffold with which to build a simple, light-driven photocatalyst based on the organisation and function of the donor side of the Photo System II reaction centre, as a model for artificial photosynthesis,. Bacterioferritin (BFR) (cytochrome b_1) has several, inherently useful design features for engineering light-driven electron transport. Among these are: (i) a di-iron binding site; (ii) a potentially redox-active tyrosine residue; and (iii) the ability to dimerise and form an inter-protein haem-binding pocket within electron tunnelling distance of the di-iron binding site (Conlan *et al.*, 2009). Illumination of the engineered BFR in which the haem has been replaced by photoactive zinc-chlorine6 (ZnCe6) and the di-iron site with two Mn ions, which bind as a weakly coupled dinuclear Mn2II,II centre results in oxidation of the dinuclear Mn cluster, with tyrosine residues possibly functioning as electron tunnelling intermediates. More recently, light-induced electron transfer from proximal tyrosine residues to the photo-oxidised ZnCe6 has been reported in this model (Hingorani *et al.*, 2014).

References

Allen, M., Willits, D., Young, M. and Douglas, T. (2003) Constrained synthesis of cobalt oxide nanomaterials in the 12 subunit protein cage from *Listeria innocua*. *Inorg. Chem.*, **42**, 6300–6305.

Altuvia, S., Almirón, M., Huisman, G., Kolter, R. and Storz, G. (1994) The dps promoter is activated by OxyR during growth and by IHF and sigma S in stationary phase. *Mol. Microbiol.*, **13**, 265–272.

Almiron, M., Link, A.J., Furlong, D. and Kolter, R.A. (1992) A novel DNA-binding protein with regulatory and protective roles in starved *Escherichia coli*. *Genes Dev.*, **6**, 2646–2654.

Andersen, Ø., Dehli, A., Standal, H., *et al.* (1995) Two ferritin subunits of Atlantic salmon (*Salmo salar*): cloning of the liver cDNAs and antibody preparation. *Mol. Mar. Biol. Biotechnol.*, **4**, 164–170.

Andrews, S.C. (2010) The Ferritin-like superfamily: Evolution of the biological iron storeman from a rubrerythrin-like ancestor. *Biochim. Biophys. Acta*, **1800**, 691–705.

Andrews, S.C., Arosio, P., Bottke, W., *et al.* (1992) Structure, function, and evolution of ferritins. *J. Inorg. Biochem.*, **47**, 161–174.

Andrews, S.C., Le Brun, N.E., Barynin, V., *et al.* (1995) Site-directed replacement of the coaxial heme ligands of bacterioferritin generates heme-free variants. *J. Biol. Chem.*, **270**, 23268–23274.

Antonyuk, S.V. and Hough, M.A. (2011) Monitoring and validating active site redox states in protein crystals. *Biochim. Biophys. Acta*, **1814**, 778–784.

Arenas-Salinas, M., Townsend, P.D., Brito, C., *et al.* (2014) The crystal structure of ferritin from Chlorobium tepidum reveals a new conformation of the 4-fold channel for this protein family. *Biochimie*, **106**, 39–47.

Baaghil, S., Lewin, A., Moore, G.R. and Le Brun, N.E. (2003) Core formation in *Escherichia coli* bacterioferritin requires a functional ferroxidase center. *Biochemistry*, **42**, 14047–14056.

Barynin, V.V., Whittaker, M.M., Antonyuk, S.V, *et al.* (2001) Crystal structure of manganese catalase from *Lactobacillus plantarum*. *Structure*. **9**, 725–738.

Bauminger, E.R., Harrison, P.M., Hechel, D., *et al.* (1993) Iron (II) oxidation and early intermediates of iron-core formation in recombinant human H-chain ferritin. *Biochem. J.*, **296**, 709–719.

Bertini, I., Lalli, D., Mangani, S., *et al.* (2012) Structural insights into the ferroxidase site of ferritins from higher eukaryotes. *J. Am. Chem. Soc.*, **134**, 6169–6176.

Bhartacharyya, A. and Grove, S.P. (2007) Differential DNA binding and protection by dimeric and dodeca-meric forms of the ferritin homolog Dps from *Deinococcus radiodurans*. *J. Mol. Biol.*, **347**, 495–508.

Bielig, H.J. and Bayer, E. (1955) Synthetisches Ferritin, ein Elsen(III)-komplex des Apoferritins. *Naturwissenschafte*, **42**, 125–126.

Bou-Abdallah, F. (2010) The iron redox and hydrolysis chemistry of the ferritins. *Biochim. Biophys. Acta*, **1800**, 719–731.

Bou-Abdallah, F., Arosio, P., Santambrogio, P., *et al.* (2002a) Ferrous ion binding to recombinant human H chain ferritin. An isothermal titration calorimetry study. *Biochemistry*, **41**, 11184–11191.

Bou-Abdallah, F., Papaefthymiou, G.C., Scheswohl, D.M., *et al.* (2002b) mu-1,2-Peroxobridged di-iron(III) dimer formation in human H-chain ferritin. *Biochem. J.*, **364**, 57–63.

Bou-Abdallah, F., Zhao, G., Mayne, H.R., Arosio, P. and Chasteen, N.D. (2005) Origin of the unusual kinetics of iron deposition in human H-chain ferritin. *J. Am. Chem. Soc.*, **127**, 3885–3893.

Bou-Abdallah, F., Zhao, G., Biasiotto, G., *et al.* (2008) Facilitated diffusion of iron(II) and dioxygen substrates into human H-chain ferritin. A fluorescence and absorbance study employing the ferroxidase center substitution Y34W. *J. Am. Chem. Soc.*, **130**, 17801–17811.

Boyd, D., Vecoli, C., Belcher, D.M., Jain, S.K. and Drysdale, J.W. (1985) Structural and functional relationships of human ferritin H and L chains deduced from cDNA clones. *J. Biol. Chem.* **260**, 11755–11761.

Bozzi, M., Mignogna, G., Stefanini, S., *et al.* (1997) A novel non-heme iron-binding ferritin related to the DNA-binding proteins of the Dps family in *Listeria* innocua. *J. Biol. Chem.*, **272**, 3259–3265.

Bradley, J.M., Moore, G.R. and Le Brun, N.E. (2014) Mechanisms of iron mineralization in ferritins: one size does not fit all. *J. Biol. Inorg. Chem.*, **19**, 775–785.

Bridges, K.R. (1987) Ascorbic acid inhibits lysosomal autophagy of ferritin. *J. Biol. Chem.*, **262**, 14773–14778.

Broadwater, J.A., Ai, J., Loehr, T.M., Sanders-Loehr, J. and Fox, B.G. (1998) Peroxodiferric intermediate of stearoyl-acyl carrier protein Δ^9 desaturase: oxidase reactivity during single turnover and implications for the mechanism of desaturation *Biochemistry*, **37**, 14664–14671.

Bunker J., Lowry, T., Davis, G., *et al.* (2005) Kinetic studies of iron deposition catalyzed by recombinant human liver heavy and light ferritins and *Azotobacter vinelandii* bacterioferritin using O_2 and H_2O_2 as oxidants. *Biophys. Chem.*, **114**, 235–244.

Carette, N., Hagen, W., Bertrand, L., *et al.* (2006) Optical and EPR spectroscopic studies of demetallation of hemin by L chain apoferritins. *J. Inorg. Biochem.*, **100**, 1426.

Castruita, M., Saito, M., Schottel, P.C., *et al.* (2006) Overexpression and characterization of an iron storage and DNA-binding Dps protein from *Trichodesmium erythraeum*. *Appl. Environ. Microbiol.*, **72**, 2918–2924.

Ceci, P., Ilari, A., Falvo, E. and Chiancone E. (2003) The Dps protein of *Agrobacterium tumefaciens* does not bind to DNA but protects it toward oxidative cleavage: x-ray crystal structure, iron binding, and hydroxyl-radical scavenging properties. *J. Biol. Chem.*, **278**, 20319–20326.

Ceci, P., Cellai, S., Falvo, E., *et al.* (2004) DNA condensation and self-aggregation of *Escherichia coli* Dps are coupled phenomena related to the properties of the N-terminus. *Nucleic Acids Res.*, **32**, 5935–5944.

Ceci, P., Ilari, A., Falvo, E., Giangiacomo, L. and Chiancone, E. (2005) Reassessment of protein stability, DNA binding, and protection of *Mycobacterium smegmatis* Dps. *J. Biol. Chem.*, **280**, 34776–34785.

Ceci, P., Mangiarotti, L., Rivetti, C. and Chiancone, E. (2007) The neutrophil-activating Dps protein of *Helicobacter pylori*, HP-NAP, adopts a mechanism different from *Escherichia coli* Dps to bind and condense DNA. *Nucleic Acids Res.*, **35**, 2247–2256.

Chasteen, N.D. and Harrison, P.M. (1999) Mineralization in ferritin: an efficient means of iron storage. *J. Struct. Biol.*, **126**, 182–194.

Chen, T., Villeneuve, T.S., Garant, K.A., Amons, R. and MacRae, T.H. (2007) Functional characterization of artemin, a ferritin homolog synthesized in *Artemia* embryos during encystment and diapauses. *FEBS J.*, **274**, 1093–1101.

Chen-Barrett, Y., Harrison, P.M., Treffry, A., *et al.* (1995) Tyrosyl radical formation during the oxidative deposition of iron in human apoferritin. *Biochemistry*, **34**, 7847–7853.

Chiancone, E. and Ceci, P. (2010a) The multifaceted capacity of Dps proteins to combat bacterial stress conditions: Detoxification of iron and hydrogen peroxide and DNA binding. *Biochim. Biophys. Acta*, **1800**, 798–805.

Chiancone, E. and Ceci, P. (2010b) Role of Dps (DNA-binding proteins from starved cells) aggregation on DNA. *Front. Biosci.*, **15**, 122–131.

Cho, K.J., Shin, H.J., Lee, J.H., *et al.* (2009) The crystal structure of ferritin from *Helicobacter pylori* reveals unusual conformational changes for iron uptake. *J. Mol. Biol.*, **390**, 83–98.

Cobessi, D., Huang, L.S., Ban, M., Pon, N.G., *et al.* (2002) The 2.6 Å resolution structure of *Rhodobacter capsulatus* bacterioferritin with metal-free dinuclear site and heme iron in a crystallographic 'special position'. *Acta Crystallogr. D*, **54**, 29–38.

Conlan, B., Cox, N., Su, J.N., *et al.* (2009) Photo-catalytic oxidation of a di-nuclear manganese centre in an engineered bacterioferritin 'reaction centre'. *Biochim. Biophys. Acta*, **1787**, 1112–1121.

Costanzo, F., Santoro, C., Colantuoni, V., *et al.* (1984) Cloning and sequencing of a full length cDNA coding for a human apoferritin H chain: evidence for a multigene family. *EMBO J.*, **3**, 23–27.

Cook, S.F. (1929) The structure and composition of hemosiderin. *J. Biol. Chem.*, **82**, 595–609.

Cooley, R.B., Arp, D.J. and Karplus, P.A. (2011) Symerythrin structures at atomic resolution and the origins of rubrerythrins and the ferritin-like superfamily. *J. Mol. Biol.*, **413**, 177–194.

Corsi, B., Cozzi, A., Arosio, P., *et al.* (2002) Human mitochondrial ferritin expressed in HeLa cells incorporates iron and affects cellular iron metabolism. *J. Biol. Chem.*, **277**, 22430–22437.

Costanzo, F., Santoro, C., Colantuoni, V., *et al.* (1984) Cloning and sequencing of a full length cDNA coding for a human apoferritin H chain: evidence for a multigene family. *EMBO J.* **3**, 23–27.

Coulter, E.D., Shenvi, N.V., Beharry, Z.M., Smith, J.J. and Prickril, B.C. (2000) Rubrerythrin-catalyzed substrate oxidation by dioxygen and hydrogen peroxide. *Inorg. Chim. Acta*, **297**, 231–241.

Crichton, R.R. (1978) Ferritin iron deposition and mobilization: molecular mechanisms and cellular consequences, in *Transport by Proteins* (eds G. Blauer and H. Sund), de Gruyter, Berlin, pp. 243–258

Crichton, R.R. (2009) *Inorganic Biochemistry of Iron Metabolism from Molecular Mechanisms to Clinical Consequences*, 3rd edition, John Wiley & Sons, Chichester, pp. 183–222.

Crichton, R.R. and Roman, F. (1978) A novel mechanism for ferritin iron oxidation and Deposition. *J. Mol. Catal.*, **4**, 75–82.

Crichton, R.R. and Declercq, J.P. (2010) X-ray structures of ferritins and related proteins. *Biochim. Biophys. Acta*, **1800**, 706–718.

Crichton, R.R., Soruco, J.-A., Roland, F., *et al.* (1997) Remarkable ability of horse spleen apoferritin to demetallate hemin and to metallate protoporphyrin IX as a function of pH. *Biochemistry*, **36**, 15049–15054.

Crow, A., Lawson, T.L., Lewin, A., Moore, G.R. and Le Brun, N.E. (2009) Structural basis for iron mineralization by bacterioferritin. *J. Am. Chem. Soc.*, **131**, 6808–6813.

Dautant, A., Meyer, J.B., Yariv, J., Précigoux, G., *et al.* (1998) Structure of a monoclinic crystal from of cyctochrome b1 (Bacterioferritin) from *E. coli*. *Acta Crystallogr. D*, **54**, 16–24.

De Domenico, I., Vaughn, M.B., Li, J., *et al.* (2006) Ferroportin-mediated mobilization of ferritin iron precedes ferritin degradation by the proteasome. *EMBO J.*, **25**, 5396–5404.

De Domenico, I., Ward, D.M. and Kaplan, J. (2009) Specific iron chelators determine the route of ferritin degradation. *Blood*, **114**, 4546–4551.

deMaré, F., Kurtz, D.M. Jr and Nordlund, P. (1996) The structure of *Desulfovibrio vulgaris* rubrerythrin reveals a unique combination of rubredoxin-like FeS4 and ferritin-like diiron domains. *Nat. Struct. Biol.*, **3**, 539–546.

de Val, N., Declercq, J.P., Lim, C.K. and Crichton, R.R. (2012) Structural analysis of haemin demetallation by L-chain apoferritins. *J. Inorg. Biochem.*, **112**, 77–84.

Dickey, L.F., Sreedharan, S., Theil, E.C., *et al.* (1987) Differences in the regulation of messenger RNA for housekeeping and specialized-cell ferritin. A comparison of three distinct ferritin complementary DNAs, the corresponding subunits, and identification of the first processed in amphibia. *J. Biol. Chem.*, **262**, 7901–7907.

Dillard, B.D., Demick, J.M., Adams, M.W. and Lanzilotta, W.N. (2011) A cryo-crystallographic time course for peroxide reduction by rubrerythrin from *Pyrococcus furiosus*. *J. Biol. Inorg. Chem.*, **16**, 949–959.

Douglas, T. and Ripoll, D.R. (1998) Calculated electrostatic gradients in recombinant human H chain ferritin. *Protein Sci.*, **1**, 1083–1091.

Douglas, T. and Stark, V.T. (2000) Nanophase cobalt oxyhydroxide mineral synthesized within the protein cage of ferritin. *Inorg. Chem.*, **39**, 1828–1830.

Douglas, T., Dickson, D.P., Betteridge, S., *et al.* (1995) Synthesis and structure of an iron(III) sulfide-ferritin bioinorganic nanocomposite. *Science*, **269**, 54–57.

Dusek, P., Dezortova, M. and Wuerfel, J. (2013) Imaging of iron. *Int. Rev. Neurobiol.*, **110**, 195–239.

Ebrahimi, K.H., Hagedoorn, P.-L. and Hagen, W.R. (2013) A conserved tyrosine in ferritin is a molecular capacitor. *ChemBioChem*, **14**, 1123–1133.

Ensign, D., Young, M. and Douglas, T. (2004) Photocatalytic synthesis of copper colloids from CuII by the ferrihydrite core of ferritin. *Inorg. Chem.*, **43**, 3441–3446.

Evans, J.E. and Browning, N.D. (2013) Enabling direct nanoscale observations of biological reactions with dynamic TEM. *Microscopy (Oxf).*, **62**, 147–156.

Fan, K., Cao, C. and Pan, Y. (2012) Magnetoferritin nanoparticles for targeting and visualizing tumour tissues. *Nat. Nanotechnol.*, **7**, 459–464.

Fan, K., Gao, L. and Yan, X. (2013) Human ferritin for tumor detection and therapy. *WIREs Nanomed Nanobiotechnol.*, **5**, 287–298.

Finn, R.D., Mistry, J., Tate, J., *et al.* (2010) The Pfam protein families database. *Nucleic Acids Res.*, **D38**, D211–D222.

Fischbach, F.A. and Anderegg, J.W. (1965) An X-ray scattering study of ferritin and Apoferritin. *J. Mol. Biol.*, **14**, 458–473.

Ford, G.C., Harrison, P.M., Rice, D.W., *et al.* (1984) Ferritin: design and formation of an iron-storage molecule. *Philos. Trans. R. Soc. Lond. B*, **304**, 551–565.

Franceschini, S., Ceci, P., Alaleona, F., Chiancone, E. and Ilari, A. (2006) Antioxidant Dps protein from the thermophilic cyanobacterium *Thermosynechococcus elongates*. *FEBS J.*, **273**, 4913–4928.

Frolow, F. and Kalb, A.J. (2001) Cytochrome *b*1-bacterioferritin, in *Handbook of Metalloproteins* (eds A.H.R. Messerschmidt, K. Poulos and K. Weighardt), Vol. 2, John Wiley & Sons, Chichester, UK, pp. 782–790.

Frolow, F., Kalb, A.J. and Yariv, Y. (1994) Structure of a unique twofold symmetric haem-binding site. *Nat. Struct. Biol.*, **1**, 453–460.

Funk, F., Lenders, J.P., Crichton, R.R. and Schneider W. (1985) Reductive mobilisation of ferritin iron. *Eur. J. Biochem.*, **152**, 167–172.

Fushinobu, S., Shoun, H. and Wakagi, T. (2003) Crystal structure of sulerythrin, a rubrerythrin-like protein from a strictly aerobic archaeon, *Sulfolobus tokodaii* strain 7, shows unexpected domain swapping. *Biochemistry*, **42**, 11707–11715.

Gálvez, N., Sánchez, P. and Domínguez-Vera, J.M.. (2005) Preparation of Cu and CuFe Prussian Blue derivative nanoparticles using the apoferritin cavity as nanoreactor. *Dalton Trans.*, 2492–2494.

Gauss, G.H., Benas, P., Wiedenheft, B., *et al.* (2006) Structure of the DPS-like protein from *Sulfolobus solfataricus* reveals a bacterioferritin-like dimetal binding site within a DPS-like dodecameric assembly. *Biochemistry*, **45**, 10815–10827.

Gerl, M. and Jaenicke, R. (1987a) Mechanism of the self-assembly of apoferritin from horse spleen. Cross-linking and spectroscopic analysis. *Eur. Biophys. J.*, **15**, 103–109.

Gerl, M. and Jaenicke, R. (1987b) Assembly of apoferritin from horse spleen: comparison of the protein in its native and reassembled state. *Biol. Chem. Hoppe Seyler*, **368**, 387–396.

Gomes, C.M., Le Gall, J., Xavier, A.V. and Teixeira, M. (2001) Could a diiron-containing four-helix-bundle protein have been a primitive oxygen reductase? *ChemBioChem*, **2**, 583–587.

Grant, R.A., Filman, D.J. Finkel, S.E. Kolter, R. and Hogle, J.M. (1998) The crystal structure of Dps, a ferritin homolog that binds and protects DNA. *Nat. Struct. Biol.*, **5**, 294–303.

Grove, A. and Wilkinson, S.P. (2005) Differential DNA binding and protection by dimeric and dodecameric forms of the ferritin homolog Dps from *Deinococcus radiodurans*. *J. Mol. Biol.*, **347**, 495–508.

Gupta, S. and Chatterji, D. (2003) Bimodal protection of DNA by *Mycobacterium smegmatis* DNA-binding protein from stationary phase cells. *J. Biol. Chem.*, **278**, 5235–5241.

Gupta, V., Gupta, R.K., Khare, G., Salunke, D.M, and Tyagi, A.K. (2009) Crystal structure of Bfr A from *Mycobacterium tuberculosis*: incorporation of selenomethionine results in cleavage and demetallation of haem. *PLoS One*, **4**, e8028.

Hainfeld, J.F. (1992) Uranium-loaded apoferritin with antibodies attached – molecular design for uranium neutron-capture therapy. *Proc. Natl Acad. Sc. USA*, **89**,11064–11068.

Hamburger, A.E., West, A.P. Jr, Hamburger, Z.A., *et al.* (2005) Crystal structure of a secreted insect ferritin reveals a symmetrical arrangement of heavy and light chains. *J. Mol. Biol.*, **349**, 558–569.

Hempstead, P.D., Hudson, A.J., Artymiuk, P.J., *et al.* (1994) Direct observation of the iron binding sites in a ferritin. *FEBS Lett.*, **350**, 258–262.

Hempstead, P.D., Yewdall, S.J., Fernie, A.R., *et al.* (1997) Comparison of the three dimensional structures of recombinant human H and horse L ferritins at high resolution. *J. Mol. Biol.*, **268**, 424–448.

Heusterspreute, M. and Crichton, R.R. (1981) Amino acid sequence of horse spleen Apoferritin. *FEBS Lett.*, **129**, 322–327.

Hingorani, K., Pace, R., Whitney, S., *et al.* (2014) Photo-oxidation of tyrosine in a bio-engineered bacterioferritin 'reaction centre' – a protein model for artificial photosynthesis. *Biochim. Biophys. Acta*, **1837**, 1821–1834.

Honarmand Ebrahimi, K., Hagedoorn, P.L., Jongejan, J.J. and Hagen, W.R. (2009) Catalysis of iron core formation in *Pyrococcus furiosus* ferritin. *J. Biol. Inorg. Chem.*, **14**, 1265–1274.

Honarmand Ebrahimi, K., Bill, E., Hagedoorn, P.L. and Hagen, W.R. (2012) The catalytic center of ferritin regulates iron storage via Fe(II)-Fe(III) displacement. *Nat. Chem. Biol.*, **8**, 941–948.

Honarmand Ebrahimi, K.H., Hagedoorn, P.L. and Hagen, W.R. (2014) Unity in the biochemistry of the iron-storage proteins ferritin and bacterioferritin. *Chem. Rev.*, **115**, 295–326.

Hosein, H.A., Strongin, D.R., Allen, M. and Douglas, T. (2004) Iron and cobalt oxide and metallic nanoparticles prepared from ferritin. *Langmuir*, **20**, 10283–10287.

Hughes, G.A. (2005) Nanostructure-mediated drug delivery. *Nanomedicine*, **1**, 22–30.

Ilari, A., Stefanini, S., Chiancone, E. and Tsernoglou, D. (2000) The dodecameric ferritin from *Listeria innocua* contains a novel intersubunit iron-binding site. *Nat. Struct. Biol.*, **7**, 38–43.

Ilari, A., Ceci, P., Ferrari, D., *et al.* (2002) Iron incorporation into *Escherichia coli* Dps gives rise to a ferritin-like microcrystalline core. *J. Biol. Chem.*, **277**, 37619–37623.

Iyer, R.B., Silaghi-Dumitrescu, R., Kurtz, D.M. Jr and Lanzilotta, W.N. (2005) High-resolution crystal structures of *Desulfovibrio vulgaris* (Hildenborough) nigerythrin: facile, redox-dependent iron movement, domain interface variability, and peroxidase activity in the rubrerythrins. *J. Biol. Inorg. Chem.*, **10**, 407–416.

Jamieson, G.N.L., Jin, W., Krebs, C., *et al.* (2002) Stoichiometric production of hydrogen peroxide and parallel formation of ferric multimers through decay of the diferric-peroxo complex, the first detectable intermediate in ferritin mineralization. *Biochemistry*, **41**, 13435–13443.

Jin, S., Kurtz, D.M. Jr, Liu, Z.J., Rose, J. and Wang, B.C. (2002) X-ray crystal structure of *Desulfovibrio vulgaris* rubrerythrin with zinc substituted into the $[Fe(SCys)_4]$ site and alternative diiron site structures. *J. Am. Chem. Soc.*, **124**, 9845–9855.

Johnson, E., Cascio, D., Sawaya, M.R., *et al.* (2005) Crystal structures of a tetrahedral open pore ferritin from the hyperthermophilic archaeon *Archaeoglobus fulgidus*. *Structure*, **13**, 637–648.

Jones, T., Spencer, R. and Walsh, C. (1978) Mechanism and kinetics of iron release from ferritin by dihydroflavins and dihydroflavin analogues. *Biochemistry*, **17**, 4011–4017.

Kawasaki, S., Ono, M., Watamura, Y., *et al.* (2007) An O_2-inducible rubrerythrin-like protein, rubperoxin, is functional as a H_2O_2 reductase in an obligatory anaerobe *Clostridium acetobutylicum*. *FEBS Lett.*, **581**, 2460–2464.

Keogh, M.J., Jonas, P., Coulthard, A., Chinnery, P.F. and Burn, J. (2012) Neuroferritinopathy: a new inborn error of iron metabolism. *Neurogenetics*, **13**, 93–96.

Keogh, M.J., Morris, C.M. and Chinnery, P.F. (2013) Neuroferritinopathy. *Int. Rev. Neurobiol.*, **110**, 91–123.

Keren, N., Aurora, R. and Pakrasi, H.B. (2004) Critical roles of bacterioferritins in iron storage and proliferation of cyanobacteria. *Plant Physiol.*, **135**, 1666–1673.

Khare, G., Gupta, V., Nangpal, P., *et al.* (2011) Ferritin structure from *Mycobacterium tuberculosis*: comparative study with homologues identifies extended C-terminus involved in ferroxidase activity. *PLoS One*, **4**, e8028.

Kidane, T.Z., Sauble, E. and Linder, M.C. (2006) Release of iron from ferritin requires lysosomal activity. *Am. J. Physiol. Cell Physiol.*, **291**, C445–C455.

Kilic, M.A., Ozlu, E. and Calis, S. (2012) A novel protein-based anticancer drug encapsulating nanosphere: apoferritin-doxorubicin complex. *J. Biomed. Nanotechnol.*, **8**, 508–514.

Kim, B.Y., Lee, K.S., Yoon, H.J., *et al.* (2009) Expression profile of the iron-binding proteins transferrin and ferritin heavy chain subunit in the bumblebee *Bombus ignites*. *Comp. Biochem. Physiol. B*, **153**, 165–170.

Kispal, G., Csere, P., Prohl, C. and Lill, R. (1999) The mitochondrial proteins Atm1p and Nfs1p are essential for biogenesis of cytosolic Fe/S proteins. *EMBO J.*, **18**, 3981–3989.

Kraulis, P.J. (1991) MOLSCRIPT: a progam to produce both detailed and schematic plots of protein structures. *J. Appl. Crystallogr.*, **24**, 946–950.

Krebs, C., Bollinger, J.M. Jr and Booker, S.J. (2011) Cyanobacterial alkane biosynthesis further expands the catalytic repertoire of the ferritin-like 'di-iron-carboxylate' proteins. *Curr. Opin. Chem. Biol.*, **15**, 291–303.

Kurtz, D.M. Jr (2006) Avoiding high-valent iron intermediates: superoxide reductase and rubrerythrin. *J. Inorg. Biochem.*, **100**, 679–693.

Kurtz, D.M. and Prickril, B.C. (1991) Intrapeptide sequence homology in rubrerythrin from *Desulfovibrio vulgaris*: identification of potential ligands to the diiron site. *Biochem. Biophys. Res. Commun.*, **181**, 337–341.

Laghaei, R., Evans, D.G. and Coalson, R.D. (2013) Metal binding sites of human H-chain ferritin and iron transport mechanism to the ferroxidase sites: a molecular dynamics simulation study. *Proteins*, **81**, 1042–1050.

Lalli, D. and Turano, P. (2013) Solution and solid-state NMR approaches to draw iron pathways in the ferritin nanocage. *Acc. Chem. Res.*, **46**, 2676–2685.

Laufberger, V. (1937) Sur la cristallisation de la ferritine. *Bull. Soc. Chim. Biol.*, **19**, 1575–1582.

Laulhère, J.P., Labouré, A.M. and Briat, J.F. (1989) Mechanism of the transition from plant ferritin to phytosiderin. *J. Biol. Chem.*, **264**, 3629–3635.

Laulhère, J.P., Labouré, A.M., Van Wuytswinkel, O., Gagnon, J. and Briat, J.F. (1992) Purification, characterization and function of bacterioferritin from the cyanobacterium *Synechocystis* P.C.C. 6803. *Biochem. J.*, **281**, 785–793.

Lawson, D.M., Treffry, A., Artymiuk, P.J., *et al.* (1991) Identification of the ferroxidase centre in ferritin. *FEBS Lett.*, **254**, 207–210.

Lawson, T.L., Crow, A., Lewin, A., *et al.* (2009) Monitoring the iron status of the ferroxidase center of *Escherichia coli* bacterioferritin using fluorescence spectroscopy. *Biochemistry*, **48**, 9031–9039.

Leahy, J.G., Batchelor, P.J. and Morcomb, S.M. (2003) Evolution of the soluble diiron monooxygenases. *FEMS Microbiol. Rev.*, **27**, 449–479.

Le Brun, N.E., Andrews, S.C., Guest, J.R., *et al.* (1995) Identification of the ferroxidase centre of *Escherichia coli* bacterioferritin. *Biochem. J.*, **312**, 385–392.

LeGall, J., Prickril, B.C., Moura, I., *et al.* (1988) Isolation and characterization of rubrerythrin, a non-heme iron protein from *Desulfovibrio vulgaris* that contains rubredoxin centers and a hemerythrin-like binuclear iron cluster. *Biochemistry*, **27**, 1636–1642.

Leidgens, S., Bullough, K.Z., Shi, H., *et al.* (2013) Each member of the poly-r(C)-binding protein 1 (PCBP) family exhibits iron chaperone activity toward ferritin. *J. Biol. Chem.*, **288**, 17791–1802.

Lescure, A.M., Proudhon, D., Pesey, H., *et al.* (1991) Ferritin gene transcription is regulated by iron in soybean cell cultures. *Proc. Natl Acad. Sci. USA*, **88**, 8222–8226.

Levi, S., Luzzago, A., Cesareni, G., *et al.*, (1988) Mechanism of ferritin iron uptake: activity of the H-chain and deletion mapping of the ferro-oxidase site. A study of iron uptake and ferro-oxidase activity of human liver, recombinant H-chain ferritins, and of two H-chain deletion mutants. *J. Biol. Chem.*, **263**, 18086–18092.

Levi, S., Girelli, D., Perrone, F., *et al.* (1998) Analysis of ferritins in lymphoblastoid cell lines and in the lens of subjects with hereditary hyperferritinemia-cataract syndrome. *Blood*, **91**, 4180–4187.

Liang, M., Fan, K., Zhou, M., *et al.* (2014) H-ferritin-nanocaged doxorubicin nanoparticles specifically target and kill tumors with a single-dose injection. *Proc. Natl Acad. Sci. USA*, **111**, 14900–14905.

Lin, X., Xie, J., Niu, G., *et al.* (2011) Chimeric ferritin nanocages for multiple function loading and multimodal imaging. *NanoLetters*, **11**, 814–819.

Linder, M.C. (2013) Mobilization of stored iron in mammals: a review. *Nutrients*, **5**, 4022–4050.

Liu, H.L., Zhou, H.N., Xing, W.M., *et al.* (2004) 2.6 Å resolution crystal structure of the bacterioferritin from *Azotobactervinelandii*. *FEBS Lett.*, **573**, 93–98.

Liu, K.E., Wang, D., Huynh, B.H., *et al.* (1994) Spectroscopic detection of intermediates in the reaction of dioxygen with the reduced methane monooxygenase/hydroxylase from *Methylococcus capsulatus* (Bath). *J. Am. Chem. Soc.*, **116**, 7465–7466.

Liu, X., Kim, K., Leighton, T. and Theil, E.C. (2006) Paired *Bacillus anthracis* Dps (mini-ferritin) have different reactivities with peroxide. *J. Biol. Chem.*, **281**, 27827–27835.

Lobréaux, S., Yewdall, S.J., Briat, J.F. and Harrison, P.M. (1992) Amino-acid sequence and predicted three-dimensional structure of pea seed (*Pisum sativum*) ferritin. *Biochem. J.*, **288**, 931–939.

Long, J.C., Sommer, F., Allen, M.D., Lu, S.F. and Merchant, S.S. (2008) FER1 and FER2 encoding two ferritin complexes in *Chlamydomonas reinhardtii* chloroplasts are regulated by iron. *Genetics*, **179**, 137–147.

Lundin, D., Poole, A.M., Sjöberg, B.M. and Högbom, M. (2012) Use of structural phylogenetic networks for classification of the ferritin-like superfamily. *J. Biol. Chem.*, **287**, 20565–20575.

Macedo, S., Romao, C.V., Mitchell, E., *et al.* (2003) The nature of the di-iron site in the bacterioferritin from *Desulfovibrio desulfuricans*. *Nat. Struct. Biol.*, **10**, 285–290.

Mancias, J.D., Wang, X., Gygi, S.P., Harper, J.W. and Kimmelman, A.C. (2014) Quantitative proteomics identifies NCOA4 as the cargo receptor mediating ferritinophagy. *Nature*, **509**, 105–109.

Marchetti, A., Parker, M.S., Moccia, L.P., *et al.* (2009) Ferritin is used for iron storage in bloom-forming marine pennate diatoms. *Nature*, **457**, 467–470.

Masuda, T., Goto, F., Yoshihara, T. and Mikami B. (2010a) Crystal structure of plant ferritin reveals a novel metal binding site that functions as a transit site for metal transfer in ferritin. *J. Biol. Chem.*, **285**, 4049–4059.

Masuda, T., Goto, F., Yoshihara, T. and Mikami, B. (2010b) The universal mechanism for iron translocation to the ferroxidase site in ferritin, which is mediated by the well conserved transit site. *Biochem. Biophys. Res. Commun.*, **400**, 94–99.

Masuda, T., Morimoto, S., Mikami, B. and Toyohara, H. (2012) The extension peptide of plant ferritin from sea lettuce contributes to shell stability and surface hydrophobicity. *Protein Sci.*, **21**, 786–796.

Mathevon, C., Pierrel, F., Oddou, J.L., *et al.* (2007) tRNA-modifying MiaE protein from *Salmonella typhimurium* is a nonheme diiron monooxygenase. *Proc. Natl Acad. Sci. USA*, **104**, 13295–13300.

May, A., Hillmann, F., Riebe, O., Fischer, R.J. and Bahl, H. (2004) A rubrerythrin-like oxidative stress protein of *Clostridium acetobutylicum* is encoded by a duplicated gene and identical to the heat shock protein Hsp21. *FEMS Microbiol. Lett.*, **238**, 249–254.

Meldrum, F.C., Heywood, B.R. and Mann, S. (1992) Magnetoferritin: in vitro synthesis of a novel magnetic protein. *Science*, **257**, 522–523.

Meldrum, F.C., Douglas, T., Levi, S., *et al.* (1995) Reconstitution of manganese oxide cores in horse spleen and recombinant ferritins. *J. Inorg. Biochem.*, **58**, 59–68.

Michaux, M.-A., Dautant, A., Gallois, B., *et al.* (1996) Structural investigation of the complexation properties between horse spleen apoferritin and metalloporphyrins. *Proteins*, **24**, 314–321.

Mignogna, G., Chiaraluce, R., Consalvi, V., *et al.* (2002) Ferritin from the spleen of the Antarctic teleost *Trematomus bernacchii* is an M-type homopolymer. *Eur. J. Biochem.*, **269**, 1600–1606.

Millonig, G., Muckenthaler, M.U. and Mueller, S. (2010) Hyperferritinaemia-cataract syndrome: worldwide mutations and phenotype of an increasingly diagnosed genetic disorder. *Hum. Genom.*, **4**, 250–262.

Mishra, M. and Imlay, J. (2012) Why do bacteria use so many enzymes to scavenge hydrogen peroxide? *Arch. Biochem. Biophys.*, **525**, 145–160.

Missirlis, F., Kosmidis, S., Brody, T., *et al.* (2007) Homeostatic mechanisms for iron storage revealed by genetic manipulations and live imaging of *Drosophila* ferritin. *Genetics*, **177**, 89–100.

Moenne-Loccoz, P., Krebs, C., Herlihy, K., *et al.* (1999) The ferroxidase reaction of ferritin reveals a diferric μ-1,2 bridging peroxide intermediate in common with other O_2-activating non-heme diiron proteins. *Biochemistry*, **38**, 5290–5295.

Murray, L.J., Naik, S.G., Ortillo, D.O., *et al.* (2007) Characterization of the arene oxidizing intermediate in ToMOH as a diiron(III) species. *J. Am. Chem. Soc.*, **129**, 14500–14510.

Nichol, H., Law, J.H. and Winzerling, J.J. (2002) Iron metabolism in insects. *Annu. Rev. Entomol.*, **47**, 535–559.

Nordlund, P., Sjöberg, B.M. and Eklund, H. (1990) Three-dimensional structure of the free radical protein of ribonucleotide reductase. *Nature*, **345**, 593–598.

Okuda, M., Iwahori, K., Yamashita, I. and Yoshimura, H. (2003) Fabrication of nickel and chromium nanoparticles using the protein cage of apoferritin. *Biotechnol. Bioeng.*, **84**, 187–194.

Peer, D., Karp, J.M., Hong, S., *et al.* (2007) Nanocarriers as an emerging platform for cancer therapy. *Nat. Nanotechnol.*, **2**, 751–760.

Pereira, A.S., Tavares, P., Lloyd, S.G., *et al.*, (1997) Rapid and parallel formation of Fe^{3+} multimers, including a trimer, during H-type subunit ferritin mineralization. *Biochemistry*. **36**, 7917–7927.

Pereira, A.S., Small, W., Krebs, C., *et al.* (1998) Direct spectroscopic and kinetic evidence for the involvement of a peroxodiferric intermediate during the ferroxidase reaction in fast ferritin mineralization. *Biochemistry*, **37**, 9871–9876.

Perls, M. (1867) Nachweis von Eisenoxyd in gewissen Pigmenten. *Virchows Arch. A*, **39**, 42–48.

Pfaffen, S., Abdulqadir, R., Le Brun, N.E. and Murphy, M.E. (2013) Mechanism of ferrous iron binding and oxidation by ferritin from a pennate diatom. *J. Biol. Chem.*, **288**, 14917–14925.

Pham, D.K. and Winzerling, J.J. (2010) Insect ferritins: Typical or atypical? *Biochim. Biophys. Acta.*, **1800**, 824–833.

Précigoux, G., Yariv, J., Gallois, B., *et al.* (1994) A crystallographic study of haem binding to ferritin. *Acta Crystallogr.*, **D50**, 739–743.

Proudhon, D., Briat, J.-F. and Lescure, A.-M. (1989) Iron induction of ferritin synthesis in soybean cell suspensions. *Plant Physiol.*, **90**, 586–590.

Ragland, M., Briat, J.F., Gagnon, J., *et al.* (1990) Evidence for conservation of ferritin sequences among plants and animals and for a transit peptide in soybean. *J. Biol. Chem.*, **265**, 18339–18344.

Ramsay, B., Wiedenheft, B., Allen, M., *et al.* (2006) Dps-like protein from the hyperthermophilic archaeon *Pyrococcus furiosus*. *J. Inorg. Biochem.*, **100**, 1061–1068.

Rice, D.W., Ford, G.C., White, J.L., *et al.* (1983) The spatial structure of horse spleen apoferritin. *Adv. Inorg. Biochem.*, **5**, 39–49.

Richter, G.W. (1978) The iron-loaded cell – the cytopathology of iron storage. A review. *Am. J. Pathol.*, **91**, 363–397.

Riebe, O., Fischer, R.J., Wampler, D.A., Kurtz, D.M. Jr and Bahl, H. (2009) Pathway for H_2O_2 and O_2 detoxification in *Clostridium acetobutylicum*. *Microbiology*, **155**, 16–24.

Romao, C.V., Louro, R., Timkovich, M., Lubben, M., *et al.* (2000) Iron-coproporphyrin III is a natural cofactor in bacterioferritin from the anaerobic bacterium *Desulfovibrio desulfuricans*. *FEBS Lett.*, **480**, 213–216.

Rosenzweig, A.C., Frederick, C.A., Lippard, S.J. and Nordlund, P. (1993) Crystal structure of a bacterial non-haem iron hydroxylase that catalyses the biological oxidation of methane. *Nature*, **366**, 537–543.

Roy, S., Saraswathi, R., Gupta, S., *et al.* (2007) Role of N and C-terminal tails in DNA binding and assembly in Dps: structural studies of *Mycobacterium smegmatis* Dps deletion mutants. *J. Mol. Biol.*, **370**, 752–767.

Roy, S., Saraswathi, R., Chatterji, D. and Vijayan, M. (2008) Structural studies on the second *Mycobacterium smegmatis* Dps: invariant and variable features of structure, assembly and function. *J. Mol. Biol.*, **375**, 948–959.

Santambrogio, P., Cozzi, A., Levi, S., *et al.* (2000) Functional and immunological analysis of recombinant mouse H- and L-ferritins from *Escherichia coli*. *Protein Expr. Purif.*, **19**, 212–218.

Sazinsky, M.H. and Lippard, S.J. (2006) Correlating structure with function in bacterial multicomponent monooxygenases and related diiron proteins. *Acc. Chem. Res.*, **39**, 558–66.

Schwartz, J.K., Liu, X.S., Tosha, T., Theil, E.C. and Solomon, E.I. (2008) Spectroscopic definition of the ferroxidase site in M ferritin: comparison of binuclear substrate vs cofactor active sites. *J. Am. Chem. Soc.*, **130**, 9441–9450.

Shanklin, J., Guy, J.E., Mishra, G. and Lindqvist, Y. (2009) Desaturases: emerging models for understanding functional diversification of diiron-containing enzymes. *J. Biol. Chem.*, **284**, 18559–18563.

Shi, H., Bencze, K.Z., Stemmler, T.L. and Philpott, C.C. (2008). A cytosolic iron chaperone that delivers iron to ferritin. *Science*, **320**, 1207–1210.

Sieker, L.C., Holmes, M., Le Trong, I., *et al.* (2000) The 1.9 Å crystal structure of the 'as isolated' rubrerythrin from *Desulfovibrio vulgaris*: some surprising results. *J. Biol. Inorg. Chem.*, **5**, 505–513.

Sirivech, S., Frieden, E. and Osaki, S. (1974) The release of iron from horse spleen ferritin by reduced flavins. *Biochem. J.*, **143**, 311–315.

Stefanini, S., Desideri, A., Vecchini, P., *et al.* (1987) Identification of the iron entry channels in apoferritin. Chemical modification and spectroscopic studies. *Biochemistry*, **28**, 378–382.

Steifel, E.I. and Watt, G.D. (1979) *Azotobacter* cytochrome b557.5 is a bacterioferritin. *Nature*, **279**, 81–83.

Stillman, T.J., Hempstead, P.D., Artymiuk, P.J., *et al.* (2001) The high-resolution X-ray crystallographic structure of the ferritin (EcFtnA) of *Escherichia coli*; comparison with human H ferritin (HuHF) and the structures of the Fe(3+) and Zn(2+) derivatives. *J. Mol. Biol.*, **307**, 587–603.

Stillman, T.J., Upadhyay, M., Norte, V.A., *et al.* (2005) Insights into the effects on metal binding of the systematic substitution of five key glutamate ligands in the ferritin of *Escherichia coli*. *J. Biol. Chem.*, **278**, 26275–26286.

Strickler-Dinglasan, P.M., Guz, N., Attardo, G. and Aksoy, S. (2006) Molecular characterization of iron binding proteins from *Glossina morsitans morsitans* (Diptera: Glossinidae). *Insect Biochem. Mol. Biol.*, **36**, 921–933.

Su, M., Cavallo, S., Stefanini, S., Chiancone, E. and Chasteen, N.D. (2005) The so-called *Listeria innocua* ferritin is a Dps protein. Iron incorporation, detoxification, and DNA protection properties. *Biochemistry*, **44**, 5572–5578.

Sun, C.J., Yang, H., Yuan, Y., *et al.* (2011) Controlling assembly of paired gold clusters within apoferritin nanoreactor for in vivo kidney targeting and biomedical imaging. *J. Am. Chem. Soc.*, **133**, 8617–8624.

Sun, S., Arosio, P., Levi, S. and Chasteen, N.D. (1993) Ferroxidase kinetics of human liver apoferritin, recombinant H chain apoferritin, and site-directed mutants. *iochemistry*, **36**, 9362–9369.

Swartz, L., Kuchinskas, M., Li, H., Poulos, T.L. and Lanzilotta, W.N. (2006) Redox-dependent structural changes in the *Azotobacter vinelandii* bacterioferritin: new insights into the ferroxidase and iron transport mechanism. *Biochemistry*, **45**, 4421–4428.

Tatur, J. and Hagen, W.R. (2005) The dinuclear iron-oxo ferroxidase center of *Pyrococcus furiosus* ferritin is a stable prosthetic group with unexpectedly high reduction potentials. *FEBS Lett.*, **579**, 4729–4732.

Tatur, J., Hagen, W.R. and Mathias, P.M. (2007) Crystal structure of the ferritin from the hyperthermophilic archaeal anaerobe *Pyrococcus furiosus*. *J. Biol. Inorg. Chem.*, **12**, 615–630.

Theil, E.C. (2011) Ferritin protein nanocages use ion channels, catalytic sites, and nucleation channels to manage iron/oxygen chemistry. *Curr. Opin. Chem. Biol.*, **15**, 304–311.

Theil, E.C (2013) Ferritin: the protein nanocage and iron biomineral in health and in disease. *Inorg. Chem.*, **52**, 12223–12233.

Theil, E.C., Liu, X.S. and Tosha, T. (2008) Gated pores in the ferritin nanocage. *Inorg. Chim. Acta*, **361**, 868–874.

Tonello, F., Dundon, W.G., Satin, B., *et al.* (1999) The *Helicobacter pylori* neutrophil activating protein is an iron-binding protein with dodecameric structure. *Mol. Microbiol.*, **34**, 238–246.

Tong, W.H., Chen. S., Lloyd, S.G., *et al.* (1996) Mechanism of assembly of the diferric cluster-tyrosyl radical cofactor of *Escherichia coli* ribonucleotide reductase from the diferrous form of the R2 subunit. *J. Am. Chem. Soc.*, **118**, 2107–2108.

Tosha, T., Ng, H.L., Bhattasali, O., Alber, T. and Theil, E.C. (2010) Moving metal ions through ferritin-protein nanocages from three-fold pores to catalytic sites. *J. Am. Chem. Soc.*, **132**, 14562–14569.

Tosha, T., Behera, R.K. and Theil, E.C. (2012) Ferritin ion channel disorder inhibits Fe(II)/O$_2$ reactivity at distant sites. *Inorg. Chem.*, **51**, 11406–11411.

Toussaint, L., Bertrand, L., Hue, L., Crichton, R.R. and Declercq, J.P. (2007) High-resolution X-ray structures of human apoferritin H-chain mutants correlated with their activity and metal-binding sites. *J. Mol. Biol.*, **365**, 440–452.

Treffry, A., Zhao, Z.W., Quail, M.A., *et al.* (1995) Iron(II) oxidation by H chain ferritin: evidence from site-directed mutagenesis that a transient blue species is formed at the dinuclear iron center. *Biochemistry*, **34**, 15204–15213.

Treffry, A., Zhao, Z.W., Quail, M.A., *et al.* (1997) Dinuclear center of ferritin: studies of iron binding and oxidation show differences in the two iron sites. *Biochemistry*, **36**, 432–441.

Turano, P., Lalli, D., Felli, I.C., Theil, E.C. and Bertini, I. (2010) NMR reveals pathway for ferric mineral precursors to the central cavity of ferritin. *Proc. Natl Acad. Sci. USA*, **107**, 545–550.

Uchida, M., Kang, S., Reichhardt, C., Harlen, K. and Douglas, T. (2010) The ferritin superfamily: Supramolecular templates for materials synthesis. *Biochim. Biophys. Acta*, **1800**, 834–845.

van Eerde, A., Wolterink-van Loo, S., van der Oost, J. and Dijkstra, B.W. (2006) Fortuitous structure determination of 'as-isolated' *Escherichia coli* bacterioferritin in a novel crystal form. *Acta Crystallogr. F Struct. Biol. Cryst. Commun.*, **62**, 1061–1066.

Van Wuytswinkel, O., Savino, G. and Briat, J.F. (1995) Purification and characterization of recombinant pea-seed ferritins expressed in *Escherichia coli*: influence of N-terminus deletions on protein solubility and core formation in vitro. *Biochem. J.*, **305**, 253–261.

Wakagi, T. (2003) Sulerythrin, the smallest member of the rubrerythrin family, from a strictly aerobic and thermoacidophilic archaeon, *Sulfolobus tokodaii* strain 7. *FEMS Microbiol. Lett.*, **222**, 33–37.

Waldo, G.S. and Theil, E.C. (1993) Formation of iron(III)-tyrosinate is the fastest reaction observed in ferritin. *Biochemistry*, **32**, 13262–13269.

Wang, D., Kim, B.Y., Lee, K.S., *et al.* (2009) Molecular characterization of iron binding proteins, transferrin and ferritin heavy chain subunit, from the bumblebee *Bombus ignitus*. *Comp. Biochem. Physiol. B*, **152**, 20–27.

Ward, R.J., Ramsey, M.H., Dickson, D.P., *et al.* (1992) Chemical and structural characterisation of iron cores of haemosiderins isolated from different sources. *Eur. J. Biochem.*, **209**, 847–850.

Ward, R.J., Ramsey, M.H., Dickson, D.P., *et al.* (1994) Further characterisation of forms of haemosiderin in iron-overloaded tissues. *Eur. J. Biochem.*, **225**, 187–194.

Ward, R.J., Legssyer, R., Henry, C. and Crichton, R.R. (2000) Does the haemosiderin iron core determine its potential for chelation and the development of iron-induced tissue damage? *J. Inorg. Biochem.*, **79**, 311–317.

Watt, G.D., Jacobs, D. and Frankel, R.B. (1988) Redox reactivity of bacterial and mammalian ferritin: is reductant entry into the ferritin interior a necessary step for iron release? *Proc. Natl Acad. Sci. USA*, **85**, 7457–7461.

Weeratunga, S.K., Lovell, S., Yao, H., *et al.* (2010) Structural studies of bacterioferritin B from *Pseudomonas aeruginosa* suggest a gating mechanism for iron uptake via the ferroxidase center. *Biochemistry*, **49**, 1160–1175.

Willies, S.C., Isupov, M.N., Garman, E.F. and Littlechild, J.A. (2009) The binding of haem and zinc in the 1.9 Å X-ray structure of *Escherichia coli* bacterioferritin. *J. Biol. Inorg. Chem.*, **14**, 201–207.

Wolf, S.G., Frenkiel, D., Arad, T., *et al.* (1999) DNA protection by stress-induced biocrystallization. *Nature*, **400**, 83–85.

Wong, K.K. and Mann, S. (1996) Biomimetic synthesis of cadmium sulfide-ferritin nanocomposites. *Adv. Mater.*, **8**, 928.

Wong, K.K., Douglas, T., Gider, S., *et al.* (1998) Biomimetic synthesis of cadmium sulfide-ferritin nanocomposites. *Chem. Mater.*, **10**, 279.

Wu, T.M., Hsu, Y.T., Sung, M.S., Hsu, Y.T. and Lee, T.M. (2009) Expression of genes involved in redox homeostasis and antioxidant defense in a marine macroalga *Ulva fasciata* by excess copper. *Aquat. Toxicol.*, **94**, 275–285.

Wustefeld, C. and Crichton, R.R. (1982) The amino acid sequence of human spleen apoferritin. *FEBS Lett.*, **150**, 43–48.

Xu, B. and Chasteen, N.D. (1991) Iron oxidation chemistry in ferritin. Increasing Fe/O_2 stoichiometry during core formation. *J. Biol. Chem.*, **266**, 19965–19970.

Yan, F., Zhang, Y., Yuan, H.K., Gregas, M.K. and Vo-Dinh, T. (2008) Apoferritin protein cages: a novel drug nanocarrier for photodynamic therapy. *Chem. Commun. (Camb).*, **14**, 4579–4581.

Yang, X., Chen-Barrett, T., Arosio, P. and Chasteen, N.D. (1998) Reaction paths of iron oxidation and hydrolysis in horse spleen and recombinant human ferritins. *Biochemistry*, **26**, 9763–9750.

Yang, X., Le Brun, N.E., Thomson, A.J., Moore, G.R. and Chasteen, N.D. (2000) The iron oxidation and hydrolysis chemistry of *Escherichia coli* bacterioferritin. *Biochemistry*, **39**, 4915–4923.

Yao, H., Jepkorir, G., Lovell, S., *et al.* (2011) Two distinct ferritin-like molecules in *Pseudomonas aeruginosa*: the product of the bfrA gene is a bacterial ferritin (FtnA) and not a bacterioferritin (Bfr). *Biochemistry*, **50**, 5236–5248.

Yasmin, S., Andrews, S.C., Moore, G.R. and Le Brun, N.E. (2011) A new role for heme, facilitating release of iron from the bacterioferritin iron biomineral. *J. Biol. Chem.*, **286**, 3473–3483.

Yun, D., Garcia-Serres, R., Chicalese, B.M., *et al.* (2007) (μ-1,2-Peroxo)diiron(III/III) complex as a precursor to the diiron(III/IV) intermediate X in the assembly of the iron radical cofactor of ribonucleotide reductase from mouse. *Biochemistry*, **46**, 1925–1932.

Zhao, G., Bou-Abdallah, F., Yang, X., *et al.* (2001) Ferroxidase kinetics of human liver apoferritin, recombinant H chain apoferritin, and site-directed mutants. *Biochemistry*, **32**, 9362–9369.

Zhao, G., Ceci, P., Ilari, A., *et al.* (2002) Iron and hydrogen peroxide detoxification properties of DNA-binding protein from starved cells. A ferritin-like DNA-binding protein of *Escherichia coli. J. Biol. Chem.*, **277**, 27689–27696.

Zhao, G., Bou-Abdallah, F., Arosio, P., *et al.* (2003) Multiple pathways for mineral core formation in mammalian apoferritin. The role of hydrogen peroxide. *Biochemistry*, **42**, 3142–3150.

Zhao, G., Su, M. and Chasteen, N.C. (2005) mu-1,2-peroxo diferric complex formation in horse spleen ferritin. A mixed H/L-subunit heteropolymer. *J. Mol. Biol.*, **352**, 467–477.

Zhao, W., Ye, J. and Zhao, J. (2007) RbrA, a cyanobacterial rubrerythrin, functions as a FNR-dependent peroxidase in heterocysts in protection of nitrogenase from damage by hydrogen peroxide in *Anabaena* sp. PCC 7120. *Mol. Microbiol.*, **66**, 1219–1230.

Zhao, Z.W., Treffry, A., Quail, M.A., *et al.* (1997) Catalytic iron(II) oxidation in the non haem ferritin of *Escherichia coli*: The early intermediate is not an iron tyrosinate. *J. Chem. Soc., Dalton Trans.*, 3977–3978.

Zhen, Z., Tang, W., Guo, C., *et al.* (2013) Ferritin nanocages to encapsulate and deliver photosensitizers for efficient photodynamic therapy against cancer. *ACS Nano.*, **7**, 6988–6996.

Zhen, Z., Tang, W., Todd, T. and Xie, J. (2014) Ferritins as nanoplatforms for imaging and drug delivery. *Expert Opin. Drug. Deliv.*, **11**, 1913–1922.

10

Cellular and Systemic Iron Homeostasis

10.1 Cellular Iron Homeostasis

10.1.1 Translational Control of Protein Synthesis

Whereas during the early 1960s there was a very good understanding of how microbial protein synthesis was regulated – essentially at the level of transcription of DNA into mRNA – there was very little information concerning the ways in which protein synthesis in eukaryotes was controlled. However, exploiting the seminal discovery that the expression of ferritin in animal cells was regulated by changes in dietary iron (Granick, 1946a,b), Hamish Munro and his collaborators, initially in Glasgow, and subsequently in Boston, would dramatically change the understanding of the control of mammalian protein synthesis at the level of translation of mRNA. Their initial observation was that ferritin biosynthesis in rat liver was indeed induced by the administration of dietary iron, however, without the incorporation of [14]C- leucine into any other liver proteins, in a process that was insensitive to the transcriptional inhibitor actinomycin D (Drysdale and Munro, 1965, 1966). Further, when mRNA from the livers of normal and iron-loaded rats were translated in a wheat germ system, a twofold increase in the amount of ferritin mRNA was found in the polyribosomal fraction from iron-loaded rats compared to controls (Zähringer et al., 1976). This led to the conclusion that iron stimulates the recruitment of ferritin mRNA to polyribosomes. Once molecular gene cloning techniques became available, it was observed that the translational regulation of both ferritin H and L mRNA depends on the presence of a conserved sequence within a hairpin loop in the 5′-untranslated region (UTR) (Aziz and Munro, 1986, 1987) This was independently confirmed by others, and the term 'iron-responsive element' (IRE) was proposed for this hairpin (Hentze et al., 1987a,b). Using gel-retardation assays, Leibold and Munro (1988) then showed that the IRE binds to a cytoplasmic protein, now termed Iron Regulatory Protein (IRP), an observation

Iron Metabolism – From Molecular Mechanisms to Clinical Consequences, Fourth Edition. Robert Crichton.
© 2016 John Wiley & Sons, Ltd. Published 2016 by John Wiley & Sons, Ltd.

which was again rapidly confirmed (Rouault *et al.*, 1988). It was subsequently shown that the binding of IRP to the IRE in the 5′-UTR of ferritin mRNA prevents formation of the small 43S pre-initiation translation complex with the 30S ribosomal subunit, a necessary prerequisite for the initiation of protein synthesis (Gray and Hentze, 1994). In the presence of iron, this IRE–IRP interaction is blocked, as we will see below, allowing translation of the mRNA which explains the initial observations in rat liver (Kühn, 2014).

At around the same time, Owen and Kühn (1987) showed that TfR1 protein expression changed inversely with iron levels in cell cultures, independent of transcription, and that this effect necessitates the presence of a strongly conserved structured region in the TfR1 mRNA 3′-UTR and is due to changes in mRNA stability (Müllner and Kuhn, 1988). Subsequent studies showed that there were no less than five IREs in this region, each of which binds IRPs with a similarly strong affinity to the ferritin IREs (Müllner *et al.*, 1989; Koeller *et al.*, 1989), and that IRP binding prevents TfR1 mRNA degradation. It was also shown that there are two IRE-binding proteins, which are now known as IRP1 and IRP2 (Müllner *et al.*, 1989).

10.1.2 The IRE/IRP System

Iron homeostasis in mammalian cells is regulated by balancing iron uptake with intracellular storage and use, and this is largely achieved at the level of protein synthesis (translation of mRNA into protein) rather than at the level of transcription (mRNA synthesis) by the IRE/IRP system. The IREs form hairpin structures in their respective mRNAs, which are recognised by the IRPs. With the demonstration that the binding of the IRPs had different effects depending on the localisation of the IRE (either in the 5′- or the 3′-UTR), it was concluded that the IRE/IRP system constituted a general post-transcriptional regulatory mechanism for controlling cellular iron homeostasis (Casey *et al.*, 1988; Müllner *et al.*, 1989). When cells are depleted of iron, the IRPs bind to the IREs (Figure 10.1). Binding to the single IRE located in the 5′-UTR of ferritin mRNA prevents translation of the mRNA, whereas binding to the IREs present in the 3′-UTR of transferrin receptor (TfR) mRNA prevents nuclease degradation. This ensures that iron uptake is stimulated while iron storage is prevented. In contrast, in iron-replete cells the IRPs no longer bind to the IREs. Ferritin mRNA is translated while transferrin receptor mRNA undergoes cleavage by an as yet uncharacterised endonuclease. As a consequence, potential iron toxicity is avoided by upregulation of the storage protein, while the unnecessary uptake of iron is suppressed. Thus, the IRPs act as iron sensors, controlling either the translation of the mRNA or its stability – hence their classification either as regulators of either of translation or turnover. As we will see in the following sections, IREs are present in the mRNAs of a number of other key players of cellular iron metabolism. These include erythroid cell δ-aminolaevulinate synthase, the first enzyme of haem biosynthesis, ferroportin, the iron exporter, and HIF2α, the transcription factor hypoxia-inducible factor 2α, all in the 5′-UTRs, whereas one of the splice variants of the divalent metal transporter DMT1 has an IRE in the 3′-UTR (Kühn, 2014).

A series of detailed studies showed that the position of the single-copy 5′-UTR IREs in mRNAs is absolutely crucial for their activity as translational regulators. They are all located within 40 nucleotides or less from the 5′ m^{7}G cap of the mRNA (see Figure 10.1), and when IRP binds the complex prevents the stable association of the small ribosomal complex (the 43S preinitiation complex) with the mRNA (Gray and Hentze, 1994; Mückenthaler *et al.*, 1998).

There are five IREs in the 3′-UTR of TfR mRNA which share the same structural features as other IREs, and at least four of these are accessible for IRP binding, although only some 250 nucleotides, including IREs B, C and D, are required for regulation. Specific cleavage in the 3′-UTR of TfR

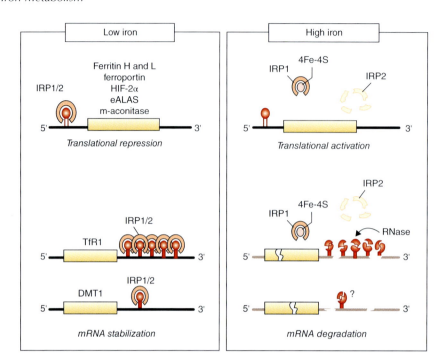

Figure 10.1 *Cellular regulation of mammalian iron homeostasis by the IRPs. IRPs bind to IREs located in either the 5′- or 3′-UTRs of specific mRNAs. During low-iron conditions, IRP1 and IRP2 bind with high affinity to 5′ IREs and to the five 3′ IREs in TfR mRNA, resulting in the translational repression of 5′ IRE-containing mRNAs and the stabilisation of the TfR mRNA. During high-iron conditions, IRPs lose their affinity for IREs, increasing the translation of 5′ IRE-containing mRNAs and mediating degradation of the TfR mRNA. Increased iron levels result in the conversion of the IRP1 RNA binding form into the [4Fe–4S] cluster c-acon form, while increased iron and/or haem levels mediate IRP2 proteasomal degradation. Reprinted with permission from Elsevier from Wallander, M.L., Leibold, E.A. and Eisenstein, R.S. (2006) Molecular control of vertebrate iron homeostasis by iron regulatory proteins. Biochim. Biophys. Acta, **1763**, 668–689*

mRNA occurs between IRE C and D, close to the previously mapped instability elements and, unlike several other unstable mRNAs, does not appear to require prior poly(A) tail shortening.

10.1.3 The IREs – Distribution and Structure

After the initial discoveries of IREs in the mRNAs of ferritins and of TfR1, they have been identified in the 5′- or 3′-UTRs of a number of other mRNAs (Figure 10.2). IREs in the 5′-UTR, which have all been shown to be regulated by iron, are present in erythroid 5-aminolaevulinate synthase mRNA (Cox *et al.*, 1991; Dandekar *et al.*, 1991), mitochondrial aconitase mRNA (Kim *et al.*, 1996; Schalinske *et al.*, 1998), subunit b of *Drosophila* succinate dehydrogenase mRNA (Kohler *et al.*, 1995; Melefors, 1996), ferroportin mRNA (Abboud and Haile, 2000; McKie *et al.*, 2000), and HIF2α mRNA (Sanchez *et al.*, 2007; Zimmer *et al.*, 2008). A splice variant of ferroportin mRNA without the IRE, is expressed in duodenum and erythroid cells (Cianetti *et al.*, 2005; Zhang *et al.*, 2009a). One of the splice variants of the divalent metal transporter DMT1 (SLC11A2) mRNA has a single IRE in its 3′-UTR (Gunshin *et al.*, 2001; Hubert and Hentze, 2002), which

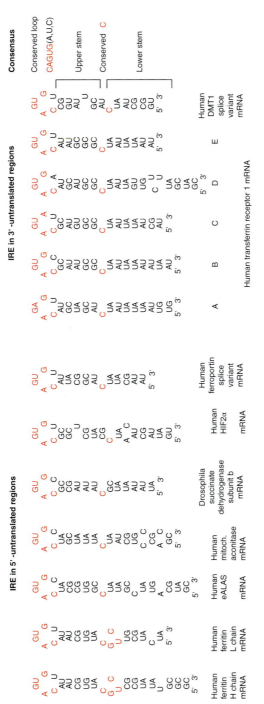

Figure 10.2 The most studied IREs in mRNAs related to iron metabolism. IREs present in different mRNAs show a conserved hairpin structure with an upper and a lower paired stem of nucleotides, at least one conserved unpaired C, and a six-base loop sequence with conserved residues CAG(A,U)G(A,U,C), in which positions 1 and 5 are paired. Reprinted with permission of the Royal Society of Chemistry from Kühn, L. C. (2014) Iron regulatory proteins and their role in controlling iron metabolism. Metallomics, **7**, 232–243

confers increased mRNA expression after iron deprivation (Gunshin *et al.*, 2001), and decreases mRNA expression in intestine-specific IRP1 knockout mice (Galy *et al.*, 2008). The IRE–IRP interaction probably results in mRNA stabilisation as for TfR1 mRNA, but this was not directly shown. An IRE was also identified in the 3′-UTR of human CDC42-binding kinase α (MRCKα, CDC42BPA) mRNA (Cmejla *et al.*, 2006), and its regulation by iron levels is thought to modulate transferrin endocytosis (Cmejla *et al.*, 2010). However, unlike the IREs of TfR1 and DMT1, which are present in all mammalian species, the MRCKα IRE is only present in the human mRNA and is absent from all others, including chimpanzee, which suggests a very recent evolutionary acquisition, albeit of limited functional importance. Recent microarray studies have identified additional 5′- and 3′-IREs in CDC14A mRNA (Sanchez *et al.*, 2006) and in a number of other potential target mRNAs (Sanchez *et al.*, 2011), although their physiological relevance needs to be established. The use of SELEX procedures (Systematic evolution of ligands by exponential enrichment – a molecular biological adaptation of combinatorial chemistry techniques for producing oligonucleotides of single-stranded RNA which specifically bind to a target ligand or ligands) has been exploited to identify mutant IREs with sequences similar to native IREs which are not found in natural mRNAs, but nonetheless bind to IRPs (Henderson *et al.*, 1994, 1996; Menotti *et al.*, 1998; Butt *et al.*, 1996; Goforth *et al.*, 2010). These studies not only allow a better definition of what is required for high-affinity binding to IRPs but also lead to the conclusion that IRP1 and IRP2 bind to distinct RNA target sequences.

The IREs present in these different mRNAs show a conserved hairpin structure with an upper and a lower paired stem of nucleotides, at least one conserved unpaired C, and a six-base loop sequence with conserved residues CAG(A,U)G(A,U,C), in which positions 1 and 5 are paired (Kühn, 2014). The two IREs in DMT1 and HIF2α mRNA have an additional nucleotide in the upper stem, and bind better to IRP1 than to IRP2 (Gunshin *et al.*, 2001; Sanchez *et al.*, 2007). All of the IREs are well conserved in vertebrates and some of the genes are also found in insects, annelids (Rothenberger *et al.*, 1990) and snails (Von Darl *et al.*, 1994). IREs have a long evolutionary history, since they made their first appearance in metazoan ferritins (Piccinelli and Samuelsson, 2007).

Unusual IRE-like structures have been found in the 3′-UTR of α-haemoglobin-stabilising protein (AHSP) mRNA (dos Santos *et al.*, 2008) and in the 5′-UTR of glycolate oxidase (HAO1) mRNA (Kohler *et al.*, 1999), although the former showed poor binding to IRPs and the latter was shown to be nonfunctional in 5′-UTR translational regulation. A novel iron-responsive element, designated IRE-Type II, was found in the 5'-UTR of the Alzheimer's amyloid precursor protein (APP) transcript (+51 to +94 from the 5'-cap site), located immediately upstream of an interleukin-1-responsive acute box domain (Rogers *et al.*, 2002). Despite an entirely different sequence and potentially very different folding, this IRE was shown to have strong *in-vitro* binding properties for IRP1, but not IRP2, and was shown to function as a translational regulatory element *in vivo* (Cho *et al.*, 2010). The potential implications of this in neurodegeneration will be discussed in detail in Chapter 14.

The three-dimensional structure of ferritin IRE bound to IRP1 has been determined using NMR (Walden *et al.*, 2006). IRP1 not only binds IREs in mRNAs, it can also (as discussed below) bind an iron–sulphur cluster, to become the cytosolic tricarboxylic acid cycle enzyme aconitase. The 2.8 Å-resolution crystal structure of the IRP1:ferritin H IRE complex shows an open protein conformation compared with that of cytosolic aconitase, the crystal structure (Dupuy *et al.*, 2006) of which is also shown in Figure 10.3. The extended, L-shaped IRP1 molecule embraces the IRE stem–loop through interactions at two sites separated by approximately 30 Å, each involving about a dozen protein–RNA bonds. Extensive conformational changes related to binding of either the IRE or an iron–sulphur cluster explain the alternate functions of IRP1 as an mRNA regulator or an enzyme.

(a) (b)

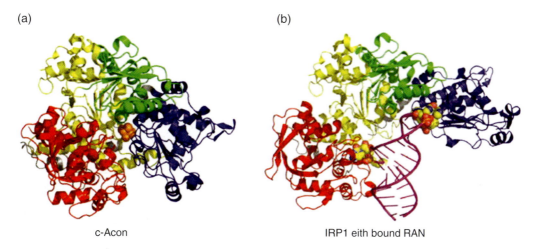

c-Acon   IRP1 eith bound RAN

Figure 10.3 *Crystal structure of c-aconitase and the IRP1–IRE complex. The crystal structures of c-aconitase (Dupuy et al., 2006) and the IRP1–IRE complex (Selezneva et al., 2006; Walden et al., 2006) are shown. (a) Cytosolic aconitase structure showing domain 1 (yellow), domain 2 (green), domain 3 (blue) and domain 4 (red) with the [4Fe–4S] cluster in the centre (orange balls). (b) IRP1–IRE complex structure shown with domains 1 to 4, as in (A). The ferritin IRE helix (purple) is shown with the two major contact sites of C8 (left) and the $A_{16}G_{17}U_{18}$ bases of the pseudotriloop shown (right) as enlarged balls. Reprinted with permission from Elsevier from Anderson, C.P., Shen, M., Eisenstein, R.S. and Leibold, E.A. (2012) Mammalian iron metabolism and its control by iron regulatory proteins.* Biochim. Biophys. Acta, **1823**, 1468–1483*

The NMR structure confirmed the mutant studies which showed a strong binding preference for loops in which residues 1 and 5 are base-paired, and also showed that conserved unpaired purines and pyrimidines at loop-positions 2 to 4 and the cytosine between the upper and lower stem are turned outwards, providing specific contact sites for conserved amino acids on the surface of IRP1, as shown in the cocrystal structure (Walden *et al.*, 2006; Selezneva *et al.*, 2013). Five amino acids make base-specific contacts (Figure 10.4), and mutagenesis studies show that four of the five contact points contribute uniquely to the overall binding affinity of the IRP1–IRE interaction. They also showed that Lys379 and Ser681, which make contact with the conserved nucleotides G16 and C8, respectively, are particularly critical for providing specificity and stability to IRP1–IRE complex formation (Selezneva *et al.*, 2013).

10.1.4   Structural Features of IRP1 and 2

There are two iron regulatory proteins, IRP1 (gene *ACO1*) and IRP2 (gene *IREB2*), both present in the cytosol, which share 56% sequence identity. However, IRP2 has a cysteine-rich 73-amino acid insertion in its N terminus, although the function of the insertion is not clear (Pantopoulos, 2004). Both, IRP1 and IRP2 are ubiquitously expressed, with IRP1 highly expressed in the kidneys, liver and brown fat, and IRP2 highly expressed in the central nervous system (Meyron-Holtz *et al.*, 2004). A lack of both IRP1 and IRP2 prevents the viability of mice beyond the blastocyst stage of embryonic development (Smith *et al.*, 2006), whereas mice with either Irp1 or Irp2 deficiency are viable and fertile, suggesting that Irp proteins can compensate for the loss of one another and are functionally redundant (Meyron-Holtz *et al.*, 2004). Conditional deletion of both *Irp1* and *Irp2* in hepatocytes compromises iron–sulphur cluster and haem synthesis, and impairs mitochondrial

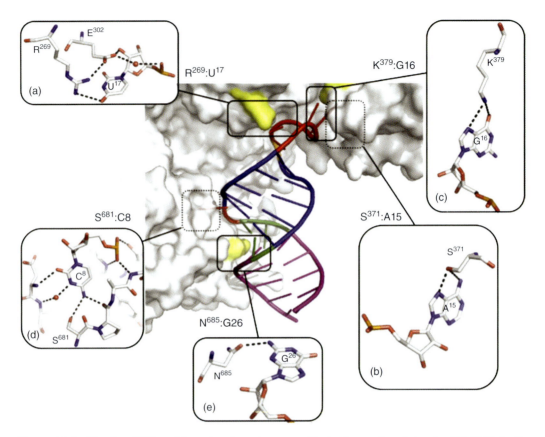

Figure 10.4 *The five IRP1 residues that form base-specific hydrogen bonds to the IRE RNA in the IRP1–IRE complexes. The IRE (cartoon) is shown as bound to the IRP1 protein (solvent-accessible surface). The amino acids Arg269, Lys379 and Asn685 are visible (yellow), while Ser371 and Ser681 are hidden from view. Details of the five base-specific contacts are shown by insets. Note that these residues are different from the four aconitase active-site arginines (Arg536, Arg541, Arg699, and Arg780) previously studied based on homology modelling (Philpott et al., 1994; Hirling et al., 1994; Butt et al., 1996). Reprinted with permission from Elsevier from Selezneva, A.I., Walden, W.E. and Volz, K.W. (2013) Nucleotide-specific recognition of iron-responsive elements by iron regulatory protein 1.* J. Mol. Biol., ***425**, 3301–3310*

functions, suggesting an essential role for IRPs in mitochondrial respiration. Induced deletion of both *Irp1* and *Irp2* in duodenal enterocytes, impairs iron absorption and promotes mucosal iron retention via a ferritin-mediated 'mucosal block'. IRP deficiency does not interfere with intestinal sensing of body iron loading and erythropoietic iron need, but rather alters the basal expression of the iron-absorption machinery (Galy *et al.*, 2013).

IRP1 was shown to be structurally related to mitochondrial aconitase (Rouault *et al.*, 1991), and when the crystal structure of human IRP1 in its aconitase form was determined (Dupuy *et al.*, 2006) it became clear that it was indeed very similar to the ~20% smaller mammalian mitochondrial aconitase (Robbins and Stout, 1989; Lauble *et al.*, 1992), despite an overall sequence identity of only 22%. Each protein is composed of four globular domains with an extended linker which joins domains 3 and 4 located on the surface of the protein (Figure 10.3). In iron-replete conditions,

IRP1 acquires a [4Fe–4S] cluster in its active cleft and displays cytosolic aconitase activity. The conversion of citrate to isocitrate in the cytosol, by enhancing NADPH generation, may favour lipid biosynthesis (Tong and Rouault, 2007). The [4Fe–4S] cluster is located in the centre of the molecule at the interface of the four domains, and the protein is in a closed conformation. The [4Fe–4S] cluster is ligated to the protein by three cysteine residues (Cys437, 503 and 506) which anchor the iron–sulphur cluster into the enzyme, while the labile fourth iron atom of the cluster binds solvent and substrate. As had been suggested for mitochondrial aconitase, access to the active site may occur through movement of domain 4 with respect to the other domains (Beinert *et al.*, 1996). IRP1 can be converted *in vitro* from the aconitase form to the RNA-binding apoprotein form (Haile *et al.*, 1992), and from the apoprotein back to the aconitase form (Emery-Goodman *et al.*, 1993; Gray *et al.*, 1993). Mutation of all three Cys residues which constitute the inactive aconitase results in a constitutively active RNA-binding protein, independent of iron levels (Hirling *et al.*, 1994). Comparisons of the aconitase and IRP1 structures (Figure 10.3) show domains 3 and 4 rotated outwards to create a large pocket which can interact with the multiple sites in the IRE described earlier, notably the conserved unpaired C and the loop nucleotides AGU (Walden *et al.*, 2006).

In contrast, IRP2 does not have the capacity to incorporate an Fe–S cluster, lacks enzymatic activity and, as we will see in more detail shortly, its non-IRE-binding form is removed by ubiquitination and degradation by the proteosome. IRP2 deficiency causes alterations in iron homeostasis in the duodenum, central nervous system and, most notably, in motor neurons of the spinal cord (La Vaute *et al.*, 2001), with accumulation of iron in the brain. The role of IRP2 in neurodegenerative disorders will be dealt with in more detail in Chapter 15.

In iron-replete conditions IRP2 is not transformed into an aconitase. It lacks a mandatory residue which is required as a catalytic base, and it does not appear to insert a [4Fe–4S] cluster. Instead, in iron-replete conditions and under increased oxygen pressure, IRP2 is rapidly ubiquitinated and degraded by proteasomes (Guo *et al.*, 1994, 1995). Unlike IRP1, IRP2 is activated by hypoxia (Hanson *et al.*, 1999; Meyron-Holz *et al.*, 2004), since low oxygen pressure prevents IRP2 degradation (Hanson *et al.*, 2003). It was initially thought that the 73-amino acid region of IRP2, which is absent in IRP1, thought to be the target of iron-dependent oxidation and ubiquitination by a specific HOIL-1 ubiquitin ligase involving a direct interaction of haem with a haem regulatory motif in IRP2, was the cause of IRP2 degradation (Iwai *et al.*, 1998; Yamanaka *et al.*, 2003; Ishikawa *et al.*, 2005). However, deletion of the 73-amino acid region, mutation of specific cysteines, or RNA-interference against HOIL-1 did not abrogate iron-dependent IRP2 degradation (Hanson *et al.*, 2003; Bourdon *et al.*, 2003; Wang *et al.*, 2004; Zumbrennen *et al.*, 2008). Instead, a short portion in the C-terminal domain was required for iron-dependent proteasomal degradation (Wang *et al.*, 2008a). Moreover, IRP1 cysteine-mutants that are unable to insert the [4Fe–4S] cluster were also found to be sensitive to iron-dependent proteasomal degradation (Clarke *et al.*, 2006; Wang *et al.*, 2007).

10.1.5 The IRE/IRP System Revisited – Iron Controls Iron

Already in 2009, Lukas Kühn proposed that 'iron controls iron' (Kühn, 2009). What this implied was that the iron content of the labile iron pool (LIP) would act as a trigger to switch the IRE/IRP system between two extremes (Figure 10.5). When iron is low, IRPs bind to IREs in mRNAs of key players of intracellular iron metabolism. This effectively blocks ferritin and ferroportin translation, thereby reducing iron storage and export while TfR1 and DMT1 mRNA are protected against degradation, thereby increasing iron uptake. The physiological effect is cumulative and tends to increase the LIP. As the LIP increases, it attains a level at which labile free iron contributes to the

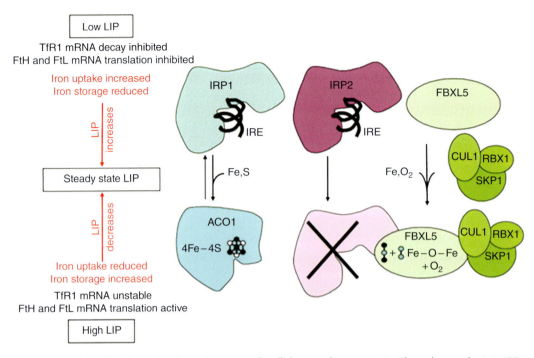

Figure 10.5 *Feedback mechanisms that control cellular iron homeostasis. The scheme depicts IRP1 and IRP2, which are active as RNA-binding proteins at low LIP levels. By binding to IREs, they inhibit the translation or degradation of mRNAs encoding proteins required for cellular iron storage and import, thereby increasing the LIP. Once it has reached a sufficiently high concentration, labile free iron then contributes to the assembly of the [4Fe–4S] cluster that inactivates RNA-binding of IRP1. Concomitantly, the insertion of a di-iron centre into a haemrythrin-like domain of FBXL5 renders this protein more stable such that it combines with additional subunits to form an E3 ubiquitin ligase complex, which then binds IRP2 and induces its degradation by the proteasomal pathway. The assembly of these two iron centres corresponds to an iron-sensing mechanism, in which free iron acts on its own level through these elaborate feedback loops. Reprinted with permission of the Royal Society of Chemistry from Kühn, L.C. (2014) Iron regulatory proteins and their role in controlling iron metabolism.* Metallomics, **7**, 232–243

assembly of the [4Fe–4S] cluster, inactivating the RNA-binding of IRP1 and reversing the physiological effects. In this context, IRP1 can be considered as a natural sensor of LIP and its activities control the LIP (Kühn, 2014). Concomitantly, the insertion of a di-iron centre into a haemerythrin-like domain of FBXL5 renders this protein more stable such that it combines with additional subunits to form an E3 ubiquitin ligase complex, which then binds IRP2 and induces its degradation by the proteasomal pathway (Salahudeen *et al.*, 2009; Vashisht *et al.*, 2009). Before discussing the role of FBXL5 as a cellular sensor of free iron levels, the reader is reminded of the ubiquitin/proteasome pathway.

Protein ubiquitylation is a post-translational modification which controls all aspects of eukaryotic cell functionality, and its defective regulation is manifested in various human diseases. The ubiquitylation process requires a set of enzymes (Figure 10.6), of which the ubiquitin ligases (E3s) are the substrate-recognition components. Modular CULLIN-RING ubiquitin ligases (CRLs) are the most prevalent class of E3s, comprising hundreds of distinct CRL complexes with the potential to recruit

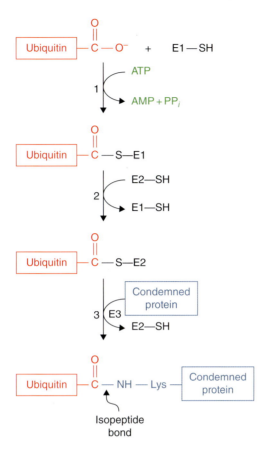

Figure 10.6   *The reactions involved in the attachment of ubiquitin to a target protein destined for proteasomal degradation. The carboxyl group of ubiquitin is coupled to the ubiquitin-activating enzyme (E1) and then transferred to the ubiquitin-conjugating enzyme (E2). The ubiquitin–protein ligase (E3) complex finally transfers the ubiquitin from E2 to the target protein. Reproduced from Voet, D. and Voet, J.G. (2011)* Biochemistry. *3rd edn, John Wiley & Sons, Hoboken, NJ, 1591 pp*

as many and even more protein substrates. Of these, the best understood at both structural and functional levels are CRL1 or SCF (SKP1/CUL1/F-box protein) complexes. The structural organisation of SCF/CRL1 complexes (Genshik *et al.*, 2013) consists of a catalytic core module composed of the scaffold proteins Cullin 1 (CUL1), and the RING finger protein RBX1 with a SKP1 (S phase kinase-associated protein 1)/FBP heterodimer bridging CUL1-RBX1 to the substrate. Substrate recognition is governed by an independent protein–protein interaction domain (PID) in the FBPs The N terminus of CUL-1 binds the adaptor Skp1, while the C terminus binds the RING finger protein Rbx1, which binds the ubiquitin-bearing E2.

The E3 ubiquitin ligase complex required for IRP2 degradation has been identified, and is composed of an SCF protein complex of FBXL5, SKP1, CUL1 and RBX1 (Figure 10.5). FBXL5 interacts directly with both IRP2 and the apo-IRP1 mutants referred to above in an iron-dependent fashion, and increases IRP2 ubiquitination *in vitro* and *in vivo*. FBXL5 is unstable and degraded by the proteasome when cellular free iron or oxygen concentrations are low in a process which involves the ubiquitin ligase HERC2 (Moroishi *et al.*, 2014). The iron- and oxygen-dependent stability of FBXL5 requires the presence of its N-terminal 199 amino acids, which was predicted to fold into a haemerythrin-like domain containing a characteristic di-iron cluster. Mutational studies of carboxylate and imidazole ligands have shown that both oxygen and iron are necessary for correct folding of this domain (Salahudeen *et al.*, 2009; Vashisht *et al.*, 2009). The structure of the di-iron centre is shown in Figure 10.7, along with the iron-containing cluster of IRP1, together with an indication of their respective sensitivity to various stimuli (Kühn, 2014). Each of these iron-containing clusters are able to sense the iron levels within the cellular LIP.

Thus, FBXL5 appears to be yet another cellular sensor for free iron levels in addition to IRP1 (Figure 10.5). However, the influence of oxygen on IRP1 inactivation and the degradation of IRP2 consequent upon the ubiquitin ligase activity of the di-iron form of FBXL5 is different. FBXL5 requires both iron and oxygen for its stability due to an uncharacterised mechanism, and IRP2 is degraded only when both are at sufficient levels (Hanson *et al.*, 1999, 2003; Meyron-Holz *et al.*, 2004). Iron sensing by this second iron centre allows cells to respond to LIP changes over a wide range of physiological conditions, and may provide an explanation for the evolutionary appearance of two IRPs. At low-oxygen conditions IRP1 activity is more easily inactivated, and even at low-iron

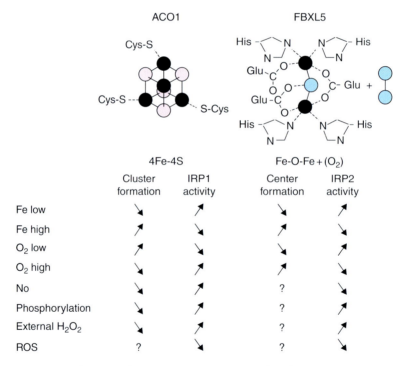

Figure 10.7 *Sensitivity of IRP1 and IRP2 to various compounds. Schematic representation of the two cellular iron-containing clusters that sense iron in cells. The [4Fe–4S] cluster associates with IRP1 (gene ACO1) and inactivates its RNA-binding properties to generate a cytoplasmic aconitase. The di-iron centre of the E3 ubiquitinase subunit FBXL5, only in the presence of sufficient dioxygen, stabilises this protein such that the RNA-binding IRP2 is ubiquitinated and degraded in proteasomes. Various conditions promote or reduce the assembly of these clusters and, accordingly, the IRP1 and IRP2 activities change, as indicated by upwards or downwards arrows. Reprinted with permission of the Royal Society of Chemistry from Kühn, L.C. (2014) Iron regulatory proteins and their role in controlling iron metabolism. Metallomics, **7**, 232–243*

conditions, because the [4Fe–4S] cluster forms readily, while FBXL5 remains unstable and IRP2 is not degraded (Figure 10.7) (Meyron-Holz *et al.*, 2004). In contrast, at high oxygen concentrations, IRP1 remains more active at low-iron conditions, whereas IRP2 is more readily degraded.

10.1.6 Metabolic Consequences of Mutations in IREs

The importance of the IRE/IRP system in cellular iron homeostasis is underlined by the effects of its dysregulation in a number of diseases. The first of these to be reported was hereditary hyper-ferritinaemia-cataract syndrome (HHCS) (Girelli *et al.*, 1995; Beaumont *et al.*, 1995), which is characterised by the combination of a marked elevation of serum ferritin levels (>1000 μg l⁻¹) and a high probability of developing early-onset bilateral cataract, which is inherited as an autosomal dominant trait due to L-ferritin deposits in the lens. The syndrome is caused by mutations within the IRE of L-ferritin which prevent the efficient binding of IRPs 1 and 2 to the IRE in L-ferritin mRNA, resulting in uncontrolled ferritin translation. Numerous mutations have subsequently been described (Cazzola and Skoda, 2000; Ismail *et al.*, 2006; Millonig *et al.*, 2010), and the degree of hyperferritinaemia and cataract severity has been shown to correlate with the *in-vitro* binding affinity of IRP for HHCS mutant IREs (Allerson *et al.*, 1999). However, a recent study (Luschieti *et al.*, 2013) has identified two new mutations, the Badalona +36C>U and Heidelberg +52G>C muta-tions within the L-ferritin IRE, which only mildly alter the binding capacity of the IRPs but are still causative for the disease. To date, 37 reported mutations causing HHCS have been identified, of which 31 are point mutations and six are deletions of different sizes (Millonig *et al.*, 2010; Luschieti *et al.*, 2013). The majority of the causative mutations are located in the hexanucleotide loop, followed by the C-bulge region, the upper stem and the lower stem of the IRE structure. Other occurrences of inherited unexplained hyperferritinaemia, but without cataracts or cataracts diagnosed in adult age, have been attributed to mutations in the promoter region, coding region or outside the IRE motif of L-ferritin (Cremonesi *et al.*, 2003; Kannengiesser *et al.*, 2009; Faniello *et al.*, 2009; Thurlow *et al.*, 2012). A mutation in the IRE of human H ferritin has been reported to cause auto-somal dominant iron overload (Kato *et al.*, 2001), while the disruption of IRE elements in the mouse FPN1 promoter alters erythropoiesis, iron homeostasis and induces age-dependent loss of retinal photoreceptors (Mok *et al.*, 2004; Iacovelli *et al.*, 2009). IRP1 has an essential role in regu-lating HIF2α translation, and it has been suggested (Zhang *et al.*, 2014) that the activation of IRP1 could repress HIF2α translation, thereby decreasing erythropoietin (EPO) expression and reducing red blood cell production in polycythaemia patients. In contrast, in the anaemia of chronic disease the inhibition of this effect could increase HIF2α translation and upregulate endogenous EPO levels (Zimmer *et al.* 2008).

10.2 Systemic Iron Homeostasis

10.2.1 Introduction

While the IRE/IRP system is involved in regulating cellular iron homeostasis, it is essential to regulate iron balance at the level of the whole organism, such that there is sufficient iron to supply iron body requirements, without generating the problems of toxicity associated with iron excess (Chapter 12). In mammals there are two other regulatory systems which maintain systemic iron metabolism in balance, involving the regulation of iron absorption from the intestinal tract, iron recycling from macrophages and, under certain circumstances, the mobilisation of iron from hepatic stores. Over the past twenty years it has become clear that the major regulator of systemic iron homeostasis relies on the regulatory circuit of the hormone hepcidin and the cellular iron exporter ferroportin (FPN1). However, as we will see, hypoxia-inducible factors (HIFs) also control the transcription of numerous genes involved in maintaining iron metabolism in equilibrium (Haase, 2013). For recent reviews of systemic iron homeostasis, see Steinbicker and Mückenthaler (2013), Ganz (2013) and Pantopoulos *et al.* (2013).

10.2.2 Hepcidin, the Key Player

The regulation of systemic iron balance is controlled to a large extent by hepcidin, an antimicrobial peptide hormone found in the circulation and produced essentially in liver (Krause *et al.*, 2000; Park *et al.*, 2001). However, while hepcidin is normally expressed at high levels in liver, in iron-loaded mice it was significantly upregulated (Pigeon *et al.*, 2001). Serendipitous inactivation of the mouse hepcidin gene was found to lead to massive iron overload in the liver and pancreas, whereas curiously the spleen, which is rich in macrophages, was not affected (Nicolas *et al.*, 2001) As we will see in Chapter 10, this corresponds very closely to what is observed in genetic haemochromatosis in humans, with increased intestinal iron absorption, increased parenchymal iron loading, but no accumulation of iron in the macrophages. It was subsequently found that when mice overexpressed hepcidin they developed severe iron-deficiency anaemia and most of them died at birth (Nicolas *et al.*, 2002), while targeted disruption of the hepcidin gene caused severe iron overload (Viatte *et al.*, 2005).

The single three-exon human hepcidin gene, located on chromosome 19 (Krause *et al.*, 2000; Park *et al.*, 2001; Pigeon *et al.*, 2001) encodes an 84-residue prepropeptide, with a 24-amino acid signal peptide which is cleaved to yield the intermediate cellular propeptide. This in turn is cleaved at a characteristic polybasic cleavage site by the prohormone convertase furin (Valore and Ganz, 2008) just to the N-terminal side of the mature, 25-residue hepcidin peptide itself (Figure 10.8A). This is the form which was first identified in human urine and plasma (Krause *et al.*, 2000; Park *et al.*, 2001; Campostrini *et al.*, 2012). Two C-terminal truncated forms of the peptide, of 22 and 20 residues, are also found in urine, probably resulting from proteolytic degradation. The antimicrobial activity of hepcidin is modest compared to its iron regulatory activity, whereas the truncated forms have antibacterial activity. Removal of the five N-terminal residues progressively decreases the iron regulatory activity and the 20-residue peptide is completely inactive, both *in vitro* and *in vivo* (Nemeth *et al.*, 2006). Unlike many other antimicrobial and antifungal peptides, the amino acid sequences of which vary widely between even closely related species, the sequence of hepcidin is highly conserved between vertebrate species (Figure 10.8), including all eight of the Cys residues which form the four disulphide bonds.

The solution structures of human and sea bass hepcidin were determined using NMR (Hunter *et al.*, 2002; Lauth *et al.*, 2005). They both form a distorted antiparallel β-sheet hairpin structure, crosslinked by four conserved disulphide bonds with connectivity Cys^7–Cys^{23}, Cys^{10}–Cys^{13}, Cys^{11}–Cys^{19} and Cys^{14}–Cys^{22}, three of which stabilise the antiparallel strands of its simple β-sheet, while the fourth was reported to link two adjacent Cys residues in an unusual vicinal disulphide bridge found at the turn of the hairpin. However, a more recent study using NMR, disulphide mapping and X-ray crystallography, has shown that this connectivity is apparently incorrect and that instead, the disulphides form a different connectivity that shares two of the disulphides from the originally proposed connectivity, 7-23 and 11-19, but the vicinal disulphide is absent, and the other two disulphide bonds are located between 10-13 and 14-22 (Jordan *et al.*, 2009).

As we will discuss in greater detail below, hepcidin acts by exerting post-translational control on the membrane concentration of its receptor, the only known cellular iron exporter, ferroportin

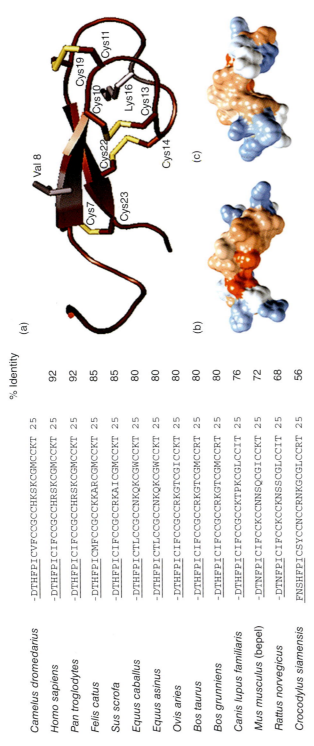

	% Identity	
Camelus dromedarius	-DTHFPICVFCCGCCHKSKCGMCCKT	25
Homo sapiens	-DTHFPICIFCCGCCHRSKCGMCCKT	25	92
Pan troglodytes	-DTHFPICIFCCGCCHRSKCGMCCKT	25	92
Felis catus	-DTHFPICMFCCGCCKKARCGMCCKT	25	85
Sus scrofa	-DTHFPICIFCCGCCRKAICGMCCKT	25	85
Equus caballus	-DTHFPICTLCCGCCNKQKCGWCCKT	25	80
Equus asinus	-DTHFPICTLCCGCCNKQKCGWCCKT	25	80
Ovis aries	-DTHFPICIFCCGCCRKGTCGICCKT	25	80
Bos taurus	-DTHFPICIFCCGCCRKGTCGMCCRT	25	80
Bos grunniens	-DTHFPICIFCCGCCRKGTCGMCCRT	25	80
Canis lupus familiaris	-DTHFPICIFCCGCCKTPKCGLCCIT	25	76
Mus musculus (bepel)	-DTNFPICIFCCKCNNSQCGICCKT	25	72
Rattus norvegicus	-DTNFPICIFCCKCCKNSSCGLCCIT	25	68
Crocodylus siamensis	FNSHFPICSYCCNCCRNKGCGLCCRT	25	56

Figure 10.8 *Left: Multiple amino acid sequence alignment of hepcidin with different mammalian hepcidin sequences. Underlined residues indicate essential amino acid sequence for binding to ferroportin. Hepcidin sequences used for the alignment were provided from Gene Bank. Right: Model structure of the camel hepcidin. (a) Ribbon model structure of Camelus dromedarius hepcidin constructed basing on the human hepcidin-25 solution NMR revisited structure (Ref. PDB: 2KEF) used as template by SWISS-MODEL program tool. Rendering of the ribbon model structure has been carried out with PyMol program. Disulfide bridges are coloured in yellow, showing connections between the conserved cysteine residues. Side chains of the Val8 and Lys16 (unique residues making the difference with human hepcidin) are shown as sticks. Two views of space-filling diagrams of hepcidin-25 indicating the hydrophobic (pink) side on b and cationic charges (blue) on c were generated with UCSF Chimera 1.6.1 program. Reproduced with permission from John Wiley & Sons from Boumaiza, M., Ezzine, A., Jaouen, M., Sari, M.A. and Marzouki, M.N. (2014) Molecular characterization of a novel hepcidin (HepcD) from Camelus dromedarius. Synthetic peptide forms exhibit antibacterial activity.* J. Pept. Sci., **20**, 680–688

(Nemeth *et al.*, 2004). Since ferroportin delivers iron to the plasma, whether from the diet, from storage depots or from recycling of effete red cells, its interaction with ferroportin effectively controls the flux of iron through the plasma and therefore the supply of iron available for the multiple requirements of iron-consuming tissues (Ganz, 2013). A single intraperitoneal injection $1-2\,\mu g\,g^{-1}$ of hepcidin in mice causes a rapid fall in serum iron to levels 80% lower than in control mice within 1 h, and serum iron remains suppressed for more than 48 h after the injection (Rivera *et al.*, 2005). Chronic overexpression of hepcidin causes iron-deficiency anaemia (Nicolas *et al.*, 2002; Roy *et al.*, 2007) by inhibiting iron absorption and preventing the mobilisation of storage iron, while hepcidin deficiency increases iron absorption and causes parenchymal iron overload, associated with the apparently paradoxical loss of macrophage iron stores (Lesbordes-Brion *et al.*, 2006; Nicolas *et al.*, 2001; Roetto *et al.*, 2003). These effects are all a reflection of the fundamental role of hepcidin in regulating iron absorption and iron release from macrophages, while heterozygous mutations in human ferroportin which interfere with hepcidin binding (Sham *et al.*, 2005, 2009) mimic hepcidin deficiency, confirming the role of hepcidin–ferroportin interactions in iron homeostasis, and suggesting that ferroportin is the sole target of hepcidin (Ganz, 2013).

An interesting connection between ferroportin and the multicopper ferroxidase ceruloplasmin has been proposed, involving the finding that ferroxidase activity is required to stabilise Fpn at the surface of cells expressing Cp-GPI (De Domenico *et al.*, 2007). In the absence of Cp, Fpn is rapidly internalised and degraded. The depletion of extracellular Fe(II) by the yeast ferroxidase Fet3p or iron chelators can maintain cell-surface Fpn in the absence of Cp, whereas in the absence of multicopper oxidases iron remains bound to Fpn. Fpn with bound iron is recognised by a ubiquitin ligase, which ubiquitinates Fpn on Lys253. The mutation of Lys253 to alanine prevents ubiquitination and maintains Fpn-iron on the cell surface in the absence of ferroxidase activity (De Domenico *et al.*, 2007). The requirement for a ferroxidase to maintain iron transport activity represents a new mechanism of regulating cellular iron export, a new function for Cp, and an explanation for brain iron overload in patients with aceruloplasminaemia. Recent data indicate that iron efflux from endothelial cells of the brain microvasculature, mediated by ferroportin, requires the action of a ferroxidase which can be either extracellular ceruloplasmin or endogenous hephaestin (McCarthy and Kosman, 2013).

10.2.3 Factors which Regulate Hepcidin Synthesis

Hepcidin is mainly synthesised and secreted by hepatocytes and circulates mostly free in the plasma but with some of it weakly bound to albumin and α-2-macroglobulin (Itkonen *et al.*, 2012; Peslova *et al.*, 2009), and it can cleared from the circulation by the kidneys (Park *et al.*, 2001; Wolff *et al.*, 2013). Other cell types and organs, such as monocytes (Theurl *et al.*, 2008), macrophages (Nguyen *et al.*, 2006), heart (Merle *et al.*, 2007), kidney (Kulaksiz *et al.*, 2005), brain (Wang *et al.*, 2008b) and adipose tissue (Bekri *et al.*, 2006), also produce hepcidin in much smaller amounts. Since hepcidin is clearly the peptide hormone which orchestrates the *fluxes* of iron through the systemic circulation (reviewed in Hentze *et al.*, 2010; Ganz and Nemeth, 2012), it is important to establish the factors which regulate hepatic hepcidin synthesis. Already in 1994, Clem Finch (Finch, 1994) defined two clear candidates: the store factor and the erythroid factor. Today, this canvas can be enlarged so as to identify five principal factors which are known to modulate systemic iron homeostasis (Figure 10.9):

  i. Iron availability, which essentially is reflected by total body iron stores and corresponds to Finch's store factor; it makes no sense to take up more dietary iron when the stores are adequate.
 ii. Inflammatory stimuli, such as microbial infections, which will provoke a withdrawal of iron from the circulation in order to starve the invading microorganisms of the iron essential for their proliferation, and hence decrease the risk of infection.

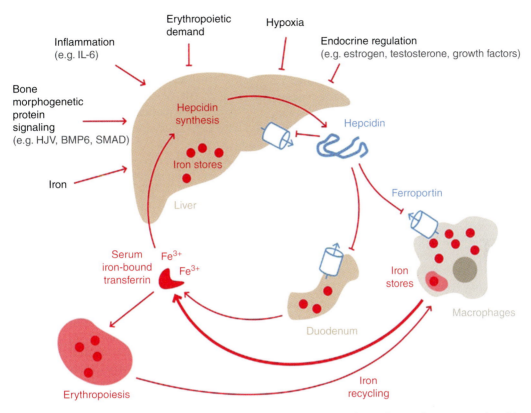

Figure 10.9 *Regulation of hepatic hepcidin production. Hepatic hepcidin synthesis is regulated by iron, bone morphogenetic protein signalling, inflammation, erythropoiesis, hypoxia, or endocrine stimuli. FPN1, which is expressed predominantly in hepatocytes, macrophages and enterocytes, is internalised and degraded following hepcidin binding. Iron is transported in the blood bound to transferrin. Most iron is required for erythropoiesis. Aging erythrocytes that exceed a lifespan of approximately 120 days are recycled in macrophages. Transferrin-iron is a critical indicator for systemic iron homeostasis and regulator of hepcidin expression. Reproduced from Steinbicker, A.U. and Mückenthaler, M.U. (2013). Out of balance – systemic iron homeostasis in iron-related disorders. Nutrients, 5, 3034–3061. This is an open access article distributed under the Creative Commons Attribution License*

iii. Erythropoietic demand – the iron requirements of the erythroid system for haemoglobin synthesis, which can increase following phlebotomy, haemolysis or the administration of EPO.

iv. Hypoxia – in conditions of hypoxia the body will increase its red cell volume, which will increase the demand for iron.

v. Endocrine signals – more recently, growth hormones have been shown to control serum iron levels and hepcidin gene expression.

10.2.3.1 Iron Availability

The level of diferric transferrin Tf-Fe$_2$ is the parameter which best represents iron stores/iron availability, and it regulates hepatic hepcidin transcription in a negative feedback loop, which is controlled by the bone morphogenic protein (BMP) signalling pathway (Figure 10.9). When Tf-Fe$_2$ levels increase, hepcidin increases, shutting down dietary iron absorption and iron release from macrophages and hepatocytes. As the systemic iron flux increases, Tf-Fe$_2$ levels drop and if they descend below a critical tipping point, hepcidin levels fall and dietary and storage iron are once again mobilised.

Much of the current knowledge regarding how hepcidin functions have derived from studies on hereditary haemochromatosis (HH), and this is discussed in Chapter 11. Three of the proteins which are known to be mutated in different genetic forms of HH, namely HFE (the gene product of the classic type I form of HH), HJV (haemojuvelin, associated with juvenile Type 2 haemochromatosis) and TfR2 (transferrin receptor 2, associated with Type 3 haemochromatosis), turn out to be intimately involved in the regulation of hepcidin by Tf-Fe$_2$. Transferrin bound iron (Tf-Fe) is monitored by an 'iron-sensing complex', consisting of the transferrin receptors TfR1 and TfR2, the former bound to Tf-Fe$_2$, together with HFE and HJV. Protein–protein interactions between these three membrane proteins are involved in transmitting increased Tf-Fe$_2$ levels and thereby inducing hepatic hepcidin transcription (Hentze *et al.*, 2004; Steinbicker and Mückenthaler, 2013; Core *et al.*, 2014), as outlined in Figure 10.10. HJV, as will be seen in Chapter 11, is a glycosylphosphatidylinositol (GPI)-linked membrane protein and a member of the repulsive guidance molecule (RGM) family (Monnier *et al.*, 2002; Samad *et al.*, 2004). Type 2 haemochromatosis patients with HJV mutations and *Hjv* knockout mice exhibit significantly reduced hepatic hepcidin expression, implicating HJV in the regulation of hepcidin synthesis (Papanikolaou *et al.*, 2004; Huang *et al.*, 2005; Niederkofler *et al.*, 2005). Since RGM proteins are known to function as BMP coreceptors this led to the recognition that BMP signalling was the major signalling pathway which controls hepcidin regulation (Babitt *et al.*, 2006). Patients with HFE-deficiency (Bolondi *et al.*, 2010) and mice with HFE or TfR2-deficiency (Corradini *et al.*, 2011) show an attenuation of BMP signalling, underlining the importance of these proteins in the HJV–BMP activation of hepcidin transcription, and biochemical evidence for a membrane-associated complex of HJV, HFE and TfR2 has been found in human hepatoma cells (D'Alessio *et al.*, 2012).

In the canonical signalling pathway, BMP ligands bind to type I and type II serine threonine kinase receptors to induce the phosphorylation of cytoplasmic SMAD1, SMAD5, and SMAD8 proteins, which then form a complex with SMAD4 and translocate to the nucleus to regulate gene transcription. In their role as BMP coreceptors, HJV and other RGM family members bind selectively to BMP ligands and receptors to enhance SMAD phosphorylation in response to BMP signals (Babitt *et al.*, 2005, 2006; Samad *et al.*, 2005). Subsequently, Bmp6, a member of the transforming growth factor-beta (TFG-β) superfamily, was identified as the major ligand which activates hepcidin levels, convincingly underlined by the observation that Bmp6 knockout mice show severe iron overload due to a failure to activate hepcidin expression (Meynard *et al.*, 2009; Andriopoulos *et al.*, 2009). Binding of Bmp6 to type I BMP receptors (Alk1, Alk2, Alk3 and Alk6) and type II BMP receptors (BMPRII, ActRIIa or ActRIIb) induces the type II receptor to phosphorylate and activate the BMP type I receptor. The BMP type I receptors Alk2 and Alk3 are expressed in the liver (Figure 10.10) (of the other BMP type I receptors, Alk1 is predominantly expressed in endothelial cells and Alk6 is not expressed in hepatocytes) (Otu *et al.*, 2007; Yu *et al.*, 2008). Mice with liver-specific deficiency of Alk2 and Alk3 respectively develop moderate to very severe iron overload, due to decreased hepcidin mRNA expression (Steinbicker *et al.*, 2011). Although it is known that BMP2, BMP4 and BMP6 are endogenous ligands for HJV in human hepatoma cells, and HJV selectively uses the BMP type II receptors BMPRII and ActRIIA (Xia *et al.*, 2008), specific roles for individual BMP type II receptors in iron metabolism have yet to be investigated. Once activated, BMP type I receptors participate in the phosphorylation of intracellular signalling molecules called receptor-associated SMAD proteins (R-SMADs) which, together with SMAD4, transfer to the hepatocyte nucleus to induce hepcidin transcription (Figure 10.10) (Babitt *et al.*, 2006).

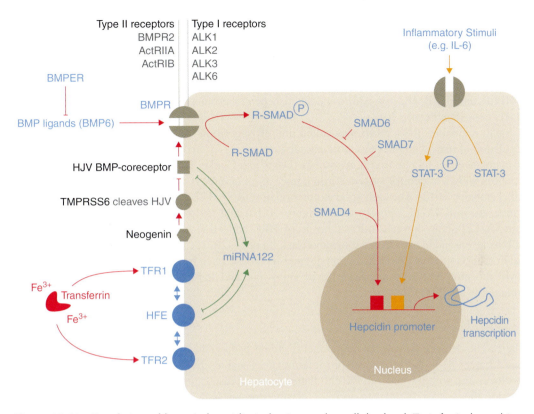

Figure 10.10   *Regulation of hepatic hepcidin induction at the cellular level. Transferrin bound iron (Tf-Fe) is monitored by an 'iron-sensing complex', which consists of the transferrin receptors (TfR) 1 and 2, HFE, and HJV. HJV is a glycosylphosphatidylinositol (GPI)-linked membrane-associated protein that functions as a BMP coreceptor, and enhances bone morphogenetic protein (BMP) signalling. Binding of one of the more than 25 known BMP ligands (such as BMP6) to type I and II BMP receptors induces the type II receptor to phosphorylate and activate the BMP type I receptor. There are four BMP type I receptors (called ALK1, ALK2, ALK3, and ALK6), and three BMP type II receptors (BMPR2, ActRIIA, and ActRIIB). The activated BMP type I receptor leads to phosphorylation of intracellular signalling molecules called receptor-associated SMAD proteins (R-SMADs). Phosphorylated R-SMADs transfer together with SMAD 4 to the hepatocyte nucleus and induce hepcidin transcription. SMAD6 and SMAD7 are inhibitory SMADs. BMPER, the BMP endothelial cell precursor-derived regulator inhibits BMP signalling and decreases hepatic hepcidin expression. MicroRNA 122 is activated by HFE or HJV and inhibits the latter in a negative feedback regulatory loop. The transmembrane serine protease (TMPRSS6, also known as Matripase 2) cleaves HJV and thereby decreases BMP-mediated hepcidin induction. Neogenin, a transmembrane protein known to interact with HJV, can also interact with TMPRSS6 to enable HJV cleavage in transfected cells. Soluble HJV is generated by proprotein convertase activity, and has been proposed to sequester BMPs. Inflammatory stimuli such as interleukin-6 (IL-6) induce hepcidin transcription via the JAK/STAT signalling pathway. A SMAD- and a STAT-binding element have been identified in the hepcidin promoter. Reproduced from Steinbicker, A.U. and Mückenthaler, M.U. (2013). Out of balance – systemic iron homeostasis in iron-related disorders. Nutrients, **5**, 3034–3061. This is an open access article distributed under the Creative Commons Attribution License*

Whereas Smad1/5/8 in association with Smad4 activate hepcidin gene expression, the inhibitory Smads Smad6 and Smad7 decrease hepcidin expression in response to a high iron load (Vujić-Spasić *et al.*, 2012; Mleczko-Sanecka *et al.*, 2010).

Another regulator of BMP signalling is the BMP-binding endothelial cell precursor-derived regulator (Bmper), which is overexpressed in hypotransferrinaemic mice (Trf(hpx/hpx)). Soluble BMPER inhibits BMP2- or BMP6-mediated hepcidin promoter activity in human HepG2 and HuH7 cells (Patel *et al.*, 2012).

Small regulatory RNA molecules called microRNAs (miRNAs) have an important role in the regulation of many cellular regulatory and disease processes, and they may also be key regulators in many facets of human iron homeostasis (Davis and Clarke, 2013). The liver-specific miR-122 has been shown to control systemic iron homeostasis in mice (Castoldi *et al.*, 2011; Castoldi and Mückenthaler, 2012). The high-level expression of miRNA-122 depends on HFE and HJV, both of which are miRNA-122 target genes (Figure 10.10) and, as a consequence, mice depleted of miRNA-122 show elevated mRNA levels of HFE and HJV, which causes increased hepcidin mRNA levels and plasma iron deficiency (Castoldi *et al.*, 2011; Castoldi and Mückenthaler, 2012). Additionally, microRNA-130a is upregulated in mouse liver by iron deficiency and targets the BMP receptor ALK2 to attenuate BMP signalling and hepcidin transcription (Zumbrennen-Bulough *et al.*, 2014).

10.2.3.2 Inflammatory Stimuli

The classic defence strategy to counteract invading pathogens with a voracious appetite for iron (see Chapter 4) is the release of pro-inflammatory signals by the innate immune system; this results in iron withdrawal from the circulation, thereby restricting the availability of this essential metal to the invader. In order to decrease plasma iron levels it is essential that hepcidin transcription should be activated. Inflammatory stimuli were shown to be potent inducers of hepcidin (Pigeon *et al.*, 2001; Nicolas *et al.*, 2002; Nemeth *et al.*, 2003, 2004) (Figure 10.9) mediated by inflammatory cytokines, of which the most important are interleukin (IL) -6 (IL-6) (Nemeth *et al.*, 2004) and IL-22 (Armitage *et al.*, 2011). The molecular mechanism by which inflammation regulates hepcidin transcription involves binding of IL-6 to the gp130–protein receptor complex, which activates JAK1/2 phosphorylation of STAT3. Translocation of phosphorylated STAT3 into the nucleus and binding to the canonical STAT3 binding site in the proximal hepcidin promoter results in an upregulation of hepcidin gene expression (Pietrangelo *et al.*, 2007; Wrighting and Andrews, 2006; Verga-Falzacappa *et al.*, 2008).

The anaemia of chronic disease (ACD), which we discuss in greater clinical detail in Chapter 11, is characterised by an increased hepcidin production, in response to a persistent inflammatory stimulus. Studies from a number of different animal models of ACD (reviewed in Steinbicker and Mückenthaler, 2013) have consistently revealed crosstalk between the inflammatory JAK/STAT pathway and the BMP signalling pathway in the control of the hepcidin response to inflammation. These data are supported by an analysis of the hepcidin promoter which showed that both a STAT-binding site and a BMP-response element are required for hepcidin stimulation by IL-6 (Verga-Falzacappa *et al.*, 2007, 2008).

10.2.3.3 Erythropoietic Demand

Although the search for the stores regulator of systemic iron homeostasis now seems to be over, the erythroid regulator, which coordinates iron turnover with erythropoietic activity, has proved elusive. In the face of increased erythropoietic demand, whether because of blood loss, administration of erythropoietin, or oxygen tension (discussed below), hepcidin should be downregulated. This is what is observed, and it was proposed that hepcidin suppression by erythropoietic drive was mediated by secreted factor(s) released by proliferating red blood cell precursors in the bone marrow (Pak *et al.*, 2006; Vokurka *et al.*, 2006). Two hepcidin suppression factors have been proposed, namely the TGF-β/BMP superfamily modulators growth and differentiation factor 15 (GDF15) and twisted gastrulation 1 (TWSG1). Both are released from erythroid precursor cells in the context of ineffective erythropoiesis in iron-loading anaemias and suppress hepcidin transcription in cellular assays (Tanno *et al.*, 2007, 2009). The role of GDF15 and TWSG1 in hepcidin suppression by erythropoietic drive in other contexts has been questioned (Ashby *et al.*, 2010), and it was recently shown that GDF15$^{-/-}$ mice respond to phlebotomy with a decrease in hepcidin levels similar to wild-type mice (Casanovas *et al.*, 2013). More recently, a new hormone and a novel erythroid regulator (Kautz *et al.*, 2014a), erythroferrone (ERFE), has been identified which mediates hepcidin suppression during stress erythropoiesis. ERFE is produced by erythroblasts in response to erythropoietin. ERFE also contributes to the recovery from anaemia of inflammation by suppressing hepcidin and increasing iron availability (Kautz *et al.*, 2014b).

10.2.3.4 *Hypoxia*

Hypoxia is known to stimulate both erythropoietin production and erythropoiesis, increasing iron requirements and lowering hepcidin levels to allow increased dietary iron absorption and release of storage iron (Figures 10.9 and 10.11). *In-vivo* studies on the exposure of humans to high altitude have confirmed substantially decreased hepcidin levels (Piperno *et al.*, 2011; Talbot *et al.*, 2012). Hypoxia-inducible factors, HIF-1 and HIF-2, are heterodimeric transcription factors composed of an alpha- and a beta-subunit, which respond to hypoxia. The alpha subunits of HIF are hydroxylated at conserved proline residues by HIF prolyl-hydroxylases (PHDs), iron- and 2-oxoglutarate-dependent dioxygenases utilising O_2 as substrate, 2-oxoglutarate as a cosubstrate, and iron (Fe^{2+}) and ascorbate as cofactors. The 4-hydroxyprolines are subsequently recognised by the protein von Hippel–Lindau (pVHL) E3 ubiquitin ligase, which targets HIF-α for degradation by the 26S proteasome through polyubiquitination (Maxwell *et al.*, 1999) in normoxic conditions. In hypoxic conditions, the PHDs are inhibited, allowing the stabilised HIF-1 and HIF-2 to regulate the transcription of a number of genes involved in iron metabolism (*Tf*, *TfR*, *ceruloplasmin*, *DMT-1*, *FPN1*). Studies in mice with liver-specific disruption of the *Vhl* gene (von Hippel–Lindau) suggested a key role for HIFs in hepcidin regulation (Peysonneaux *et al.*, 2007), although a direct transcriptional activity of HIFs on the hepcidin promoter is not supported by biochemical data (Volke *et al.*, 2009). Whereas HIF directly regulates renal and hepatic EPO synthesis under hypoxia, when erythropoiesis was inhibited pharmacologically, hepcidin gene expression was no longer suppressed despite profound elevations in serum EPO; this indicated that EPO by itself is not directly involved in the regulation of the hepcidin gene (Liu *et al.*, 2012). Stabilisation of HIF by inhibitors of PHDs significantly reduces hepcidin mRNA levels (Braliou *et al.*, 2008)

It is thus likely that the inhibitory effects of hypoxia on hepcidin expression are primarily triggered by an increased erythropoietic drive. Consistent with this view, hepatic HIF2α has been shown to inhibit hepcidin expression via an EPO-mediated increase in the level of erythropoiesis (Mastrogiannaki *et al.*, 2012). Studies in hepatoma cells suggest that hypoxia downregulates hepcidin expression by inhibiting SMAD4 signalling (Chaston *et al.*, 2011). Hypoxia has been shown to increase TMPRSS6 transcription (Lakhal *et al.*, 2011), mediated by an hypoxic responsive element in the TMPRSS6 promoter (Maurer *et al.*, 2012), although the loss of Hfe, TfR2 and Tmprss6 in mice does not affect the hypoxic response of hepcidin (Lee *et al.*, 2012).

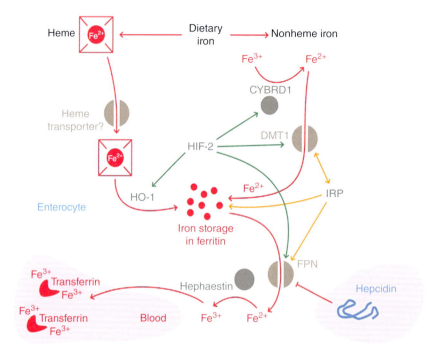

Figure 10.11 *Iron absorption in the intestine. In the human diet, iron is present as haem or non-haem iron. Absorption of haem iron (Fe²⁺) is incompletely understood and likely mediated by a haem transporter. Intracellularly, iron is released from haem by hemoxygenase-1 (HO-1). Non-haem iron (Fe³⁺) is reduced by the membrane-associated ferric reductase CYBRD1 (DCYTB) for transport into the intestinal enterocyte by the divalent metal transporter (DMT1). Within the enterocyte, iron can be stored in ferritin or exported into the bloodstream by the iron exporter ferroportin (FPN1, SLC40A1). FPN expression is controlled by hepcidin. Hephaestin, a multicopper oxidase is required to incorporate two Fe³⁺ into one transferrin (Tf) molecule. Hypoxia-inducible factor 2 (HIF-2) controls CYBRD1, DMT1, FPN, and HO-1 mRNA expression (depicted in green), and iron regulatory proteins (IRPs) post-transcriptionally control the expression of DMT1, ferritin, and FPN (depicted in orange). Reproduced from Steinbicker, A.U. and Mückenthaler, M.U. (2013). Out of balance – systemic iron homeostasis in iron-related disorders.* Nutrients, **5**, *3034–3061. This is an open access article distributed under the Creative Commons Attribution License*

10.2.3.5   Endocrine Signals

Both, growth hormones and sex hormones have been found to control hepcidin levels. Growth hormone increases hepcidin levels when administered to fasting subjects but in healthy volunteers it has the opposite effect, presumably stimulating erythropoiesis (Troutt *et al.*, 2012). Other growth factors also decrease liver hepcidin production (Goodnough *et al.*, 2012). Oestrogen administration reduces hepcidin production (Ikeda *et al.*, 2012), and an oestrogen response element was identified in the hepcidin promoter (Ikeda *et al.*, 2012; Hou *et al.*, 2012). Testosterone promotes the association of the androgen receptor with Smad1 and Smad4 to reduce their binding to BMP-Re in men (Guo *et al.*, 2013). Glucose has also been shown to affect serum hepcidin levels (Aigner *et al.*, 2013) and mice heterozygous for BMP type 1 receptor Alk3 show abnormal glucose metabolism (Scott *et al.*, 2009).

The presence of an IRE within the 5′-UTR of HIF2α mRNA suggests a further iron- and oxygen-dependent mechanism for translational regulation of its expression via IRP1 and IRP2. It has recently been shown that the disruption of mouse IRP1, but not IRP2, leads to profound HIF2α-dependent abnormalities in erythropoiesis and systemic iron metabolism in juvenile mice (Wilkinson and Pantopoulos, 2013).

10.3 Integration of Iron Homeostatic Systems

The interplay between the three regulatory systems, the IRF/IRP system, the HIF system and the ultimate key orchestrator of systemic iron homeostasis, the hepcidin/ferroportin system, is slowly beginning to be understood. Since FPN expression is controlled by hepcidin, the transfer of iron from the diet is essentially under the control of hepcidin and the induction of its transcription by the various factors, as described earlier. Hypoxia-inducible factor 2 (HIF-2) exerts transcriptional control over CYBRD1, DMT1, FPN, and HO-1 mRNA expression, while the IRPs act post-transcriptionally to control the expression of DMT1, ferritin, FPN and, as indicated above, possibly also to regulate HIF-2.

References

Abboud, S. and Haile, D.J. (2000) A novel mammalian iron regulated protein involved in intracellular iron metabolism. *J. Biol. Chem.*, **275**, 19906–19912.

Aigner, E., Felder, T.K., Oberkofler, H., *et al.* (2013) Glucose acts as a regulator of serum iron by increasing serum hepcidin concentrations. *J. Nutr. Biochem.*, **24**, 112–117.

Allerson, C.R., Cazzola, M. and Rouault, T.A. (1999) Clinical severity and thermodynamic effects of iron-responsive element mutations in hereditary hyperferritinemia-cataract syndrome. *J. Biol. Chem.*, **274**, 26439–26447.

Anderson, C.P., Shen, M., Eisenstein, R.S. and Leibold, E.A. (2012) Mammalian iron metabolism and its control by iron regulatory proteins. *Biochim. Biophys. Acta*, **1823**, 1468–1483.

Andriopoulos, B., Jr, Corradini, E., Xia, Y., *et al.* (2009) BMP6 is a key endogenous regulator of hepcidin expression and iron metabolism. *Nat. Genet.*, **41**, 482–487.

Armitage, A.E., Eddowes, L.A., Gileadi, U., *et al.* (2011) Hepcidin regulation by innate immune and infectious stimuli. *Blood*, **118**, 4129–4139.

Ashby, D.R., Gale, D.P., Busbridge, M., *et al.* (2010) Erythropoietin administration in humans causes a marked and prolonged reduction in circulating hepcidin. *Haematologica*, **95**, 505–508.

Aziz, N. and Munro, H.N. (1986) Both subunits of rat liver ferritin are regulated at a translational level by iron induction. *Nucleic Acids Res.*, **14**, 915–927.

Aziz, N. and Munro, H.N. (1987) Iron regulates ferritin mRNA translation through a segment of its 5' untranslated region. *Proc. Natl Acad. Sci. USA*, **84**, 8478–8482.

Babitt, J.L., Zhang, Y., Samad, T.A., *et al.* (2005) Repulsive guidance molecule (RGMa), a DRAGON homologue, is a bone morphogenetic protein co-receptor. *J. Biol. Chem.*, **280**, 29820–29827.

Babitt, J.L., Huang, F.W., Wrighting, D.M., *et al.* (2006) Bone morphogenetic protein signaling by hemojuvelin regulates hepcidin expression. *Nat. Genet.*, **38**, 531–539.

Beaumont, C., Leneuve, P., Devaux, I., *et al.* (1995) Mutation in the iron responsive element of the L ferritin mRNA in a family with dominant hyperferritinaemia and cataract. *Nature Genet.*, **11**, 444–446.

Beinert, H., Kennedy, M.C. and Stout, D.C. (1996) Aconitase as iron-sulfur protein, enzyme, and iron-regulatory protein. *Chem. Rev.*, **96**, 2335–2374.

Bekri, S., Gual, P., Anty, R., *et al.* (2006) Increased adipose tissue expression of hepcidin in severe obesity is independent from diabetes and NASH. *Gastroenterology*, **131**, 788–796.

Bolondi, G., Garuti, C., Corradini, E., *et al.* (2010) Altered hepatic BMP signaling pathway in human HFE hemochromatosis. *Blood Cells Mol. Dis.*, **45**, 308–312.

Boumaiza, M., Ezzine, A., Jaouen, M., Sari, M.A. and Marzouki, M.N. (2014) Molecular characterization of a novel hepcidin (HepcD) from *Camelus dromedarius*. Synthetic peptide forms exhibit antibacterial activity. *J. Pept. Sci.*, **20**, 680–688.

Bourdon, E., Kang, D.K., Ghosh, M.C., *et al.* (2003) The role of endogenous haem synthesis and degradation domain cysteines in cellular iron-dependent degradation of IRP. *Blood Cells Mol. Dis.*, **31**, 247–255.

Braliou, G.G., Verga Falzacappa, M.V., Chachami, G., *et al.* (2008) 2-Oxoglutarate-dependent oxygenases control hepcidin gene expression. *J. Hepatol.*, **48**, 801–810.

Butt, J., Kim, H.Y., Basilion, J.P., *et al.* (1996) Differences in the RNA binding sites of iron regulatory proteins and potential target diversity. *Proc. Natl Acad. Sci. USA*, **93**, 4345–4349.

Campostrini, N., Traglia, M., Martinelli, N., *et al.*, (2012) Serum levels of the hepcidin-20 isoform in a large general population: the Val Borbera study. *J. Proteomics*, **76**, Spec. No. 28–35.

Casanovas, G., Vujić Spasić, M., Casu, C., *et al.* (2013) The murine growth differentiation factor 15 is not essential for systemic iron homeostasis in phlebotomized mice. *Haematologica*, **98**, 444–447.

Casey, J.L., Hentze, M.W., Koeller, D.M., *et al.* (1988) Iron responsive elements: regulatory RNA sequences that control mRNA levels and translation. *Science*, **240**, 924–928.

Castoldi, M. and Mückenthaler, M. (2012) Regulation of iron homeostasis by microRNAs. *Cell. Mol. Life Sci.*, **69**, 3945–3952.

Castoldi, M., Vujić Spasić, M., Altamura, S., *et al.* (2011) The liver-specific microRNA miR-122 controls systemic iron homeostasis in mice. *J. Clin. Invest.*, **121**, 1386–1396.

Cazzola, M. and Skoda, R.C. (2000) Translational pathophysiology: a novel molecular mechanism of human disease. *Blood*, **95**, 3280–3288.

Chaston, T.B., Patak, P., Pourvali, K., *et al.* (2011) Hypoxia inhibits hepcidin expression in HuH7 hepatoma cells via decreased SMAD4 signaling. *Am. J. Physiol.*, **300**, C888–C895.

Cho, H.H., Cahill, C.M., Vanderburg, C.R., *et al.* (2010) Selective translational control of the Alzheimer amyloid precursor protein transcript by iron regulatory protein-1. *J. Biol. Chem.*, **285**, 31217–31232.

Cianetti, L., Segnalini, P., Calzolari, A., *et al.* (2005) Expression of alternative transcripts of ferroportin-1 during human erythroid differentiation. *Haematologica*, **90**, 1595–1606.

Clarke, S.L., Vasanthakumar, A., Anderson, S.A., *et al.* (2006) Iron-responsive degradation of iron-regulatory protein 1 does not require the Fe-S cluster. *EMBO J.*, **25**, 544–553.

Cmejla, R., Petrak, J. and Cmejlova, J. (2006) A novel iron responsive element in the 3'UTR of human MRCKalpha. *Biochem. Biophys. Res. Commun.*, **341**, 158–166.

Cmejla, R., Ptackova, P., Petrak, J., *et al.* (2010) Human MRCKalpha is regulated by cellular iron levels and interferes with transferrin iron uptake. *Biochem. Biophys. Res. Commun.*, **395**, 163–167.

Core, A.B., Canali, S. and Babitt, J.L. (2014) Hemojuvelin and bone morphogenetic protein (BMP) signaling in iron homeostasis. *Front. Pharmacol.*, **5**, 104.

Corradini, E., Schmidt, P.J., Meynard, D., *et al.* (2011) BMP6 treatment compensates for the molecular defect and ameliorates hemochromatosis in Hfe knockout mice. *Gastroenterology*, **139**, 1721–1729.

Cox, T.C., Bawden, M.J., Martin, A. and May, B.K. (1991) Human erythroid 5-aminolevulinate synthase: promoter analysis and identification of an iron-responsive element in the mRNA. *EMBO J.*, **10**, 1891–1902.

Cremonesi, L., Paroni, R., Foglieni, B., *et al.* (2003) Scanning mutations of the 5'UTR regulatory sequence of L-ferritin by denaturing high-performance liquid chromatography: identification of new mutations. *Br. J. Haematol.*, **121**, 173–179.

D'Alessio, F., Hentze, M.W. and Mückenthaler, M.U. (2012) The hemochromatosis proteins HFE, TfR2, and HJV form a membrane-associated protein complex for hepcidin regulation. *J. Hepatol.*, **57**, 1052–1060.

Dandekar, T., Stripecke, R., Gray, N.K., *et al.* (1991) Identification of a novel iron-responsive element in murine and human erythroid delta-aminolevulinic acid synthase mRNA. *EMBO J.*, **10**, 1903–1909.

Davis, M. and Clarke, S. (2013) Influence of microRNA on the maintenance of human iron metabolism. *Nutrients*, **5**, 2611–2628.

De Domenico, I., Ward, D.M., di Patti, M.C., *et al.* (2007) Ferroxidase activity is required for the stability of cell surface ferroportin in cells expressing GPI-ceruloplasmin. *EMBO J.*, **26**, 2823–2831.

dos Santos, C.O., Dore, L.C., Valentine, E., *et al.* (2008) An iron responsive element-like stem-loop regulates alpha-hemoglobin-stabilizing protein mRNA. *J. Biol. Chem.*, **283**, 26956–26964.

Drysdale, J.W. and Munro, H.N. (1965) Failure of actinomycin D to prevent induction of liver apoferritin after iron administration. *Biochim. Biophys. Acta*, **103**, 185–188.

Drysdale, J.W. and Munro, H.N. (1966) Regulation of synthesis and turnover of ferritin in rat liver. *J. Biol. Chem.*, **241**, 3630–3637.

Dupuy, J., Volbeda, A., Carpentier, P., *et al.* (2006) Crystal structure of human iron regulatory protein 1 as cytosolic aconitase. *Structure*, **14**, 129–139.

Emery-Goodman, A., Hirling, H., Scarpellino, L., Henderson, B. and Kühn, L.C. (1993) Iron regulatory factor expressed from recombinant baculovirus: conversion between the RNA-binding apoprotein and Fe-S cluster containing aconitase. *Nucleic Acids Res.*, **21**, 1457–1461.

Faniello, M.C., Di Sanzo, M., Quaresima, B., *et al.* (2009) Bilateral cataract in a subject carrying a C to A transition in the L ferritin promoter region. *Clin. Biochem.*, **42**, 911–914.

Finch, C. (1994) Regulators of iron balance in humans. *Blood*, **84**, 1697–1702.

Galy, B., Ferring-Appel, D., Kaden, S., Gröne, H.J. and Hentze, M.W. (2008) Iron regulatory proteins are essential for intestinal function and control key iron absorption molecules in the duodenum. *Cell Metab.*, **7**, 79–85.

Galy, B., Ferring-Appel, D., Becker, C., Gretz, N., Grone, H.J., Schumann, K., *et al.* (2013) Iron regulatory proteins control a mucosal block to intestinal iron absorption. *Cell Rep.*, **3**, 844–857.

Ganz, T. (2013) Systemic iron homeostasis. *Physiol. Rev.*, **93**, 1721–1741.

Ganz, T. and Nemeth, E. (2012) Hepcidin and iron homeostasis. *Biochim. Biophys. Acta*, **1823**, 1434–1443.

Genshik, P., Sumara, I. and Lechner, E. (2013) The emerging family of CULLIN3-RING ubiquitin ligases (CRL3s): cellular functions and disease implications. *EMBO J.*, **32**, 2307–2320.

Girelli, D., Corrocher, R., Bisceglia, L., *et al.* (1995) Molecular basis for the recently described hereditary hyperferritinemia-cataract syndrome: a mutation in the iron-responsive element of ferritin L-subunit gene (the 'Verona mutation'). *Blood*, **86**, 4050–4053.

Goforth, J.B., Anderson, S.A., Nizzi, C.P. and Eisenstein, R.S. (2010) Multiple determinants within iron-responsive elements dictate iron regulatory protein binding and regulatory hierarchy. *RNA*, **16**, 154–169.

Goodnough, J.B., Ramos, E., Nemeth, E. and Ganz, T. (2012) Inhibition of hepcidin transcription by growth factors. *Hepatology*, **56**, 291–299.

Granick, S. (1946a) Protein apoferritin and ferritin in iron feeding and absorption. *Science*, **103**, 107.

Granick, S. (1946b) Ferritin IX; Increase of the protein apoferritin in the gastrointestinal mucosa as a direct response to iron feeding; the function of ferritin in the regulation of iron absorption. *J. Biol. Chem.*, **164**, 737–746.

Gray, N.K. and Hentze, M.W. (1994) Iron regulatory protein prevents binding of the 43S translation pre-initiation complex to ferritin and eALAS mRNAs. *EMBO J.*, **13**, 3882–3891.

Gray, N.K., Quick, S., Goosen, B., *et al.* (1993) Recombinant iron-regulatory factor functions as an iron-responsive-element-binding protein, a translational repressor and an aconitase. A functional assay for translational repression and direct demonstration of the iron switch. *Eur. J. Biochem.*, **218**, 657–667.

Gunshin, H., Allerson, C.R., Polycarpou-Schwartz, M., *et al.* (2001) Iron-dependent regulation of the divalent metal ion transporter. *FEBS Lett.*, **509**, 309–316.

Guo, B., Yu, Y. and Leibold, E.A. (1994) Iron regulates cytoplasmic levels of a novel iron-responsive element-binding protein without aconitase activity. *J. Biol. Chem.*, **269**, 24252–24260.

Guo, B., Phillips, J.D., Yu, Y. and Leibold, E.A. (1995) Iron regulates the intracellular degradation of iron regulatory protein 2 by the proteasome. *J. Biol. Chem.*, **270**, 21645–21651.

Guo, W., Bachman, E., Li, M., *et al.* (2013) Testosterone administration inhibits hepcidin transcription and is associated with increased iron incorporation into red blood cells. *Aging Cell*, **12**, 280–291.

Haase, V.H. (2013) Regulation of erythropoiesis by hypoxia-inducible factors. *Blood Rev.*, **27**, 41–53.

Haile, D.J., Rouault, T.A., Tang, C.K., *et al.* (1992) Reciprocal control of RNA-binding and aconitase activity in the regulation of the iron-responsive element binding protein: role of the iron-sulfur cluster. *Proc. Natl Acad. Sci. USA*, **89**, 7536–7540.

Hanson, E.S., Foot, L.M. and Leibold, E.A. (1999) Hypoxia post-translationally activates iron-regulatory protein 2. *J. Biol. Chem.*, **274**, 5047–5052.

Hanson, E.S., Rawlins, M.L. and Leibold, E.A. (2003) Oxygen and iron regulation of iron regulatory protein 2. *J. Biol. Chem.*, **278**, 40337–40342.

Henderson, B.R., Menotti, E., Bonnard, C. and Kühn, L.C. (1994) Optimal sequence and structure of iron-responsive elements. Selection of RNA stem-loops with high affinity for iron regulatory factor. *J. Biol. Chem.*, **269**, 17481–17489.

Henderson, B.R., Menotti, E. and Kühn, L.C. (1996) Iron regulatory proteins 1 and 2 bind distinct sets of RNA target sequences. *J. Biol. Chem.*, **271**, 4900–4908.

Hentze, M.W., Caughman, S.W., Rouault, T.A., *et al.* (1987a) Identification of the iron-responsive element for the translational regulation of human ferritin mRNA. *Science*, **238**, 1570–1573.

Hentze, M.W., Rouault, T.A., Caughman, S.W., *et al.* (1987b) A cis-acting element is necessary and sufficient for translational regulation of human ferritin expression in response to iron. *Proc. Natl Acad. Sci. USA*, **84**, 6730–6734.

Hentze, M.W., Mückenthaler, M.U. and Andrews, N.C. (2004) Balancing acts: molecular control of mammalian iron metabolism. *Cell*, **117**, 285–297.

Hentze, M.W., Mückenthaler, M.U., Galy, B. and Camaschella, C. (2010) Two to tango: regulation of mammalian iron metabolism. *Cell*, **142**, 24–38.

Hirling, H., Henderson, B.R. and Kühn, L.C. (1994) Mutational analysis of the [4Fe-4S]-cluster converting iron regulatory factor from its RNA-binding form to cytoplasmic aconitase. *EMBO J.*, **13**, 453–461.

Hou, Y., Zhang, S., Wang, L., *et al.* (2012) Estrogen regulates iron homeostasis through governing hepatic hepcidin expression via an estrogen response element. *Gene*, **511**, 398–403.

Huang, F.W., Pinkus, J.L., Pinkus, G.S., Fleming, M.D. and Andrews, N.C. (2005) A mouse model of juvenile hemochromatosis. *J. Clin. Invest.*, **115**, 2187–2191.

Hubert, N. and Hentze, M.W. (2002) Previously uncharacterized isoforms of divalent metal transporter (DMT)-1: implications for regulation and cellular function. *Proc. Natl Acad. Sci. USA*, **99**, 12345–12350.

Hunter, H.N., Fulton, D.B., Ganz, T. and Vogel, H.J. (2002) The solution structure of human hepcidin, a peptide hormone with antimicrobial activity that is involved in iron uptake and hereditary hemochromatosis. *J. Biol. Chem.*, **277**, 37597–37603.

Iacovelli, J., Mlodnicka, A.E., Veldman, P., *et al.* (2009) Brain and retinal ferroportin 1 dysregulation in polycythaemia mice. *Brain Res.*, **1289**, 85–95.

Ikeda, Y., Tajima, S., Izawa-Ishizawa, Y., *et al.* (2012) Estrogen regulates hepcidin expression via GPR30-BMP6-dependent signaling in hepatocytes. *PLoS One*, **7**, e40465.

Ishikawa, H., Kato, M., Hori, H., *et al.* (2005) Involvement of haem regulatory motif in haem-mediated ubiquitination and degradation of IRP2. *Mol. Cell*, **19**, 171–181.

Ismail, A.R., Lachlan, K.L., Mumford, A.D., *et al.* (2006) Hereditary hyperferritinemia cataract syndrome: ocular, genetic, and biochemical findings. *Eur. J. Ophthalmol.*, **16**, 153–160.

Itkonen, O., Stenman, U.H., Parkkinen, J., *et al.* (2012) Binding of hepcidin to plasma proteins. *Clin. Chem.*, **58**, 1158–1160.

Iwai, K., Drake, S.K., Wehr, N.B., *et al.* (1998) Iron-dependent oxidation, ubiquitination, and degradation of iron regulatory protein 2: implications for degradation of oxidized proteins. *Proc. Natl Acad. Sci. USA*, **95**, 4924–4928.

Jordan, J.B., Poppe, L., Haniu, M., *et al.* (2009) Hepcidin revisited, disulfide connectivity, dynamics, and structure. *J. Biol. Chem.*, **284**, 24155–24167.

Kannengiesser, C., Jouanolle, A.M., Hetet, G., *et al.* (2009) A new missense mutation in the L ferritin coding sequence associated with elevated levels of glycosylated ferritin in serum and absence of iron overload. *Haematologica*, **94**, 335–339.

Kato, J., Fujikawa, K., Kanda, M., *et al.* (2001) A mutation, in the iron-responsive element of H ferritin mRNA, causing autosomal dominant iron overload. *Am. J. Hum. Genet.*, **69**, 191–197.

Kautz, L., Jung, G., Valore, E.V., *et al.* (2014a) Identification of erythroferrone as an erythroid regulator of iron metabolism. *Nat. Genet.*, **46**, 678–684.

Kautz, L., Jung, G., Nemeth, E. and Ganz, T. (2014b) Erythroferrone contributes to recovery from anemia of inflammation. *Blood*, **124**, 2569–2574.

Kim, H.-Y., LaVaute, T., Iwai, K., Klausner, R.D. and Rouault, T.A. (1996) Identification of a conserved and functional iron-responsive element in the 5'-untranslated region of mammalian mitochondrial aconitase. *J. Biol. Chem.*, **271**, 24226–24230.

Koeller, D.M., Casey, J.L., Hentze, M.W., *et al.* (1989) A cytosolic protein binds to structural elements within the iron regulatory region of the transferrin receptor mRNA. *Proc. Natl Acad. Sci. USA*, **86**, 3574–3578.

Kohler, S.A., Henderson, B.R. and Kühn, L.C. (1995) Succinate dehydrogenase b mRNA of *Drosophila melanogaster* has a functional iron-responsive element in its 5'-untranslated region. *J. Biol. Chem.*, **270**, 30781–30786.

Kohler, S.A., Menotti, E. and Kühn, L.C. (1999) Molecular cloning of mouse glycolate oxidase. High evolutionary conservation and presence of an iron-responsive element-like sequence in the mRNA. *J. Biol. Chem.*, **274**, 2401–2407.

Krause, A., Neitz, S., Magert, H.J., *et al.* (2000) LEAP-1, a novel highly disulfide-bonded human peptide, exhibits antimicrobial activity. *FEBS Lett.*, **480**, 147–150.

Kühn, L.C. (2009) How iron controls iron. *Cell Metab.*, **10**, 439–441.

Kühn, L.C. (2014) Iron regulatory proteins and their role in controlling iron metabolism. *Metallomics*, **7**, 232–243.

Kulaksiz, H., Theilig, F., Bachmann, S., *et al.* (2005) The iron-regulatory peptide hormone hepcidin: expression and cellular localization in the mammalian kidney. *J. Endocrinol.*, **184**, 361–370.

Lakhal, S., Schodel, J., Townsend, A.R., *et al.* (2011) Regulation of type II transmembrane serine proteinase TMPRSS6 by hypoxia-inducible factors: new link between hypoxia signaling and iron homeostasis. *J. Biol. Chem.*, **286**, 4090–4097.

Lauble, H., Kennedy, M.C., Beinert, H. and Stout, C.D. (1992) Crystal structures of aconitase with isocitrate and nitroisocitrate bound. *Biochemistry*, **31**, 2735–2748.

Lauth, X., Babon, J.J., Stannard, J.A., *et al.* (2005) Bass hepcidin synthesis, solution structure, antimicrobial activities and synergism, and in vivo hepatic response to bacterial infections. *J. Biol. Chem.*, **280**, 9272–9282.

LaVaute, T., Smith, S., Cooperman, S., Iwai, K., Land, W., Meyron-Holtz, E., *et al.* (2001). Targeted deletion of the gene encoding iron regulatory protein-2 causes misregulation of iron metabolism and neurodegenerative disease in mice. *Nat. Genet.*, **27**, 209–214.

Lee, P., Hsu, M.H., Welser-Alves, J., *et al.* (2012) 2-Oxoglutarate-dependent oxygenases control hepcidin gene expression. *J. Hepatol.*, **48**, 801–810.

Leibold, E.A. and Munro, H.N. (1988) Cytoplasmic protein binds in vitro to a highly conserved sequence in the 5' untranslated region of ferritin heavy- and light-subunit mRNAs. *Proc. Natl Acad. Sci. USA*, **85**, 2171–2175.

Lesbordes-Brion, J.C., Viatte, L., Bennoun, M., *et al.* (2006) Targeted disruption of the hepcidin 1 gene results in severe hemochromatosis. *Blood*, **105**, 4861–4864.

Liu, Q., Davidoff, O., Niss, K. and Haase, V.H. (2012) Hypoxia-inducible factor regulates hepcidin via erythropoietin-induced erythropoiesis. *J. Clin. Invest.*, **122**, 4635–4644.

Luschieti, S., Tolle, G., Aranda, J., *et al.* (2013) Novel mutations in the ferritin-L iron-responsive element that only mildly impair IRP binding cause hereditary hyperferritinaemia cataract syndrome. *Orphanet. J. Rare Dis.*, **8**, 30.

Mastrogiannaki, M., Matak, P., Mathieu, J.R., *et al.* (2012) Hepatic HIF-2 down-regulates hepcidin expression in mice through epo-mediated increase in erythropoiesis. *Haematologica*, **97**, 827–834.

Maurer, E., Gutschow, M. and Stirnberg M. (2012) Matriptase-2 (TMPRSS6) is directly up-regulated by hypoxia inducible factor-1: identification of a hypoxia-responsive element in the TMPRSS6 promoter region. *Biol. Chem.*, **393**, 535–540.

Maxwell, P.H. Wiesener, M.S., Chang, G.W., *et al.* (1999) The tumour suppressor protein VHL targets hypoxia-inducible factors for oxygen-dependent proteolysis. *Nature*, **399**, 271–275.

McCarthy, R.C. and Kosman, D.J. (2013) Ferroportin and exocytoplasmic ferroxidase activity are required for brain microvascular endothelial cell iron efflux. *J. Biol. Chem.*, **288**, 17932–17940.

McKie, A.T., Marciano, P., Rolfs, A., *et al.* (2000) A novel duodenal iron-regulated transporter, IREG1, implicated in the basolateral transfer of iron to the circulation. *Mol. Cell*, **5**, 299–309.

Melefors, O. (1996) Translational regulation in vivo of the *Drosophila melanogaster* mRNA encoding succinate dehydrogenase iron protein via iron responsive elements. *Biochem. Biophys. Res. Commun.*, **221**, 437–441.

Menotti, E., Henderson, B.R. and Kühn, L.C. (1998) Translational regulation of mRNAs with distinct IRE sequences by iron regulatory proteins 1 and 2. *J. Biol. Chem.*, **273**, 1821–1824.

Merle, U., Fein, E., Gehrke, S.G., Stremmel, W. and Kulaksic, H. (2007) The iron regulatory peptide hepcidin is expressed in the heart and regulated by hypoxia and inflammation. *Endocrinology*, **148**, 2663–2668.

Meynard, D., Kautz, L., Darnaud, V., *et al.* (2009) Lack of the bone morphogenetic protein BMP6 induces massive iron overload. *Nat. Genet.*, **41**, 478–481.

Meyron-Holtz, E.G., Ghosh, M.C. and Rouault, T.A. (2004) Mammalian tissue oxygen levels modulate iron-regulatory protein activities *in vivo*. *Science*, **306**, 2087–2090.

Millonig, G., Mückenthaler, M.U. and Mueller, S. (2010) Hyperferritinaemia-cataract syndrome: worldwide mutations and phenotype of an increasingly diagnosed genetic disorder. *Hum Genomics*, **4**, 250–262.

Mleczko-Sanecka, K., Casanovas, G., Ragab, A., *et al.* (2010) SMAD7 controls iron metabolism as a potent inhibitor of hepcidin expression. *Blood*, **115**, 2657–2665.

Mok, H., Mendoza, M., Prchal, J.T., Balogh, P. and Schumacher, A. (2004) Dysregulation of ferroportin 1 interferes with spleen organogenesis in polycythaemia mice. *Development*, **131**, 4871–4881.

Monnier, P.P., Sierra, A., Macchi, P., *et al.* (2002) RGM is a repulsive guidance molecule for retinal axons. *Nature*, **419**, 392–395.

Moroishi, T., Yamauchi, T., Nishiyama, M. and Nakayama, K.I. (2014) HERC2 targets the iron regulator FBXL5 for degradation and modulates iron metabolism. *J. Biol. Chem.*, **289**, 16430–16441.

Mückenthaler, M., Gray, N.K. and Hentze, M.W. (1998) IRP-1 binding to ferritin mRNA prevents the recruitment of the small ribosomal subunit by the cap-binding complex eIF4F. *Mol. Cell*, **2**, 383–388.

Müllner, E.W. and Kuhn, L.C. (1988) A stem-loop in the 3' untranslated region mediates iron-dependent regulation of transferrin receptor mRNA stability in the cytoplasm. *Cell*, **53**, 815–825.

Müllner, E.W., Neupert, B. and Kuhn, L.C. (1989) A specific mRNA binding factor regulates the iron-dependent stability of cytoplasmic transferrin receptor mRNA. *Cell*, **58**, 373–382.

Nemeth, E., Valore, E.V., Territo, M., *et al.* (2003) Hepcidin, a putative mediator of anemia of inflammation, is a type II acute-phase protein. *Blood*, **101**, 2461–2463.

Nemeth, E., Rivera, S., Gabayan, V., *et al.* (2004) IL-6 mediates hypoferremia of inflammation by inducing the synthesis of the iron regulatory hormone hepcidin. *J. Clin. Invest.*, **113**, 1271–1276.

Nemeth, E., Preza, G.C., Jung, C.L., *et al.* (2006) The N-terminus of hepcidin is essential for its interaction with ferroportin: structure-function study. *Blood*, **103**, 328–333.

Nguyen, N.B., Callaghan, K.D., Ghio, A.J., *et al.* (2006) Hepcidin expression and iron transport in alveolar macrophages. *Am. J. Physiol. Lung Cell. Mol. Physiol.*, **291**, L417–L425.

Nicolas, G., Bennoun, M., Devaux, I., *et al.* (2001) Lack of hepcidin gene expression and severe tissue iron overload in upstream stimulatory factor 2 (USF2) knockout mice. *Proc. Natl Acad. Sci. USA*, **98**, 8780–8785.

Nicolas, G., Chauvet, C., Viatte, L., *et al.* (2002) The gene encoding the iron regulatory peptide hepcidin is regulated by anemia, hypoxia, and inflammation. *J. Clin. Invest.*, **110**, 1037–1044.

Niederkofler, V., Salie, R. and Arber, S. (2005) Hemojuvelin is essential for dietary iron sensing, and its mutation leads to severe iron overload. *J. Clin. Invest.*, **115**, 2180–2186.

Otu, H.H., Naxerova, K., Ho, K., *et al.* (2007) Restoration of liver mass after injury requires proliferative and not embryonic transcriptional patterns. *J. Biol. Chem.*, **282**, 11197–11204.

Owen, D. and Kuhn, L.C. (1987) Noncoding 3' sequences of the transferrin receptor gene are required for mRNA regulation by iron. *EMBO J.*, **6**, 1287–1293.

Pak, M., Lopez, M.A., Gabayan, V., Ganz, T. and Rivera, S. (2006) Suppression of hepcidin during anemia requires erythropoietic activity. *Blood*, **108**, 3730–3735.

Pantopoulos, K. (2004) Iron metabolism and the IRE/IRP regulatory system: an update. *Ann. N. Y. Acad. Sci.*, **1012**, 1–13.

Pantopoulos, K., Porwal, S.K., Tartakoff, A. and Devireddy, L. (2013) Mechanisms of mammalian iron homeostasis. *Biochemistry*, **51**, 5705–5724.

Papanikolaou, G., Samuels, M.E., Ludwig, E.H., *et al.* (2004) Mutations in HFE2 cause iron overload in chromosome 1q-linked juvenile hemochromatosis. *Nat. Genet.*, **36**, 77–82.

Park, C.H., Valore, E.V., Waring, A.J. and Ganz, T. (2001) Hepcidin, a urinary antimicrobial peptide synthesized in the liver. *J. Biol. Chem.*, **276**, 7806–7810.

Patel, N., Masaratana, P., Diaz-Castro, J., *et al.* (2012) BMPER protein is a negative regulator of hepcidin and is up-regulated in hypotransferrinemic mice. *J. Biol. Chem.*, **287**, 4099–4106.

Peslova, G., Petrak, J., Kuzelova, K., *et al.* (2009) Hepcidin, the hormone of iron metabolism, is bound specifically to alpha-2-macroglobulin in blood. *Blood*, **113**, 6225–6236.

Peyssonnaux, C., Zinkernagel, A.S., Schuepbach, R.A., *et al.* (2007) Regulation of iron homeostasis by the hypoxia-inducible transcription factors (HIFs). *J. Clin. Invest.*, **117**, 1926– 1932.

Philpott, C.C., Klausner, R.D. and Rouault, T.A. (1994) The bifunctional iron-responsive element binding protein/cytosolic aconitase: the role of active-site residues in ligand binding and regulation. *Proc. Natl Acad. Sci. USA*, **91**, 7321–7325.

Piccinelli, P. and Samuelsson, T. (2007) Evolution of the iron-responsive element. *RNA*, **13**, 952–966.

Pietrangelo, A., Dierssen, U., Valli, L., *et al.* (2007) STAT3 is required for IL-6-gp130-dependent activation of hepcidin in vivo. *Gastroenterology*, **132**, 294–300.

Pigeon, C., Ilyin, G., Courselaud, B., *et al.* (2001) A new mouse liver-specific gene, encoding a protein homologous to human antimicrobial peptide hepcidin, is overexpressed during iron overload. *J. Biol. Chem.*, **276**, 7811–7819.

Piperno, A., Galimberti, S., Mariani, R., *et al.* (2011) Modulation of hepcidin production during hypoxia-induced erythropoiesis in humans in vivo: data from the HIGHCARE project. *Blood*, **117**, 2953–2959.

Rivera, S., Nemeth, E., Gabayan, V., *et al.* (2005) Synthetic hepcidin causes rapid dose-dependent hypoferremia and is concentrated in ferroportin-containing organs. *Blood*, **106**, 2196–2199.

Robbins, A.H. and Stout, C.D. (1989) The structure of aconitase. *Proteins*, **5**, 289–312.

Roetto, A., Papanikolaou, G., Politou, M., *et al.* (2003) Mutant antimicrobial peptide hepcidin is associated with severe juvenile hemochromatosis. *Nat. Genet.*, **33**, 21–22.

Rogers, J.T., Randall, J.D., Cahill, C.M., *et al.* (2002) An iron-responsive element type II in the 5'-untranslated region of the Alzheimer's amyloid precursor protein transcript. *J. Biol. Chem.*, **277**, 45518–45528.

Rothenberger, S., Müllner, E.W. and Kuhn, L.C. (1990) The mRNA-binding protein which controls ferritin and transferrin receptor expression is conserved during evolution. *Nucleic Acids Res.*, **18**, 1175–1179.

Rouault, T.A., Hentze, M.W., Caughman, S.W., Harford, J.B. and Klausner, R.D. (1988) Binding of a cytosolic protein to the iron-responsive element of human ferritin messenger RNA. *Science*, **241**, 1207–1210.

Rouault, T.A., Stout, C.D., Kaptain, S., Harford, J.B. and Klausner, R.D. (1991) Structural relationship between an iron-regulated RNA-binding protein (IRE-BP) and aconitase: functional implications. *Cell*, **64**, 881–883.

Roy, C.N., Mak, H.H., Akpan, I., *et al.* (2007) Hepcidin antimicrobial peptide transgenic mice exhibit features of the anemia of inflammation. *Blood*, **109**, 4038–4044.

Salahudeen, A.A., Thompson, J.W. and Ruiz, J.C. (2009) An E3 ligase possessing an iron-responsive haem-rythrin domain is a regulator of iron homeostasis. *Science*, **326**, 722–726.

Samad, T.A., Srinivasan, A., Karchewski, L.A., *et al.* (2004) DRAGON: a member of the repulsive guidance molecule-related family of neuronal- and muscle-expressed membrane proteins is regulated by DRG11 and has neuronal adhesive properties. *J. Neurosci.*, **24**, 2027–2036.

Samad, T.A., Rebbapragada, A., Bell, E., *et al.* (2005) DRAGON, a bone morphogenetic protein co-receptor. *J. Biol. Chem.*, **280**, 14122–14129.

Sanchez, M., Galy, B., Dandekar, T., *et al.* (2006) Iron regulation and the cell cycle: identification of an iron-responsive element in the 3'-untranslated region of human cell division cycle 14A mRNA by a refined microarray-based screening strategy. *J. Biol. Chem.*, **281**, 22865–22874.

Sanchez, M., Galy, B., Mückenthaler, M.U. and Hentze, M.W. (2007) Iron-regulatory proteins limit hypoxia-inducible factor-2alpha expression in iron deficiency. *Nat. Struct. Mol. Biol.*, **14**, 420–426.

Sanchez, M., Galy, B., Schwanhaeusser, B., *et al.* (2011) Iron regulatory protein-1 and -2: transcriptome-wide definition of binding mRNAs and shaping of the cellular proteome by iron regulatory proteins. *Blood*, **118**, e168–e179.

Schalinske, K.L., Chen, O.S. and Eisenstein, R.S. (1998) Iron differentially stimulates translation of mitochondrial aconitase and ferritin mRNAs in mammalian cells. Implications for iron regulatory proteins as regulators of mitochondrial citrate utilization. *J. Biol. Chem.*, **273**, 3740–3746.

Scott, G.J., Ray, M.K., Ward, T., *et al.* (2009) Abnormal glucose metabolism in heterozygous mutant mice for a type I receptor required for BMP signaling. *Genesis*, **47**, 385–391.

Sham, R.L., Phatak, P.D., West, C., *et al.* (2005) Autosomal dominant hereditary hemochromatosis associated with a novel ferroportin mutation and unique clinical features. *Blood Cells Mol. Dis.*, **34**, 157–161.

Sham, R.L., Phatak, P.D., Nemeth, E. and Ganz, T. (2009) Hereditary hemochromatosis due to resistance to hepcidin: high hepcidin concentrations in a family with C326S ferroportin mutation. *Blood*, **114**, 493–494.

Selezneva, A.I., Walden, W.E. and Volz, K.W. (2013) Nucleotide-specific recognition of iron-responsive elements by iron regulatory protein 1. *J. Mol. Biol.*, **425**, 3301–3310.

Smith, S.R., Ghosh, M.C., Ollivierre-Wilson, H., Hang Tong, W. and Rouault, T.A. (2006) Complete loss of iron regulatory proteins 1 and 2 prevents viability of murine zygotes beyond the blastocyst stage of embryonic development. *Blood Cells Mol. Dis.*, **36**, 283–287.

Steinbicker, A.U. and Mückenthaler, M.U. (2013) Out of balance – systemic iron homeostasis in iron-related disorders. *Nutrients*, **5**, 3034–3061.

Steinbicker, A.U., Bartnikas, T.B., Lohmeyer, L.K., *et al.* (2011) Perturbation of hepcidin expression by BMP type I receptor deletion induces iron overload in mice. *Blood*, **118**, 4224–4230.

Talbot, N.P., Lackhal, S., Smith, T.G., *et al.* (2012) Regulation of hepcidin expression at high altitude. *Blood*, **119**, 857–860.

Tanno, T., Bhanu, N.V., Oneal, P.A., *et al.* (2007) High levels of GDF15 in thalassemia suppress expression of the iron regulatory protein hepcidin. *Nat. Med.*, **13**, 1096–1101.

Tanno, T., Porayette, P., Sripichai, O., *et al.* (2009) Identification of TWSG1 as a second novel erythroid regulator of hepcidin expression in murine and human cells. *Blood*, **114**, 181–186.

Theurl, I., Theurl, M., Seifert, M., *et al.* (2008) Autocrine formation of hepcidin induces iron retention in human monocytes. *Blood*, **111**, 2392–2399.

Thurlow, V., Vadher, B., Bomford, A., *et al.* (2012) Two novel mutations in the L ferritin coding sequence associated with benign hyperferritinaemia unmasked by glycosylated ferritin assay. *Ann. Clin. Biochem.*, **49**, 302–305.

Tong, W.H. and Rouault, T.A. (2007) Metabolic regulation of citrate and iron by aconitases: role of iron-sulfur cluster biogenesis. *Biometals*, **20**, 549–564.

Troutt, J.S., Rudling, M., Persson, L., *et al.* (2012) Circulating human hepcidin-25 concentrations display a diurnal rhythm, increase with prolonged fasting, and are reduced by growth hormone administration. *Clin. Chem.*, **58**, 1225–1232.

Valore, E.V. and Ganz, T. (2008) Posttranslational processing of hepcidin in human hepatocytes is mediated by the prohormone convertase furin. *Blood Cells Mol. Dis.*, **40**, 132–138.

Vashisht, A.A., Zumbrennen, K.B., Huang, X., *et al.* (2009) Control of iron homeostasis by an iron-regulated ubiquitin ligase. *Science*, **326**, 718–721.

Verga Falzacappa, M.V., Vujić Spasić, M., Kessler, R., *et al.* (2007) STAT3 mediates hepatic hepcidin expression and its inflammatory stimulation. *Blood*, **109**, 353–358.

Verga Falzacappa, M.V., Casanovas, G., Hentze, M.W. and Muckenthaler, M.U. (2008) A bone morphogenetic protein (BMP)-responsive element in the hepcidin promoter controls HFE2-mediated hepatic hepcidin expression and its response to IL-6 in cultured cells. *J. Mol. Med.*, **86**, 531–540.

Viatte, L., Lesbordes-Brion, J.C., Lou, D.Q., *et al.* (2005) Deregulation of proteins involved in iron metabolism in hepcidin-deficient mice. *Blood*, **105**, 4861–4864.

Voet, D. and Voet, J.G. (2004) *Biochemistry*. 3rd edn, John Wiley & Sons, Hoboken, NJ, 1591 pp.

Vokurka, M., Krijt, J., Sulc, K. and Necas, E. (2006) Hepcidin mRNA levels in mouse liver respond to inhibition of erythropoiesis. *Physiol. Res.*, **55**, 667–674.

Volke, M., Gale, D.P., Maegdefrau, U., *et al.* (2009) Evidence for a lack of a direct transcriptional suppression of the iron regulatory peptide hepcidin by hypoxia-inducible factors. *PLoS One*, **4**, e7875.

Von Darl, M., Harrison, P.M. and Bottke, W. (1994) Expression in *Escherichia coli* of a secreted invertebrate ferritin. *Eur. J. Biochem.*, **222**, 367–376.

Vujić Spasić, M., Sparla, R., Mleczko-Sanecka, K., *et al.* (2013) Smad6 and Smad7 are co-regulated with hepcidin in mouse models of iron overload. *Biochim. Biophys. Acta*, **1832**, 76–84.

Walden, W.E., Selezneva, A.I., Dupuy, J., *et al.* (2006) Structure of dual function iron regulatory protein 1 complexed with ferritin IRE-RNA. *Science*, **314**, 1903–1908.

Wallander, M.L., Leibold, E.A. and Eisenstein, R.S. (2006) Molecular control of vertebrate iron homeostasis by iron regulatory proteins. *Biochim. Biophys. Acta*, **1763**, 668–689.

Wang, J., Chen, G., Muckenthaler, M., *et al.* (2004) Iron-mediated degradation of IRP2, an unexpected pathway involving a 2-oxoglutarate-dependent oxygenase activity. *Mol. Cell. Biol.*, **24**, 954–965.

Wang, J., Fillebeen, C., Chen, G., *et al.* (2007) Iron-dependent degradation of apo-IRP1 by the ubiquitin-proteasome pathway. *Mol. Cell. Biol.*, **27**, 2423–2430.

Wang, J., Chen, G., Lee, J. and Pantopoulos, K. (2008a) Iron-dependent degradation of IRP2 requires its C-terminal region and IRP structural integrity. *BMC Mol. Biol.*, **9**, 15.

Wang, Q., Du, F., Qian, Z.M., *et al.* (2008b) Lipopolysaccharide induces a significant increase in expression of iron regulatory hormone hepcidin in the cortex and substantia nigra in rat brain. *Endocrinology*, **149**, 3920–3925.

Wilkinson, N. and Pantopoulos, K. (2013) IRP1 regulates erythropoiesis and systemic iron homeostasis by controlling HIF2α mRNA translation. *Blood*, **122**, 1658–1668.

Wolff, F., Deleers, M., Melot, C., Gulbis, B. and Cotton, F. (2013) Hepcidin-25: Measurement by LC-MS/MS in serum and urine, reference ranges and urinary fractional excretion. *Clin. Chim. Acta*, **423**, 99–104.

Wrighting, D.M. and Andrews, N.C. (2006) Interleukin-6 induces hepcidin expression through STAT3. *Blood*, **108**, 3204–3209.

Xia, Y., Babitt, J.L., Sidis, Y., *et al.* (2008) Hemojuvelin regulates hepcidin expression via a selective subset of BMP ligands and receptors independently of neogenin. *Blood*, **111**, 5195–5204.

Yamanaka, K., Ishikawa, H., Megumi, Y., *et al.* (2003) Identification of the ubiquitin-protein ligase that recognizes oxidized IRP2. *Nat. Cell Biol.*, **5**, 336–340.

Yu, P.B., Hong, C.C., Sachidanandan, C., *et al.* (2008) Dorsomorphin inhibits BMP signals required for embryogenesis and iron metabolism. *Nat. Chem. Biol.*, **4**, 33–41.

Zähringer, J., Baliga, S. and Munro, H.N. (1976) Novel mechanism for translational control in regulation of ferritin synthesis by iron. *Proc. Natl Acad. Sci. USA*, **73**, 857–861.

Zhang, D.L., Hughes, R.M., Ollivierre-Wilson, H., Ghosh, M.C. and Rouault, T.A. (2009) A ferroportin transcript that lacks an iron-responsive element enables duodenal and erythroid precursor cells to evade translational repression. *Cell Metab.*, **9**, 461–473.

Zhang, D.L., Ghosh, M.C. and Rouault, T.A. (2009) The physiological functions of iron regulatory proteins in iron homeostasis – an update. *Front. Pharmacol.*, **5**, 124.

Zhang, D.L., Ghosh, M.C. and Rouault, T.A. (2014) The physiological functions of iron regulatory proteins in iron homeostasis – an update. *Front. Pharmacol.*, **5**, 124.

Zimmer, M., Ebert, B.L., Neil, C., *et al.* (2008) Small-molecule inhibitors of HIF-2a translation link its 5'-UTR iron-responsive element to oxygen sensing. *Mol. Cell*, **32**, 838–848.

Zumbrennen, K.B., Hanson, E.S. and Leibold, E.A. (2008) HOIL-1 is not required for iron-mediated IRP2 degradation in HEK293 cells. *Biochim. Biophys. Acta*, **1783**, 246–252.

Zumbrennen-Bulough, K.B., Wu, Q., Core, A.B., *et al.* (2014) MicroRNA-130a is up-regulated in mouse liver by iron deficiency and targets the bone morphogenetic protein (BMP) receptor ALK2 to attenuate BMP signaling and hepcidin transcription. *J. Biol. Chem.*, **289**, 23796–23808.

11

Iron Deficiency, Iron Overload and Therapy

Having seen just how important a role hepcidin plays in orchestrating systemic iron homeostasis, it clearly comes as no surprise that hepcidin deregulation can cause severe iron-related diseases, as illustrated in Figure 11.1 (Finberg, 2013; Steinbicker and Mückenthaler, 2013). If the iron homeostatic balance is disturbed the outcome will be two major classes of disease – anaemia and haemochromatosis. Elevated levels of hepcidin, resulting in decreased ferroportin expression, will trap iron within enterocytes, hepatocytes and macrophages. These are the conditions which prevail in the anaemia of chronic disease (ACD) and in iron-resistant iron-deficiency anaemia (IRIDA). In marked contrast, if hepcidin levels are inappropriately low, allowing the overexpression of ferroportin, then iron absorption from the gut will be increased, causing iron overload. This is what is seen in primary haemochromatosis, which will be referred to as *hereditary haemochromatosis* (HH), and in secondary haemochromatosis (genetic dysfunction of erythropoiesis), which we will describe as *acquired iron overload*.

11.1   Iron-deficiency Anaemia (IDA)

11.1.1   Introduction – The Size of the Problem

Iron deficiency is a deficit in total body iron which occurs when the iron requirement, essentially for the production of red blood cells, exceeds the iron supply, with major consequences for human health as well as social and economic development (WHO, 2008). Iron deficiency can occur both with or without anaemia, as reviewed in Denic and Agarwal (2007). The prevalence of different anaemia subtypes is shown in Figure 11.2. About 50% of anaemias arise from nutritional iron deficiency, and 42% are caused by inflammation and infection. The remaining 8% of anomies develop

Iron Metabolism – From Molecular Mechanisms to Clinical Consequences, Fourth Edition. Robert Crichton.
© 2016 John Wiley & Sons, Ltd. Published 2016 by John Wiley & Sons, Ltd.

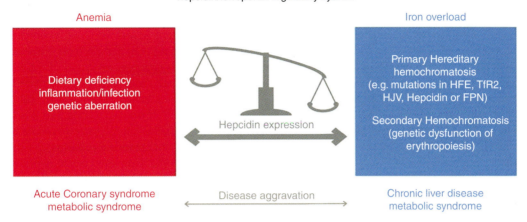

Figure 11.1 *Alterations of systemic iron homeostasis caused by imbalances of the hepcidin/ ferroportin regulatory system. Reproduced with permission from Elsevier from Steinbicker, A.U. and Muckenthaler, M. (2013) Out of balance – systemic iron homeostasis in iron-related disorders. Nutrients, 5, 3034–3061. This is an open access article distributed under the Creative Commons Attribution License*

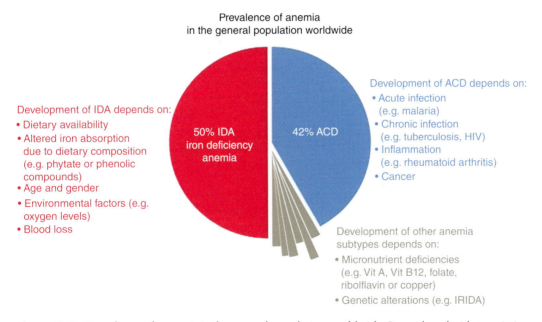

Figure 11.2 *Prevalence of anaemia in the general population worldwide. Reproduced with permission from Elsevier from Steinbicker, A.U. and Muckenthaler, M. (2013) Out of balance – systemic iron homeostasis in iron-related disorders. Nutrients, 5, 3034–3061. This is an open access article distributed under the Creative Commons Attribution License*

due to nutritional deficiencies (such as vitamin A, vitamin B_{12}, folate, riboflavin, or copper), or are caused by genetic defects (Steinbicker and Mückenthaler, 2013).

Iron-deficiency anaemia (IDA) is the most common and widespread nutritional disorder in the world. It not only affects an enormous number of children and women in developing countries, but is the only nutrient deficiency which is also significantly prevalent in industrialised countries, where iron deficiency is the most common nutritional deficiency and is by far the most common haematological disorder encountered by the general practitioner. It occurs at all stages of the life cycle, but is more prevalent in pregnant women and young children. Although its prevalence is reduced in all age and gender groups in the USA compared to global values (Clark, 2008), some 10 million people are iron-deficient in the USA, including five million who have IDA. The World Health Organization (WHO, 2008; McLean *et al.*, 2009) estimates that the global prevalence of anaemia (defined as having haemoglobin levels that are below recommended thresholds) for the world's population is 24.8%, which corresponds to 1.62 billion people. Estimated anaemia prevalence is 47.4% in pre-school-aged children, 41.8% in pregnant women, and 30.2% in non-pregnant women. This corresponds to 293 million pre-school-aged children, 56 million pregnant women and 468 million non-pregnant women, who are affected. The highest prevalence in pre-school children is in Africa (67.6%) and South-East Asia (65.5%). The prevalence of anaemia for pregnant women is slightly lower; although its distribution by region follows the same trend as is observed for pre-school-aged children, while in non-pregnant women the prevalence of anaemia is slightly lower than in pregnant women. The global prevalence of anaemia in men is only 12.7%.

The main cause of IDA is iron deficiency, but in the developing world – particularly in poor areas – this is frequently exacerbated by infectious diseases such as malaria, HIV/AIDS, hookworm infestation, schistosomiasis, other infections such as tuberculosis, deficiencies of other important nutrients such as folate, vitamin B_{12} and vitamin A, or genetically inherited disorders such as thalassaemia which affect red blood cells. IDA has important consequences for human health and, in particular for childhood development. Both, anaemic women and their children are at greater risk of mortality during the perinatal period. The mental and physical development of children is delayed and/or impaired by IDA (Beard, 2007; Lozoff, 2011), while the work capacity and productivity of manual workers is greatly reduced.

11.1.2 Causes of IDA

The major causes of IDA are discussed briefly here, and can be enumerated as follows: increased iron demand in women during pregnancy and post-partum lactation; blood loss; diet and malabsorption of iron; malaria and hookworm (Miller, 2015).

Pregnant women are particularly susceptible to IDA, due to the considerable iron demands of pregnancy. While there are net savings early in pregnancy due to the cessation of menstruation, iron requirements rise to a maximum of 3–8 mg per day during the third trimester. The net cost of a singleton pregnancy is estimated to range from 480 to 1200 mg, with nearly 300 mg being transferred to the foetus (Lee and Okam, 2011; Cao and O'Brien, 2013). This means that, to accommodate the iron demands of pregnancy, women would need to have about 500 mg of storage iron at the outset, but only 20% of women of reproductive age are estimated to have this reserve, and approximately 40% of women worldwide enter pregnancy with no iron reserves (Baker and Greer, 2010). Maternal IDA during pregnancy and perinatal care can have devastating effects on both mother and child, resulting in reduced foetal brain maturation, paediatric cognitive defects as well as maternal depression, on top of the direct effects of anaemia (Black *et al.*, 2011; Miller, 2013). This has led to an ongoing debate on iron supplementation during pregnancy which is troubled, to say the least, by the difficulty in assessing maternal iron status during pregnancy, compromised by variability in maternal plasma volume expansion, leading to the apparent physiological anaemia of pregnancy due to haemodilution (Cao and O'Brien, 2013). Whereas some national authorities recommend prenatal iron supplementation for all pregnant women while others recommend daily iron supplementation only in the second half of pregnancy, there are some who advocate using iron supplementation only in women with haemoglobin concentrations clearly below that considered as indicative of anaemia either at the outset or after 28 weeks of pregnancy (reviewed in Cao and O'Brien, 2013). In many circumstances, particularly in developing countries, multiple micronutrient deficiencies exist and it may be necessary to add additional micronutrients to iron supplements. Increased demands for iron, not met by adequate iron intake, occur in premature infants, during any period associated with increased growth and during pregnancy. During gestation, the foetus stores about 250 mg of iron and draws on these stores during breastfeeding, because breast milk supplies only about 0.15 mg of absorbed iron per day, whereas requirements for absorbed iron are about 0.55 mg per day. This means that low-birthweight infants and those whose mothers are iron-deficient during pregnancy are at high risk of developing iron deficiency while being breastfed.

The majority of cases of iron deficiency and IDA in industrialised countries result from chronic blood loss, mostly via the intestinal tract. Chronic gastrointestinal bleeding can be caused by a number of diseases (Annibale *et al.*, 2001; Nainz and Weiss, 2006), and increased bleeding from gastrointestinal lesions in patients taking aspirin, warfarin or nonsteroidal anti-rheumatics may also result in IDA (James *et al.*, 2005). Worldwide, blood loss from menstruation or hookworm infection have the greatest impact. Organs which may be involved in the development of IDA, mostly involving blood loss, are: the uterus (increased menstrual blood loss, iron transfer to the foetus during pregnancy); the oesophagus (varicose veins in patients with liver cirrhosis); the stomach and bulbus duodeni (hiatus hernia, aspirin and detrimental effects of other nonsteroidal anti-inflammatory drugs, peptic ulcer, carcinoma, partial gastrectomy); the small intestine (hookworm, celiac disease, diverticulosis, morbus Crohn, angiodysplasia); the colon and rectum (carcinoma, diverticulosis, angiodysplasia, varices, colitis); and, rarely, the kidneys or lungs. Functional iron deficiency may also occur in patients undergoing treatment with erythropoietic agents. However, there are also nonbleeding gastrointestinal conditions responsible for IDA, due for example to gastrointestinal iron malabsorption caused by underlying diseases, such as coeliac disease, atrophic gastritis or gastritis associated with *Helicobacter pylori* infection (Cardenas *et al.*, 2006). Gastric acid secretion is required to maintain ferric iron in solution, and impaired iron absorption due to achlorhydria is an important cause of iron deficiency, particularly in elderly people. Many subjects with unexplained IDA have *H. pylori* infection and, since *H. pylori* impairs gastric acid secretion, eradication of the *H. pylori* infection can restore normal haemoglobin levels (Hershko *et al.*, 2007).

Nutritional iron deficiency occurs when physiological requirements can no longer be met from dietary iron absorption. As we saw in Chapter 8, in most non-vegetarian diets more than one-third of the total daily intake is supplied by dietary haemoglobin and myoglobin, although haem iron only accounts for 10–15% of dietary iron content. In contrast, populations consuming monotonous plant-based diets with little meat, in which most of the iron is non-haem, will often absorb less than 10% of total dietary iron. (Zimmermann and Hurrell, 2007). The diet of a given population strongly affects iron bioavailability and, as a rule of thumb, recommended iron intakes in diets which are poor in vitamin C and in animal protein will be around three times that of diets rich in vitamin C and in animal protein (FAO/WHO, 2003). Whereas phytates, polyphenolics and other plant constituents found in vegetarian diets inhibit non-haem-iron absorption, vitamin C, citric acid and other organic acids facilitate non-haem-iron absorption. An appropriately planned and well-balanced vegetarian diet is compatible with adequate iron status. (Craig, 2009; Saunders *et al.*, 2013). However, vegetarians who eat a restrictive, macrobiotic vegetarian diet are more susceptible to IDA than those in the former group. Western vegetarians who consume a variety of foods have a better iron status than those in developing countries who consume a limited diet based on unleavened, unrefined cereals. However, poor diet is also a cause of iron deficiency in some socioeconomic groups in developed countries. Female blood donors in particular may develop iron deficiency.

In most tropical regions of the world, IDA and malaria coexist, with malaria causing intravascular haemolysis and urinary blood loss. In humans, iron deficiency appears to protect against severe malaria, while iron supplementation enhances the risk of infection and disease. The immune response to *Plasmodium* infection suppresses erythropoietin (Burgmann *et al.*, 1996) and has a direct effect on erythropoiesis (Skorokhod *et al.*, 2010). Hepcidin is upregulated during the blood-stage of the disease, which probably explains the iron deposition in macrophages, and the inhibition of dietary iron absorption that is observed. The parasite requires iron for its proliferation, both during the clinically silent liver stage of growth and in the disease-associated phase of erythrocyte infection, although how the protozoan acquires iron from its mammalian host remains unclear. There is clearly a complex interplay between iron, malaria and hepcidin, which needs to be better understood before treating IDA in malaria-endemic regions (Okebe *et al.*, 2011; Miller, 2013; Spottiswoode *et al.*, 2014).

Hookworm infection is one of the world's most common neglected tropical diseases and a leading cause of IDA in low- and middle-income countries (Bungiro and Cappello, 2011; Periago and Bethony, 2012; Miller, 2013). There are two hookworm species responsible for human hookworm disease, *Necator americanus* and *Ancylostoma duodenale*, which affect approximately 700 million people, with *N. americanus* being the predominant species. Both are found in tropical regions, based on their requirement of moist soil for survival, and are introduced into the soil by the faecal contamination of soil in regions where sanitation is absent or inadequate. Unlike other pathogens, hookworms are well-evolved, multicellular parasites which establish long-term infections in their human hosts with an insidious, pathogenesis in the form of IDA (Periago and Bethony, 2012). Treatment with antihelminthic drugs can cause a reversal of IDA, even without additional iron supplements (Bhargava *et al.*, 2003).

11.1.3 Clinical Stages and Diagnosis of IDA

The essential characteristic of iron deficiency is that the amount of iron released from macrophage and hepatocyte stores, together with dietary iron supply, is insufficient to supply the needs of iron for erythropoiesis. Iron deficiency and ultimately anaemia develop in several stages, which can be assessed by measuring a number of biochemical indices (Crichton *et al.*, 2008). The sequential depletion of iron within different compartments indicating the corresponding stages of iron depletion, together with the corresponding changes in iron-related measurements, are indicated in Figure 11.3. During the first stage of *latent iron deficiency*, during which all iron stores will be mobilised (Verloop, 1970), there is evidence of iron deficiency without anaemia; that is, the haemoglobin levels remain normal (Beutler and Waalen, 2006). This may be 'diagnostically silent' as the laboratory parameters will remain within normal limits, although serum ferritin concentration and bone marrow iron stores (ferritin and haemosiderin) will gradually be decreased. Due to a higher need for haemoglobin production, iron absorption may already be increased, and signs of 'functional iron deficiency' may be observed such as increased zinc protoporphyrin levels (Hershko *et al.*, 1985).

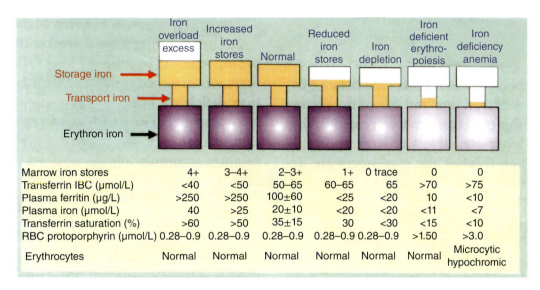

	Iron overload excess	Increased iron stores	Normal	Reduced iron stores	Iron depletion	Iron deficient erythro-poiesis	Iron deficiency anaemia
Marrow iron stores	4+	3–4+	2–3+	1+	0 trace	0	0
Transferrin IBC (µmol/L)	<40	<50	50–65	60–65	65	>70	>75
Plasma ferritin (µg/L)	>250	>250	100±60	<25	<20	10	<10
Plasma iron (µmol/L)	40	>25	20±10	<20	<20	<11	<7
Transferrin saturation (%)	>60	>50	35±15	30	<30	<15	<10
RBC protoporphyrin (µmol/L)	0.28–0.9	0.28–0.9	0.28–0.9	0.28–0.9	0.28–0.9	>1.50	>3.0
Erythrocytes	Normal	Normal	Normal	Normal	Normal	Normal	Microcytic hypochromic

Figure 11.3 *Schematic illustration of various iron parameters in iron overload and deficiency conditions. Reproduced with permission from UNI-MED, Bremen from Crichton, R., Danielson B.G. and Geisser, P. (2008)* Iron Therapy With Special Emphasis on Intravenous Administration, *4th edition*

The second phase, *iron-deficient erythropoiesis*, corresponds to exhaustion of the iron stores such that a lack of iron limits the production of haemoglobin and other iron-containing proteins. The haemoglobin concentration is still normal (since changes are insufficient for detection by standard clinical methods). However, other diagnostic criteria for iron deficiency are now easily recognizable, namely decreased serum ferritin, low serum iron, high serum transferrin (and as a result decreased transferrin saturation) and increased plasma levels of soluble transferrin receptor (Mast *et al.*, 1998; Skikne *et al.*, 1990).

In the third stage, *iron-deficiency anaemia*, the haemoglobin concentration decreases. Initially, the mean corpuscular volume (MCV) and mean corpuscular haemoglobin (MCH) are still normal. In the chronic phase, with a further decrease of haemoglobin, the MCV and MCH can become very low, together with the appearance of pathological erythroblasts in the bone marrow and a pathological morphology of red cells in the peripheral blood. A continuous shortage of iron may profoundly affect the production of haemoglobin while the impact on muscular myoglobin is less pronounced (Celsing *et al.*, 1988). *Functional iron deficiency* occurs when erythropoiesis is stimulated by recombinant erythropoietin and iron cannot be mobilised fast enough from stores to match the increased demand of the bone marrow.

Two main categories of laboratory measurements for the identification of iron deficiency can be distinguished: definitive measurements which evaluate tissue iron status, and screening methods, which detect iron-deficient erythropoiesis (reviewed in Beutler *et al.*, 2003a; Cook, 2005). The optimal diagnostic approach is to measure the serum ferritin (SF) as an index of iron stores and the serum transferrin receptor (sTfR) as a surrogate marker of bone marrow iron stores and therefore of iron-deficient erythropoiesis.

Serum ferritin is a widely available and well-standardised measurement which has proved to be the single most reliable index of iron status (Mei *et al.*, 2005), and low SF is diagnostic of IDA. In healthy individuals, SF is proportional to body iron stores: 1 µg l^{-1} SF corresponds to 8–10 mg body iron, or 120 µg storage iron per kg body weight (Finch *et al.*, 1986). However, ferritin is an acute-phase protein and in acute or chronic inflammation the SF level increases independent of iron status. The distinction between anaemia of chronic disease and IDA is difficult because an increased SF concentration in itself does not exclude IDA in the presence of inflammation. It is therefore advisable – particularly in surveys in developing countries with a high frequency of infection – to include a marker of inflammation such as C-reactive protein or α1-acid glycoprotein (Wieringa *et al.*, 2002). SF is also unreliable in patients with malignancy, hyperthyroidism, liver disease or heavy alcohol intake (Wieringa *et al.*, 2002; Umbreit, 2005).

When iron deficiency is suspected, measures of iron-deficient erythropoiesis, such as the transferrin iron saturation, mean corpuscular haemoglobin concentration, erythrocyte zinc protoporphyrin, percentage of hypochromic erythrocytes or reticulocyte haemoglobin concentration, can improve the diagnosis (Cook, 2005; Zimmermann and Hurrell, 2007).

Measurements of transferrin saturation reflect the balance of iron flowing into and out of the plasma iron pool, and once this value drops below 15%, iron-deficient erythropoiesis is clearly present. However, despite the advantage of low cost and wide availability, transferrin saturation undergoes marked diurnal variations and is affected by many clinical disorders (Cook, 2005; Umbreit, 2005). The examination of peripheral blood smears is reliable in experienced hands, but is not cost-effective in routine clinical practice. The MCV is a reliable indicator of iron deficiency, but is one of the last parameters to change with the onset of iron-deficient erythropoiesis. The percentage of hypochromic erythrocytes is also a relatively late indicator of iron-deficient erythropoiesis. Reticulocyte haemoglobin content is a sensitive indicator, which falls within a few days of the onset of iron-deficient erythropoiesis (Mast *et al.*, 2002; Ullrich *et al.*, 2005), but its use is limited. Falsely elevated values can occur when the MCV is elevated or in thalassaemia (Mast *et al.*, 2002). Erythrocyte zinc protoporphyrin can be measured directly on a drop of blood with a portable haematofluorometer (Metzgeroth *et al.*, 2005), and is a simple and precise measurement of iron-deficient erythropoiesis. It is a useful screening test in field surveys, particularly in children (Zimmermann *et al.*, 2005). However, zinc protoporphyrin increases with lead poisoning, particularly in urban and industrial settings (Zimmermann *et al.*, 2006), and falsely elevated values can occur in patients with elevated serum bilirubin or on regular haemodialysis. However, changes in these measurements with iron deficiency are indistinguishable from those seen in patients with the anaemia of chronic disease (see below). This is because, as was seen in Chapter 10, inflammatory disorders increase circulating hepcidin concentrations, blocking iron release from enterocytes and cells of the reticuloendothelial system, and resulting in iron-deficient erythropoiesis.

The serum transferrin receptor (sTfR) is a soluble 85 kDa form, constituting the extracellular domain of the transferrin receptor lacking the first 100 amino acids (Kogho *et al.*, 1986). Ferrokinetic studies have shown that sTfR is directly correlated with the total mass of erythroid precursors over the complete spectrum of haematological disorders, ranging from marrow aplasia to thalassaemia major (Huebers *et al.*, 1990). The only other determinant of sTfR, other than the erythroid precursor mass, is tissue iron status (Skikne *et al.*, 1990); hence, sTfR levels are increased by enhanced erythropoiesis and iron deficiency (Cook, 2005; Skikne *et al.*, 1990).

The single best measure to assess stores noninvasively is the serum ferritin concentration. In the range of 20 to 200 µg l^{-1}, there is a quantitative relationship between serum ferritin and iron stores: each 1 µg l^{-1} is indicative of 8 mg of storage iron. Careful phlebotomy studies have shown that serum ferritin concentrations decrease until stores are exhausted, which is indicated by a serum ferritin of around 12 µg l^{-1}. However, alcohol consumption, infection, inflammation, neoplasia and hepatic dysfunction may all spuriously raise the serum ferritin concentration relative to stores and, therefore, result in a misleadingly high serum ferritin concentration. The size of stores can also be assessed invasively by measurements of the iron content of bone marrow or liver biopsies, but these methods are unsuitable for routine use (Crichton, 2013).

Because the sTfR concentration remains normal in patients with the anaemia of chronic disease (Ferguson *et al.*, 1992) and is not substantially influenced by the acute-phase response (Cook, 2005), it is an invaluable addition to the SF measurement. The ratio sTfR to SF is a quantitative estimate of total body iron (Punnonen *et al.*, 1997), and the log(sTfR/SF) is directly proportional to the amount of stored iron in iron-replete patients and the tissue iron deficit in iron deficiency (Malope *et al.*, 2001; Cook *et al.*, 2003). This ratio may be even more sensitive than other laboratory tests for iron deficiency in elderly people (Rimon *et al.*, 2002). As Jim Cook tactfully pointed out (Beutler *et al.*, 2003a), "Use of the receptor/ferritin ratio can eliminate the need for bone marrow examination to detect iron deficiency in patients with chronic inflammatory joint or bowel disease who are usually reluctant to undergo this unpleasant procedure".

However, it is clear that the assay cannot be used in individuals with inflammation because the SF might be too high, independent of iron stores. Although it has only been validated for adults, the ratio is also used in children (Asobayire *et al.*, 2001; Cook *et al.*, 2005; Zimmermann *et al.*, 2005; Moretti *et al.*, 2006; Worwood, 2002). Because the sTfR/log ferritin ratio, often referred to as the sTfR index, theoretically takes advantage of the reciprocal relationship of iron deficiency on the two variables (increase of sTfR and decrease of ferritin concentrations), its use as the criterion for IDA continues to be advanced (Skikne *et al.*, 2011; Oustamanolakis *et al.*, 2011), although a recent meta-analysis demonstrated that sTfR rather than the sTfR index might have greater clinical value (Braga *et al.*, 2014).

11.1.4 Therapeutic Approaches

The therapeutic management of IDA must include both treatment of the underlying cause, for example gastrointestinal blood loss, and correction of the deficiency. Treatment of IDA uncomplicated by other disorders is rather simple and inexpensive in most subjects, and entails either oral or intravenous iron supplementation (Brugnara, 2003; Swanson, 2003; Clark, 2008; Crichton *et al.*, 2008). Simple ferrous salts are widely used for oral iron therapy, since these are the cheapest, and of these ferrous sulphate is the most common. A common daily dose is 150–200 mg of iron per day or, in children 3–5 mg of iron per kg body weight. The best absorption is obtained when the iron is given between meals, otherwise the interactions with foodstuffs will seriously decrease the absorption. However, the major obstacle to successful oral iron therapy is the nausea and epigastric discomfort that occurs 30–60 min after taking iron. These side effects can be reduced by using iron formulations which permit a slow release of iron, of which the least toxic is ferrous fumarate. Alternatively, iron complexes such as iron–polymaltose complex, which do not interact with foodstuffs or other medication (Geisser, 1990, 2007), can be used. Parenteral iron therapy is indicated for uncontrolled blood loss, intolerance to oral iron, intestinal malabsorption and poor adherence to an oral regime. A number of iron complexes are now available for parenteral iron therapy (Geisser and Burckhardt, 2011; Crichton *et al.*, 2008) which can be administered intramuscularly or intravenously, although the latter route is preferred. After the anaemia has been corrected, iron should be continued for at least four to six months until SF concentrations have reached 50 µg l^{-1} or the transferrin saturation exceeds 30% (Crichton *et al.*, 2008). The oral administration of ferrous salts may lead to high transferrin saturation levels and, thus, the formation of non-transferrin-bound iron, a potentially toxic form of iron with a propensity to induce oxidative stress. Intravenous iron preparations used for the treatment of IDA may also induce oxidative and/or nitrosative stress. The potential of various iron formulations to induce oxidative and nitrosative stress has been recently reviewed (Koskenkorva-Frank *et al.*, 2013), and the metabolism of various intravenous iron preparations and possible points of iron-induced oxidative/nitrosative stress are illustrated in Figure 11.4.

However, the mainstay of IDA treatment and prevention remains iron fortification of staple foodstuffs, which is considered to be the most cost-effective method for providing additional iron for populations with a high prevalence of IDA (Lynch, 2011). The WHO/FAO Guidelines on Food Fortification with Micronutrients (Allen *et al.*, 2006) has defined three categories of fortification: (i) market-driven fortification of products such as breakfast cereals, initiated by manufacturers, common in industrialised societies (Dary, 2002); (ii) targeted fortification, designed to meet the needs of specific groups; and (iii) mass fortification involving the addition of micronutrients to foods commonly consumed by the general population. The first of these has been widely practised in the developed world (e.g. the fortification of wheat flour in Canada, UK and USA since the 1940s), while menstruating and pregnant women have been a particular target for fortification programmes (Fernández-Gaxiola and De-Regil, 2011). In the underdeveloped world, iron is often provided with other micronutrients to reduce anaemia in schoolchildren (Ahmed *et al.*, 2010; Best *et al.*, 2011; Lemaire *et al.*, 2011). As a general rule, correcting the anaemia and replenishing iron stores should be the cut-off for fortification, to avoid iatrogenic iron overload, particularly with intravenous therapy.

11.1.5 Anaemia of Chronic Disease (ACD), Iron Refractory IDA (IRIDA) and Anaemia of Chronic Kidney Disease (CKD)

Anaemia of chronic disease (ACD) occurs as a consequence of chronic infection, inflammation or neoplasia, Hepcidin activation by cytokines causes low serum iron levels and transferrin saturation, although serum ferritin levels are high due to inflammation (Weiss and Goodnough, 2005; Weinstein *et al.*, 2002). Oral iron supplementation is ineffective because the elevated hepcidin levels impair intestinal iron absorption. There is also impaired erythropoiesis and a reduced biological activity of erythropoietin. Thus, the diversion of iron from the circulation into the reticuloendothelial system and the resulting iron limitation for erythropoiesis are central for the development of ACD. In the general Western population, ACD is the second most prevalent anaemia after IDA (Weiss, 2002, 2009), and within the hospital population it is the most frequent, occurring in patients with acute or chronic activation of the immune system. In affected individuals, infections, malignancies, autoimmune disorders, chronic kidney disease and chronic rejection after solid organ transplantation are the conditions most commonly associated with ACD (Weiss and Goodnough, 2005). Erythropoiesis-stimulating agents and/or intravenous iron injections are frequently used for the treatment of ACD, as are red blood cell transfusions as well as treatment of the underlying disease (Weiss and Goodnough, 2005; Weiss and Gordeuk, 2005; Roy, 2010). The possibility of directly decreasing hepcidin levels has been explored experimentally, using anti-hepcidin antibodies (Sasu *et al.*, 2010), or the Spiegelmer NOX-H94 (Schwoebel *et al.*, 2013), both of which bind to hepcidin, or inhibitors of bone morphogenetic protein (BMP) expression, such as LDN-193189 (Steinbicker *et al.*, 2011; Theurl *et al.*, 2011). More recently, LDN-193189 has been shown to improve the therapeutic efficacy of erythropoiesis-stimulating agents in a rat model of ACD (Theurl *et al.*, 2014).

Iron-refractory anaemia is a hereditary recessive anaemia due to a defect in the *TMPRSS6* gene encoding Matriptase-2. As we saw in Chapter 9, Matriptase-2 cleaves Haemojuvelin (HJV) and decreases hepcidin induction. Hallmarks of the disease are microcytic hypochromic anaemia, low transferrin saturation and normal/high serum hepcidin values (De Falco *et al.*, 2013). Some

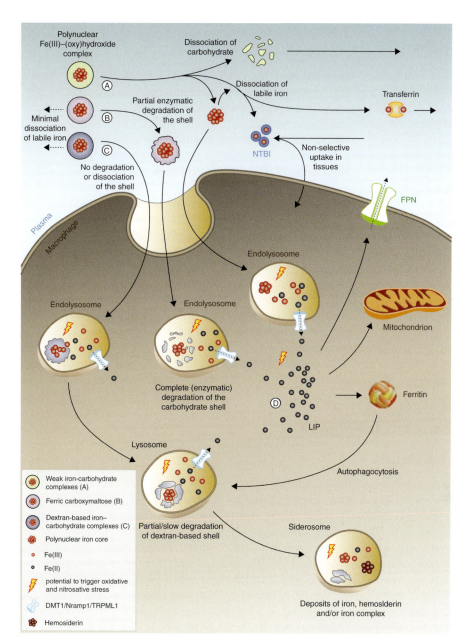

Figure 11.4 *Model depicting the metabolism of various intravenous iron preparations and possible points of iron-induced oxidative/nitrosative stress. (A) Metabolism of weaker iron–carbohydrate complexes (e.g. iron sucrose and sodium ferric gluconate). (B) Metabolism of ferric carboxymaltose. (C) Metabolism of dextran-based iron–carbohydrate complexes. (D) Metabolism of iron released from the iron–carbohydrate complexes: tightly bound by transferrin. When H_2O_2 diffuses into the lysosomes, Fenton-mediated production of $HO^•$ or high-valent iron forms may take place and lead to peroxidation of membranes and membrane rupture. Rupture of lysosomes and/or nonspecific uptake of NTBI can also rapidly increase the LIP concentration, which may lead to cell damage and proceed to apoptosis or to necrosis. Abbreviations: DMT1, divalent metal transporter 1; FPN, ferroportin; LIP, labile iron pool; Nramp1, natural resistance-associated macrophage protein 1; MPS, mononuclear phagocyte system; NTBI, non-transferrin-bound iron; TRPML1, transient receptor potential cation channel, mucolipin subfamily, member 1. Reprinted with permission from Elsevier from Koskenkorva-Frank, T.S., Weiss, G., Koppenol, W.H. and Burckhardt, S. (2013) The complex interplay of iron metabolism, reactive oxygen species, and reactive nitrogen species: insights into the potential of various iron therapies to induce oxidative and nitrosative stress. Free Radic. Biol. Med., 65, 1174–1194*

40 different Matriptase-2 mutations have been reported, affecting all functional domains of the large ectodomain of the protein. In patients with IRIDA, serum hepcidin is inappropriately high for the low iron status and accounts for the poor response to oral iron treatment, in contrast to current treatment based on parenteral iron administration. In the future, manipulation of the hepcidin pathway with the aim of suppressing it might become an alternative therapeutic approach (De Falco *et al.*, 2013).

Anaemia is a common complication of chronic kidney disease (CKD), and has a negative effect on the cardiovascular prognosis, the patient's quality of life and, ultimately, their survival (Mircescu *et al.*, 2013). CKD patients are prone to iron deficiency due to increased blood loss (Eschbach *et al.*, 1977), increased iron utilisation from erythropoiesis-stimulating agent (ESA) therapy (Van Wyck, 1989), and poor dietary iron absorption (Markowitz *et al.*, 1997). ESAs and iron are the cornerstones of therapy for this disease (KDIGO, 2012; Besarab and Coyne, 2010). While ESAs improve the quality of life and reduce transfusion requirements, they have not been demonstrated to improve other adverse outcomes associated with anaemia of CKD, such as cardiovascular disease and mortality, in prospective randomised controlled trials (KDIGO, 2012). Since excess levels of hepcidin are thought to contribute to anaemia in CKD patients by decreasing iron availability, hepcidin-lowering agents might represent an interesting therapeutic approach. BMP inhibitors have been shown to lower hepcidin levels in rodents (Babitt *et al.*, 2007; Yu *et al.*, 2008; Steinbicker *et al.*, 2011; Theurl *et al.*, 2011), and the BMP inhibitor LDN-193189 has been shown to mobilise iron for incorporation into red blood cells in a CKD model in rats (Sun *et al.*, 2013).

11.2 Hereditary Iron Overload

11.2.1 Introduction

Disorders of iron overload are characterised by an excessive accumulation of iron in various tissues, resulting progressively in tissue damage caused by the iron-generated production of highly reactive free radicals and, ultimately, organ failure (for reviews, see Pietrangelo, 2010; Steinbicker and Mückenthaler, 2013; Bardou-Jocquet *et al.*, 2014). As was pointed out in Chapter 7, the incapacity of the human body to excrete iron compared to most other mammals means, as was originally suggested by McCance and Widdowson (1937), that iron balance in humans is primarily determined by iron absorption. Iron-loading syndromes are a heterogeneous collection of disorders, which can be broadly divided into disorders that are *hereditary*, which may require pedigree studies and genetic counselling, and those that are *acquired*, in which an external cause may need to be identified and, where possible, eliminated (Pietrangelo, 2007). In what follows, hereditary haemochromatosis including the so-called 'ferroportin disease' (Pietrangelo, 2007) will first be discussed, followed by the hereditary iron-loading anaemias such as thalassaemia. Aceruloplasminaemia and Friedreich's ataxia will be discussed in Chapter 15.

11.2.2 Hereditary Haemochromatosis (HH)

The term 'haemochromatos' was first used in 1889 by von Recklinghausen (1889) to describe the dark tissue staining in liver which he attributed to haem, but which is now known to be due to heavy deposits of haemosiderin, with accompanying cirrhosis and massive organ damage. The association between diabetes mellitus and pigmentation of the liver and pancreas had already been noted by Trousseau in 1865 (Trousseau, 1865), but it was in his monumental review of all of the cases published in the world literature some seventy years later that Sheldon (1935) advanced the view that haemochromatosis was multivisceral and resulted from an inborn error of metabolism. The pioneering work of Marcel Simon in Rennes then led to the recognition that the disease was transmitted in a recessive manner, and that the gene was located on chromosome 6 close to the HLA-A locus (Simon *et al.*, 1977). The gene was finally located to a novel member of the major histocompatability complex (MHC) class I family of proteins (Feder *et al.*, 1996), and the pathogenic mutation (C282Y) was subsequently found to be present in the majority of haemochromatosis patients throughout the world. Subsequently, mutations in a number of other iron metabolism genes were discovered, which also led to iron overload (Camaschella *et al.*, 2004), with many phenotypic features characteristic of classic haemochromatosis. These include transferrin receptor 2 (*TfR2*) (Camaschella *et al.*, 2000), hepcidin (*HAMP*) (Roetto *et al.*, 2003), haemojuvelin (*HJV*) (Papanikolaou *et al.*, 2004) and the iron exporter, ferroportin (*FPN*) (Montosi *et al.*, 2001; Njajou *et al.*, 2001). All of these haemochromatoses have the same pathological origin, namely a genetic disruption of hepcidin action (Pietrangelo, 2007, 2010).

11.2.3 Causes of HH

For several of the hereditary forms of ion-overload disorders a common pathogenic mechanism can be discerned, which involves the entry of iron into the bloodstream in excess of requirements for erythropoiesis, first increasing transferrin saturation, and then leading to accumulation of iron in the parenchymal cells of liver, heart and endocrine glands. The outcome is haemochromatosis, characterised by cirrhosis, hypogonadism, cardiomyopathy, arthropathy and skin pigmentation, although erythropoiesis is not impaired. Whereas elevated levels of hepcidin cause IDAs like ACD and IRIDA, low levels of hepcidin cause the iron overload of haemochromatosis. Haemochromatosis is thus a well-defined syndrome characterised by normal iron-driven erythropoiesis, but with increased iron export from enterocytes, hepatocytes and macrophages due to low levels of hepcidin and overexpression of ferroportin. In metabolic studies of patients with haemochromatosis, dietary iron absorption exceeded iron loss by approximately 3 mg per day (Smith *et al.*, 1969).

What then are the causes of the low levels of hepcidin that result in haemochromatosis? Hepcidin insufficiency can be caused by mutations in the gene for hepcidin, *HAMP* (Roetto *et al.*, 2003), or by mutations which hamper the interaction of hepcidin with ferroportin (Sham *et al.*, 2005; Lok *et al.*, 2009). However, most cases of haemochromatosis arise from mutations in the genes which regulate hepcidin synthesis, including *HFE* (Feder *et al.*, 1996), which accounts for more than 80% of cases of haemochromatosis, *TfR2* (Camaschella *et al.*, 2000) and *HJV* (Papanikolaou *et al.*, 2004). In mice, the loss or disruption of *HFE* (Ahmad *et al.*, 2002), *TfR2* (Kawabata *et al.*, 2005), *HJV* (Huang *et al.*, 2005; Niederkofler *et al.*, 2005), or ferroportin (*FPN*) (Mok *et al.*, 2004), or of four other genes that regulate its biology, namely Bmp6 (Andriopoulos *et al.*, 2009; Meynard *et al.*, 2009), Smad4 (Wang *et al.*, 2005), neogenin (Lee *et al.*, 2010), C/EBP alpha (Courselaud *et al.*, 2002), or indeed of hepcidin (Viatte *et al.*, 2005), cause iron overload but not organ disease. In humans, loss of TfR2, HJV and hepcidin itself or FPN mutations result in full-blown haemochromatosis. In marked contrast, unlike these rare instances, while homozygotes for C282Y polymorphism in HFE are numerous, they are only predisposed to haemochromatosis, as will be discussed below.

HH is characterised by four basic features (Pietrangelo, 2006): (i) its hereditary origin (usually autosomal recessive, although the ferroportin disease is autosomal dominant); (ii) an early and progressive increase in serum transferrin saturation levels, from the normal physiological value of ~30% to complete saturation, accompanied by the appearance of highly toxic nontransferrin-bound iron (NTBI) (see Chapter 5), which has been shown to play a major role in the pathogenesis of iron overload and toxicity (Brissot and Loréal, 2002), and to be rapidly cleared from plasma by the liver (Wright *et al.*, 1986); (iii) progressive parenchymal iron deposits involving endocrine glands, heart, articulations and liver, with increasing probability of severe tissue damage; and (iv) no impairment of erythropoiesis and a satisfactory response to therapeutic phlebotomy.

11.2.4 Types of Haemochromatosis

11.2.4.1 HFE-related (Type 1) Haemochromatosis

This is the classical and most widely prevalent form of HH, the most frequent human genetic disorder in people of European descent, with an allele frequency of one in eight, which means that it is more common than cystic fibrosis, muscular dystrophy and phenylketonuria combined (Pietrangelo, 2010). The *HFE* gene located on chromosome 6 encodes a 348-residue type I transmembrane glycoprotein, HFE, which is homologous to class I MHC molecules and associates with the class I light chain β2-microglobulin (β2m) (Feder *et al.*, 1996), although its definite role at the membrane remains unclear. Unlike classical class I MHC molecules, which function in the immune system by presenting peptide antigens to T cells, HFE does not bind peptides or perform any known immune function, most likely because its ancestral peptide binding groove is too narrow and too shallow to allow classic antigen presentation (Lebron *et al.*, 1998). Most HH patients are homozygous for the *C282Y* mutation (substitution of a Cys for Tyr due to a single base change, 845 G to A), which disrupts a disulphide bond, preventing association with β2m and the stabilisation, intracytoplasmic transport and expression of HFE on the cell surface and on endosomal membranes, where it interacts with TfR1 (Feder *et al.*, 1997; Waheed *et al.*, 1997). A second mutation, *H63D*, which is also a common HFE variant, does not prevent β2m association, cell-surface expression, and nor does it impair HFE–TfR1 interaction (Feder *et al.*, 1997; Waheed *et al.*, 1997), which can lead to iron overload when present in the homozygous state (Jouanolle *et al.*, 1997). The mutation prevalence of *C282Y* is high in Caucasian populations (Deugnier *et al.*, 2002; Adams *et al.*, 2005) ; 10% of subjects are heterozygous, three to five subjects per thousand are homozygous, but almost absent in the non-Caucasian populations (Merryweather-Clarke *et al.*, 1997). The *C282Y* mutation seems to be of Celtic rather than Viking origin, which is supported by the mutation date of before 4000 BC (Distante *et al.*, 2004; Olson *et al.*, 2011). Other genotypes than *C282Y* homozygosity cannot explain overt haemochromatosis: *C282Y* heterozygosity, *H63D* heterozygosity or homozygosity and compound heterozygosity *C282Y/H63D* do not result in clinically significant iron overload in the absence of cofactors accounting for disturbed iron metabolism (alcoholism or metabolic syndrome) (Gochee *et al.*, 2002; Walsh *et al.*, 2006). Despite *C282Y* homozygosity predisposing to haemochromatosis, the phenotypic expression of *C282Y* homozygosity is quite variable, and the full-blown form of the disease (especially with cirrhosis) is rare (Olynyk *et al.*, 1999; Beutler *et al.*, 2002; Waalen *et al.*, 2005; Allen *et al.*, 2008). This is outlined schematically in Figure 11.5, in which five stages can be distinguished in a classification proposed by the French Haute Authorité de Santé (HAS) (Brissot and de Bels, 2006; Deugnier *et al.*, 2008) as the basis for its clinical recommendations on the management of *HFE* haemochromatosis. At the outset, as expected, 100% of *C282Y* homozygous patients have the unexpressed genetic predisposition, which decreases to 75% by stage 1, corresponding to increased transferrin saturation (>45%) only, and falls to 50% in stage 2, with both increased transferrin saturation and increased serum ferritin (>200 μg l^{-1} in women and >300 μg l^{-1} in men). An estimated 25% will reach stage 3, accompanied by an impaired functional prognosis (chronic fatigue and arthralgias), while less than 10% will progress to stage 4, with organ damage life-threatening disorders, including diabetes, cardiomyopathy, liver cirrhosis and hepatocellular carcinoma (HCC). Clearly, while

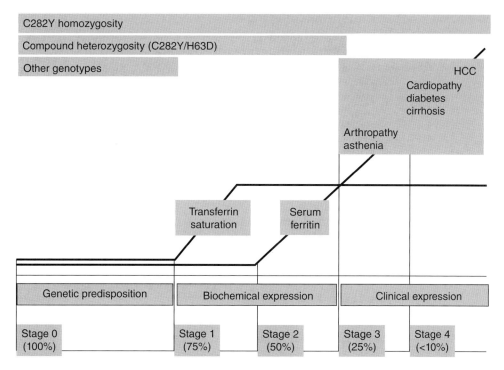

Figure 11.5 *Natural course, phenotype and penetrance of C282Y homozygosity. A five-stage classification was recently proposed by the French Haute Authorité de Santé (HAS) (Brissot and De Bel, 2006) as the basis for its clinical recommendations on the management of HFE haemochromatosis. Stage 0 corresponds to unexpressed genetic predisposition, stage 1 to increased transferrin saturation (>45%) only, stage 2 to increase in both transferrin saturation and serum ferritin (>200 μg l[-1] in women and >300 μg l[-1] in men), stage 3 to symptoms resulting in impaired functional prognosis (chronic fatigue and arthralgias), and stage 4 to organ damage with life-threatening disorders, especially diabetes, cardiomyopathy, liver cirrhosis and hepatocellular carcinoma (HCC). The approximate percentage of patients at each stage (%) clearly indicates incomplete penetrance of C282Y homozygosity. Reproduced from Deugnier, Y., Brissot, P. and Loréal, O. (2008) Iron and the liver: Update 2008. J. Hepatol., **48** (Suppl. 1), S113–S123. This is an open access article distributed under the Creative Commons Attribution License*

C282Y homozygosity is a necessary factor, other modifying factors impacting upon iron metabolism or hepcidin secretion must be involved in the expression of the disease. There is no lack of suggestions, including diet (Kaltwasser *et al.*, 1998; van der A *et al.*, 2006), alcohol (Loréal *et al.*, 1992; Bridle *et al.*, 2006), hepatic dysfunction (Detivaud *et al.*, 2005) and metabolic syndrome (Lainé *et al.*, 2005; Bekri *et al.*, 2006; Desgrippes *et al.*, 2013). Gender-related genetic factors (Moirand *et al.*, 1997; Deugnier *et al.*, 2002; Beutler *et al.*, 2002; Adams *et al.*, 2005) or genes associated with iron metabolism have also been proposed (Lee *et al.*, 2002; Merryweather-Clarke *et al.*, 2003; Jacolet *et al.*, 2004; Le Gac *et al.*, 2004a; Milet *et al.*, 2007), although in the latter case the evidence is more convincing in mouse models (Levy *et al.*, 2000; Bensaid *et al.*, 2004; Tolosano *et al.*, 2005) than in humans.

It has recently been shown (Wu *et al.*, 2014) that HFE associates with BMP receptor type I (Alk3), inhibiting Alk3 ubiquitination and proteasomal degradation and increasing Alk3 protein expression and accumulation on the cell surface of hepatocytes. As a consequence, transcription of the iron-hormone hepcidin is activated. The two HFE mutants associated with HH, HFE *C282Y* and HFE *H63D*, regulated ALK3 protein ubiquitination and trafficking differently, but both failed to increase ALK3 cell-surface expression.

11.2.4.2 Juvenile (Type 2) Haemochromatosis

The first description of the rare Type 2 haemochromatosis (Lamon *et al.*, 1979) identified two of its characteristics, namely the usually young age at diagnosis and an almost equal distribution between the sexes. We now recognise that there are two distinct forms: Type 2A haemochromatosis due to mutations in the hemojuvelin (*HJV*) gene (Papanikolaou *et al.*, 2004), located on chromosome 1, and the much rarer type 2B haemochromatosis due to mutations in the hepcidin (*HAMP*) gene (Roetto *et al.*, 2003) itself, located on chromosome 19. Both forms are autosomal recessive diseases. Type 2 haemochromatosis is a particularly severe form of the disease, usually affecting young male or female patients (15–20 years old), often associated with cardiomyopathy and central endocrine impact (impotence/amenorrhoea). Iron overload is massive and liver fibrosis is frequent, although cardiac and endocrine manifestations predominate. When associated with HFE haemochromatosis, mutations in the promoter region of *HAMP* have been described as a worsening factor of iron overload (Island *et al.*, 2009).

11.2.4.3 TfR2-related (Type 3) Haemochromatosis

TfR2-related, or Type 3 haemochromatosis is an autosomal recessive disease caused by mutations of the transferrin receptor 2 gene (TFR2) located on chromosome 7. It can be considered as an 'intermediate' disease between juvenile and HFE haemochromatosis, since its clinical picture mimics HFE haemochromatosis but the patients are usually younger and iron overload more severe (Camaschella *et al.*, 2000; Roetto *et al.*, 2001; Girelli *et al.*, 2002; Le Gac *et al.*, 2004b; Piperno *et al.*, 2004; Majore *et al.*, 2006; Hsiao *et al.*, 2007; Bardou-Jacquet *et al.*, 2013). The age of onset is usually described as young adulthood (30–40 years old), although several reports of children with type 3 haemochromatosis have suggested that particular genotypes or cofactors could result in an earlier onset and a more severe disease (Gérolami *et al.*, 2008; Bardou-Jacquet *et al.*, 2013). The most common TfR2 mutation associated with haemochromatosis is the nonsense mutation (Y250X) which truncates TfR2 at residue 250 (Camaschella *et al.*, 2000; Biasiotto *et al.*, 2008; Radio *et al.*, 2014), although mutations are scattered throughout the gene (Figure 11.6). Cardiac and endocrine dysfunctions are less frequent in the TfR2-related disease than in juvenile haemochromatosis.

11.2.4.4 Ferroportin Disease

Ferroportin disease is a clinically and genetically heterogeneous iron overload syndrome: unlike other types of haemochromatosis, its inheritance is autosomal dominant. Although rare, it is more frequent than types 2 and 3 haemochromatosis and has been reported worldwide (Beutler *et al.*, 2003b; Subramanian *et al.*, 2005; Barton *et al.*, 2007). Hyperferritinaemia, a normal to low transferrin saturation and macrophage cell iron storage, presenting as hepatic and spleen iron overload, are the characteristic features of *classical* ferroportin disease (Pietrangelo, 2004). Increased transferrin saturation and hepatocellular iron overload, in addition to hyperferritinaemia and macrophage iron loading, is considered characteristic for the *non-classical* phenotype (Pietrangelo, 2004; Zoller and Cox, 2005). This form is more rare, and is similar to types 1 and 3 haemochromatosis.

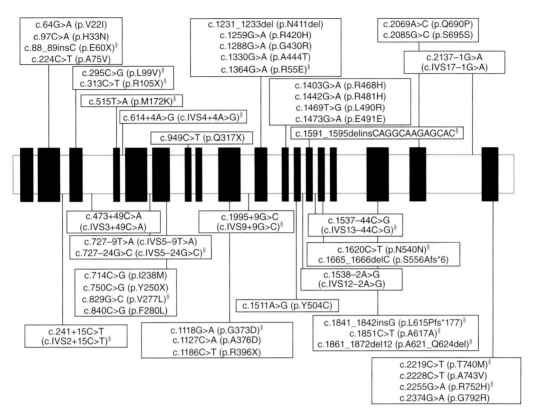

Figure 11.6 *Graphic review of TFR2 variants. The pathogenic mutations were reported in bold character. Reproduced with permission from Elsevier from Radio, F.C., Majore, S., Binni, F., et al. (2014) TFR2-related hereditary hemochromatosis as a frequent cause of primary iron overload in patients from Central-Southern Italy.* Blood Cells Mol. Dis., **52**, 83–87

The clinical heterogeneity of the disease can be explained by a genotype–phenotype correlation, where most mutations (e.g. A77D, D157G, V162del, N174I, Q182H, Q248H, and G323V) are associated with *classical* ferroportin disease (Drakesmith *et al.*, 2005; Schimanski *et al.*, 2005; De Domenico *et al.*, 2008; Lok *et al.*, 2009), which is pathologically distinct from haemochromatosis (Pietrangelo, 2004). Here, macrophage iron overload results from cellular iron export deficiency, that is, a loss of ferroportin function (Schimanski *et al.*, 2005). Distinct mutations (e.g. N144H, Y64N, C326Y/S, S338R, Y501C) have been found in patients who present with the *non-classical* phenotype (Drakesmith *et al.*, 2005; Wallace *et al.*, 2007; Sham *et al.*, 2009; Letocart *et al.*, 2009), which result in a haemochromatosis syndrome by rendering ferroportin resistant to inactivation by hepcidin and cause a gain of iron export function: this results in the hyperabsorption of dietary iron and hepatocellular iron overload (Mayr *et al.*, 2010; Pietrangelo, 2010). The location of some of ferroportin mutations in the structural model described in Chapter 6 are shown in Figure 11.7 (Le Gac *et al.*, 2013).

11.2.5 Therapy of Hereditary Haemochromatosis

Before therapy, the first step involves diagnosis – typically plasma iron and transferrin saturation are increased (except in classical ferroportin disease), as are serum ferritin levels, the most

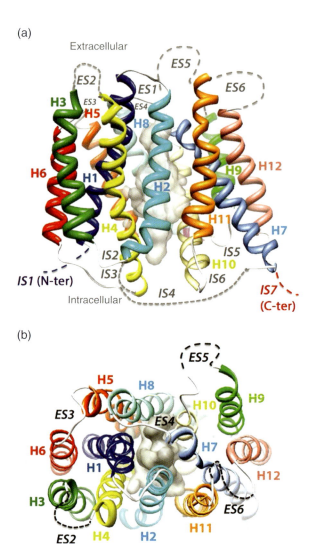

Figure 11.7 *Disease-associated mutations in ferroportin. Disease-associated mutations are reported on the model of the 3D structure of human ferroportin. The nonmodelled extracellular and intracellular loops are represented as dashed lines. Amino acids for which mutations are associated with a loss-of-function are coloured in red (likely affecting the fold), orange (likely affecting the iron export function), and blue (possibly affecting interaction with Jak2), whereas those for which mutations are reported as gain-of-function are shown in green. p.Tyr302 and p.Tyr303 are shown as references, as well as the rough positions of p.Lys229 and p.Lys269 within the large nonmodelled IS4. Note that this figure only represents positions of residues that have been clearly associated to clinical mutations and that have been the target of functional characterisations. Reproduced with permission from John Wiley & Sons from Le Gac, G., Ka, C., Joubrel. R., et al. (2013) Structure–function analysis of the human ferroportin iron exporter (SLC40A1): effect of hemochromatosis type 4 disease mutations and identification of critical residues.* Hum. Mutat., **34**, 1371–1380

frequent surrogate marker for tissue iron overload. The next step is to confirm that the elevated serum ferritin is related to iron overload by assessing potential confounding factors, such as alcohol consumption, metabolic syndrome, inflammation and acute or chronic liver injury resulting in hepatocyte damage. Once the elevated serum ferritin has been shown to truly reflect iron overload, the next step is to identify if there is a hereditary character to the overload and to assess body iron stores to quantify the iron overload. Thanks to advances in molecular genetics, which allow identification of the mutations involved in hereditary iron overload disorders, and also to improvements in imaging which allow the noninvasive diagnosis of hepatic iron overload, the task of the clinician confronted with the suspicion of tissue iron excess has been greatly facilitated.

If serum transferrin saturation is elevated, *HFE*-related haemochromatosis is the most likely diagnosis in the Caucasian population, and should thus be confirmed by *HFE* C282Y testing before further exploration. Lack of C282Y homozygosity requires further evaluation of the origins of iron overload. The hepatic iron content (HIC) is a reliable reflection of overall iron content in the organism (Angelucci *et al.*, 2000), and magnetic resonance imaging (MRI) has become the reference technique for assessing HIC, replacing liver biopsy because it is noninvasive. The use of MRI to estimate tissue iron was conceived during the 1980s (Stark *et al.*,1983), and it has become a practical reality during the past decade (for reviews, see Wood, 2011, 2014; Baksi and Pennell, 2014; Hernando *et al.*, 2014; Schönnagel *et al.*, 2013). The technique can used to estimate hepatic, spleen and cardiac iron in patients with haemochromatosis and transfusional siderosis, and has largely replaced liver biopsy for liver iron quantification. MRI can be used to distinguish between classic ferroportin disease, characterised by hepatocyte, splenic macrophage and bone marrow macrophage iron retention and the nonclassic form, associated with liver iron overload but normal spleen and bone marrow iron content (Pietrangelo *et al.*, 2006).

Subsequent to the finding of elevated transferrin saturation, and if *HFE* testing is negative, other *HFE* genotypes must be considered. Compound C282Y/H63D heterozygosity does not result in clinically relevant iron overload (Walsh *et al.*, 2006), and H63D homozygosity, C282Y heterozygosity and H63D heterozygosity may not explain abnormal serum iron and ferritin levels in the absence of an associated cause of impaired iron metabolism (Deugnier *et al.*, 2008).

When increased transferrin saturation is observed in a non-C282Y homozygous patient, non-*HFE* haemochromatosis is an option provided that liver disease and haematological disease have been ruled out, and liver iron excess has been established using MRI. In young patients with severe iron excess resulting in cardiac and endocrine symptoms, *HJV* or *HAMP* juvenile haemochromatosis is the first likelihood (although some cases of early and severe disease in *TfR2* haemochromatosis have been reported). Mild and late symptoms, mainly related to joints and liver, would result in a search for non-classical ferroportin disease, *TfR2* haemochromatosis and rare mutations in the *HFE* gene (Deugnier *et al.*, 2008).

In the event that the hyperferritinaemia is accompanied by only slightly increased, normal or low transferrin saturation, classical ferroportin disease is indicated, which is associated with a massive iron loading of the reticuloendothelial macrophages. The use of abdominal MRI is a useful tool for identifying this macrophage iron signature of classic ferroportin disease, characterised by a suggestive low MRI signal in both liver and spleen, allowing the differentiation of this disorder from haemochromatosis (Pietrangelo *et al.*, 2006). While ferroportin disease should be suspected in all cases of hyperferritinaemia, a differential diagnosis should also consider the rare condition of familial hyperferritinaemia congenital cataract syndrome (Beaumont *et al.*, 1995; Girelli *et al.*, 1995), which is not associated with tissue iron overload, aceruloplasminaemia

(Yoshida *et al.*, 1995; Hellman and Gitlin, 2002) and dysmetabolic hepatosiderosis (Moirand *et al.*, 1997) present in dyslipidaemic patients.

The treatment of all types of haemochromatosis involves blood-letting (phlebotomy), with the goal during the initial phase of iron-depletion to induce a mildly iron-deficient state. The removal of one unit (400–500 ml) of whole blood (containing 200–250 mg of iron) can usually restore safe iron levels (serum ferritins less than 20–50 µg l^{-1} and transferrin saturation of less than 30%) within one to two years. Thereafter, this is followed up by maintenance therapy, typically involving the removal of two to four units of blood per year, in order to keep serum ferritin levels between 50 and 100 µg l^{-1}. Lower serum ferritin values need to be avoided, since they can depress hepcidin secretion and result in increased iron absorption (Pietrangelo, 2010). Phlebotomy should only be replaced by other iron-removal strategies (e.g. chelation therapy) if it is nontolerated or contraindicated.

Chelation therapy may also be used, instead of phlebotomy, for example in Type 1 patients where there is poor venous access or patient unwillingness (Phatak *et al.*, 2010), and in combination with phlebotomy in Type 2 patients (Santos *et al.*, 2010). In classical ferroportin disease, while phlebotomy remains the standard treatment it is often less well tolerated than in haemochromatosis patients (Le Lan *et al.*, 2011). In the case of classic ferroportin disease, phlebotomy is also an effective therapy, but aggressive weekly phlebotomy is not tolerated in some patients, with manifestation of slight anaemia and low transferrin saturation being rapidly reached. These patients can usually be iron-depleted, but the therapeutic target of serum ferritin <30 µg l^{-1} used for classical haemochromatosis should be avoided due to the risk of anaemia. Some benefits may accrue from adjuvant therapy with erythropoietin.

Therapeutic approaches involving the normalisation of hepcidin levels in order to lower serum iron levels are being pursued in animal models of haemochromatosis (Figure 11.8) (reviewed in Ganz, 2013; Schmidt and Fleming, 2014). Constitutive overexpression of hepcidin in Hfe$^{(-/-)}$ mice greatly decreased iron loading (Nicolas *et al.*, 2003), leading to IDA in some animals (Figure 11.8b). By analogy to hormone deficiency disorders such as type 1 diabetes, iron loading in HH might be treated by hormone replacement therapy, and minihepcidins have been shown to reverse iron loading in mice deficient in hepcidin (Preza *et al.*, 2011) and to prevent liver iron loading in iron-depleted hepcidin null mice (Ramos *et al.*, 2012) although, as expected, high doses of the peptide led to anaemia, highlighting the narrowness of the therapeutic window. Bmp6 administration to Hfe$^{(-/-)}$ mice increased liver hepcidin mRNA and reduced serum iron and transferrin saturation (Figure 11.8c) without however improving liver, heart and pancreas iron levels (Corradini *et al.*, 2010). As we saw earlier, mutations in the *Tmprss6* gene coding for matripase 2 leads to IRIDA with overexpression of hepcidin, and an IRIDA phenotype is observed in mice lacking Tmprss6 (Finberg *et al.*, 2008). Since Tmprss6 cleaves HJV from the cell membrane and dampens hepcidin expression, targeting *Tmprss6* may be an effective therapeutic strategy. Heterozygous loss of *Tmprss6* in Hfe$^{(-/-)}$ mice (Figure 11.9a) reduced the systemic iron overload, whereas homozygous loss caused systemic iron deficiency and elevated the hepatic expression of hepcidin (Finberg *et al.*, 2011). Suppressing *Tmprss6* in Hfe$^{(-/-)}$ mice either with siRNA treatment (Schmidt *et al.*, 2013) or by the use of antisense oligonucleotides (Guo *et al.*, 2013) leads to an overexpression of hepcidin (Figure 11.9b), decreased transferrin saturation and liver iron while increasing spleen iron concentration, indicating a redistribution of iron from hepatocytes to macrophages in the spleen. More recent data indicate that siRNA suppression of Tmprss6, in conjunction with oral iron chelation therapy, may prove superior for the treatment of anaemia and secondary iron loading seen in β-thalassaemia intermedia (Schmidt *et al.*, 2015).

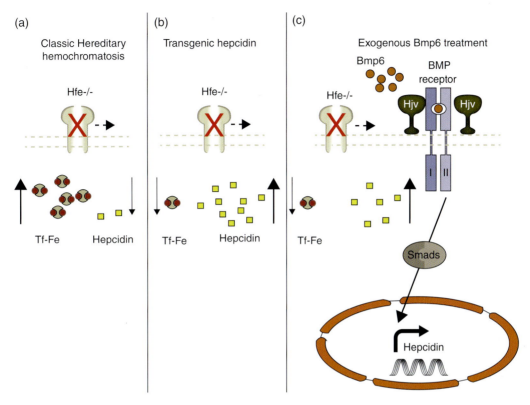

Figure 11.8 *Interventions in a mouse model of hemochromatosis* (Hfe$^{-/-}$). *(a) Genetic ablation of the Hfe protein* (Hfe$^{-/-}$) *leads to diminished hepcidin production and elevated iron uptake and distribution. Transgenic overexpression of hepcidin (b) greatly diminishes tissue iron loading and leads to a microcytic, hypochromic anaemia. Application of supraphysiological amounts of BMP6 (c) initiates hepcidin production through stimulation of the Bmp/Hjv/Smad signalling pathway, leading to diminished available iron. Tf-Fe, transferrin-bound iron. Reprinted with permission from Elsevier from Schmidt, P.J. and Fleming, M.D. (2014) Modulation of hepcidin as therapy for primary and secondary iron overload disorders: preclinical models and approaches.* Hematol. Oncol. Clin. North Am., ***28,*** *387–401*

11.3 Acquired Iron Overload

11.3.1 Introduction – Causes of Acquired Iron Overload

Acquired iron overload is most commonly encountered in the context of haematological diseases in which iron overload is a long-term consequence of repeated blood transfusions. By far the most common monogenic diseases are the haemoglobinopathies, principally the thalassaemias and sickle cell diseases (Porter and Garbowski, 2014; Williams and Weatherall, 2012). These represent between 300 000 and 400 000 babies born with a serious haematological disorder each year. The pathophysiological consequences of transfusional iron overload (TIO) are best understood in thalassaemia major (TM), and broadly reflect the distribution of excess storage iron to the heart, endocrine tissues and the liver. Hepatic iron overload results from both the downregulation of hepcidin production by erythroid factors, such as growth differentiation factor 15 (GDF15), which

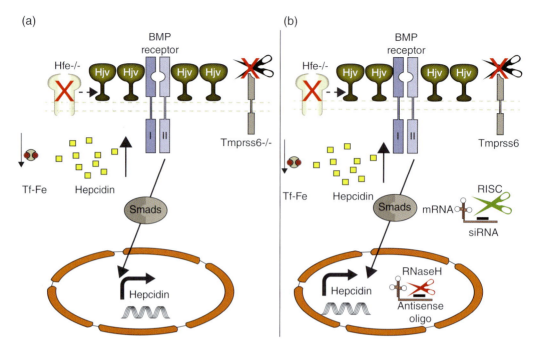

Figure 11.9 *Modulation of hepcidin expression through genetic or pharmacological targeting of Tmprss6. Loss of all endogenous Tmprss6 protein (a) leads to elevated levels of Hjv, the Bmp coreceptor, on the cell membrane. Significant hepcidin expression causes suppressed iron levels and a hypochromic, microcytic anaemia, even in a mouse lacking Hfe. (b) Targeting of Tmprss6 through pharmacological means. Targeting of Tmprss6 siRNA to the liver in lipid nanoparticle-formulated siRNAs, or by antisense oligonucleotide technology, leads to diminished* Tmprss6 *mRNA expression through classic RNA-induced silencing complex (RISC)-mediated (cytoplasmic) or RnaseH-mediated (nucleus) suppression, respectively. Suppression of Tmprss6 causes elevated levels of Hjv to remain on the cell membrane, triggering heightened hepcidin expression and ameliorating the* Hfe[−/−] *phenotype. Reprinted with permission from Elsevier from Schmidt, P.J. and Fleming, M.D. (2014) Modulation of hepcidin as therapy for primary and secondary iron overload disorders: preclinical models and approaches.* Hematol. Oncol. Clin. North Am., **28***, 387–401*

is produced in excess (Tanno *et al.*, 2007), and multiple blood transfusions (Porter and Garbowski, 2014). Long-term transfusions are the cornerstone of therapeutic management of TM in children, but regular transfusions are also required, much as in patients with sickle cell anaemia. The transfusion of red blood cells is also mandatory in myelodysplastic syndromes and leukaemias.

In TM, blood transfusions typically begin during the first year of life. Current transfusion recommendations in TM aim to keep the pretransfusion haemoglobin level at approximately 9.5 g dl^{-1} and to maintain an average haemoglobin of 12 g dl^{-1}, which usually amounts to an iron load rate of 0.3–0.5 mg kg^{-1} per day (Porter, 2009). This regimen has been selected to balance the beneficial effects of the suppression of ineffective erythropoiesis and dietary iron absorption with the iron accumulated from transfusion. Transfusional suppression of the endogenous bone marrow activity can be assessed by monitoring circulating transferrin receptors, which show more suppression when the pretransfusion haemoglobin level exceeds 10 g dl^{-1} (Cazzola *et al.*, 1997). In contrast, in sickle cell disease (SCD) the age of commencing blood transfusion, the transfusional iron load rate and the nature of the transfusion regimen itself all affect the rate and extent of iron overload, and often differ considerably from TM. The net iron accumulation from transfusion in SCD is slower than in TM, first because of differences in transfusion practice between these conditions and second because SCD patients tend to be in negative iron balance in the absence of transfusion. This is due to the considerable intravascular haemolysis leading to urinary iron loss, which may reach as much as 15 mg per day (ca. 0.2 mg kg^{-1} per day, which is comparable to the average SCD transfusional iron loading rate. In other forms of transfusional iron overload, the rates of iron loading again vary considerably; for example, a mean of 0.4 mg kg^{-1} per day was found in transfusion-dependent Diamond–Blackfan anaemia patients, and of 0.28 mg kg^{-1} per day in myelodysplastic syndrome (Porter *et al.*, 2008). In many cases, such as chronic haemolytic disorders, iron-loading anaemias and myelodysblastic syndrome variants, such as refractory anaemia with ring sideroblasts, an excess gastrointestinal absorption of iron is observed prior to transfusion as a consequence of ineffective erythropoiesis.

The iron overload found in sub-Saharan Africa, also termed Bantu siderosis, is particularly frequent among Africans who drink traditional beer brewed in nongalvanised steel drums, and this disorder was originally attributed exclusively to dietary excess of iron. Segregation analysis led to the conclusion that an unidentified iron-loading gene may confer susceptibility to the disease (Gordeuk *et al.*, 1992), and subsequently a mutation was found in the ferroportin 1 (*SCL40A1*) gene leading to increased intestinal iron absorption. This indicated that ferroportin may be the modifier gene in this disorder (Gordeuk *et al.*, 2003; McNamara *et al.*, 2005).

11.3.2 Mechanisms of Iron Toxicity

In contrast to HH, iron deposition in transfusional iron-overload patients primarily affects cells of the mononuclear phagocytic system (MPS) system, loading the bone marrow and reticuloendothelial system first, with liver parenchymal, endocrine, and cardiac iron loading later, in that order. The pattern of excess iron distribution reflects the pattern of nontransferrin-bound iron (NTBI) uptake by these tissues. As noted in Chapter 6, in severely iron-loaded patients, when a state of iron overload occurs, the capacity for transferrin to bind iron is exceeded, and 'free' or NTBI is found in serum, which is highly toxic and causes tissue iron loading. NTBI is found in serum when the transferrin saturation exceeds 45%, occurs in 80% of patients with TM, and its presence correlates with the appearance of oxidation products and reduced plasma antioxidant capacity (De Luca *et al.*, 1999; Cighetti *et al.*, 2002). The interactions between transferrin iron and NTBI are outlined in Figure 11.10 (Brissot *et al.*, 2012). The enhanced labile iron pool (LIP) leads to decreased expression of the Transferrin Receptor1 (TfR1) through the IRE–IRP system, but it has no effect on cellular NTBI uptake. One component of NTBI, the so-called labile plasma iron (LPI), found when transferrin saturation exceeds 75%, is iron chelatable, capable of redox cycling (Esposito *et al.*, 2003) and may represent a marker of toxicity, due to its potential for generating reactive oxygen radicals *in vivo* (Le Lan *et al.*, 2005). The direct capture of LPI has been suggested as a way to avoid the dangerous accumulation of cellular iron and to prevent the resultant adverse consequences (Cabantchik *et al.*, 2005).

The pathological mechanisms and consequences of acquired iron overload are summarised in Figure 11.11. In iron overload resulting from repeated blood transfusions or long-term increased iron absorption, iron enters the labile iron pool (LIP) and once it exceeds a critical concentration it can redox cycle to generate reactive oxygen species (ROS) (in particular, the hydroxyl radical, as discussed in Chapter 11). This will cause lipid peroxidation and organelle damage, leading to cell death and fibrogenesis mediated by transforming growth factor-beta 1 (TGFβ1). ROS also damage

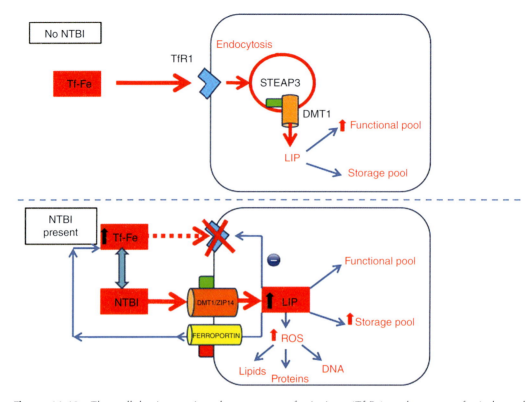

Figure 11.10 *The cellular interactions between transferrin iron (Tf-Fe) and non-transferrin-bound iron (NTBI). The enhanced labile iron pool (LIP) leads to decreased expression of the transferrin receptor 1 (TfR1) through the IRE–IRP system, but it has no effect on cellular NTBI uptake. Reproduced with permission from Elsevier from Brissot, P., Ropert, M., Le Lan, C. and Loréal, O. (2012) Non-transferrin bound iron: a key role in iron overload and iron toxicity. Biochim. Biophys. Acta, **1820**, 403–410*

DNA, and directly activate caspases thereby accelerating apoptotic death. Paradoxically, ROS may also have antiapoptotic effects by activating NF-κB, which may contribute to myelodysplastic syndrome (MDS) transformation and to iron-mediated neoplasia, such as hepatoma. An important, but often neglected, mechanism of toxicity from iron overload is that of the increased risk of infection, which is the second commonest cause of death in TM. This may reflect the increased levels of NTBI in plasma, which will be more available to microorganisms than transferrin iron.

11.3.3 Evaluation of Iron Overload

As in HH, transfusional iron-overload patients usually present with liver disease, cardiomyopathy, diabetes, endocrinopathies and skin pigmentation. The tissue iron load can be estimated by determining serum ferritin levels, by chemical analysis of liver iron, or by measuring liver iron and cardiac iron by noninvasive methods. The liver accounts for approximately 70–80% of the total-body iron stores in iron-overloaded patients. As a result, changes in liver iron accurately predict the balance between transfusional burden and iron-removal therapies (Brittenham *et al.*, 1994; Angelucci *et al.*, 2000). Liver iron is often considered the 'gold standard' for estimating body iron

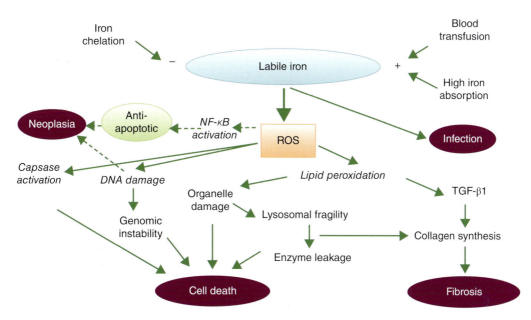

Figure 11.11   *Pathological mechanisms and consequences of iron overload. In iron overload resulting from repeated blood transfusions or long-term increased iron absorption, the labile iron pool generates a variety of ROS, principally hydroxyl radicals. ROS increase lipid peroxidation and organelle damage, leading to cell death and fibrogenesis mediated by transforming growth factor beta 1 (TGF-β1). ROS also damage DNA, risking genomic instability, mutagenesis, and cell death or neoplasia. ROS directly activate caspases, thereby accelerating apoptotic death. Paradoxically, ROS may also have antiapoptotic effects by activating NF-κB (dashed lines), which may contribute to MDS transformation and to iron-mediated neoplasia such as hepatoma. Reproduced from Porter, J.B. and Garbowski, M. (2014) The pathophysiology of transfusional iron overload.* Hematol. Oncol. Clin. North Am., **28**, 683–701

stores, and has been shown to correlate with total body iron stores (Angelucci *et al.*, 2002). It can be measured chemically by liver biopsy, but this can be inaccurate on account of fibrosis, cirrhosis or an uneven distribution of iron. Noninvasive techniques have become increasingly prevalent in modern medicine, and since tissue iron is paramagnetic measuring the magnetic properties of liver can be used to quantify liver iron. The first devices to accomplish this were superconducting quantum interference devices (SQUIDs), which used superconducting magnetic coils (Brittenham *et al.*, 2001; Fischer *et al.*, 2003; Nielsen *et al.*, 2002). Although reasonably accurate, these devices are expensive, require specialised expertise for measurement acquisition and device maintenance, and can only quantitate iron in the liver and spleen. MRI can also be used to quantify iron overload; it does not measure liver iron directly but rather the effect of liver iron on water protons as they diffuse in the magnetically inhomogeneous environment caused by iron deposition. The principles are simple. The scanner transmits energy into the body in the form of microwaves, waits for a period of time, and then actively recalls this energy as microwaves that are received by an antenna or 'coil'. The longer the scanner waits before recalling an echo, the less energy returns. This process is known as relaxation, and is characterised by the relaxation rates R2 and R2* (measured in Hz). These rates are simply the mathematical inverse of the characteristic relaxation times, T2 and T2* (measured in milliseconds) (Wood, 2014). The higher the iron concentration, the higher the relaxation rates and the shorter the relaxation times. Both, R2 and R2* are suitable for estimates of liver iron concentration in clinical practice if performed using validated acquisition and analysis protocols (Pennell, 2005; St Pierre *et al.*, 2005), and are equally effective in evaluating chronic response to iron chelation therapy (Wood *et al.*, 2014). In a study of TM patients, all those who died were found to have liver iron concentrations >15 mg g^{-1} dry weight (Brittenham *et al.*, 1994), and this level has subsequently been regarded as an index of high risk of death from cardiac disease. In other studies this level was also found to be associated with fibrosis and cirrhosis (Angelucci *et al.*, 2002). This compares with the upper limits of 7 mg g^{-1} found in carriers of genetic haemochromatosis.

Although liver iron content is an excellent surrogate for total iron balance, it has a limited ability to predict risk in extrahepatic organs. The endocrine glands and the heart develop pathologic iron overload exclusively through uptake of NTBI, although the mechanism by which this uptake occurs remains controversial; some studies have implicated L-type calcium channels (Oudit *et al.*, 2006). Direct measurement of cardiac iron by endomyocardial biopsy is inappropriate. However, reproducible, sensitive and accurate noninvasive measures of cardiac iron have been developed using the MRI T2* technique (Anderson *et al.*, 2001; Westwood *et al.*, 2003). The gradient echo imaging for calculating T2* (Anderson *et al.*, 2001) for documenting myocardial iron overload involves a short imaging time and allows completion of the procedure in one breath-hold, thereby decreasing movement artefacts. T2* values greater than 20 ms are considered normal. All patients with TM having T2* values in this range had a normal ejection fraction (Figure 11.12a). As T2* declined to less than 20 ms, there was an increasing prevalence of myocardial dysfunction, with a particularly high prevalence for T2* values less than 10 ms. In a recent multicentre study the breath-hold myocardial T2 technique has been found to be transferable between scanners with good intersite and local interstudy reproducibility (He et al., 2008). T2* values of less than 20 ms were found to correlate with the presence of cardiac dysfunction, detected by echocardiography, 24-h monitoring or the need for cardiac therapy, and can be conveniently used to monitor changes in cardiac iron during intensive chelation therapy (Anderson *et al.*, 2002). Calibration curves for the MRI parameters R2 and R2* (or their reciprocals, T2 and T2*) have been developed for the liver and heart, and the techniques have been shown to be highly reproducible within and across machines; they have also been chemically validated in both the liver and the heart (Wood, 2007). Figure 11.12b presents the probability of developing clinical heart failure over a one-year interval, based on initial cardiac T2* (Kirk *et al.*, 2009). A cardiac T2* <6 ms was associated with a near-50% likelihood of developing heart failure over one year.

11.3.4 Chelation Therapy for Acquired Iron Overload

There are three groups of patients for whom, because of the underlying disease, phlebotomy is contraindicated, and therefore iron chelation therapy is mandatory (Beutler *et al.*, 2003a). These are: (i) TM patients; (ii) patients with nontransfusion-dependent but nonetheless severe genetic diseases of haemoglobin synthesis (thalassaemia intermedia) who become iron loaded because of increased iron absorption, but who are too anaemic to undergo phlebotomy; and (iii) regularly transfused patients with sickle cell anaemia, myelodysplasia, myelofibrosis, red cell aplasia, aplastic anaemia, congenital dyserythropoeitic anaemia and congenital sideroblastic anaemia, for example. Iron chelators are used to remove iron from the body to prevent damage to liver, endocrine organs and, in particular, the heart. In TM, about 100–200 ml of pure red cells per kg per year are transfused (this corresponds to 0.32–0.64 mg kg^{-1} per day of iron) (Beutler *et al.*, 2003a). In thalassaemia intermedia, iron absorption is about five- to tenfold the normal amount (ca. 0.1 mg kg^{-1} per day). The primary aim of chelation therapy is to remove iron from the body at a rate which is either

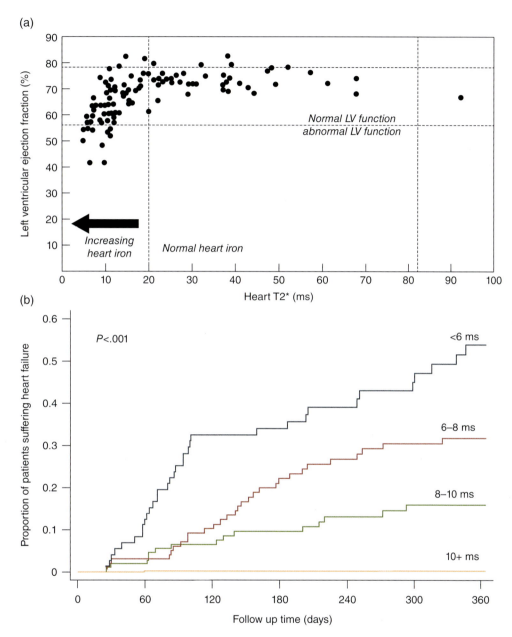

Figure 11.12 *(a) Plot of left ventricular ejection fraction (%) versus heart T2* (in ms). A T2* >20 ms indicates that the heart is free of cardiac iron. An ejection fraction >56% is considered normal. As heart iron increases (T2* declines), the prevalence of abnormal function increases. (b) Probability of developing clinical heart failure over a one-year interval, based on initial cardiac T2*. Cardiac T2* <6 ms was associated with a near-50% likelihood of developing heart failure over one year. Reprinted from Wood, J.C. (2014) Use of magnetic resonance imaging to monitor iron overload.* Hematol. Oncol. Clin. North Am., **28**, *747–764*

greater than the transfusional iron input (reduction therapy) or equal to the iron input (maintenance therapy) (Cappellini, 2007).

Thus, the iron overload and resulting clinical consequences in patients receiving chronic blood transfusions requires lifelong chelation therapy, with the overall aim being to maintain a 'safe' iron status at all times. Ideally, chelation therapy should be administered to prevent iron accumulation and iron-related complications. including hepatic, endocrinological and cardiac dysfunction. The age at which iron chelation is started in patients with TM is a key factor in their survival (Brittenham *et al.*, 1994; Borgna-Pignatti *et al.*, 2006; Davis *et al.*, 2004), since transfusion is generally initiated just after birth. The aim of effective chelation therapy, as noted earlier, is particularly to try and chelate the plasma NTBI and LPI, as these are the most toxic forms of iron (Cabantchik *et al.*, 2005).

There are currently three iron chelators approved for clinical use, namely desferrioxamine (DFO, Desferal®; DFO; Novartis Pharma AG, Basel, Switzerland), deferiprone (DFP, Ferriprox®; DFP; Apotex Inc., Toronto, ON, Canada) and deferasirox (DFX, Exjade®; Novartis Pharma AG, Basel, Switzerland), the structures of which are shown in Figure 11.13 (reviewed in Poggiali *et al.*, 2012; Seth, 2014). Before chelation therapy became available on a routine basis, chronically transfused patients died from cardiac iron overload in their teens and twenties (Engle *et al.*, 1964), whereas since the introduction of DFO in the early 1970s the life expectancy of such patients has improved dramatically (Borgna-Pignatti *et al.*, 2006). DFO was developed more than 40 years ago, and the wealth of clinical experience in iron-overloaded patients has established a role for iron

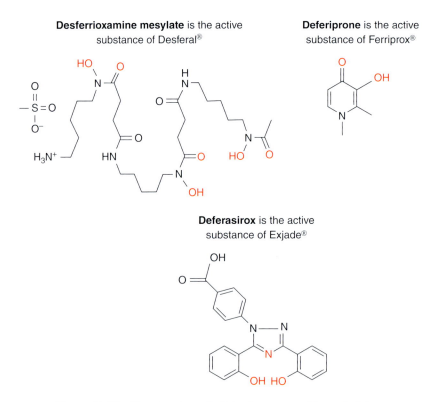

Figure 11.13 The structure of clinically approved iron chelators

chelators in the improvement in both the quality of life and overall survival of patients (Olivieri *et al.*, 1994; Olivieri and Brittenham, 1997). DFO (Figure 11.13) is a hexadentate chelator, with one molecule binding one atom of iron. However, it is not active by oral administration and its effectiveness is further limited by its short half-life (20–30 min). This means that DFO must be administered by slow subcutaneous infusion, using a battery-operated pump over an 8- to 12-h period, five to seven times per week, at a standard dose of 40 mg kg^{-1} per day (Porter, 2001). Therapy is usually begun in children after 10–20 transfusions, or when serum ferritin levels reach 1000 µg l^{-1}. This demanding therapeutic regime leads to poor patient compliance, and a large number of patients fail to obtain the full benefits of therapy and die prematurely (Brittenham *et al.*, 1994; Wonke, 2001). The probability of survival to 25 years of age in poorly chelated TM patients was only one-third that of patients who were well chelated by DFO (Brittenham *et al.*, 1994). If compliance was defined as more than 250 infusions a year, Gabutti and Piga (1996) found that 95% of compliant patients were alive at 30 years of age compared to only 12% of noncompliant patients. It seems that the number of days a patient was receiving chelation was more important than the overall dose. However, because it is impossible to achieve 24-h chelation coverage with DFO, the harmful effects of toxic NTBI cannot be prevented and, indeed, it was found that levels of LPI rebounded as soon as DFO infusion was stopped (Cabantchik *et al.*, 2005).

Since the greatest challenges with DFO are the demanding regime and the poor patient compliance with the therapy, it comes as no surprise that the search began for more convenient chelators, which would be active by oral administration. There are currently two oral iron chelators licensed for the treatment of iron overload, DFP and DFX.

DFP is a small lipophilic bidentate iron chelator of the 3-hydroxypyrid-4-one family, which binds to iron in a 3:1 ratio, and was first tested in clinical trials during the 1980s. It is available in The European Union, Canada, and more recently was approved for use in the USA. Since its half-life is 3–4 h it is administered at 75 mg kg^{-1} per day, fractionated in three doses. Like DFO, it cannot provide 24-h chelation coverage, and LPI levels have been shown to rebound between doses (Cabantchik *et al.*, 2005). DFO can enter myocytes and capture LPI in specific organelles of cardiomyocytes and macrophages. It also mobilises iron from iron-loaded cells and donates it to pre-erythroid cells for haemoglobin synthesis, both in the presence and absence of transferrin. The most serious adverse effects associated with DFP are agranulocytosis and neutropenia, with an incidence of 0.2 and 2.8 per 100 patient–years, respectively (Cohen *et al.*, 2003). Retrospective studies have demonstrated reduced cardiac morbidity and mortality (Piga *et al.*, 2003; Borgna-Pignatti *et al.*, 2006) and lower myocardial iron deposition (Anderson *et al.*, 2002) among patients treated with DFP than among those treated with DFO. A large clinical study showed that DFP treatment resulted in an improvement in T2* in patients with all degrees of cardiac iron loading (Berdoukas *et al.*, 2009). The combination of DFO and DFP is currently the most effective means of reducing cardiac iron loading, and should be started in patients with significant cardiac siderosis. It has been suggested that, when administered simultaneously, DFP can shuttle iron from sites inaccessible to DFO, and experimental evidence of this effect has been demonstrated in animal models of iron overload (Link *et al.*, 2001) and in the removal of NTBI from the plasma of patients with TM (Evans *et al.*, 2010). However, such a regime is clearly impractical, and a sequential use of DFO and DFP is usually adopted. The efficacy of such combined therapy has been borne out in clinical trials (Tanner *et al.*, 2007, 2008; Pantalone *et al.*, 2011).

DFX (Figure 11.13) is quite similar to the tridentate chelator, desferrithiocin, which was shown to be orally active, and extremely effective in reducing liver iron in rats loaded with 3,5,5-trimethylhexanoylferrocene (Jin *et al.*, 1989; Nick *et al.*, 2003). However, the compound proved to be toxic in animals, although as we will see later, a number of desferrithiocin derivatives and molecules have ultimately been brought to clinical trials (for a recent review, see Bergeron *et al.*, 2014). In the search for a safe tridentate chelator, the bis-hydroxyphenyltriazoles, a completely new chemical class of iron chelators, was discovered by a combination of rational design, intuition and experience (Acklin, 2000). After evaluating more than 40 derivatives of the triazole series, and more than 700 chelators from various other chemical classes, using vigorous selection criteria with a focus on tolerability, the tridentate chelator 4-[(3,5-bis-(2-hydroxyphenyl)-1,2,4)triazol-1-yl]-benzoic acid (ICL670) emerged as the most promising compound, combining oral effectiveness with low toxicity (Nick *et al.*, 2002, 2003). Because of its poor solubility in water, DFX is usually administered as a suspension in fruit juice, and is metabolised predominantly to glucuronides, which still bind iron. Iron excretion is dose-dependent and almost entirely faecal (Nisbet-Brown *et al.*, 2003; Galanello *et al.*, 2003), thereby avoiding the potential for renal damage observed with desferrithiocin. DFX has a plasma half life of 11–19 h (Nisbet-Brown *et al.*, 2003; Galanello *et al.*, 2003) and can therefore be used as a once-daily oral iron chelator.

The efficacy and safety were initially evaluated in patients with beta-thallasaemia (Nisbet-Brown *et al.*, 2003; Cappellini *et al.*, 2006), and subsequently in a wide range of patients with a number of other anaemias including myeloplastic syndromes, sickle cell disease, aplastic anaemia and Diamond–Blackfan anaemia (reviewed in Poggiali *et al.*, 2012). DFX is currently approved in many countries worldwide for the treatment of chronic transfusional iron overload in patients aged 2 years and older. Since DFX is detectable in the blood within the therapeutic range over a 24-h period, it offers complete chelation coverage with standard dosing and can provide a sustained reduction in LPI (Daar *et al.*, 2009). It is typically well tolerated, with adverse events generally being mild. The efficacy of DFX was shown to be similar to that of DFO in reducing liver iron concentration and serum ferritin levels in a large randomised trial in patients with TM (Cappellini *et al.*, 2006), and its ability to remove hepatic iron has been confirmed in a number of other studies (Porter *et al.*, 2008; Taher *et al.*, 2009; Deugnier *et al.*, 2011; Cassinerio *et al.*, 2015). A number of studies have been carried out on the effects of DFX treatment on cardiac function and myocardial iron overload. In an early study, while DFX was effective in patients with mild to moderate iron stores it failed to remove cardiac iron in patients with severe hepatic iron burdens (Wood *et al.*, 2010). While most later studies gave positive outcomes (Pennell *et al.*, 2012, 2015; Cassinerio *et al.*, 2012, 2015), further studies are needed to better delineate the effect of DFX on cardiac iron overload and iron-related cardiac dysfunction. In a consensus statement from the American Heart Association (Pennell *et al.*, 2013) it was stated that: "The current knowledge on the efficacy of removal of cardiac iron by the 3 commercially available iron chelators is summarised for cardiac iron overload without overt cardiac dysfunction. Evidence from well-conducted randomised controlled trials shows superior efficacy of deferiprone versus deferoxamine, the superiority of combined deferiprone with deferoxamine versus deferoxamine alone, and the equivalence of deferasirox versus deferoxamine". The combination of DFX with DFO has not been extensively studied, although preliminary studies seem promising (Lal *et al.*, 2013; Cassinerio *et al.*, 2014), and such an approach needs to be considered in situations where monotherapy is not able to remove the cardiac overload.

A number of oral iron chelators are currently under development. Re-engineering the desferri-thiocin pharmacophore in order to overcome toxicological problems while maintaining iron-clearing efficacy has led to three ligands being evaluated in human clinical trials, including a novel oral once-daily iron chelator, FBS0701 (Rienhoff *et al.*, 2010; Neufeld *et al.*, 2012). An α-ketohydroxypyridine analogue of DFP, LINAII (1-(N-acetyl-6-aminohexyl)-3-hydroxy-2-methylpyridin-4-one) has shown promising results in an animal model of thalassaemia (Chansiw *et al.*, 2014).

The primary use of chelation has been transfusional iron overload. There is now an increasing body of evidence for the benefits of iron chelation in other conditions, including myelodysplasia, pre-stem cell transplantation, neurodegenerative diseases and potentially in the treatment of malignancies (Yamasaki *et al.*, 2011; Raza *et al.*, 2014). A particularly exciting development is the recognition that local iron overload in particular brain regions is clearly associated with a growing number of neurodegenerative diseases, and already chelation therapy is showing encouraging results.

11.3.5 Other Therapeutic Approaches

As for hereditary haemochromatosis, the potential to modulate hepcidin activity as a treatment modality to treat transfusional iron overload is beginning to be explored in preclinical animal models (Schmidt and Fleming, 2014). The most likely application is in untransfused patients with chronic anaemia and iron overload. Some of the strategies described for HH have been applied to two mouse models of β-thalassaemia intermedia with the genotypes $Hbb^{th3/+}$ and $Hbb^{th1/th1}$ (Skow *et al.*, 1983; Yang *et al.*, 1995), which display many of the key characteristics of the human disease. Transferrin therapy was found to ameliorate the disease and to significantly increase hepcidin expression (Li *et al.*, 2010). However, whether transferrin therapy is effective because it promotes or inhibits iron delivery to the erythron is unclear.

Gardenghi *et al.* (2010) transplanted $Hbb^{th3/+}$ hematopoietic stem cells into mice transgenically expressing hepcidin in a tetracycline-inducible manner. A moderate overexpression of hepcidin in this $Hbb^{th3/+}$ model reduces iron overload, improves anaemia, and decreases splenomegaly. However, in several animals the anaemia actually became worse and these animals expressed higher levels of hepcidin than their counterparts, which experienced improvement in the anaemia, once again illustrating the delicate balance between iron restriction and desirable effects.

Similar to the studies described earlier, which validated *Tmprss6* as a target to moderate murine $Hfe^{-/-}$ HH, Nai *et al.* (2012) showed that a targeted deletion of *Tmprss6* not only decreased iron loading but also *uniformly* ameliorated the anaemia and ineffective erythropoiesis in $Hbb^{th3/+}$ mice. Importantly, this would suggest that, unlike the induction of endogenous hepcidin through other means or potentially the administration of hepcidin mimetics, complete inhibition of this target should not have the untoward effects of excessively iron-restricted erythropoiesis.

Using methodologies described earlier, Schmidt *et al.* (2013) and Guo *et al.* (2013) used LNP-formulated siRNAs and ASOs, respectively, targeted against *Tmprss6* mRNA to enhance hepcidin expression in the $Hbb^{th3/+}$ thalassaemia model. Both groups had qualitatively similar results, demonstrating that suppression of Tmprss6 expression in $Hbb^{th3/+}$ mice significantly induces liver-expressed hepcidin and diminishes tissue and serum iron levels. More importantly, both treatments substantially improved the anaemia by altering RBC survival and ineffective erythropoiesis. The improvement in RBC survival was probably a consequence of decreased accumulation of erythrocyte membrane-associated α-globin precipitates. A reduction in splenomegaly and ineffective erythropoiesis was confirmed by the restoration of proper splenic architecture and diminution of serum erythropoietin.

While the application of these experimental therapies have been limited to mouse models of HH and β-thalassaemia intermedia, their extension to the much more frequent β-TM would represent a major breakthrough, particularly since in these patients – although the baseline hepcidin levels are grossly elevated – they may still be inappropriately low considering the systemic iron burden (Origa *et al.*, 2007). In these patients, hepcidin levels are increased pre- and post-transfusion, whereas erythropoiesis and GDF15 are decreased (Pasricha *et al.*, 2013). Thus, a desirable goal would call for a compromise between erythropoiesis and iron absorption, which might be achieved with a hepcidin mimetic. Furthermore, the combination of these therapies, together with state-of-the-art iron chelation strategies, may open the possibility to further decrease the burden of iron loading and its complications in both transfusion-dependent and transfusion-independent β-thalassaemias (Schmidt and Fleming, 2014).

References

Adams, P.C., Reboussin, D.M., Barton, J.C., *et al.* (2005) Hemochromatosis and iron-overload screening in a racially diverse population. *N. Engl. J. Med.*, **352**, 1769–1778.

Ahmad, K.A., Ahmann, J.R., Migas, M.C., *et al.* (2002) Decreased liver hepcidin expression in the Hfe knockout mouse. *Blood Cells Mol. Dis.*, **29**, 361–366.

Ahmed, F., Khan, M.R., Akhtaruzzaman, M., *et al.* (2010) Long-term intermittent multiple micronutrient supplementation enhances hemoglobin and micronutrient status more than iron + folic acid supplementation in Bangladeshi rural adolescent girls with nutritional anemia. *J. Nutr.*, **140**, 1879–1886.

Acklin, P. (2000) A molecular-mechanics approach for the prediction of the geometry of high-spin Fe^{III} complexes with oxygen and nitrogen as coordinating atoms. *Helv. Chim. Acta*, **83**, 677–686.

Allen, K.J., Gurrin, L.C., Constantine, C.C., *et al.* (2008) Iron-overload-related disease in HFE hereditary hemochromatosis. *N. Engl. J. Med.*, **358**, 221–230.

Allen, L., De Benoist, B., Dary, O. and Hurrell, R. (2006) *Guidelines on food fortification with micronutrients.* WHO/FAO, Geneva.

Anderson, L., Holden, S., Davis, B., *et al.* (2001) Cardiovascular T2-star (T2*) magnetic resonance for the early diagnosis of myocardial iron overload. *Eur. Heart J.*, **22**, 2171–2179.

Anderson, L.J., Wonke, N., Prescott, E., *et al.* (2002) Comparison of effects of oraldeferiprone and subcutaneous desferrioxamine on myocardial iron concentrations and ventricular function in beta-thalassaemia. *Lancet*, **360**, 516–520.

Andriopoulos, B. Jr, Corradini, E., Xia, Y., *et al.* (2009) BMP6 is a key endogenous regulator of hepcidin expression and iron metabolism. *Nat. Genet.*, **41**, 482–487.

Angelucci, E., Brittenham, G.M., McLaren, C.E., *et al.* (2000) Hepatic iron concentration and total body iron stores in thalassemia major. *N. Engl. J. Med.*, **343**, 327–331.

Angelucci, E., Muretto, P., Nicolucci, A., *et al.* (2002) Effects of iron overload and hepatitis C virus positivity in determining progression of liver fibrosis in thalassemia following bone marrow transplantation. *Blood*, **100**, 17–21.

Annibale, B., Capurso, G., Christolini, A., *et al.* (2001) Gastrointestinal causes of refractory iron deficiency anemia in patients without gastrointestinal symptoms. *Am. J. Med.*, **111**, 439–445.

Asobayire, F.S., Adou, P., Davidsson, I., *et al.* (2001) Prevalence of iron deficiency with and without concurrent anemia in population groups with high prevalences of malaria and other infections: a study in Côte d'Ivoire. *Am. J. Clin. Nutr.*, **74**, 776–782.

Babitt, J.L., Huang, F.W., Xia, Y., *et al.* (2007) Modulation of bone morphogenetic protein signaling in vivo regulates systemic iron balance. *J. Clin. Invest.*, **117**, 1933–1939.

Baker, R.D. and Greer, F.R., Committee on Nutrition American Academy of Pediatrics (2010) Diagnosis and prevention of iron deficiency and iron-deficiency anemia in infants and young children (0–3 years of age). *Pediatrics*, **126**, 1040–1050.

Baksi, A.J. and Pennell, D.J. (2014) T2* imaging of the heart: methods, applications, and outcomes. *Top. Magn. Reson. Imaging*, **23**, 13–20.

Bardou-Jacquet, E., Cunat, S., Beaumont-Epinette, M.P., *et al.* (2013) Variable age of onset and clinical severity in transferrin receptor 2 related haemochromatosis: novel observations. *Br. J. Haematol.*, **162**, 278–281.

Bardou-Jacquet, E., Ben Ali, Z., Beaumont-Epinette, M.-P., *et al.* (2014) Non-HFE hemochromatosis: pathophysiological and diagnostic aspects. *Clin. Res. Hepatol. Gastroenterol.*, **38**, 143–154.

Barton, J.C., Acton, R.T., Lee, P.I. and West, C. (2007) SLC40A1 Q248H allele frequencies and Q248H-associated risk of non-HFE iron overload in persons of sub-Saharan African descent. *Blood Cells Mol. Dis.*, **39**, 206–211.

Beard, J. (2007) Recent evidence from human and animal studies regarding iron status and infant development. *J. Nutr.*, **137**, 524S–530S.

Beaumont, C., Leneuve, P., Devaux, I., *et al*. (1995) Mutation in the iron responsive element of the L ferritin mRNA in a family hyperferritinaemia and cataract. *Nat. Genet.*, **11**, 444–446.

Bekri, S., Gual, P., Anty, R., *et al*. (2006) Increased adipose tissue expression of hepcidin in severe obesity is independent from diabetes and NASH. *Gastroenterology*, **131**, 788–796.

Bensaid, M., Fruchon, S., Mazères, C., *et al*. (2004) Multigenic control of hepatic iron loading in a murine model of hemochromatosis. *Gastroenterology*, **126**, 1400–1408.

Berdoukas, V., Chouliaras, G., Moraitis, P., *et al*. (2009) The efficacy of iron chelator regimes in reducing cardiac and hepatic iron in patients with thalassaemia major: a clinical observational study. *J. Cardiovasc. Magn. Reson.*, **11**, 20.

Bergeron, R.J., Wiegand, J., McManis, J.S. and Bharti, N. (2014) Desferrithiocin: a search for clinically effective iron chelators. *J. Med. Chem.*, **57**, 9259–9291.

Besarab, A. and Coyne, D.W. (2010) Iron supplementation to treat anemia in patients with chronic kidney disease. *Nat. Rev. Nephrol.*, **6**, 699–710.

Best, C., Neufingerl, N., Del Rosso, J.M., *et al*. (2011) Can multi-micronutrient food fortification improve the micronutrient status, growth, health, and cognition of schoolchildren? A systematic review. *Nutr. Rev.*, **69**, 186–204.

Beutler, E. and Waalen, J. (2006) The definition of anemia: what is the lower limit of normal of the blood hemoglobin concentration? *Blood*, **107**, 1747–1750.

Beutler, E., Felitti, V.J., Koziol, J.A., *et al*. (2002) Penetrance of 845G→ A (C282Y) HFE hereditary haemochromatosis mutation in the USA. *Lancet*, **359**, 211–218.

Beutler, E., Hoffbrand, A.V. and Cook, J.D. (2003a) Iron Deficiency and Overload. *Hematology, Am. Soc. Hematol. Educ. Program*, 40–61.

Beutler, E., Barton, J.C. and Felitti, V.J. (2003b) Ferroportin 1 (SCL40A1) variant associated with iron overload in African-Americans. *Blood Cells Mol. Dis.*, **31** (3), 305–309.

Bhargava, A., Jukes, M., Lambo, J., *et al*. (2003) Anthelmintic treatment improves the hemoglobin and serum ferritin concentrations of Tanzanian schoolchildren. *Food Nutr. Bull.*, **24** (4), 332–342.

Biasiotto, G., Camaschella, C., Forni, G.L., *et al*. (2008) New TFR2 mutations in young Italian patients with hemochromatosis. *Haematologica*, **93**, 309–310.

Black, M.M., Quigg, A.M., Hurley, K.M. and Pepper, M.R. (2011) Iron deficiency and iron-deficiency anemia in the first two years of life: strategies to prevent loss of developmental potential. *Nutr. Rev.*, **69** (Suppl. 1), S64–S70.

Borgna-Pignatti, C., Cappellini, M.D., De Stafano, P., *et al*. (2006) Cardiac morbidity and mortality in deferoxamine- or deferiprone-treated patients with thalassemia major. *Blood*, **107**, 3733–3737.

Braga, F., Infusino, I., Dolci, A. and Panteghini, M. (2014) Soluble transferrin receptor in complicated anemia. *Clin. Chim. Acta*, **431**, 143–147.

Bridle, K., Cheung, T.K., Murphy, T., *et al*. (2006) Hepcidin is down-regulated in alcoholic liver injury: implications for the pathogenesis of alcoholic liver disease. *Alcohol Clin. Exp. Res.*, **30**, 106–112.

Brissot, P. and Loréal, O. (2002) Role of non-transferrin-bound iron in the pathogenesis of iron overload and toxicity. *Adv. Exp. Med. Biol.*, **509**, 45–53.

Brissot, P. and de Bels, F. (2006) Current approaches to the management of haemochromatosis. *Hematology*, **36**, 1295–1300.

Brissot, P., Ropert, M., Le Lan, C. and Loréal, O. (2012) Non-transferrin bound iron: a key role in iron overload and iron toxicity. *Biochim. Biophys. Acta*, **1820**, 403–410.

Brittenham, G.M., Griffith, P.M., Nienhaus, A.W., *et al*. (1994) Efficacy of deferoxamine in preventing complications of iron overload in patients with thalassemia major. *N. Engl. J. Med.*, **331**, 567–573.

Brittenham, G.M., Sheth, S., Allen, C.J. and Farrell, D.E. (2001) Noninvasive methods for quantitative assessment of transfusional iron overload in sickle cell disease. *Semin. Hematol.*, **38**, 37–56.

Brugnara, C. (2003) Iron deficiency and erythropoiesis: new diagnostic approaches. *Clin. Chem.*, **49**, 1573–1578.

Bungiro, F. and Cappello, M. (2011) Twenty-first century progress toward the global control of human hookworm infection. *Curr. Infect. Dis. Rep.*, **13**, 210–217.

Burgmann, H., Looareesuwan, S., Kapiotis, S., *et al*. (1996) Serum levels of erythropoietin in acute *Plasmodium falciparum* malaria. *Am. J. Trop. Med. Hyg.*, **54**, 280–283.

Cabantchik, Z.I., Breuer, W., Zanninelli, G. and Cianciuli, P. (2005) LPI-labile plasma iron in iron overload. *Best Pract. Res. Clin. Haematol.*, **18**, 277–287.

Camaschella, C., Roetto, A., Cali, A., *et al*. (2000) The gene TFR2 is mutated in a new type of haemochromatosis mapping to 7q22. *Nat. Genet.*, **25**, 14–15.

Camaschella, C., Roetto, A. and De Gobbi, M. (2004) New insights into iron homeostasis through the study of non-HFE hereditary haemochromatosis. *Best Pract. Res. Clin. Haematol.*, **18**, 235–250.

Cao, C. and O'Brien, K.O. (2013) Pregnancy and iron homeostasis: an update. *Nutr. Rev.*, **71**, 35–51.

Cappellini, M.D. (2007) Exjade® (deferasirox, ICL670) in the treatment of chronic iron overload associated with blood transfusion. *Ther. Clin. Risk Manag.*, **3**, 291–299.

Cappellini, M.D., Cohen, A., Piga, A., *et al.* (2006) A phase 3 study of deferasirox (ICL670), a once-daily oral iron chelator, in patients with beta-thalassemia. *Blood*, **107**, 3455–3462.

Cardenas, V.M., Mulla, Z.D., Ortiz, M. and Graham, D.Y. (2006) Iron deficiency and *Helicobacter pylori* infection in the United States. *Am. J. Epidemiol.*, **163**, 127–134.

Cassinerio, E., Roghi, A., Pedrotti, P., *et al.* (2012) Cardiac iron removal and functional cardiac improvement by different iron chelation regimens in thalassemia major patients. *Ann. Hematol.*, **91**, 1443–1449.

Cassinerio, E., Orofino, N. and Roghi, A., *et al.* (2014) Combination of deferasirox and deferoxamine in clinical practice: an alternative scheme of chelation in thalassemia major patients. *Blood Cells Mol. Dis.*, **53**, 164–167.

Cassinerio, E., Roghi, A., Orofino, N., *et al.* (2015) A 5-year follow-up in deferasirox treatment: improvement of cardiac and hepatic iron overload and amelioration in cardiac function in thalassemia major patients. *Ann. Hematol.*, **94**, 939–945.

Cazzola, M., Borgna-Pignatti, C., Locatelli, F., *et al.* (1997) A moderate transfusion regimen may reduce iron loading in beta-thalassemia major without producing excessive expansion of erythropoiesis. *Transfusion*, **37**, 135–140.

Celsing, F., Ekblom, B., Sylven, C., *et al.* (1988) Effects of chronic iron deficiency anaemia on myoglobin content, enzyme activity, and capillary density in the human skeletal muscle. *Acta Med. Scand.*, **223**, 451–457.

Chansiw, N., Pangjit, K., Phisalaphong, C., *et al.* (2014) Effect of a novel oral active iron chelator: 1-(N-acetyl-6-aminohexyl)-3-hydroxy-2-methylpyridin-4-one (CM1) in iron-overloaded and non-overloaded mice. *Asian Pac. J. Trop. Med.*, **7S1**, S155–S161.

Cighetti, G., Duca, L., Bertone, L., *et al.* (2002) Oxidative status and malondialdehyde in beta-thalassaemia patients, *Eur. J. Clin. Invest.*, **32**, 55–60.

Clark, S.F. (2008) Iron deficiency anemia. *Nutr. Clin. Pract.*, **23**, 128–141.

Cohen, A.R., Galanello, R., Piga, A., *et al.* (2003) Safety and effectiveness of long-term therapy with the oral iron chelator deferiprone. *Blood*, **102**, 1583–1587.

Cook, J.D. (2005) Diagnosis and management of iron-deficiency anaemia. *Best Pract. Res. Clin. Haematol.*, **18**, 319–332.

Cook, J.D., Flowers, C.H. and Skikne, B.S. (2003) The quantitative assessment of body iron. *Blood*, **101**, 3359–3364.

Cook, J.D., Boy, E., Flowers, C.H. and Daroca Mdel, C. (2005) The influence of high-altitude living on body iron. *Blood*, **106**, 1441–1446.

Corradini, E., Schmidt, P.J., Meynard, D., *et al.* (2010) BMP6 treatment compensates for the molecular defect and ameliorates hemochromatosis in Hfe knockout mice. *Gastroenterology*, **139**, 1721–1729.

Courselaud, B., Pigeon, C., Inoue, Y., *et al.* (2002) C/EBPalpha regulates hepatic transcription of hepcidin, an antimicrobial peptide and regulator of iron metabolism. *Cross-talk between C/EBP pathway and iron metabolism. J. Biol. Chem.*, **277**, 41163–41170.

Craig, W.J. (2009) Health effects of vegan diets. *Am. J. Clin. Nutr.*, **89**, 1627S–1633S.

Crichton, R.R. (2013) Iron, in *Biochemical, Physiological, Molecular Aspects of Human Nutrition*, 3rd edition (eds M.H. Stipanuk and M.A. Caudill), Saunders-Elsevier, St Louis, pp. 801–827.

Crichton, R.R., Danielson, B.G. and Geisser, P. (2008) *Iron Therapy with Special Emphasis on Intravenous Administration*, 4th edition. UNI-MED Verlag AG, Bremen, pp. 128.

Daar, S., Pathare, A., Nick, H., *et al.* (2009) Reduction in labile plasma iron during treatment with deferasirox, a once-daily oral iron chelator, in heavily iron-overloaded patients with beta-thalassaemia. *Eur. J. Haematol.*, **82**, 454–457.

Dary, O. (2002) Staple food fortification with iron: a multifactorial decision. *Nutr. Rev.*, **60**, S34–S41.

Davis, B.A., O'Sullivan, C., Jarritt, P.H. and Porter, J.B. (2004) Value of sequential monitoring of left ventricular ejection fraction in the management of thalassemia major. *Blood*, **104**, 263–269.

De Domenico, I., Nemeth, E., Nelson, J.M., *et al.* (2008) The hepcidin-binding site on ferroportin is evolutionarily conserved. *Cell Metab.*, **8**, 146–156.

De Falco, L., Sanchez, M., Silvestri, L., *et al.* (2013) Iron refractory iron deficiency anemia. *Haematologica*, **98**, 845–853.

De Luca C, Filosa A, Grandinetti M. *et al.* (1999) Blood antioxidant status and urinary levels of catecholamine metabolites in beta-thalassemia, *Free Radic. Res.*, **30**, 453–462.

Denic, S. and Agarwal, M.M. (2007) Nutritional iron deficiency: an evolutionary perspective. *Nutrition*, **23**, 603–614.

Desgrippes, R., Lainé, F., Morcet, J., *et al.* (2013) Decreased iron burden in overweight C282Y homozygous women: Putative role of increased hepcidin production. *Hepatology*, **57**, 1784–1792.

Detivaud, L., Nemeth, E., Boudjema, K., *et al.* (2005) Hepcidin levels in humans are correlated with hepatic iron stores, hemoglobin levels, and hepatic function. *Blood*, **106**, 746–748.

Deugnier, Y., Jouanolle, A.M., Chaperon, J., *et al.* (2002) Gender-specific phenotypic expression and screening strategies in C282Y-linked haemochromatosis: a study of 9396 French people. *Br. J. Haematol.*, **118**, 1170–1178.

Deugnier, Y., Brissot, P. and Loréal, O. (2008) Iron and the liver: Update 2008. *J. Hepatol.*, **48** (Suppl. 1), S113–S123.

Deugnier, Y., Turlin, B., Ropert, M., *et al.* (2011) Improvement in liver pathology of patients with β-thalassemia treated with deferasirox for at least 3 years. *Gastroenterology*, **141**, 1202–1211,

Distante, S., Robson, K.J., Graham-Campbell, J., *et al.* (2004) The origin and spread of the HFE-C282Y haemochromatosis mutation. *Hum. Genet.*, **115**, 269–279.

Drakesmith, H., Schimanski, L.M., Ormerod, E., *et al.* (2005) Resistance to hepcidin is conferred by hemochromatosis-associated mutations of ferroportin. *Blood*, **106**, 1092–1097.

Engle, M.A., Erlandson, M. and Smith, C.H. (1964) Late cardiac complications of chronic, severe, refractory anemia with hemochromatosis. *Circulation*, **30**, 698–705.

Eschbach, J.W., Cook, J.D., Scribner, B.H., *et al.* (1977) Iron balance in hemodialysis patients. *Ann. Intern. Med.*, **87**, 710–713.

Esposito, B.P., Breuer, W., Sirankapracha, P. *et al.* (2003) Labile plasma iron in iron overload: redox activity and susceptibility to chelation, *Blood*, **102**, 2670–2677.

Evans, P., Kayyali, R., Hider, R.C., Eccleston, J. and Porter, J.B. (2010) Mechanisms for the shuttling of plasma non-transferrin-bound iron (NTBI) onto deferoxamine by deferiprone. *Transl. Res.*, **156**, 55–67.

FAO/WHO (2003) *Diet, Nutrition and Prevention of Chronic Diseases: report of a joint WHO/FAO expert consultation*. WHO technical report series: 916. WHO, Geneva.

Feder, J.N., Gnirke, A., Thomas, W., *et al.* (1996) A novel MHC class I-like gene is mutated in patients with hereditary haemochromatosis. *Nat. Genet.*, **13**, 399–408.

Feder, J.N., Tsuchihashi, Z., Irrinki, A., *et al.* (1997) The hemochromatosis founder mutation in HLA-H disrupts beta2-microglobulin interaction and cell surface expression. *J. Biol. Chem.*, **272**, 14025–14028.

Ferguson, B.J., Skikne, B.S., Simpson, K.M., *et al.* (1992) Serum transferrin receptor distinguishes the anemia of chronic disease from iron deficiency anemia, *J. Lab. Clin. Med.*, **119**, 385–390.

Fernández-Gaxiola, A.C. and De-Regil, L.M. (2011) Intermittent iron supplementation for reducing anaemia and its associated impairments in menstruating women. *Cochrane Database Syst. Rev.*, **7**, CD009218. doi: 10.1002/14651858.

Finberg, K.E. (2013) regulation of systemic iron homeostasis. *Curr. Opin. Hematol.*, **20**, 208–214.

Finberg, K.E., Heeney, M.M., Campagna, D.R., *et al.* (2008) Mutations in TMPRSS6 cause iron-refractory iron deficiency anemia (IRIDA). *Nat. Genet.*, **40**, 569–571.

Finberg, K.E., Whittlesey, R.L. and Andrews, N.C. (2011) Tmprss6 is a genetic modifier of the Hfe-hemochromatosis phenotype in mice. *Blood*, **117**, 4590–4599.

Finch, C.A., Belotti, V., Stray, S., *et al.* (1986) Plasma ferritin determination as a diagnostic tool. *West. J. Med.*, **145**, 657–663.

Fischer, R., Longo, D.F., Nielsen, P., *et al.* (2003) Monitoring long-term efficacy of iron chelation therapy by deferiprone and desferrioxamine in patients with beta-thalassaemia major: application of SQUID biomagnetic liver susceptometry. *Br. J. Haematol.*, **121**, 938–948.

Gabutti, V. and Piga, A. (1996) Results of long-term iron-chelating therapy. *Acta Haematol.*, **95**, 26–36.

Galanello, R., Piga, A., Alberti, D., *et al.* (2003) Safety, tolerability, and pharmacokinetics of ICL670, a new orally active iron-chelating agent in patients with transfusion-dependent iron overload due to beta-thalassemia. *J. Clin. Pharmacol.*, **43**, 565–572.

Ganz, T. (2013) Systemic iron homeostasis. *Physiol. Rev.*, **93**, 1721–1741.

Gardenghi, S., Ramos, P., Marongui, M.F., *et al.* (2010) Hepcidin as a therapeutic tool to limit iron overload and improve anemia in β-thalassemic mice. *J. Clin. Invest.*, **120**, 4466–4477.

Geisser, P. (1990) In vitro studies on interactions of iron salts and complexes with food-stuffs and medicaments. *Arzneim.-Forsch.*, **40**, 754–760.

Geisser, P. (2007) Safety and efficacy of iron(III)-hydroxide polymaltose complex: a review of over 25 years' experience. *Arzneim.-Forsch.*, **57**, 439–452.

Geisser, P. and Burckhardt, S. (2011) The pharmacokinetics and pharmacodynamics of iron preparations. *Pharmaceutics*, **3**, 12–33.

Gérolami, V., Le Gac, G. Mercier, L., *et al.* (2008) Early-onset haemochromatosis caused by a novel combination of TFR2 mutations(p.R396X/c.1538-2 A→G) in a woman of Italian descent. *Haematologica*, **93**, e45–e46.

Girelli, D., Corrocher, R., Bisceglia, L., *et al.* (1995) Molecular basis for the recently described hereditary hyperferritinaemia-cataract syndrome: a mutation in the iron-responsive element of ferritin L-subunit gene (the Verona mutation). *Blood*, **86**, 4050–4053.

Girelli, D., Bozzini, C., Roetto, A, *et al.* (2002) Clinical and pathologic findings in hemochromatosis type 3 due to a novel mutation in transferrin receptor 2 gene. *Gastroenterology*, **122**, 1295–1302.

Gochee, P.A., Powell, L.W., Cullen, D.J., *et al.* (2002) A population-based study of the biochemical and clinical expression of the H63D hemochromatosis mutation. *Gastroenterology*, **122**, 646–651.

Gordeuk, V., Mukiibi, J., Hasstedt, S.J., *et al.* (1992) Iron overload in Africa. Interaction between a gene and dietary iron content. *N. Engl. J. Med.*, **326**, 95–100.

Gordeuk, V., Caleffi, A., Corradini, E., *et al.* (2003) Iron overload in Africans and African-Americans and a common mutation in the SCL40A1 (ferroportin 1) gene. *Blood Cells Mol. Dis.*, **31**, 299–304.

Guo, S., Casu, C., Gardenghi, S., *et al.* (2013) Reducing TMPRSS6 ameliorates hemochromatosis and β-thalassemia in mice. *J. Clin. Invest.*, **123**, 1531–1541.

He, T., Kirk, P., Firmin, D.N., *et al.* (2008) Multi-center transferability of a breath-hold T2 technique for myocardial iron assessment. *J. Cardiovasc. Magn. Reson.*, **10**, 11–15.

Hellman, N.E. and Gitlin, J.D. (2002) Ceruloplasmin metabolism and function. *Annu. Rev. Nutr.*, **22**, 439–458.

Hernando, D., Levin, Y.S., Sirlin, C.B. and Reeder, S.B. (2014) Quantification of liver iron with MRI: state of the art and remaining challenges. *J. Magn. Reson. Imaging*, **40**, 1003–1021.

Hershko, C., Konijn, A.M., Link, G., *et al.* (1985) Combined use of zinc protoporphyrin (ZPP), mean corpuscular volume and haemoglobin measurements for classifying microcytic RBC disorders in children and young adults. *Clin. Lab. Haematol.*, **7**, 259–269.

Hershko, C., Ianculovich, M. and Souroujon, M. (2007) A hematologist's view of unexplained iron deficiency anemia in males: impact of *Helicobacter pylori* eradication. *Blood Cells Mol. Dis.*, **38**, 45–53.

Hsiao, P.J., Tsai, K.B., Shin, S.J., *et al.* (2007) A novel mutation of transferrin receptor 2 in a Taiwanese woman with type 3 hemochromatosis. *J. Hepatol.*, **47**, 303–306.

Huang, F.W., Pinkus, J.L., Pinkus, G.S., Fleming. M.D. and Andrews, N.C. (2005) A mouse model of juvenile hemochromatosis. *J. Clin. Invest.*, **115**, 2187–2191.

Huebers, H., Beguin, Y., Pootrakul, P., *et al.* (1990) Intact transferrin receptors in human plasma and their relation to erythropoiesis. *Blood*, **75**, 102–107.

Island, M., Jouanolle, A.M., Mosser, A., *et al.* (2009) A new mutation in the hepcidin promoter impairs its BMP response and contributes to a severe phenotype in HFE related hemochromatosis. *Haematologica*, **94**, 720–724.

Jacolet, S., Le Gac, G., Scotet, V., *et al.* (2004) HAMP as a modifier gene that increases the phenotypic expression of the HFE pC282Y homozygous genotype. *Blood*, **103**, 2835–2840.

James, M.W., Chen, C.M., Goddard, W.P., *et al.* (2005) Risk factors for gastrointestinal malignancy in patients with iron-deficiency anaemia. *Eur. J. Gastroenterol. Hepatol.*, **17**, 1197–1203.

Jin, Y., Baquet, A., Florence, A., Crichton, R.R and Schneider, J.-J. (1989) Desferrithiocin and desferrioxamine B. Cellular pharmacology and storage iron mobilization. *Biochem. Pharmacol.*, **38**, 3233–3240.

Jouanolle, A.M., Fergelot, P., Gandon, G., *et al.* (1997) A candidate gene for hemochromatosis: frequency of the C282Y and H63D mutations. *Hum. Genet.*, **100**, 544–547.

Kaltwasser, J.P., Werner, E., Schalk, K., *et al.* (1998) Clinical trial on the effect of regular tea drinking on iron accumulation in genetic haemochromatosis. *Gut*, **43**, 699–704.

Kawabata, H., Fleming, R.E., Gui, D., *et al.* (2005) Expression of hepcidin is down-regulated in TfR2 mutant mice manifesting a phenotype of hereditary hemochromatosis. *Blood*, **105**, 376–381.

KDIGO (Kidney Disease: Improving Global Outcomes) Anemia Work Group. (2012) KDIGO Clinical Practice Guideline for Anemia in Chronic Kidney Disease. *Kidney Int.*, **2**, 279–335.

Kirk, P., Roughton, M., Porter, J.B., *et al.* (2009) Cardiac T2* magnetic resonance for prediction of cardiac complications in thalassemia major. *Circulation*, **120**, 1961–1968.

Kohgo, Y., Nishisato, T., Kondo, H., *et al.* (1986) Circulating transferrin receptor in human serum. *Br. J. Haematol.*, **64**, 277–281.

Koskenkorva-Frank, T.S., Weiss, G., Koppenol, W.H. and Burckhardt, S. (2013) The complex interplay of iron metabolism, reactive oxygen species, and reactive nitrogen species: insights into the potential of various iron therapies to induce oxidative and nitrosative stress. *Free Radic. Biol. Med.*, **65**, 1174–1194.

Lainé, F., Jouannolle, A.M., Morcet, J., *et al.* (2005) Phenotypic expression in detected C282Y homozygous women depends on body mass index. *J. Hepatol.*, **43**, 1055–1059.

Lal, A., Porter, J., Sweeters, N., *et al.* (2013) Combined chelation therapy with deferasirox and deferoxamine in thalassemia. *Blood Cells Mol. Dis.*, **50**, 99–104.

Lamon, J.M., Marynick, S.P., Roseblatt, R. and Donnelly, S. (1979) Idiopathic hemochromatosis in a young female. *A case study and review of the syndrome in young people. Gastroenterology*, **76**, 178–183.

Lebron, J.A., Bennett, M.J., Vaughn, D.E., *et al.* (1998) Crystal structure of the hemochromatosis protein HFE and characterization of its interaction with transferrin receptor. *Cell*, **93**, 111–123.

Lee, A.I. and Okam, M.M. (2011) Anemia in pregnancy. *Hematol. Oncol. Clin. North Am.*, **25**, 241–259.

Lee, D.H., Zhou, L.J., Zhou, Z., *et al.* (2010) Neogenin inhibits HJV secretion and regulates BMP-induced hepcidin expression and iron homeostasis. *Blood*, **115**, 3136–3145.

Lee, P., Gelbart, T., West, C., Halloran, C. and Beutler, E. (2002) Seeking candidate mutations that affect iron homeostasis. *Blood Cells Mol. Dis.*, **29**, 471–487.

Le Gac, G., Scotet, V., Ka, C., *et al.* (2004a) The recently identified type 2A juvenile haemochromatosis gene (HJV), a second candidate modifier of the C282Y homozygous phenotype. *Hum. Mol. Genet.*, **13** (17), 1913–1918.

Le Gac, G., Mons, F., Jacolot, S., *et al.* (2004b) Early onset hereditary hemochromatosis resulting from a novel TFR2 gene nonsense mutation (R105X) in two siblings of north French descent. *Br. J. Haematol.*, **125**, 674–678.

Le Gac, G., Ka, C., Joubrel, R., *et al.* (2013) Structure–function analysis of the human ferroportin iron exporter (SLC40A1): effect of hemochromatosis type 4 disease mutations and identification of critical residues. *Hum. Mutat.*, **34**, 1371–1380.

Le Lan, C., Loréal, O., Cohen, T. *et al.* (2005) Redox active plasma iron in C282Y/C282Y hemochromatosis, *Blood*, **105**, 4527–4531.

Le Lan, C., Mosser, A., Ropert, M., *et al.* (2011) Sex and acquired cofactors determine phenotypes of ferroportin disease. *Gastroenterology*, **140**, 1199–1207.

Lemaire, M., Islam, Q.S., Shen, H., *et al.* (2011) Iron-containing micronutrient powder provided to children with moderate-to-severe malnutrition increases hemoglobin concentrations but not the risk of infectious morbidity: a randomized, double-blind, placebo-controlled, noninferiority safety trial. *Am. J. Clin. Nutr.*, **94**, 585–593.

Letocart, E., Le Gac, G., Majore, S., *et al.* (2009) A novel missense mutation in SLC40A1 results in resistance to hepcidin and confirms the existence of two ferroportin-associated iron overload diseases. *Br. J. Haematol.*, **147**, 379–385.

Levy, J.E., Montross, L.K. and Andrews, N.C. (2000) Genes that modify the hemochromatosis phenotype in mice. *J. Clin. Invest.*, **105**, 1209–1216.

Li, H., Rybicki, A.C., Suzuka, S.M., *et al.* (2010) Transferrin therapy ameliorates disease in beta-thalassemic mice. *Nat. Med.*, **16**, 177–182.

Link, G., Konijn, A.M., Breuer, W., Cabantchik, Z.I. and Hershko, C. (2001) Exploring the 'iron shuttle' hypothesis in chelation therapy: effects of combined deferoxamine and deferiprone treatment in hypertransfused rats with labeled iron stores and in iron-loaded rat heart cells in culture. *J. Lab. Clin. Med.*, **138**, 130–138.

Lok, C.Y., Merryweather-Clarke, A.T., Viprakasit, V., *et al.* (2009) Iron overload in the Asian community. *Blood*, **114**, 20–25.

Loréal, O., Deugnier, Y., Moirand R., *et al.* (1992) Liver fibrosis in genetic hemochromatosis. Respective roles of iron and non-iron-related factors in 127 homozygous patients. *J. Hepatol.*, **16**, 122–127.

Lozoff, B. (2011) Iron deficiency and child development. *Food Nutr. Bull.*, **28**, S560–S571.

Lynch, S.R. (2011) Why nutritional iron deficiency persists as a worldwide problem. *J. Nutr.*, **141**, 763S–768S.

Majore, S., Milano, F., Binni, F., *et al.* (2006) Homozygous p.M172K mutation of the TFR2 gene in an Italian family with type 3 hereditary hemochromatosis and early onset iron overload. *Haematologica*, **91**, ECR33.

Malope, B.I., MacPhail, A.P., Alberts, M. and Hiss, D.C. (2001) The ratio of serum transferrin receptor and serum ferritin in the diagnosis of iron status. *Br. J. Haematol.*, **115**, 84–89.

Markowitz, G.S., Kahn, G.A., Feingold, R.E., *et al.* (1997) An evaluation of the effectiveness of oral iron therapy in hemodialysis patients receiving recombinant human erythropoietin. *Clin. Nephrol.*, **48**, 34–40.

Mast, A.E., Blinder, M.A., Gronowski, A.M., *et al.* (1998) Clinical utility of the soluble transferrin receptor and comparison with serum ferritin in several populations. *Clin. Chem.*, **44**, 45–51.

Mast, A.E., Blinder, M.A., Lu, Q., *et al.* (2002) Clinical utility of the reticulocyte hemoglobin content in the diagnosis of iron deficiency. *Blood*, **99**, 1489–1491.

Mayr, R., Janecke, A.R., Schranz, M., *et al.* (2010) Ferroportin disease: a systematic meta-analysis of clinical and molecular findings. *J. Hepatol.*, **53**, 941–949.

McCance, R.A. and Widdowson, E.M. (1937) Absorption and excretion of iron. *Lancet, ii*, **680–684**.

McLean, E., Cogswell, M., Egli, I., Wojdyla, D. and de Benoist, B. (2009 Worldwide prevalence of anaemia, WHO Vitamin and Mineral Nutrition Information System, 1993–2005. *Public Health Nutr.*, **12**, 444–454.

McNamara, L., Gordeuk, V. and McPhail, A.P. (2005) Ferroportin (Q248H) mutations in African families with dietary iron overload. *J. Gastroenterol. Hepatol.*, **20**, 1855–1858.

Mei, Z., Cogswell, M.E., Parvanta, I., *et al.* (2005) Hemoglobin and ferritin are currently the most efficient indicators of population response to iron interventions: an analysis of nine randomized controlled trials. *J. Nutr.*, **135**, 1974–1980.

Merryweather-Clarke, A.T., Pointon, J.J., Shearman, J.D. and Robson, K.J.H. (1997) Global prevalence of putative haemochromatosis mutations. *J. Med. Genet.*, **34**, 275–278.

Merryweather-Clarke, A.T., Cadet, E., Bomford, A., *et al.* (2003) Digenic inheritance of mutations in HAMP and HFE results in different types of haemochromatosis. *Hum. Mol. Genet.*, **12**, 2241–2247.

Metzgeroth, G., Adelberger, V., Dorn-Beineke, A., *et al.* (2005) Soluble transferrin receptor and zinc protoporphyrin – competitors or efficient partners? *Eur. J. Haematol.*, **75**, 309–317.

Meynard, D., Kautz, L., Darnaud, V., *et al.*(2009) Lack of the bone morphogenetic protein BMP6 induces massive iron overload. *Nat. Genet.*, **41**, 478–481.

Milet, J., Dehais, V., Bourgain, C., *et al.* (2007) Common variants in the BMP2, BMP4, and HJV genes of the hepcidin regulation pathway modulate HFE hemochromatosis penetrance. *Am. J. Hum. Genet.*, **81**, 799–807.

Miller, J.L. (2013) Iron deficiency anemia: a common and curable disease. *Cold Spring Harb. Perspect. Med.*, **3**, p. ii.

Mircescu, G., Crichton, R.R. and Geisser, P. (2013) Iron Therapy in Renal Anaemia, UNI-MED Verlag AG, Bremen, pp. 151.

Moirand, R., Adams, P.C., Bicheler, V., Brissot, P. and Deugnier, Y. (1997) Clinical features of genetic hemochromatosis in women compared with men. *Ann. Intern. Med.* **127**, 105–110.

Mok, H., Jelinek, J., Pai, S., *et al.* (2004) Disruption of ferroportin 1 regulation causes dynamic alterations in iron homeostasis and erythropoiesis in polycythaemia mice. *Development*, **131**, 1859–1868.

Montosi, G., Donovan, A., Totaro, A., *et al.* (2001) Autosomal-dominant hemochromatosis is associated with a mutation in the ferroportin (SLC11A3) gene. *J. Clin Invest.*, **108**, 619–623.

Moretti, D., Zimmermann, M.B., Mutayya, S., *et al.* (2006) Extruded rice fortified with micronized ground ferric pyrophosphate reduces iron deficiency in Indian schoolchildren: a double-blind randomized controlled trial. *Am. J. Clin. Nutr.*, **84**, 822–829.

Nai, A., Pagani, A., Mandelli, G., *et al.* (2012) Deletion of TMPRSS6 attenuates the phenotype in a mouse model of β-thalassemia. *Blood*, **119**, 5021–5029.

Nainz, M. and Weiss, G. (2006) Molecular and clinical aspects of iron homeostasis: From anemia to hemochromatosis. *Wien. Klin. Wochenschr.*, **118**, 442–462.

Neufeld, E.J., Galanello, R., Viprakasit, V., *et al.* (2012) A phase 2 study of the safety, tolerability, and pharmacodynamics of FBS0701, a novel oral iron chelator, in transfusional iron overload. *Blood*, **119**, 3263–3268.

Nick, H., Wong, A., Acklin, P., *et al.* (2002) ICL670A: preclinical profile. *Adv. Exp. Med. Biol.*, **509**, 185–203.

Nick, H., Acklin, P., Lattmann, R., *et al.* (2003) Development of tridentate iron chelators: from desferrithiocin to ICL670. *Curr. Med. Chem.*, **10**, 1065–1076.

Nicolas, G., Viatte, E.V., Lou, D.Q. *et al.* (2003) Constitutive hepcidin expression prevents iron overload in a mouse model of hemochromatosis, *Nat. Genet.*, **34**, 97–101.

Niederkofler, V., Salie, R. and Arber, S. (2005) Hemojuvelin is essential for dietary iron sensing, and its mutation leads to severe iron overload. *J. Clin. Invest.*, **115**, 2180–2186.

Nielsen, P., Engelhardt, E., Düllmann, J. and Fischer, R. (2002) Non-invasive liver iron quantification by SQUID-biosusceptometry and serum ferritin iron as new diagnostic parameters in hereditary hemochromatosis. *Blood Cells Mol. Dis.*, **29**, 451–458.

Nisbet-Brown, E., Olivieri, N.F., Giardina, P.J., *et al.* (2003) Effectiveness and safety of ICL670 in iron-loaded patients with thalassaemia: a randomised, double-blind, placebo-controlled, dose-escalation trial. *Lancet*, **361**, 1597–1602.

Njajou, O.T., Vaessen, N., Joosse, M., *et al.* (2001) A mutation in SLC11A3 is associated with autosomal dominant hemochromatosis. *Nat. Genet.*, **28**, 213–214.

Okebe, J.U., Yahav, D., Shbita, R. and Paul, M. (2011) Oral iron supplements for children in malaria-endemic areas. *Cochrane Database Syst. Rev.*, **5**, CD006589.

Olivieri, N.F. and Brittenham, G.M. (1997) Iron-chelating therapy and the treatment of thalassemia. *Blood*, **89**, 739–761.

Olivieri, N.F., Nathan, D.G., MacMillan, J.H. and Wayne, A.S. (1994) Survival in medically treated patients with homozygous beta-thalassemia. *N. Engl. J. Med.*, **331**, 574–578.

Olson, K.S., Konar, J., Dufva, I.H., Ricksten, A. and Raha-Chowdhury, R. (2011) Was the C282Y mutation an Irish Gaelic mutation that the Vikings helped disseminate? HLA haplotype observations of hemochromatosis from the west coast of Sweden. *Eur. J. Haematol.*, **86**, 75–82.

Olynyk, J.K., Cullen, D.J., Aquilia, S., *et al.* (1999) A population-based study of the clinical expression of the haemochromatosis gene. *N. Engl. J. Med.*, **341**, 718–724.

Origa, R., Galanello, R., Ganz, T., *et al.* (2007) Liver iron concentrations and urinary hepcidin in beta-thalassemia. *Haematologica*, **92**, 583–588.

Oudit, G.Y., Trivieri, M.G., Khaper, N., Liu, P.P. and Backx, P.H. (2006) Role of L-type Ca^{2+} channels in iron transport and iron-overload cardiomyopathy. *J. Mol. Med. (Berl).*, **84**, 349–364.

Oustamanolakis, P., Koutroubakis, I.E. and Kouroumalis, E.A. (2011) Diagnosing anemia in inflammatory bowel disease: beyond the established markers. *J. Crohns Colitis*, **5**, 381–391.

Pantalone, G.R., Maggio, A., Vitrano, A., *et al.* (2011) Sequential alternating deferiprone and deferoxamine treatment compared to deferiprone monotherapy: main findings and clinical follow-up of a large multi-center randomized clinical trial in β-thalassemia major patients. *Hemoglobin*, **35**, 206–216.

Papanikolaou, G.G., Samuels, M.E., Ludwig, E.H., *et al.* (2004) Mutations in HFE2 cause iron overload in chromosome 1q-linked juvenile hemochromatosis. *Nat. Genet.*, **36**, 77–82.

Pasricha, S.R., Frazer, D.M., Bowden, D.K. and Anderson, G.J. (2013) Transfusion suppresses erythropoiesis and increases hepcidin in adult patients with β-thalassemia major: a longitudinal study. *Blood*, **122**, 124–133.

Pennell, D.J. (2005) T2* magnetic resonance and myocardial iron in thalassemia. *Ann. N.Y. Acad. Sci.*, **1054**, 373–378.

Pennell, D.J., Porter, J.B., Cappellini, M.D., *et al.* (2012) Deferasirox for up to 3 years leads to continued improvement of myocardial T2* in patients with β-thalassemia major. *Haematologica*, **97**, 842–848.

Pennell, D.J., Udelson, J.E., Arai, A.E., *et al.* (2013) Cardiovascular function and treatment in β-thalassemia major: a consensus statement from the American Heart Association. *Circulation*, **128**, 281–308.

Pennell, D.J., Porter, J.P., Piga, A., *et al.* (2015) Sustained improvements in myocardial T2* over 2 years in severely iron-overloaded patients with beta thalassemia major treated with deferasirox or deferoxamine. *Am. J. Hematol.*, **90**, 91–96.

Periago, M.V. and Bethony, J.M. (2012) Hookworm virulence factors: making the most of the host. *Microbes Infect.*, **14**, 1451–1464.

Phatak, P., Brissot, P., Wurster, M., *et al.* (2010) A phase 1/2, dose-escalation trial of deferasirox for the treatment of iron overload in HFE-related hereditary hemochromatosis. *Hepatology*, **52**, 1671–1779.

Pietrangelo A. (2004) The ferroportin disease. *Blood Cells Mol. Dis.*, **32**, 131–138.

Pietrangelo, A. (2006) Hereditary hemochromatosis. *Annu. Rev. Nutr.*, **26**, 251–270.

Pietrangelo, A. (2007) Hemochromatosis: An endocrine liver disease. *Hepatology*, **46**, 1291–1301.

Pietrangelo, A. (2010) Hereditary hemochromatosis: pathogenesis, diagnosis, and treatment. *Gastroenterology*, **139**, 393–408, 408.e1–e2.

Pietrangelo, A., Corradini, E., Ferrara, F., *et al.* (2006) Magnetic resonance imaging to identify classic and nonclassic forms of ferroportin disease. *Blood Cells Mol. Dis.*, **37**, 192–196.

Piga, A., Gaglioti, C., Fogliacco, E. and Tricta, F. (2003) Comparative effects of deferiprone and deferoxamine on survival and cardiac disease in patients with thalassemia major: a retrospective analysis. *Haematologica*, **88**, 489–496.

Piperno, A., Roetto, A., Mariani, R., *et al.* (2004) Homozygosity for transferrin receptor-2 Y250X mutation induces early iron overload. *Haematologica*, **89**, 359–360.

Poggiali, E., Cassinerio, E., Zanaboni, L. and Cappellini, M.D. (2012) An update on iron chelation therapy. *Blood Transfus.*, **10**, 411–422.

Porter, J.B. (2001) Practical management of iron overload. *Br. J. Haematol.*, **115**, 239–252.

Porter, J.B. (2009) Blood transfusion: quality and safety issues in thalassemia, basic requirements and new trends. *Hemoglobin*, **33** (Suppl. 1), S28–S36.

Porter, J.B. and Garbowski, M. (2014) The pathophysiology of transfusional iron overload. *Hematol. Oncol. Clin. North Am.*, **28**, 683–701.

Porter, J.B., Galanello, R., Saglio, G., *et al.* (2008) Relative response of patients with myelodysplastic syndromes and other transfusion-dependent anaemias to deferasirox (ICL670): a 1-yr prospective study. *Eur. J. Haematol.*, **80**, 168–176.

Preza, G.C., Ruchala, P., Pinon, R., *et al.* (2011) Minihepcidins are rationally designed small peptides that mimic hepcidin activity in mice and may be useful for the treatment of iron overload. *J. Clin. Invest.*, **121** (12), 4880–4888.

Punnonen, K., Irjala, K. and Rajamaki, A. (1997) Serum transferrin receptor and its ratio to serum ferritin in the diagnosis of iron deficiency. *Blood*, **89**, 1052–1057.

Radio, F.C., Majore, S., Binni, F., *et al.* (2014) TFR2-related hereditary hemochromatosis as a frequent cause of primary iron overload in patients from Central-Southern Italy. *Blood Cells Mol. Dis.*, **52**, 83–87.

Ramos, E., Ruchala, P., Goodnough, J.B., *et al.* (2012) Minihepcidins prevent iron overload in a hepcidin-deficient mouse model of severe hemochromatosis. *Blood*, **120**, 3829–3836.

Raza, M., Chakraborty, S., Choudhury, M., Ghosh, P.C. and Nag, A. (2014) Cellular iron homeostasis and therapeutic implications of iron chelators in cancer. *Curr. Pharm. Biotechnol.*, **15** (12), 1125–1140.

Rienhoff, H.Y. Jr, Viprakasit, V., Tay, L., *et al.* (2010) A phase 1 dose-escalation study: safety, tolerability, and pharmacokinetics of FBS0701, a novel oral iron chelator for the treatment of transfusional iron overload. *Haematologica*, **96**, 521–525.

Rimon, E., Levy, S., Sapir, A., *et al.* (2002) Diagnosis of iron deficiency anemia in the elderly by transferrin receptor-ferritin index. *Arch. Intern. Med.*, **162**, 445–449.

Roetto, A., Papanikolaou, G., Politou, M., *et al.* (2003) Mutant antimicrobial peptide hepcidin is associated with severe juvenile hemochromatosis. *Nat. Genet.*, **33**, 21–22.

Roy, C.N. (2010) Anemia of inflammation. *Hematology Am. Soc. Hematol. Educ. Program*, **2010**, 276–280.

Santos, P.C., Cançado, R.D., Pereira, A.C., *et al.* (2010) HJV hemochromatosis, iron overload, and hypogonadism in a Brazilian man: treatment with phlebotomy and deferasirox. *Acta Haematol.*, **124**, 204–205.

Sasu, B.J., Cooke, K.S., Arvedson, T.L., *et al.* (2010) Antihepcidin antibody treatment modulates iron metabolism and is effective in a mouse model of inflammation-induced anemia. *Blood*, **115**, 3616–3624.

Saunders, A.V., Craig, W.J., Baines, S.K. and Posen, J.S. (2013) Iron and vegetarian diets. *Med. J. Aust.*, **199**, S11–S16.

Schimanski, L.M., Drakesmith, H., Merryweather-Clarke, A.T., *et al.* (2005) In vitro functional analysis of human ferroportin (FPN) and hemochromatosis-associated FPN mutations. *Blood*, **105**, 4096–4102.

Schmidt, P.J. and Fleming, M.D. (2014) Modulation of hepcidin as therapy for primary and secondary iron overload disorders: preclinical models and approaches. *Hematol. Oncol. Clin. North Am.*, **28**, 387–401.

Schmidt, P.J., Toudjarska, I., Sendamarai, A.K., *et al.* (2013) An RNAi therapeutic targeting Tmprss6 decreases iron overload in Hfe(-/-) mice and ameliorates anemia and iron overload in murine β-thalassemia intermedia. *Blood*, **121**, 1200–1208.

Schmidt, P.J., Racie, T., Westerman, M., *et al.* (2015) Combination therapy with a Tmprss6 RNAi-therapeutic and the oral iron chelator deferiprone additively diminishes secondary iron overload in a mouse model of β-thalassemia intermedia. *Am. J. Hematol.*, **90**, 310–313.

Schönnagel, B.P., Fischer, R., Nielsen, P., *et al.* (2013) Iron quantification in iron overload disease using MRI. *Rofo*, **185**, 621–627.

Schwoebel, F., van Eijk, L.T., Zboralski, D., *et al.* (2013) The effects of the anti-hepcidin Spiegelmer NOX-H94 on inflammation-induced anemia in cynomolgus monkeys. *Blood*, **121**, 2311–2315.

Seth, S. (2014) Iron chelation: an update. *Curr. Opin. Hematol.*, **21**, 179–185.

Sham, R.L., Phatak, P.D., West, C., *et al.* (2005) Autosomal dominant hereditary hemochromatosis associated with a novel ferroportin mutation and unique clinical features. *Blood Cells Mol. Dis.*, **34**, 157–161.

Sham, R.L., Phatak, P.D., Nemeth, E. and Ganz, T. (2009) Hereditary hemochromatosis due to resistance to hepcidin: high hepcidin concentrations in a family with C326S ferroportin mutation. *Blood*, **114**, 493–494.

Sheldon, J.H. (1935) *Haemochromatosis*. Oxford University Press, London.

Simon, M., Bourel, M., Genetet, B. and Fauchet, B. (1977) Idiopathic hemochromatosis. Demonstration of recessive transmission and early detection by family HLA typing. *N. Engl. J. Med.*, **297**, 1017–1021.

Skikne, B.S., Flowers, C.H. and Cook, J.D. (1990) Serum transferrin receptor: a quantitative measure of tissue iron deficiency. *Blood*, **75**, 1870–1876.

Skikne, B.S., Punnonen, K., Caldron, P.H., *et al.* (2011) Improved differential diagnosis of anemia of chronic disease and iron deficiency anemia: a prospective multicenter evaluation of soluble transferrin receptor and the sTfR/log ferritin index. *Am. J. Hematol.*, **86**, 923–927.

Skorokhod, O.A., Caione, L., Marrocco, T., *et al.* (2010) Inhibition of erythropoiesis in malaria anemia: role of hemozoin and hemozoin-generated 4-hydroxynonenal. *Blood*, **116**, 4328–4337.

Skow, L.C., Burkhart, B.A., Johnson, F.M., *et al.* (1983) A mouse model for beta-thalassemia. *Cell*, **34**, 1043–1052.

Smith, P.M., Godfrey, B.E. and Williams, R. (1969) Iron absorption in idiopathic haemochromatosis and its measurement using a whole-body counter. *Clin. Sci.*, **37**, 519–531.

Spottiswoode, N., Duffy, P.E. and Drakesmith, H. (2014) Iron, anemia and hepcidin in malaria. *Front. Pharmacol.*, **5**, 125.

Stark, D.D., Bass, N.M., Moss, A.A., *et al.* (1983) Nuclear magnetic resonance imaging of experimentally induced liver disease. *Radiology*, **148**, 743–751.

Steinbicker, A.U. and Muckenthaler, M. (2013) Out of balance – systemic iron homeostasis in iron-related disorders. *Nutrients*, **5**, 3034–3061.

Steinbicker, A.U., Sachidanandan, C., Vonner, A.J., *et al.* (2011) Inhibition of bone morphogenetic protein signaling attenuates anemia associated with inflammation. *Blood*, **117**, 4915–4923.

St Pierre, T.J., Clark, P.R. and Chua-Anusom, W. (2005) Measurement and mapping of liver iron concentrations using magnetic resonance imaging. *Ann. N.Y. Acad. Sci.*, **1054**, 379–385.

Subramanian, V.N., Wallace, D.F., Dixon, J.L., Fletcher, L.M. and Crawford, D.H. (2005) Ferroportin disease due to the A77D mutation in Australia. *Gut*, **54**, 1048–1049.

Sun, C.C., Vaja, V., Chen, S., *et al.* (2013) A hepcidin lowering agent mobilizes iron for incorporation into red blood cells in an adenine-induced kidney disease model of anemia in rats. *Nephrol. Dial. Transplant.*, **28**, 1733–1743.

Swanson, C.A. (2003) Iron intake and regulation: implications for iron deficiency and iron overload. *Alcohol*, **30**, 99–102.

Taher, A., El-Beshlawy, A., Elalfy, M.S., *et al.* (2009) Efficacy and safety of deferasirox, an oral iron chelator, in heavily iron-overloaded patients with beta-thalassaemia: the ESCALATOR study. *Eur. J. Haematol.*, **82**, 458–465.

Tanner, M.A., Galanello, R.. Dessi, C., *et al.* (2007) A randomized, placebo-controlled, double-blind trial of the effect of combined therapy with deferoxamine and deferiprone on myocardial iron in thalassemia major using cardiovascular magnetic resonance. *Circulation*, **115**, 1876–1884.

Tanner, M.A., Galanello, R.. Dessi, C., *et al.* (2008) Combined chelation therapy in thalassemia major for the treatment of severe myocardial siderosis with left ventricular dysfunction. *J. Cardiovasc. Magn. Reson.*, **10**, 12.

Tanno, T., Bhanu, N.V., Oneal, P.A., *et al.* (2007) High levels of GDF15 in thalassemia suppress expression of the iron regulatory protein hepcidin. *Nat. Med.*, **13**, 1096–1101.

Theurl, I., Schroll, A., Sonnweber, T., *et al.* (2011) Pharmacologic inhibition of hepcidin expression reverses anemia of chronic inflammation in rats. *Blood*, **118**, 4977–4984.

Theurl, M., Nairz, M., Schroll, A., *et al.* (2014) Hepcidin as a predictive factor and therapeutic target in erythropoiesis-stimulating agent treatment for anemia of chronic disease in rats. *Haematologica*, **99**, 1516–1524.

Tolosano, E., Fagoonee, S., Garuti, C., *et al.* (2005) Haptoglobin modifies the hemochromatosis phenotype in mice. *Blood*, **105**, 3353–3355.

Trousseau, A. (1865) 'Glycosurie, diabète sucré'. *Clinique Médicale de l'Hôtel-Dieu de Paris*, **2**, 663–698.

Ullrich, C., Wu, A., Armsby, C., *et al.* (2005) Screening healthy infants for iron deficiency using reticulocyte hemoglobin content. *J. Am. Med. Assoc.*, **294**, 924–930.

Umbreit, J. (2005) Iron deficiency: A concise review. *Am. J. Hematol.*, **78**, 225–231.

Van der A, D.L., Peeters, P.H., Grobbee, D.E., *et al.* (2006) HFE mutations and risk of coronary heart disease in middle-aged women. *Eur. J. Clin. Invest.*, **36**, 682–690.

Van Wyck, D.B. (1989) Iron deficiency in patients with dialysis-associated anemia during erythropoietin replacement therapy: strategies for assessment and management. *Semin. Nephrol.*, **9**, 21–24.

Verloop, M.C. (1970) Iron depletion without anemia: a controversial subject. *Blood*, **36**, 657–671.

Viatte, L., Nicolas, G., Lou, D.Q., *et al.* (2005) Chronic hepcidin induction causes hyposideremia and alters the pattern of cellular iron accumulation in hemochromatotic mice. *Blood*, **107**, 2952–2958.

von Recklinghausen, F.D. (1889) Über Hämochromatose. *Taggeblatt Versamml. Deutscher Naturforscher und Aertzte, Heidelberg*, **62**, 324–325.

Waalen, J., Nordestgaard, B.G. and Beutler, E. (2005) The penetrance of hereditary hemochromatosis. *Blood Cells Mol. Dis.*, **29**, 418–432.

Waheed, A., Parkkila, S., Zhou, X.Y., *et al.* (1997) Hereditary hemochromatosis: effects of C282Y and H63D mutations on association with beta2-microglobulin, intracellular processing, and cell surface expression of the HFE protein in COS-7 cells. *Proc. Natl Acad. Sci. USA*, **94**, 12384–12389.

Wallace, D.F., Dixon, J.L., Ramm, G.A., *et al.* (2007) A novel mutation in ferroportin implicated in iron overload. *J. Hepatol.*, **46**, 921–926.

Walsh, A., Dixon, J.L., Ramm, G.A., *et al.* (2006) The clinical relevance of compound heterozygosity for the C282Y and H63D substitutions in hemochromatosis. *Clin. Gastroenterol. Hepatol.*, **4**, 1403–1410.

Wang, R.H., Li, C., Xu, X., *et al.* (2005) A role of SMAD4 in iron metabolism through the positive regulation of hepcidin expression. *Cell Metab.*, **2**, 399–409.

Weinstein, D.A., Roy, C.N., Fleming, M.D., *et al.* (2002) Inappropriate expression of hepcidin is associated with iron refractory anemia: implications for the anemia of chronic disease. *Blood*, **100**, 3776–3781.

Weiss, G. (2002) Pathogenesis and treatment of anaemia of chronic disease. *Blood Rev.*, **16**, 87–96.

Weiss, G. (2009) Iron metabolism in the anemia of chronic disease. *Biochim. Biophys. Acta*, **1790**, 682–693.

Weiss, G. and Goodnough, L.T. (2005) Anemia of chronic disease. *N. Engl. J. Med.*, **352**, 1011–1023.

Weiss, G. and Gordeuk, V. (2005) Benefits and risks of iron therapy for chronic anaemias. *Eur. J. Clin. Invest.*, **35** (Suppl. 3), 36–45.

Westwood, M.A., Anderson, L.J., Firmin, D.N., *et al.* (2003) Interscanner reproducibility of cardiovascular magnetic resonance T2* measurements of tissue iron in thalassemia. *J. Magn. Reson. Imaging*, **18**, 616–620.

WHO (2008) Worldwide prevalence of anaemia 1993–2005: WHO Global Database on anaemia (eds B. de Benoist, E. McLean, I. Egli and M. Cogswell), part of the Vitamin and Mineral Nutrition Information System (VMNIS) (http://www.who.int/vmnis).

Wieringa, F.T., Dijkhuizen, M.A., West, C.E., *et al.* (2002) Estimation of the effect of the acute phase response on indicators of micronutrient status in Indonesian infants. *J. Nutr.*, **132**, 3061–3066.

Williams, T.N. and Weatherall, D.J. (2012) World distribution, population genetics, and health burden of the hemoglobinopathies. *Cold Spring Harb. Perspect. Med.*, **2**, a011692.

Wonke, B. (2001) Clinical management of beta-thalassemia major. *Semin. Hematol.*, **38**, 350–359.

Wood, J.C. (2007) Magnetic resonance imaging measurement of iron overload. *Curr. Opin. Hematol.*, **14**, 183–190.

Wood, J.C. (2011) Impact of iron assessment by MRI. *Hematology Am. Soc. Hematol. Educ. Program*, **2011**, 443–450.

Wood, J.C. (2014) Use of magnetic resonance imaging to monitor iron overload. *Hematol. Oncol. Clin. North Am.*, **28**, 747–764.

Wood, J.C., Kang, B.P., Thompson, A., *et al.* (2010) The effect of deferasirox on cardiac iron in thalassemia major: impact of total body iron stores. *Blood*, **116**, 537–543.

Wood, J.C., Zhang, P., Rienhoff, H., *et al.* (2014) R2 and R2* are equally effective in evaluating chronic response to iron chelation. *Am. J. Hematol.*, **89**, 505–508.

Worwood, M. (2002) Serum transferrin receptor assays and their application. *Ann. Clin. Biochem.*, **39**, 221–230.

Wright, T.L., Brissot, P., Ma, W.L. and Weisinger, R.A. (1986) Characterization of non-transferrin-bound iron clearance by rat liver. *J. Biol. Chem.*, **261**, 10909–10914.

Wu, X.G., Wang, Y., Wu, Q., *et al.* (2014) HFE interacts with the BMP type I receptor ALK3 to regulate hepcidin expression. *Blood*, **124**, 1335–1343.

Yamasaki, T., Terai, S. and Sakaida, I. (2011) Deferoxamine for advanced hepatocellular carcinoma. *N. Engl. J. Med.*, **365**, 576–578.

Yang, B., Kirby, S., Lewis, J., *et al.* (1995) A mouse model for beta-thalassemia. *Proc. Natl Acad. Sci. USA*, **92**, 11608–11612.

Yoshida, K., Furihata, K., Takeda, S., *et al.* (1995) A mutation in the ceruloplasmin gene is associated with systemic hemosiderosis in humans. *Nat. Genet.*, **9**, 267–272.

Yu, P.B., Hong, C.C., Sachidanandan, C., *et al.* (2008) Dorsomorphin inhibits BMP signals required for embryogenesis and iron metabolism. *Nat. Chem. Biol.*, **4**, 33–41.

Zimmermann, M.B. and Hurrell, R.F. (2007) Nutritional iron deficiency. *Lancet*, **370**, 511–520.

Zimmermann, M.B., Molinari, L., Staubli-Asobayire, F., *et al.* (2005) Serum transferrin receptor and zinc protoporphyrin as indicators of iron status in African children. *Am. J. Clin. Nutr.*, **81**, 615–623.

Zimmermann, M.B., Muthayya, S., Moretti, D., *et al.* (2006) Iron fortification reduces blood lead levels in children in Bangalore, India. *Pediatrics*, **117**, 2014–2021.

Zoller, H. and Cox, T.M. (2005) Hemochromatosis: genetic testing and clinical practice. *Clin. Gastroenterol. Hepatol.*, **3**, 945–958.

12

Iron and Immunity

12.1 Introduction

Mankind has evolved a sophisticated network of genes and proteins to monitor iron levels, as well as a range of receptors and effector molecules to identify and destroy invading pathogens. However, changes in iron homeostasis, either from unneeded iron supplements or inherited defects of iron metabolism, may impair the ability of humans to combat bacterial insults. In this chapter the influence of changes of iron metabolism in mammals to impair the ability of cells to respond to inflammation and infection will be discussed.

Iron and immunity are closely linked in three main ways: (i) many of the genes/proteins involved in iron homeostasis play a vital role in controlling iron fluxes, such that bacteria are prevented from utilising iron for growth; (ii) cells of the innate immune system, monocytes, macrophages, microglia and lymphocytes, are able to combat bacterial insults by carefully controlling their iron fluxes, which are mediated by hepcidin and ferroportin, while lymphocytes play an important role in adaptive immunity; and (iii) a variety of effector molecules, such as toll-like receptors, NF-κB, hypoxia factor-1 and haem oxygenase, orchestrate the inflammatory response by mobilising a variety of cytokines, neurotrophic factors, chemokines and reactive oxygen species (ROS) and reactive nitrogen species. Pathological conditions in which iron loading or depletion occur, may adversely affect the ability of these cells to respond to the bacterial insult.

The immune system can be divided into two interactive systems, namely innate and adaptive immunity. Innate immunity is characterised by the immune system's ability to rapidly mobilise a response to an invading pathogen, toxin or allergen by distinguishing self from non-self. *Innate immunity* is present at birth, the effector cells being mostly myeloid cells, neutrophils, monocytes, macrophages and glial cells, particularly microglia, which release immunoactive substances such as cytokines, neurotrophic factors, chemokines and ROS and reactive nitrogen species upon stimulation. *Adaptive immunity* is involved in the elimination of pathogens during the late phase of infection, and is elicited by B and T lymphocytes, which utilise immunoglobulins and T-cell receptors, respectively, as antigen receptors to recognise 'non-self' molecules. These receptors are generated through DNA rearrangements and respond to a wide range of potential antigens. Adaptive immunity is acquired in later life.

12.1.1 Innate Immunity

A wide number of cells constitute the innate immune system. These include cells in the blood (granulocytes, neutrophils, basophils and eosinophils), in the tissues (macrophages and microglia), in the skin, nose and intestine (dendritic cells), and in the mucous membranes (mast cells). Dendritic cells are very important in the process of antigen presentation, and serve as a link between the innate and adaptive immune systems. Mast cells are a type of innate immune cell that reside in connective tissue and in the mucous membranes. They are intimately associated with wound healing and defence against pathogens, as well as allergy and anaphylaxis. When activated, mast cells rapidly release characteristic granules that are rich in histamine and heparin, along with various hormonal mediators, as well as chemokines or chemotactic cytokines, into the environment. Histamine dilates blood vessels, causing the characteristic signs of inflammation, and recruits neutrophils and macrophages (Figure 12.1). During infection, multiple host mechanisms act to decrease the availability of iron to the invading microbes.

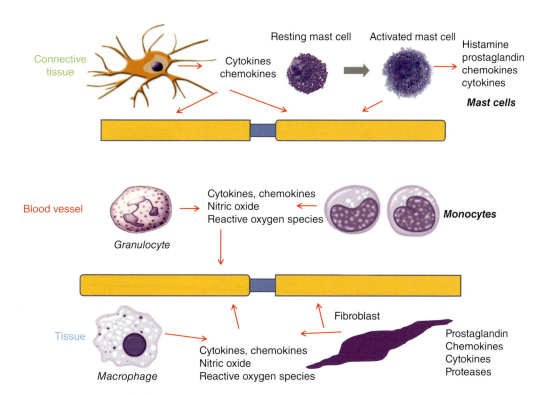

Figure 12.1 *Cells of the innate immune system. An original illustration, drawn by R.J. Ward*

Neutrophils represent 50–60% of the total circulating leukocytes, and are the first line of defence at the site of an infection. A normal healthy adult produces more than 100 billion neutrophils per day in the bone marrow, and up to 10 times more per day during acute inflammation. Similarly, eosinophils release a wide number of toxic proteins and free radicals upon stimulation by pathogens. When activated by pathogens, basophils release histamine which can play an important role in allergy. Neutrophils will recognise pathogen invasion or cell damage with intracellular or surface-expressed pattern recognition receptors (PRRs) via receptors such as NOD-like receptors and the cytoplasmic helicase retinoic acid-inducible gene protein 1, RIG-I-like receptors. These receptors will detect, either directly or indirectly, pathogen-associated molecular patterns (PAMPS), such as bacterial and viral nucleic acids, fungal β-glucan and α-mannan cell-wall components, microbial lipoproteins and carbohydrates, or damage-associated molecular patterns (DAMPS) such as ATP, interleukin (IL)-1α, uric acid, nuclear protein HMGB1, and cytoplasmic proteins S100A8 and S100A9, released from injured cells. (Figure 12.2).

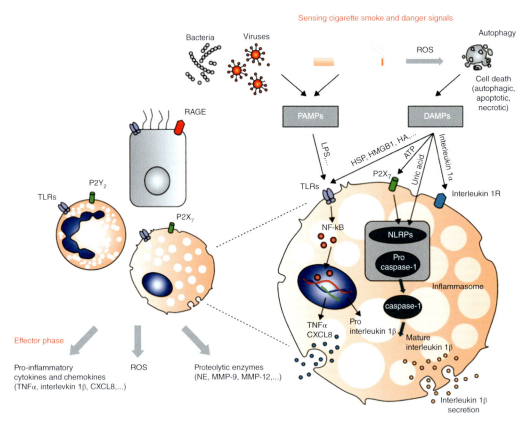

Figure 12.2 *Afferent and efferent parts of innate immune responses, where epithelial cells, macrophages and neutrophils are activated via oxidative stress and by triggering pattern recognition receptors. Reprinted with permission from John Wiley & Sons from Brusselle, G.G., Joos, G.F. and Bracke, K.R. (2011) New insights into the immunology of chronic obstructive pulmonary disease.* Lancet, **378**, 1015–1026

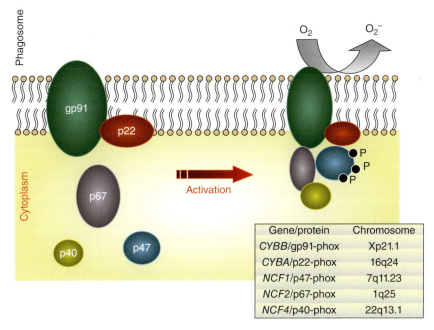

Gene/protein	Chromosome
CYBB/gp91-phox	Xp21.1
CYBA/p22-phox	16q24
NCF1/p47-phox	7q11.23
NCF2/p67-phox	1q25
NCF4/p40-phox	22q13.1

Figure 12.3 *The NADPH oxidase system. Schematic representation of the NADPH oxidase system with its components: gp91^phox and p22^phox cell membrane-bound forming the cytochrome b_{558}; and p67^phox, p47^phox and p40^phox in the cytoplasm of phagocytes. The activation occurs with phosphorylation of p47^phox followed by assembly of all components with cytochrome b_{558}, which reduces molecular oxygen (O_2) to superoxide (O_2^-). Reprinted with permission from John Wiley & Sons from de Oliveira-Junior, E.B., Bustamante, J., Newburger, P.E. and Condino-Neto, A. (2011) The human NADPH oxidase: primary and secondary defects impairing the respiratory burst function and the microbicidal ability of phagocytes. Scand. J. Immunol., **73**, 420–427*

Neutrophils recruited to the site of infection or inflammation secrete iron-sequestering lactoferrin from their secondary granules, thereby making iron unavailable for microbes. Both, neutrophils and epithelia will synthesis siderocalin (lipocalin-2, neutrophil gelatinase-associated lipocalin), a protein which has the ability to bind certain siderophores released by the invading microbes to chelate the host iron. The enzyme myeloperoxidase (MPO), most abundantly expressed in neutrophils, is a lysosomal protein stored in azurophilic granules which will also be released into the extracellular space during degranulation. MPO produces hypochlorous acid (HOCl) from hydrogen peroxide (H_2O_2) and chloride anions (Cl^-) during the neutrophil's respiratory burst, and requires haem as a cofactor. In addition, MPO can oxidise tyrosine to tyrosyl radicals using H_2O_2 as an oxidising agent. Since both hypochlorous acid and the tyrosyl radical are cytotoxic, it is essential for them to be detoxified. Hypochlorous acid is removed by the interaction between taurine and hypochlorous acid, producing taurine hypochlorite, thereby reducing toxicity. In addition to secretion from the granules after engulfing the toxic molecule into a phagosome, the enzyme NADPH oxidase (Nox) will also be stimulated. This is a unique multiprotein complex which transfers electrons across biological membranes and ultimately produces large amounts of superoxide via the reduction of molecular oxygen (Figure 12.3). Nox-derived ROS are involved in a variety of physiological processes, such as host defence and signal transduction (see Chapter 13). The Nox system is made up of two cell membrane-bound components, gp91*^phox* and p22*^phox*, which together form cytochrome b_{558}, and three cytosolic components, p67^{phox}, p47^{phox} and p40^{phox}. Upon the stimulation and activation of low-molecular-weight G proteins, Rac1 and Rac2, phosphorylation of p47^{phox} initiates migration of the cytoplasmic elements to the plasma membrane. The catalytic component gp91^{phox} facilitates electron transfer, with electrons from cytoplasmic NADPH going initially to flavin adenine dinucleotide, then via the NOX haem groups and finally across the membrane, where they are transferred to oxygen (Hernandes and Britto, 2012). Superoxide is the primary product of electron transfer, together with other downstream ROS products such as hydrogen peroxide, which can generate hydroxyl radicals via Fenton chemistry. Finally, activation of inflammatory gene transcription factors and post-translational processing will occur, for example NF-κB, AP1, CREB c/EBP and IRF.

After a few hours the concentration of iron bound to transferrin declines (hypoferraemia) due to the release of proinflammatory cytokines evoking an acute phase response. IL-6 will increase the transcription of the iron-regulatory hormone hepcidin, as well as increasing the synthesis of proteins involved in the scavenging and sequestration of iron in tissues, such as ceruloplasmin, siderocalin, haptoglobin, haemopexin and ferritin. Hepcidin can then bind to macrophage ferroportin, inducing endocytosis and degradation. Therefore, iron within the macrophages which recycle aged erythrocytes will be trapped in cytoplasmic ferritin, resulting in hypoferraemia and anaemia of chronic disease. Iron sequestration and hypoferraemia may be protective, as illustrated by the increased susceptibility of patients with hepcidin deficiency and iron overload to infections with highly iron-dependent microbes, such as *Yersinia* and *Vibrio* species (Frank *et al.*, 2011; Bergmann *et al.*, 2001; Barton and Acton, 2009).

12.2 The Key Role of Macrophages

12.2.1 Overview

Macrophages play an important role both in systemic iron homeostasis and in protecting humans from invading pathogens. In their role as phagocytic scavenger cells, they are responsible for acquiring iron from senescent erythrocytes (by erythrophagocytosis) and subsequently for its storage either within ferritin or its release via the iron exporter ferroportin into the circulation to be recycled for future erythropoiesis. Red blood cells, when destined for recycling, alter various parameters for their specific identification. These include an increase in cell density accompanied by a decrease in mean corpuscular volume, a decrease in lipid content of the cell wall, a progressive loss of sialic acid from the cell-surface glycoproteins, and an accumulation of lipid peroxidation products in the red cell membranes. The phagocytosis of the erythrocyte is different from that of intracellular pathogens in that it does not involve an inflammatory response. Subsequent to internalisation, the phagosome matures via the fusion of membranes of other vesicular compartments (early and late endosomes, plus lysosomes) such that a number of other proteins, such as hydrolases, are recruited to the membrane and the interior of the erythrophagosome where the haemoglobin will be degraded. Proteolysis of the globin releases the haem, which is degraded via haem oxygenase (predominantly HO-1), NADPH-cytochrome c reductase, and biliverdin reductase to release iron into the cytoplasm for eventual export by ferroportin.

Macrophages are also responsible for detecting, engulfing and destroying pathogens. Macrophages are the most efficient phagocytes, and can phagocytose substantial numbers of bacteria or other cells or microbes. The binding of bacterial molecules to receptors on the surface of a macrophage triggers it to engulf and destroy the bacteria through the generation of a 'respiratory burst', causing the release of ROS. Pathogens also stimulate the macrophage to produce chemokines, which summon other cells to the site of infection. The microbe or dead cell is engulfed into a phagosome, which will then fuse with a lysosome to form a phagolysosome such that the lysosomal enzymes can destroy the invader.

When macrophages are exposed to endotoxins, the bacterium or other foreign particle will be internalised within an intracellular compartment known as a *phagosome*. The multicomponent enzyme, NADPH oxidase, is assembled within the membrane of the phagosome (as described above) and activates the 'respiratory burst' of phagocytic microbial killing. Inside the phagosome this enzyme will generate superoxide, which will then undergo dismutation to hydrogen peroxide, leading to the formation of Fe^{2+}-catalysed hydroxyl radical production via Fenton chemistry. Myeloperoxidase will facilitate the production of hypochlorous acid from the reaction between hydrogen peroxide and chloride ions, which in the presence of iron will also generate more hydroxyl radicals. Changes in the total iron content of the macrophage will alter NADPH oxidase activity; in iron deficiency and iron overload it is decreased and increased, respectively, which may compromise the efficacy of these macrophages to combat invading organisms. (Ward *et al.*, 2009). The recognition of the bacteria by PRRs will elicit an inflammatory response via toll-like receptors (TLRs), such that macrophages will transcriptionally induce inducible nitric oxide synthase (iNOS), which can react with superoxide to form peroxynitrite, both of which will form part of the cytotoxic armoury. Iron loading and depletion will alter the extent of nitric oxide (NO) release, decreasing and enhancing iNOS activity, respectively (Figure 12.3b) (Ward *et al.*, 2009).

Alterations in intraphagosomal iron content will be an important determinant of bacterial growth or destruction. NRAMP1 plays an important role in controlling such iron levels, although it remains unclear whether Nramp1 functions in a similar fashion to DMT1 (Nramp2) by moving iron and other divalent metals along a proton gradient – that is, out of the phagosomes and into the cytoplasm (Forbes and Gros, 2003) or in the opposite direction, namely into the phagosome (Techau *et al.*, 2007) to elicit the generation of hydroxyl radical, via the Fenton–Haber–Weiss reaction, with antimicrobial activity.

Nramp1 (Slc11a1), a phagosomal divalent metal ion transporter, probably transports iron as well as manganese out of the phagosomal compartment into the cytosol, thereby inhibiting the growth of intra-phagosomal pathogens. Mice with wild-type Nramp1 are able to restrict early intramacrophage multiplication of various organisms such as *Salmonella*, *Leishmania* and *Mycobacterium*, after which adaptive immunity would develop to control such infections. Mice with inactive Nramp1 showed an uncontrolled growth of such organisms, which was associated with death. Mice or humans deficient in Nramp1 have an increased susceptibility to infections with *Mycobacterium bovis* (BCG), *Leishmania donovani* and *Salmonella typhimurium* (Vidal *et al.*, 1995). It remains unclear whether polymorphism of Nramp1 is associated with susceptibility to tuberculosis or leprosy in specific populations or geographical areas (Wang and Cherayil, 2009).

Peyssonnaux *et al.* (2006) showed that the infection of mouse bone marrow-derived macrophages or neutrophils with the extracellular pathogens *Pseudomonas aeruginosa* and group A *Streptoccocus* induced hepcidin mRNA expression in macrophages. Sow *et al.* (2007) also showed high levels of expression of hepcidin mRNA and protein in RAW264.7 macrophages and a human THP-1 monocytic cell line, infected with the intracellular pathogens *Mycobacterium avium* and *Mycobacterium tuberculosis*, as well as interferon (IFN)-γ that was localised to the mycobacteria-containing phagosome. It was of interest that the phagocytosis of latex beads in combination with IFN-γ, or interleukin (IL)-1β and IL-6 in RAW 264.7 macrophages in the absence of *M. avium* infection, did not induce the expression of hepcidin mRNA. This would indicate that a component of mycobacterium rather than simply phagocytosis alone had induced hepcidin mRNA. These results may indicate that the release of hepcidin from infected macrophages may be an important factor in mediating local antimicrobial activity and inhibiting iron recycling from dead cells by adjacent macrophages. Macrophages show a strong TLR4-dependent suppression of ferroportin mRNA (Liu *et al.*, 2005) and protein (Liu *et al.*, 2005; Yang *et al.*, 2002), the former being independent of hepcidin and the latter being IL-6- and hepcidin-dependent. Mice with defects in nuclear factor (NF)-κB signalling respond to lipopolysaccharide (LPS) with hypoferraemia and the downregulation of ferroportin 1 (FPN1) (Liu *et al.*, 2005), indicating that TLR4-mediated signalling which suppresses ferroportin, is possibly independent of the NF-κB pathway.

Increasing or decreasing the macrophage iron content either impaired or enhanced microbial survival (Nairz *et al.*, 2007). In general, iron-deficient macrophages, as seen in hereditary haemochromatosis, will show a lower susceptibility to bacterial infection which is associated with a lower LPS-induced increase of both tumour necrosis factor alpha (TNFα) and IL-6, as well as abnormalities in TLR4 response (TRAM and TRIF adaptor proteins) (Wang *et al.*, 2009). Hepcidin levels are not increased despite the high iron loading in the liver. In contrast, iron-overloaded macrophages, as occur in thalassaemia, will show a greater susceptibility to bacterial infection. Circulating hepcidin levels are elevated in thalassaemia, thus enhancing macrophage iron levels. Studies of NF-κB activation in iron-loaded macrophages from rats loaded *in vivo* with iron dextran, showed that NF-κB was activated almost twofold in the iron-loaded macrophages by comparison to control macrophages prior to stimulation with LPS + TNFα (Ward *et al.*, 2009), and no significant increase in the activation of this transcription factor occurred after stimulation (Figure 12.4). In contrast, unstimulated iron-depleted macrophages, isolated from rats fed an iron-deficient diet for four weeks, showed a lower NF-κB, activation, although a significant activation was evident after LPS + IFN-γ stimulation.

Iron uptake and efflux from the macrophages is controlled by a number of genes, principally transferrin receptors, DMT1, ferroportin and hepcidin with intracellular control via iron regulatory proteins (IRPs), namely IRP-1 and IRP-2. Transferrin and its receptors play an important role during the infection of macrophages with bacterial pathogens. The expression of transferrin receptor 1 (TfR1) can be modulated by bacterial infection; intracellular bacteria such as *Mycobacterium tuberculosis* and *Ehrlichia* can actively recruit TfR1 to the bacterial-containing vacuole (Pan *et al.*, 2010). It is suggested that some bacterial products can also affect IRP-1 binding affinities either directly or indirectly (and hence TfR1 expression) through intermediates of inflammation (Pan *et al.*, 2010). Furthermore it has not yet been proven whether iron released within the endosome can actually be utilised by the bacteria within the phagosome. It has been shown that iron delivered by transferrin can be utilised by *M. tuberculosis*, although a small portion of this iron will be delivered to the cytosol (Olakanmi *et al.*, 2002). It was of note that siderophores released by the bacteria could not remove iron from transferrin. In contrast, *Francisella tularensis* actively upregulated TfR1, thereby increasing the low-molecular-weight iron content. *Francisella* was also shown to activate iron acquisition events, with the upregulation of both DMT1 and STEAP3, so increasing the low-molecular-weight iron pool, as well as IRP-1 and IRP-2 (Pan *et al.*, 2010). In contrast, wild type *Salmonella typhimurium* does not require the upregulation of TfR1 for successful intracellular survival, with no increases in any of the iron genes and no changes in the low-molecular-weight iron pool. The infection of RAW264.7 murine macrophages with *S. typhimurium* increased ferroprotin expression, thereby lowering the low-molecular-weight iron pool. In parallel, the expression of HO-1 and the siderophore-binding peptide lipocalin 2 was enhanced following pathogen entry. When IFN-γ was added to murine macrophages infected with *S. typhimurium* there was a significant reduction of iron uptake via TfR1 and an upregulation of ferroportin, which resulted in an increased iron efflux. The expressions of both HO-1 and lipocalin 2 were also elevated following bacterial invasion (Nairz *et al.*, 2008).

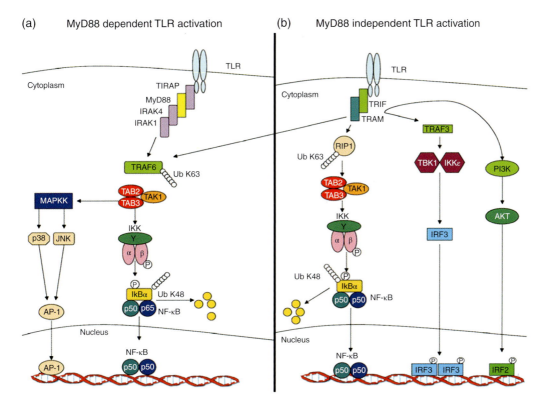

Figure 12.4   *TLR-mediated signaling. (a) The Myd88-mediated pathway is shared by all the TLRs with the exception of TLR3. MyD88 recruits TRAF6 and members of the IRAK family. TRAF6, along with Uev1A and Ubc13, activates the TAK1 complex by a K63 linked ubiquitination. The TAK1 complex then activates the IKK complex that consists of IKKα, IKKβ and IKKγ, that further catalyses IκB protein phosphorylation. This in turn facilitates IκB protein degradation in a proteasome-dependent manner, which allows NF-κB translocation to the nucleus. In parallel to activating the IKK complex, TAK1 activates the MAPK pathway which culminates in AP-1 activation. The combination of AP-1 and NF-κB controls inflammatory responses mediated by inflammatory cytokines. (b) The MyD88-independent pathway initiates when TRIF associates with TRAF3, which binds to TBK1 and IKKε. This binding culminates in IRF3 phosphorylation that facilitates IRF3 dimerisation and translocation into the nucleus and transcription regulation. TRIF can also interact with TRAF6 which, along with RIP1, mediates NF-κB activation. TRIF can also induce IRF2 translocation to the nucleus and transcription through the PI3K–AKT pathway. Reprinted with permission from Elsevier from Okun, E., Griffioen, K.J., Lathia, J.D., et al. (2009) Toll-like receptors in neurodegeneration. Brain Res. Rev., 59, 278–292*

12.2.2   Macrophage Phenotypes

During the past few years it has become clear that macrophages can be classified into specific phenotypes which are dependent upon their activation state; these are termed M1 and M2 phenotypes. These different phenotypes show distinct iron-handling mechanisms with respect to the expression of various iron genes, as well their ability to respond to infection and inflammation. Approximately 60% of iron-related genes are differentially expressed in M1 versus M2 macrophages (Recalcati *et al.*, 2010). Macrophages can be broadly divided into two groups: pro-inflammatory M1 macrophages and anti-inflammatory M2 macrophages. More recently, several novel macrophage subsets have been identified including Mhem, Mox and M4 macrophages. Of these M2 macrophages, Mhem and Mox express high levels of HO-1, which has been recognised as having major immunomodulatory and anti-inflammatory properties that have been demonstrated in HO-1-deficient mice and human cases of genetic HO-1 deficiency (Naito *et al.*, 2014). The M1 phenotype expresses lower levels of ferroportin and HO-1 than the M2 phenotype, and consequently M2 macrophages have a greater capacity for iron export (Cairo *et al.*, 2010; Corna *et al.*, 2010). This fact has clinical implications, as a greater capacity to chelate iron from specific brain regions in Parkinson disease patients having low systemic inflammation has been identified (Bastida *et al.*, 2016). M2 macrophages also take up haem–haemopexin and haemoglobin–haptoglobin complexes, using CD163 and CD91 receptors, respectively, both of which are highly expressed under M2 conditions (Figure 12.1).

The macrophage phenotype is of importance in neurodegenerative diseases since it is thought that the M1 type is predominant in these pathologies, and indicative of an active progressive inflammatory process, though this has not yet been investigated. Interestingly, it has been reported that in certain cancers, a M2 phenotype predominates, which could possibly promote tumour growth. Such observations indicate that iron is tightly bound in M1 phenotypes but in M2 phenotype it can be more rapidly released. Therefore, an ability to switch between the two phenotypes could be an interesting avenue for future therapeutic studies.

12.2.3   Microglia

Microglia, a subset of the glial cells of the brain (the other two being oligodendrocytes and astrocytes), are the resident macrophage population in the central nervous system (CNS) and are regarded as the resident immunocompetent effector cells of innate immunity in the brain. It is thought that microglia originate from circulating monocytes or precursor cells that colonise the nervous system primarily during embryonic and foetal periods of development (reviewed by Chan *et al.*, 2007). In the adult brain, under normal conditions, the blood–brain barrier prevents molecules from gaining access to the vascular lumen. However, molecules of the systemic innate immune system are able to stimulate immune cells of the brain as well as the neuronal populations. Microglia can be classified into at least two morphologically distinguishable configurations: highly branched with long processes; or round, amoeboid 'resting' cells.

Microglia are antigen-presenting cells as they express proteins of the major histocompatability (MHC)-II complex and are, thereby, potential partners for interaction with infiltrating T lymphocytes. They express a wide array of characteristic immune-cell receptors, such as chemokine and cytokine receptors and receptors of the complement-factor family. The primary role of microglia is to maintain normal CNS function, as well as to continually search for alterations in homeostasis through their constant scanning dynamic ramification. They are involved in the maintenance of synapses, the microglia ramifications interacting directly with termini, spines, astrocytic processes and the synaptic clef (reviewed by London *et al.*, 2013). Microglia can recognise neuronal activity and will facilitate synapse elimination, pruning or maturation, thereby preserving the neuronal networks. Under physiological CNS conditions, the microglia display constant motility of the highly branched cellular processes. *In-vivo* studies of microglia indicate that soluble ATP as well as connexion hemi-channels play an important role in baseline microglia motion, with the microglial processes contacting and pausing on active synapses, indicating a role for microglial motility in synaptic remodelling and function. Microglia processes are capable of rapid extension (1.25 μm min^{-1}) towards sites of acute CNS damage. This appears to be dependent upon extracellular ATP sensed via microglia P2Y12 receptors and associated outwards potassium current downstream intracellular signalling through PI3 kinase and Akt phosphorylation. In addition, integrin-β_1 activation is also involved in P2Y12-mediated chemoattraction. Nitric oxide and glutamate may also be an additional guidance cue for the directed movement of microglia. LPS activation induces microglia to retract their processes in response to ATP, sensed by the adenosine 2A receptor (Parkhurst and Gan, 2010). The rapid convergence of microglia processes to the site of injury indicates that microglia may provide a physical barrier to protect healthy tissue. A variety of receptors are present on microglia which are involved in activating these cells; these include puringeric receptors of the P1, P2X and P2Y receptor family, which bind to purines released either from neurotransmitters or from damaged or dying cells. The P2X7 receptor, P2X7R, is able to drive morphological microglia activation and proliferation in the absence of other stimuli when overexpressed *in vitro*. Activation of this receptor decreases the microglia potential for glutamate transport, which may be important in excitotoxic injury. The blockade of P2X7R impairs the microglial release of IL-1β in response to LPS or amyloid-Aβ. TLRs are expressed by microglia which, when activated, initiate a downstream signalling cascade that ultimately will release a variety of mostly proinflammatory cytokines.

One of the key issues currently under debate is the mechanisms involved in shifting microglia between a beneficial and a detrimental immune phenotype. This may be dependent on a finely regulated balance between released molecules activating/repressing the expression of specific membrane receptors, and specific timing after the insult.

When challenged, microglia are capable of acquiring diverse and complex phenotypes, which permits them to participate in the cytotoxic response, immune regulation and injury resolution. This is characterised into four main phenotypes: (i) classically activated M1 with cytotoxic properties; (ii) M2a, an alternate activation which is involved in repair and regeneration; (iii) M2b, with an immunoregulatory phenotype; or (iv) M2c, with an acquired deactivating phenotype. Agents which stimulate these different phenotypes *in vitro* are TLR-4 agonist LPS, IFN-γ and TNFα for M1; IL-4 and IL-13 for M2a; immune complexes and TLR agonists, and IL-1R ligands for M2b; and IL-10, TGF-β and glucocorticoids for M2c. In ground-breaking studies, Chhor *et al.* (2013) characterised the expression of a number of phenotype markers in primary microglia after stimulation with LPS, IL-1β, IL-4, IL-10, TNFα and IFN-γ at varying time intervals. The proinflammatory stimuli, LPS, IL-1β and TNFα increased the gene expression of the M1 markers Cox-2 and iNOS, in addition to the release of CXCL1/KC, TNFα, IL-6 and IL-1β proteins. In addition, there was an increased expression of immunomodulatory M2b markers, IL-1RN and SOCS3, and decreases in M2a repair/regeneration markers. IL-10 was the only stimulus to induce gene expression of IL-4Ra at 12 h, which was sustained for a further 36 h, although IL-6, CXCL1 and CCL2 also increased, albeit at a lower level to that of LPS stimulation. IL-4 increased the gene expression of only M2a repair and regeneration phenotype markers, arginase (Arg1) and CD206, and did not increase gene expression for either M2b or M1 phenotype markers.

Microglia are considered to be primary mediators of neuroinflammation, and as such have a vast repertoire of PPRs as well as TLRs and phagocytic receptors to collectively sense and eliminate microbes. In the healthy adult brain they exist in a non-activated state, displaying a ramified morphology and minimal expression of surface antigens (Figure 12.5). When injury is inflicted on the CNS, such as neurodegenerative diseases, stroke or traumatic brain injuries, the microglia are rapidly activated to a reactive phenotype and release cytotoxic proinflammatory molecules, including oxygen radicals, NO, glutamate, cytokines and prostaglandins which can have a detrimental effect on other neural cells. It seems that their activation also involves NF-κB, which may involve neuronal–microglial interactions (Kaltschmidt and Kaltschmidt, 2000). Microglia have been implicated in many neurological diseases, including Alzheimer's disease, Parkinson's disease and multiple sclerosis (Kreutzberg, 1996; McGeer and McGeer, 1999; Graeber and Streit, 2010).

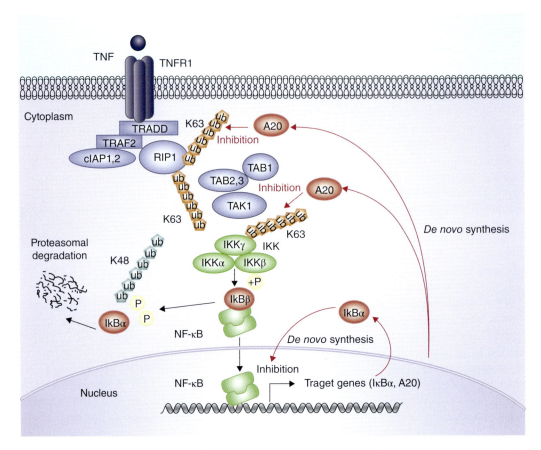

Figure 12.5 *IκBα-dependent and A20-dependent negative feedback loops in the canonical NF-κB pathway. Canonical activation of NF-κB by TNF is mediated via the recruitment of TRADD, TRAF2 and cIAP1 and cIAP2, together with RIP1, to the receptor. K63-linked polyubiquitination of RIP1 results in further recruitment of the IKK complex to the activated receptor and IKK activation. IKK phosphorylates IκBα, which triggers its K48-linked polyubiquitination and subsequent degradation by the proteasome. These events allow the translocation of NF-κB into the nucleus and activation of gene transcription. Strongly induced NF-κB target genes include those that encode the negative regulators IκBα and A20. After protein synthesis, IκBα binds to nuclear NF-κB complexes and inhibits their function by shuttling NF-κB back into the cytosol. In addition, the ubiquitin-editing enzyme A20 deubiquitinates RIP1 and IKK-γ, which leads to the disassembly of proximal NF-κB-activating complexes and shutting down of the inflammatory response. Reprinted with permission from Nature Publishing Group from Ruland J. (2011) Return to homeostasis: downregulation of NF-κB responses.* Nat. Immunol., **12**, 709–714

The control of iron homeostasis within microglia remains undefined. It is of interest that both microglia and iron deposits accumulate at the site of damage in many neurodegenerative diseases such as Alzheimer's and Parkinson's; however, whether these accumulations are a cause or effect of the disease is currently unknown. In preliminary studies it has been shown that transferrin receptor 1 and ferroportin were significantly downregulated in response to LPS treatment, while the divalent metal ion transporter, DMT1 showed no change in expression under control conditions and after LPS treatment in N9 microglia cells (Figure 12.5). Hepcidin, the iron regulatory peptide,

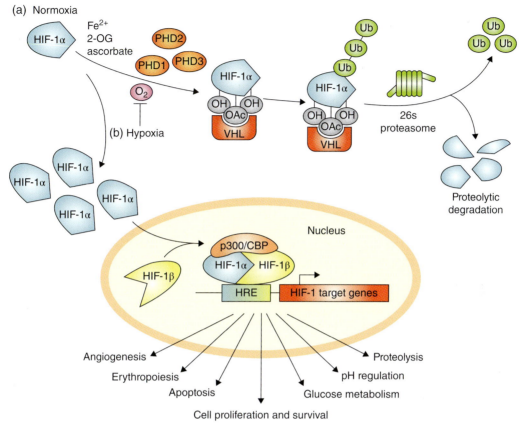

HIF-1α regulation by proline hydroxylation
Expert reviews in molecular medicine 2005 published by cambridge university press

Figure 12.6 *HIF-1α regulation by proline hydroxylation. Reprinted with permission from Cambridge University Press from Carroll, V.A. and Ashcroft, M. (2005) Targeting the molecular basis for tumour hypoxia. Expert Rev. Mol. Med., **7**, 1–16*

was not expressed. In response to LPS stimulation, microglia release cytokines such as IL-6 and NO, similar to that seen with macrophages (Figure 12.6a). Glutamate was also released which is not evident in LPS-stimulated macrophages (Figure 12.6b). However, it is as yet unknown whether iron accumulates in these activated microglia, which may contribute to the increased iron stores in specific brain regions of Parkinson's and Alzheimer's disease patients.

12.3 Effect of Iron Status on Phagocytic Cell Function

12.3.1 Iron Deficiency

Defence mechanisms that are impaired by iron deficiency include lymphocyte mitogenic response, and granulocyte functions, such as phagocytosis, respiratory burst and myeloperoxidase activity and, as a consequence, impaired bactericidal activity. In iron-deficient rats both the oxidative burst and myeloperoxidase were depressed in granulocytes (Murakawa *et al.*, 1987), while in iron-deficient children there were significantly decreased levels of IL-6, together with a diminished oxidative burst after phorbol myristate acetate (PMA) stimulation in neutrophils and monocytes. In addition, phagocytic activity was decreased in both monocytes and neutrophils (Ekiz *et al.*, 2005). Significantly lower levels of T lymphocytes as well as CD4+ cells were observed in iron-deficient children (Mullick *et al.*, 2006), although in a more recent study no association was observed between iron status and differential white blood cell counts in children (Onabanjo *et al.*, 2012). Humoral immunity, assessed by the measurement of immunoglobulin (Ig)G, IgA, IgM and subgroups of IgG, were not altered in one study of iron-deficient children, which confirmed the results of earlier studies (Ekiz *et al.*, 2005). Impaired DNA synthesis, as a result of iron deficiency, may also lead to subsequent alterations in the level of programmed cell death (apoptosis). Iron-deficient children showed reduced neutrophil and monocyte responses in terms of early and late percentages of apoptosis compared to controls (Berrak *et al.*, 2007). In another study of iron deficiency, the low levels of IL-6 detected may be due to T-cell dysfunction. In other studies of macrophages depleted of iron *in vivo* by an iron-deficient diet there were significant changes in the production of the respiratory burst (Ward *et al.*, 2011).

Expression of the hepcidin gene (*HAMP*) is downregulated by anaemia, but upregulated by high iron levels during infection and inflammation. Hepcidin is mainly expressed in the liver, and it remains uncertain whether the protein is present in macrophages. Hepcidin mRNA expression has been identified in these cells but there are no reports of protein concentrations. Monocyte hepcidin mRNA expression was significantly induced within 3 h after stimulation with LPS or IL-6, and interestingly hepcidin mRNA expression was significantly higher in monocytes of patients with anaemia of chronic disease than in controls (Theurl *et al.*, 2008). In patients with anaemia of chronic disease, monocyte hepcidin mRNA levels were significantly correlated with serum IL-6 concentrations, and increased monocyte hepcidin mRNA levels were associated with a decreased expression of the iron exporter ferroportin and iron retention in these cells (Theurl *et al.*, 2008). The exact proportion of hepcidin in the serum contributed to by macrophages, if any, is unknown. In contrast, in the study of Sow *et al.* (2007), the stimulation of macrophages with the inflammatory cytokines IL-6 and IL-β did not induce hepcidin mRNA expression. However, when the mouse RAW264.7 macrophage cell line and mouse bone marrow-derived macrophages were stimulated with mycobacteria and IFN-γ, synergistically high levels of hepcidin mRNA and protein were induced. Similar results were obtained using the human THP-1 monocytic cell line. Interestingly, the authors found that hepcidin inhibited *M. tuberculosis* growth *in vitro* and caused structural damage to the mycobacteria, which suggested that hepcidin localises to the phagosome of infected, IFN-γ-activated cells and has antimycobacterial activity. It remains unclear whether such cells can synthesise hepcidin, which would then interact with ferroportin within the same cell.

12.3.2   Iron Overload

There is a close correlation between the availability of iron and bacterial virulence, iron being essential for bacterial growth. Therefore, excess iron in the host may increase the risk of infection. One main cause for increased vulnerability to infections in iron-overloaded patients is abnormalities of neutrophil function. For example, in early studies Van Asbeck (1984) identified impaired phagocytic function in monocytes and granulocytes from patients with iron overload. Hereditary hyperferritinaemia-cataract syndrome (HHCS) is an autosomal dominant trait associated with mutations in the iron responsive element (IRE) of the ferritin light-chain (L-ferritin) gene. Patients typically show elevated serum ferritin concentrations without iron overload, and a bilateral cataract. Hyperferritinaemia can be associated with granulocyte dysfunction in patients with β-thalassaemia and in haemodialysis patients. The effect of increased L-ferritin levels on granulocyte function in patients with HHCS is unknown. Hyperferritinaemia in patients with IRE 39C→T-positive HHCS is associated with an activation of polymorphonucleocytes (PMNLs) but not with any disturbance of fundamental PMNL function.

12.4   Effect of Phagocytic Cell Function on Iron Metabolism

12.4.1   The IRE–Iron Regulatory Protein (IRP) System

Nitric oxide, superoxide and hydrogen peroxide produced by activated phagocytic cells may also alter iron homeostasis within the cell via IRP1–IRE and IRP2IRE binding, thereby altering the uptake and efflux of iron from the cell. However, published results have shown high variability which would appear to be dependent on the dose as well as the method of administration – exogenous or endogenous. IRP1 function is influenced by superoxide and H_2O_2 (discussed in greater detail in Chapter 13). Intracellular superoxide generation will result in IRP1 deactivation with associated changes in TfR and ferritin expression. Extracellular hydrogen peroxide induces the cells to rapidly increase the mRNA binding of IRP1, possibly acting via membrane-transduced signalling rather than via oxidative stress or direct interaction with IRP1 (Koskenkorva-Frank *et al.*, 2013). The effect on IRP2 is variable, with one report showing that IRP2 is not affected by exogenous H_2O_2, but a recent study indicating an increase in the IRE-binding activity of IRP2. This variance was thought due to the stabilisation of HIF-1α resulting from the oxidation of Fe(II) to Fe(III), which would prevent assembly of the Fe–O–Fe centre of FBXL5 (Koskenkorva-Frank *et al.*, 2013). *In-vitro* H_2O_2 exposure leads to IRP-dependent transient inhibition of ferritin synthesis and the upregulation of TfR, but also to an IRP-independent increased capacity to store iron in ferritin. Nontoxic H_2O_2 concentrations (<5 μM comparable to inflammatory conditions) stimulate TfR mRNA translation without affecting IRP–IRE binding activity. Higher H_2O_2 doses, however, promote proteasomal degradation of ferritin (Koskenkorva-Frank *et al.*, 2013).

NO has a high affinity for iron, particularly Fe^{2+} such that it reacts with several iron-containing proteins, such as ribonucleotide reductase, haem-containing proteins, ferrochelatase and other [Fe–S] proteins including mitochondrial aconitase and Complexes I and II of the electron transport chain, thereby affecting their activity. NO will target the IRP–IRE regulatory network, and can activate the mRNA-binding activity of IRP1 by depleting intracellular iron and interacting with the [4Fe–4S] cluster of IRP1. NO will upregulate ferritin and FPN transcriptions, possibly via the NF-E2-related factor 2 (Nrf2)/antioxidant-responsive element (ARE) pathway, by stimulating binding of Nrf2 to the AREs present in the promoter region of the ferritin and FPN genes. Recently, this mechanism was shown to be partly responsible for the protective effect of NO against infections with intracellular pathogens through increased cellular iron egress, thereby limiting iron availability for intramacrophageal bacteria. Peroxynitrite is also capable of disrupting [Fe–S] clusters, particularly aconitase via [4Fe–4S]-cluster disassembly, but whether it is able to activate IRP1 remains unclear. Again, this would appear to be due to the different experimental conditions utilised.

The production of NO by the stimulated macrophages is a central antimicrobial effector pathway. However, if the cells become loaded with iron as a result of changes in iron fluxes, their ability to release NO is impaired (Zhang *et al.*, 1998). Furthermore, these studies showed that the ability of the cells to inhibit the germination of spores from the fungus *Rhizopus* (a NO-dependent process) was impaired (Zhang *et al.*, 1998).

In conclusion, it is becoming apparent that it is hepcidin rather than the IRP–IRE system that plays the most important role in dictating the regulating cellular iron efflux and influx.

NRAMP1 has been shown to lower phagosomal iron concentrations which will in turn influence the survival and growth of several intracellular pathogens, including *Mycobacterium bovis* and *Leishmania donovani*. Polymorphisms of the *NRAMP1* gene have been linked to an altered susceptibility to some pathogens.

Ferroportin expression plays an important role in controlling iron release from enterocytes and macrophages. The post-translational regulation of ferroportin expression is by the hepatocyte-derived peptide hormone hepcidin, which will bind to ferroportin and induce its internalisation and lysosomal degradation. Mechanisms which regulate ferroportin expression include both transcriptional and post-transcriptional events, since ferroportin mRNA contains a 5′ IRE. Iron regulatory proteins, which influence ferroportin translation, are also affected at the level of expression of its mRNA by the iron status of the cell, oxidation, ROS and reactive nitrogen species, all of which will increase the IRP-1 RNA binding activity (Ward and Kaplan, 2012). Ferroportin will also be an important determinant of intracellular pathogen growth; for example, when its expression was increased *S. typhimurium* growth in macrophages was inhibited (Wang and Cherayil, 2009). The elevation of FPN levels in HeLa cells and J774 macrophages led to a significant inhibition of intracellular *Salmonella* growth. However, the hepcidin-induced downregulation of FPN had an opposite effect. The activation of macrophages, either by bacterial infection or IFN-γ, is associated with a transcriptional upregulation of FPN, indicating that FPN-mediated iron efflux may be part of the phagocyte's antimicrobial repertoire. Therefore, the ability of the cell to alter its FPN expression or function will influence the growth of pathogens inside the macrophage by altering iron availability.

Hepcidin is strongly induced during infections and inflammation, leading to intracellular iron sequestration. In both humans and mice, this is indirect and mediated by the macrophage production of cytokines IL-6 and IL-1 (Lee *et al.*, 2005; Nemeth *et al.*, 2004) as well as STAT3. Silvestri *et al.* (2007) showed that the proximal 165 bp of the hepcidin promoter is critical for hepcidin activation in response to exogenously administered IL-6. A STAT3 binding motif located at position –64/–72 of the promoter is required for high basal-level hepcidin mRNA expression. Therefore, STAT3 is also a key effector of baseline hepcidin expression during inflammatory conditions. Stress pathways signalling through the cellular endoplasmic reticulum unfolded protein response will also induce hepcidin expression (Wessling-Resnick, 2010).

The absence of functional HFE protein results in a failure of normal iron sensing leading to low hepcidin levels, and an elevated FPN expression in macrophages. Although it was predicted that Hfe knockout mice (*hfe-/hfe-*, comparable to type1 haemochromatosis) would inhibit the growth of *Salmonella* in cells and would be relatively resistant to infection, the HFE-deficient mice had higher numbers of *Salmonella* organisms in the systemic tissues. The reason for this was possibly a less-robust inflammatory response, leading to an inefficient clearance of the pathogen. This was confirmed by the fact that peritoneal macrophages from *hfe*-deficient mice produced lower levels of proinflammatory cytokines, such as TNFα and IL-6. Further studies indicated that *hfe* deficiency affected the responses of TLR-4 receptors only. This was associated with a subset of TLR, the TRAM and TRIF adaptor proteins that are recruited to the TLR-4 cytoplasmic domain in response to LPS. It was concluded that this diminished inflammatory response was caused by low intracellular iron levels. However, in other studies Nairz *et al.* (2009) reported contrasting results in *hfe* knockout mice, in that the mice were relatively resistant to *Salmonella* infection and their inflammatory response was not impaired, while de Domenico *et al.* (2011) showed that the binding of hepcidin to FPN activated signals that suppressed LPS-induced TNFα and IL-6 mRNA and protein expression. Hepcidin-deficient mice had exaggerated inflammatory responses following LPS administration.

Such animal studies suggested that *hfe* deficiency can influence the course of infection in two ways: (i) a direct effect on bacterial growth resulting from iron deprivation; or (ii) an indirect effect secondary to the attenuated pathogen-induced inflammatory response. The net outcome is a poor control of bacterial multiplication in *hfe*-deficient mice.

Studies of the ability of Type 1 haemochromatosis patients to combat infection have shown that they are susceptible to certain bacterial infections, particularly *Vibrio vulnificus* septicaemia and hepatic abscesses caused by *Yersinia enterocolitica*. This may be caused by elevated serum iron concentrations, or possibly impaired inflammatory responses. It was shown that peripheral monocytes from HH patients secrete reduced amounts of TNFα in response to LPS. In Type 4 HH, associated with dominant inactivating mutations in the *FPN* gene, patients show an increased risk of tuberculosis, which may be caused by the growth of bacteria within macrophages because of the high intracellular accumulation of iron.

12.5   Effector Molecules of the Innate Immune System

12.5.1   Toll-like Receptors

Toll-like receptors (TLRs) are the major pattern recognition receptors (PRRs) in the cell, and play an important role as mediators of the detection and responses of immune cells to invading pathogens. There are at least 13 mammalian TLRs, which are integral membrane proteins with a leucine-rich extracellular domain and a cytoplasmic domain similar to that of the IL-1 receptor. The TLRs initiate downstream signalling through kinases to activate transcription factors such as AP-1 and NF-κB (Figure 12.4). TLRs are expressed in a variety of mammalian immune-related cell types such as B cells, mast cells, natural killer (NK) cells, regulatory T cells, macrophages, monocytes, dendritic cells, neutrophils and basophils, as well as non-immune cells such as epithelial and endothelial cells. TLRs are also present in the brain, where they have been detected on microglia, astrocytes and oligodendrocytes, and possibly also on neurons.

Each TLR by itself or in combination with other TLRs recognises distinct IRP-1 function pathogen-associated molecular patterns (PAMPs), which include lipids, lipoproteins, nucleic acids and proteins. The expression of TLRs is rapidly altered in response to pathogens, cytokines and environmental stressors. With the exception of TLR-3, all TLRs engage the adaptor MyD88 either directly or in combination with the adaptor TIRAP/Mal.

All TLRs sense microbial infection and trigger a multitude of antimicrobial and inflammatory responses. A subset of TLR-induced signals is dedicated to the control of adaptive immunity (Iwasaki and Medzhitov, 2004).

12.5.2   NF-κB

IKKβ/NF-κB is an essential mediator of immunity and inflammation in immune cells. NF-κB remains inactive in the cytoplasm in a quiescent state, where it is bound to the inhibitory protein IκBα. Various pathogenic insults will activate IKKβ, which include LPS, double-stranded (ds) DNA, mitogens and cytokines. IKKβ is activated via phosphorylation at Ser177 and Ser181, which will induce phosphorylation, ubiqitination and subsequent proteasomal degradation of its substrate Iκbα. NF-κB will then be released to translocate to the nucleus, where it mediates the transcription of large numbers of target genes (Figure 12.5).

The transcriptional products of NF-κB in immune cells include many cytokines and their receptors, immune modulators, adhesion molecules and survival and apoptotic factors, which will produce a transient, robust inflammation. The importance of this transcription factor is emphasised by the fact that a lack of the genes that encode IKKβ or NF-κB subunit p65 is embryologically lethal. Various factors will influence the activation of NF-κB, such as iron ROS and oxygen, although it is clear that such changes are very cell-specific; for example, iron will activate NF-κB in macrophages but not in other cells. It has been reported that hepcidin expression in macrophages is partly dependent on NF-κB.

12.5.3 Hypoxia-Inducible Factor 1 (HIF 1)

Prolyl hydroxylases (PHDs), which require both iron and oxygen for optimal activity, are well-known transcription factors that originally were thought to regulate responses to hypoxia but which are now known also to regulate key proteins of iron metabolism. PHDs are involved in oxygen sensing and require both iron and oxygen to hydroxylate specific proline residues in hypoxia-inducible transcription factors (HIFs). A reduction of either iron or oxygen leads to inactivation of the PHDs and activation of the HIFs, which bind to hypoxic response elements (HREs) within promoters, leading to increased gene expression. Therefore, the exposure of cells to low oxygen tension or low iron levels will result in the activation of a similar set of genes (Simpson and McKie, 2015).

HIF-1α is induced by bacterial infection, hypoxia and iron deficiency, and regulates the production of key immune effector molecules. HIFs are heterodimeric transcription factors consisting of an unstable α-subunit and a stable β-subunit. Under normoxic conditions, HIF-1α is hydroxylated on specific proline residues, at amino acid residues 402 and 564, which results in polyubiquitinylation of the HIF-1α protein by von Hippel–Lindau (VHL) tumour suppressor protein, and its degradation by the proteasome (Figure 12.6). HIF-1α, which is transcriptionally controlled by the transcription factor NF-κB, regulates many of the genes of iron homeostasis, including HO-1, Nramp1, erythropoietin, DcytB, ferroportin and TfR1 during infection and inflammation. Such changes induced in TfR1 expression may be involved in modulating iron retention in inflammatory macrophages, thereby contributing to the development of hypoferraemia in the early phases of inflammation and infection. This would precede the downregulation of macrophage ferroportin by hepcidin (Tacchini *et al.*, 2008). HIF also induces the protease furin, with the subsequent release of a soluble circulating form of haemojuvelin, which may downregulate hepcidin during hypoxia or exercise (Silvestri *et al.*, 2008). Since HIF-1α plays an important role in immunity, the myeloid-specific disruption of its function will result in an increased susceptibility to infection and impaired cell-mediated inflammation (Cramer and Johnson, 2003). Mice lacking HIF-1α in their myeloid cell lineage show a decreased bactericidal activity and are unable to restrict the systemic spread of infection from an initial insult. In contrast, activation of the HIF-1α pathway (via the deletion of VHL tumour suppressor protein or pharmacological inducers) supported myeloid cell production of defence factors and improved bactericidal capacity (Peyssonnaux *et al.*, 2006). Bayele *et al.* (2007) showed that HIF-1α regulates allelic variation in Nramp1 expression by binding directly to the microsatellite during macrophage activation. Targeted HIF-1α ablation in murine macrophages attenuated Nramp1 expression and responsiveness to *S. typhimurium* infection.

Since HIF-1α regulates glycolysis in monocyte and neutrophils under both normoxic and hypoxic conditions, any changes in glycolysis, such as decreased ATP production, will also reduce HIF-1α activity and therefore inhibit the inflammatory response. A functional inactivity of HIF-1α will inhibit monocytic cell mobility and invasiveness in peritoneal macrophages (Peyssonaux and Johnson, 2004).

Recently, it has been shown that there are HREs which bind to HIF-2α in the promoters of the iron metabolism genes *DcytB* and *ferroportin*, while an IRE has been found within the 5′ region of the HIF-2 mRNA, indicating that HIF-2 may itself be regulated by iron status (Simpson and McKie, 2015).

12.5.4 Haem Oxygenase

Haem oxygenases (HO) are a family of ubiquitously expressed enzymes which regulate the catabolism of haem, leading to the formation of equimolar amounts of carbon monoxide (CO), ferrous iron (Fe^{2+}) and biliverdin, which is subsequently converted to bilirubin, a potent endogenous antioxidant with recently recognised anti-inflammatory properties (Chung *et al.*, 2009). HO exists in two distinct, catalytically active isoforms: HO-1 and HO-2. HO-1 is an inducible 32-kDa protein, while HO-2 is a constitutively synthesised 36-kDa protein. HO-1 is capable of blocking innate and adaptive immune responses by modifying the activation, differentiation, maturation and/or polarisation of numerous immune cells, including endothelial cells, monocytes/macrophages and dendritic cells. Although several transcriptional factors and signalling cascades are involved in HO-1 regulation, the two main pathways – the Nrf2/Bach1 system and the IL-10/HO-1 axis – exist in monocytes/macrophages (Naito *et al.*, 2014). HO-1 is present in high levels in the spleen (where senescent and abnormal red blood cells are destroyed) and in the liver. Its transcription can be induced by iron and by oxidative stress (Figure 12.7).

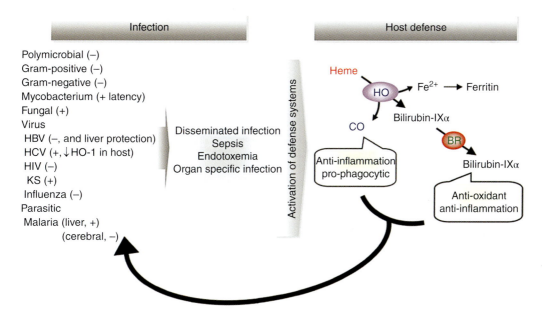

Figure 12.7 *The HO-1 pathway and its effect on microbial infections. Microbial infections that may involve the HO-1 pathway include those due to bacteria (polymicrobial, Gram-positive and Gram-negative); mycobacteria; fungi; viruses including hepatitis B virus (HBV), hepatitis C virus (HCV), HIV (and its complication Kaposi's sarcoma, KS) and influenza; and the parasitic species leading to malaria (both the exoerythrocytic liver stage and the erythrocytic blood stage). These microbes may lead to either disseminated disease (which may result in sepsis) or organ-specific infections. Microbial infections typically lead to an induction of HO-1, which degrades haem to generate carbon monoxide (CO), biliverdin-IXα (subsequently reduced to biliverdin-IXα) and iron. These metabolites have a number of properties including the anti-inflammatory and pro-phagocytic effects of CO, and the antioxidant and anti-inflammatory properties of biliverdin/bilirubin. The properties of HO-1, and the products of haem catabolism, then have an ability to suppress (–) the microbial response or promoter (+) microbial survival. Reprinted from Chung, S.W., Hall, S.R. and Perrella, M.A. (2009) Role of haem oxygenase-1 in microbial host defence. Cell. Microbiol., **11**, 199–207*

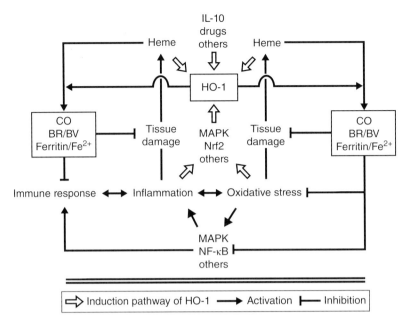

Figure 12.8 *Induction of HO-1 and subsequent production of haem degradation products exert potent antioxidative, anti-inflammatory and antiapoptotic functions for the tissue homeostasis. HO-1 can be expressed by a number of stimuli mainly via MAPK-dependent Nrf2 activation. These inducers of HO-1 include free haem, inflammatory mediators, oxidative stress, IL-10, and some inflammatory drugs. HO-1, once expressed under pathological conditions, can degrade free haem into biliverdin (BV), CO, and Fe^{2+}. BV is converted into bilirubin (BR) by BV reductase. The iron is rapidly sequestered by ferritin. Haem degradation products have been shown to modulate inflammatory response, perhaps by reducing oxidative stress, blocking MAPK pathways, and suppressing NF-κB activity. From Pae, H.O. and Chung, H.T. (2009) Haem oxygenase-1: its therapeutic roles in inflammatory diseases.* Immune Networks, **9**, *12–19. This is an open-access article distributed under the terms of the Creative Commons Attribution License*

The overexpression of HO-1 enhances the destruction of haem, which will induce a two- to threefold increased induction of ferritin, with compensatory increases in transferrin receptor expression and haem synthesis. Such results would indicate that the cytoprotective effects of HO-1, when induced or overexpressed, may relate to an elevated expression of ferritin, thereby reducing the low-molecular-weight iron pool (Lanceta *et al.*, 2013). The therapeutic roles of HO-1 in inflammatory diseases are summarised in Figure 12.8. HO-1-deficient animals are susceptible to oxidant-induced tissue damage after exposure to Gram-negative bacteria. HO-1 activity can have both beneficial and detrimental consequences for the host, depending on the infecting microbe. For example, during microbial sepsis CO derived from HO-1 has an important role as an antimicrobial agent without inhibiting the inflammatory response, while other beneficial or adverse effects of HO-1 activation were evident in mycobacterial and fungal infections (Chung *et al.*, 2009). Mutations which induce a loss-of-function in the HO-1 gene cause a rare and lethal disease in children, with severe anaemia and intravascular haemolysis, as well as damage to the endothelia and kidneys. Kovtunovych *et al.* (2014) showed that macrophages engaged in the recycling of red cells were depleted from the tissues of Hmox1(–/–) mice, which resulted in intravascular haemolysis and severe damage to the endothelial system, kidneys and other organs. In general, the basal and induced expression of HO-1 is very variable among the normal human population because of the highly polymorphic $(GT)n$ fragment in the promoter.

The levels of haemolysis in the blood are increased in both thalassaemia and sickle cell anaemia patients, the latter being much higher. As a consequence, the induction of liver HO is greater in sickle cell anaemia than thalassaemia patients. Such HO-1 induction will stimulate ferritin synthesis as well as upregulate ferroportin expression, resulting in a release of iron from macrophages, although there would appear to be an opposite effect in hepatocytes (Porter, 2009). However, recent microarray analyses of liver biopsy samples from these two groups of patients showed that HO-1 mRNA was threefold higher in transfused sickle cell anaemia patients than in thalassaemia subjects. Such divergent results clearly require further investigation to ascertain the various mechanisms involved in these two diseases.

Interestingly, there would appear to be differences in the HO-1 activity in the different phenotypes of macrophages, with the M2 phenotype showing the greater induction, indicating its role in immunomodulation.

12.5.5 DMT1, Nramp1

The exact function of DMT1/Nramp1 as an iron and divalent cation transporter remains controversial. It can function either to increase transphagosomal Fe^{2+}, thereby catalysing the Haber–Weiss/Fenton reaction to generate the hydroxyl radicals essential for macrophage bactericidal activity or, alternatively, it may efflux iron from the phagosome, depriving the intraphagosomal bacterium of Fe^{2+} and other divalent cations. NRAMP1 will decrease intracellular iron availability, thereby stimulating the production of NO, which is a potent antimicrobial effector. NRAMP1 is expressed exclusively in circulating phagocytes, where it localises to the late endosomal/lysosomal compartment and is recruited to the phagosomal membrane when infection/inflammation occurs. In NRAMP1 knockout mice, various alterations in iron homeostasis were identified after acute and chronic induction of haemolytic anaemia. Untreated knockout mice showed increased serum transferrin saturation and splenic iron content with a higher duodenal ferroportin (Fpn) and DMT1 expression. The hepatocyte iron content and hepcidin mRNA levels were dramatically lower in knockout mice, indicating that hepcidin levels were regulated by low stores of hepatocyte iron, despite the increased transferrin saturation (Soe-Lin *et al.*, 2009). The authors concluded that Nramp1 promotes efficient haemoglobin iron recycling in macrophages. The NRAMP1-G169D mutation resulted in increased susceptibility to intracellular pathogens.

12.6 Adaptive Immunity

The adaptive immune response provides the vertebrate immune system with the ability to both recognise and remember specific pathogens. Adaptive immune response takes many days to become activated. The mechanism allows a small number of genes to generate a vast number of different antigen receptors which are expressed on B and T lymphocytes. These cells utilise immunoglobulins and T-cell receptors, respectively, as antigen receptors to recognise 'non-self'. The receptors are generated through DNA rearrangement and respond to a wide number of potential antigens. This information will be inherited in all of the progeny, which includes memory B cells and memory T cells, to give long-lived specific immunity molecules. The B cells play an important role in the humoral immune response and are involved in the creation of antibodies that circulate in the blood and lymph. There are five types of antibody: IgA, IgD, IgE, IgG and IgM. The T cells are intimately involved in cell-mediated immune responses.

The induction of an *adaptive immune response* begins when a pathogen is ingested by an immature dendritic cell in the infected tissue, which will then become an activated dendritic cell (*antigen*-presenting cell) and migrate through the lymph to the regional lymph nodes to interact with recirculating naive *lymphocytes*. The receptors on the immature dendritic cell can identify common features of many pathogens, such as bacterial cell wall proteoglycans. The dendritic cells' functions are not to destroy pathogens but rather to carry the pathogen antigens to peripheral lymphoid organs and present them to T lymphocytes. It is noteworthy that many pathogenic bacteria have evolved a protective capsule that enables them to conceal recognition molecules, which avoids their recognition and phagocytosis. Furthermore, *viruses* carry no invariant molecules similar to those of bacteria and are rarely recognised directly by macrophages.

T cells and B cells interact with antigen-presenting cells to become activated, after which they proliferate and migrate to the site of inflammation. B cells will produce antibodies that target extracellular pathogens. T-cell populations include $CD8^+$ cytotoxic T cells that lyse infected cells and $CD4^+$ T-helper cells that secrete a wide range of cytokines and activate other components of the immune response. After an antigen has been encountered by the adaptive immune system, a potent lasting memory response is generated such that, on subsequent exposure, there will be an immediate response.

12.6.1 $CD8^+$ Lymphocytes and Cytotoxicity

Naïve cytotoxic T cells (killer T cells or cytotoxic lymphocytes) are activated when their T-cell receptor strongly interacts with a peptide-bound MHC class 1 molecule. Once activated, the cytotoxic T cell undergoes clonal expansion, where it gains functionality and divides rapidly such that a donor army of armed effector cells is produced. These cells will then search out other cells bearing the unique MHC class 1 peptide, whereupon granzyme will be released and enter the cells to induce apoptosis.

12.6.2 $CD4^+$ Lymphocytes

$CD4^+$ lymphocytes (helper cells) are immune response mediators that orchestrate the immune response. Helper T cells express T-cell receptors which can recognise antigen-bound MHC class II molecules. $CD4^+$ T-helper cells can be induced to differentiate specific lineages according to the local cytokine milieu, towards T-helper type 1 (Th1), Th2, Th17 and regulatory T-cell (T_{reg}) phenotypes.

12.7 Immune Function and other Factors

12.7.1 Iron Supplementation and Immune Function

There have been numerous discussions on ways to prevent iron deficiency worldwide, preferably by the oral administration of fortified foods such as milk and flour. However, there has been considerable debate as to the interaction between iron status, iron supplementation and susceptibility to infection. Early studies showed the benefit of iron supplementation in reducing rates of respiratory infections in infants, while later reports indicated a deleterious effect on susceptibility to malaria (Oppenheimer, 2001).

The idea that iron supplementation may enhance educational achievements still remains an enigma. Some reports have identified a lower standardised mathematics score among iron-deficient, school-aged children (as identified by two of the following being abnormal for age and gender;

transferrin saturation, free erythrocyte protoporphyrin or serum ferritin) (Halterman *et al.*, 2001). However, in other studies (Dissanayake *et al.*, 2009) iron status did not play a major role in the educational performance and intelligence of school-going adolescents. Such associations need to be validated, and those nutritionists who advocate the wide-scale administration of iron supplements to otherwise healthy individuals with a normal iron status to enhance concentration and educational achievements, should be cautious as such supplementation could induce immune dysfunction.

12.7.2 Immune Function in the Elderly Population

There is an increasing awareness that alterations in the peripheral immune system are associated with changes in neuronal function. During the past few years several reports have been made identifying changes in various blood biomarkers such as cytokines, chemokines and oxidative stress markers being indicative of neurological conditions, such as depression (Gimeno *et al.*, 2009), mild cognitive impairment (Magaki *et al.*, 2008), dementia (Engelhart *et al.*, 2004; Guerreiro *et al.*, 2007) and Alzheimer's disease (Ray *et al.*, 2007). As yet, there have been few studies of the iron status of such individuals. In one study of 582 Italian subjects aged >65 years, elevated proinflammatory markers were associated with anaemia and a low iron status, but not with higher urinary hepcidin (Ferrucci *et al.*, 2010).

12.7.3 Iron Overload and Immune Function

Two principal types of iron-overloading syndromes occur in humans, namely parenchymal iron overload (as seen in hereditary haemochromatosis) and reticuloendothelial iron loading (which is apparent in thalassaemia).

Type 1 haemochromatosis is associated with an increased susceptibility to pathogens such as *Yersinia enterocolitica* and *Vibrio vulnificus* (Wang *et al.*, 2009), as well as an abnormal innate immune response to oral infection with *S. typhimurium*. However, the low intracellular iron is likely to induce an inhibitory effect on both the *Salmonella*- and LPS-induced upregulation of the proinflammatory cytokines such as TNFα (Gordeuk *et al.*, 1992) and IL-6. This abnormal cytokine response was related to impaired TLR-4 signalling, via a reduction of a TRAM/TRIF-dependent response (Wang *et al.*, 2009). In addition, a decreased phagocytosis of erythrocyte-derived iron (decreased by 50%) as well as an increase in the release of low-molecular-weight iron (twofold increase) by comparison to control monocytes has also been reported in HH cells (Moura *et al.*, 1998). When *hfe* fails to function normally, FPN expression is elevated because of low levels of circulating hepcidin. Mice with a homozygous disruption of the *hfe* gene show low hepcidin levels, elevated macrophage FPN, and high serum and liver iron levels (Wang *et al.*, 2009). Altered responses to bacterial infection have been reported, for example when –*hfe*/–*hfe* macrophages were infected with *M. tuberculosis* there was a defect in their ability to acquire iron from exogenous transferrin and lactoferrin in comparison to macrophages similarly infected, but from normal controls (Olakanmi *et al.*, 2007), whereas HIV-1-infected macrophages (–*hfe*/–*hfe*) did not induce Nef-mediated iron and ferritin accumulation, in contrast to wild-type *hfe*-expressing macrophages (Drakesmith *et al.*, 2005). These results suggest that such *hfe*-mutated macrophages may be better equipped to protect against HIV-1 infection, thereby enhancing survival. Mice lacking both *hfe* alleles are protected from septicaemia with *S. typhimurium*, which is paralleled by an enhanced production of lipocalin-2, thereby reducing iron availability for *Salmonella* growth (Nairz *et al.*, 2009). In most studies (Roy *et al.*, 2004), *hfe*-deficient mice induced hepcidin after an LPS challenge, which was paralleled by hypoferraemia. The cytokine-induced inflammatory activation of hepcidin appears to occur independently of haemojuvelin (Niederkofler *et al.*, 2005).

Abnormalities in the relative proportions of the T lymphocyte subpopulations have been reported in HH patients, namely imbalances of the relative proportions of CD4+ and CD8+ T lymphocytes with abnormally high CD4/CD8 ratios as well as reduced percentages of CD28+ as well as functional abnormalities in CD8+ T lymphocytes (Porto and De Sousa, 2007). However, it remains unclear as to whether such changes in the numbers and functionality of these lymphocytes precede or occur after the development of iron overload. Various knockout mice models of spontaneous iron overload have been created, which show the modifying effect of components of the adaptive immune system, namely a MHC class 1-dependent effect, on the iron overload phenotype (Porto and De Sousa, 2007).

12.7.4 Thalassaemia

Infections are among the major complications in thalassaemic patients, caused by bloodborne viral infections associated with multiple transfusions, as well as defective chemotaxis and phagocytosis by neutrophils and macrophages, together with decreased killer cell activity (see Section 12.3.2, Iron overload).

12.8 Concluding Remarks

Lastly, over the past few years the importance of the gastrointestinal system and the immune system has become apparent. Immediately following birth, the gastrointestinal tract becomes colonised with a complex community of bacteria, which contributes to the development of the immune system. Under normal conditions the gut immune system is able to differentiate between innocuous antigens, including food protein and commensals, and harmful antigens such as pathogens. However in some subjects an intolerance to gluten proteins may develop (celiac disease), which results in a proinflammatory T-cell-mediated immune response with the production of anti-gluten and anti-tissue transglutaminase antibodies. This adaptive immune response, combined with the activation of innate inflammatory cells, will induce the destruction of the small intestinal mucosa (Galipeau and Verdu, 2014). Furthermore, in other clinical conditions such as alcoholic liver disease, changes in the gut flora induced by the excessive consumption of alcohol are thought to have adverse effects both on liver and brain function, with endotoxins being released into the systemic circulation. Clearly the expression, '…you are what you eat' may have wider connotations for health.

References

Barton, J.C. and Acton, R.T. (2009) Hemochromatosis and *Vibrio vulnificus* wound infections. *J. Clin. Gastroenterol.*, **43**, 890–893.

Bastida, A.-M., Ward, R.J., Piccini, P., *et al.* (2016) Brain iron chelation in Parkinson's disease patients. *Net. Comm.* (in press). Systemic inflammation influences the ability of deferiprone to chelate iron from specific brain regions in Parkinson's Disease patients. BIOIRON abstract.

Bayele, H.K., Peyssonnaux, C., Giatromanolaki, A., *et al.* (2007) HIF-1 regulates heritable variation and allele expression phenotypes of the macrophage immune response gene SLC11A1 from a Z-DNA forming microsatellite. *Blood*, **110**, 3039–3048.

Bergmann, T.K., Vinding, K. and Hey H. (2001) Multiple hepatic abscesses due to *Yersinia enterocolitica* infection secondary to primary haemochromatosis. *Scand. J. Gastroenterol.*, **36**, 891–895.

Berrak, S.G., Angaji, M., Turkkan, E., *et al.* (2007) The effects of iron deficiency on neutrophil/monocyte apoptosis in children. *Cell Prolif.*, **40**, 741–754.

Brusselle, G.G., Joos, G.F. and Bracke, K.R. (2011) New insights into the immunology of chronic obstructive pulmonary disease. *Lancet*, **378**, 1015–1026.

Cairo, G., Locati, M. and Mantivani, G. (2010) Control of iron homeostasis as a key component of macrophage polarization. *Haematologica*, **95**, 1801–1803.

Carroll, V.A. and Ashcroft, M. (2005) Targeting the molecular basis for tumour hypoxia. *Expert Rev. Mol. Med.*, **7**, 1–16.

Chan, W.Y,. Kohsaka, S. and Rezaie, P. (2007) The origin and cell lineage of microglia: new concepts. *Brain Res. Rev.*, **53**, 344–354.

Chhor, V., Le Charpentier, T., Lebon, S., *et al.* (2013) Characterization of phenotype markers and neuronotoxic potential of polarised primary microglia in vitro. *Brain Behav. Immun.*, **32**, 70–85.

Chung, S.W., Hall, S.R. and Perrella, M.A. (2009) Role of haem oxygenase-1 in microbial host defence. *Cell Microbiol.*, **11**, 199–207.

Corna, G., Campana, L., Pignatti, E., *et al.* (2010) Polarization dictates iron handling by inflammatory and alternatively activated macrophages. *Haematologica*, **295**, 1814–1822.

Cramer, T. and Johnson, R.S. (2003) A novel role for the hypoxia inducible transcription factor HIF-1alpha: critical regulation of inflammatory cell function. *Cell Cycle*, **2**, 192–193.

De Domenico, I., Ward, D.M. and Kaplan, J. (2011) Hepcidin and ferroportin: the new players in iron metabolism. *Semin. Liver Dis.*, **31**, 272–279.

Dissanayake, D.S., Kumarasiri, P.V., Nugegoda, D.B. and Dissanayake, D.M. (2009) The association of iron status with educational performance and intelligence among adolescents. *Ceylon Med. J.*, **54**, 75–79.

Drakesmith, H., Chen, N., Ledermann, H., Screaton, G., Townsend, A. and Xu X.N. (2005) HIV-1 Nef downregulates the hemochromatosis protein HFE, manipulating cellular iron homeostasis. *Proc. Natl Acad. Sci. USA*, **102**, 11017–11022.

Ekiz, C., Agaoglu, L., Karakas, Z., *et al.* (2005) The effect of iron deficiency anemia on the function of the immune system. *Hematol. J.*, **5**, 579–583.

Engelhart, M.J., Geerlings, M.I., Meijer, J., *et al.* (2004) Inflammatory proteins in plasma and the risk of dementia: the Rotterdam study. *Arch. Neurol.*, **61**, 668–672.

Ferrucci, L., Semba, R.D., Guralnik, J.M., *et al.* (2010) Proinflammatory state, hepcidin, and anemia in older persons. *Blood*, **115**, 3810–3816.

Forbes, J.R. and Gros, P. (2003) Iron, manganese and cobalt transporter by Nramp1 (Slc11a1) and Nramp2 (Slc11a2) expressed at the plasma membrane. *Blood*, **102**, 884–892.

Frank, K.M., Schneewind, O. and Shieh, W.J. (2011) Investigation of a researcher's death due to septicemic plague. *N. Engl. J. Med.*, **364**, 2563–2564.

Galipeau, H.J. and Verdu, E.F. (2014) Gut microbes and adverse food reactions: Focus on gluten-related disorders. *Gut Microbes*, **5**, 594–605.

Gimeno, D., Kivimäki, M., Brunner, E.J., *et al.* (2009) Associations of C-reactive protein and interleukin-6 with cognitive symptoms of depression: 12-year follow-up of the Whitehall II study. *Psychol. Med.*, **39**, 413–423.

Gordeuk, V.R, Ballou, S., Lozanski, G. and Brittenham, G.M. (1992) Decreased concentrations of tumor necrosis factor-alpha in supernatants of monocytes from homozygotes for hereditary hemochromatosis. *Blood*, **79**, 1855–1860.

Graeber, M.B. and Streit, W.J. (2010) Microglia: biology and pathology. *Acta Neuropathol.*, **119**, 89–105.

Guerreiro, R.J., Santana, I., Brás, J.M., *et al.* (2007) Peripheral inflammatory cytokines as biomarkers in Alzheimer's disease and mild cognitive impairment. *Neurodegen. Dis.*, **4**, 406–412.

Halterman, J.S., Kaczorowski, J.M., Aligne, C.A., *et al.* (2001) Iron deficiency and cognitive achievement among school-aged children and adolescents in the United States. *Pediatrics*, **107**, 1381–1386.

Hernandes, M.S. and Britto, L.R. (2012) NADPH oxidase and neurodegeneration. *Curr. Neuropharmacol.*, **10**, 321–327.

Iwasaki, A. and Medzhitov, R. (2004) Toll-like receptor control of the adaptive immune responses. *Nat. Immunol.*, **5**, 987–995.

Kaltschmidt, B. and Kaltschmidt, C. (2000) Constitutive NF-kappa B activity is modulated via neuron-astroglia interaction. *Exp. Brain Res.*, **130**, 100–104.

Kovtunovych, G., Ghosh, M.C., Ollivierre, W., *et al.* (2014) Wild-type macrophages reverse disease in heme oxygenase 1-deficient mice. *Blood*, **124**, 1522–1530.

Koskenkorva-Frank, T.S., Weiss, G., Koppenol, W.H. and Burckhardt, S. (2013) The complex interplay of iron metabolism, reactive oxygen species, and reactive nitrogen species: insights into the potential of various iron therapies to induce oxidative and nitrosative stress. *Free Radic. Biol. Med.*, **65**, 1174–1194.

Kreutzberg, G.W. (1996) Microglia: a sensor for pathological events in the CNS. *Trends Neurosci.*, **19**, 312–318.

Lanceta, L., Li, C., Choi, A.M. and Eaton, J.W. (2013) Haem oxygenase-1 overexpression alters intracellular iron distribution. *Biochem. J.*, **449**, 189–194.

Lee, P., Peng, H., Gelbart, T., Wang, L. and Beutler, E. (2005) Regulation of hepcidin transcription by interleukin-1 and interleukin-6. *Proc. Natl Acad. Sci. USA*, **102**, 1906–1910.

Liu, X.B., Nguyen, N.B., Marquess, K.D., Yang, F. and Haile, D.J. (2005) Regulation of hepcidin and ferroportin expression by lipopolysaccharide in splenic macrophages. *Blood Cells Mol. Dis.*, **35**, 47–56.

London, A., Cohen, M. and Schwartz, M. (2013) Microglia and monocyte-derived macrophages: functionally distinct populations that act in concert in CNS plasticity and repair. *Front. Cell Neurosci.*, **8**, 7–34.

Magaki, S., Yellon, S.M., Mueller, C. and Kirsch, W.M. (2008) Immunophenotypes in the circulation of patients with mild cognitive impairment. *J. Psychiatr. Res.*, **42**, 240–246.

McGeer, E.G. and McGeer, P.L. (1999) Brain inflammation in Alzheimer disease and the therapeutic implications. *Curr. Pharm. Des.*, **5**, 821–836.

Moura, E., Noordermeer, M.A., Verhoeven, N., Verheul, A.F. and Marx, J.J. (1998) Iron release from human monocytes after erythrophagocytosis in vitro: an investigation in normal subjects and hereditary hemochromatosis patients. *Blood*, **92**, 2511–2519.

Mullick, S., Rusia, U., Sikka, M. and Faridi, M.A. (2006) Impact of iron deficiency anaemia on T lymphocytes and their subsets in children. *Indian J. Med. Res.*, **124**, 647–654.

Murakawa, H., Bland, C.E., Willis, W.T. and Dallman, P.R. (1987) Iron deficiency and neutrophil function: different rates of correction of the depressions in oxidative burst and myeloperoxidase activity after iron treatment. *Blood*, **69**, 1464–1468.

Nairz, M., Theurl, I., Ludwiczek, S., *et al.* (2007) The co-ordinated regulation of iron homeostasis in murine macrophages limits the availability of iron for intracellular *Salmonella typhimurium*. *Cell. Microbiol.*, **9**, 2126–2140.

Nairz, M., Fritsche, G., Brunner, P., *et al.* (2008) Interferon-gamma limits the availability of iron for intramacrophage *Salmonella typhimurium*. *Eur. J. Immunol.*, **38**, 1923–1936.

Nairz, M., Theurl, I., Schroll, A., *et al.* (2009) Absence of functional Hfe protects mice from invasive *Salmonella enterica* serovar *Typhimurium* infection via induction of lipocalin-2. *Blood*, **114**, 3642–3651.

Naito, Y., Takagi, T. and Higashimura, Y. (2014) Heme oxygenase-1 and anti-inflammatory M2 macrophages. *Arch. Biochem. Biophys.*, **15** (564), 83–88.

Nemeth, E., Rivera, S., Gabayan, V., *et al.* (2004) IL-6 mediates hypoferremia of inflammation by inducing the synthesis of the iron regulatory hormone hepcidin. *J. Clin. Invest.*, **113**, 1271–1276.

Niederkofler, V., Salie, R. and Arber, S. (2005) Hemojuvelin is essential for dietary iron sensing, and its mutation leads to severe iron overload. *J. Clin. Invest.*, **115**, 2180–2186.

Okun, E., Griffioen, K.J., Lathia, J.D., *et al.*, (2009) Toll-like receptors in neurodegeneration. *Brain Res. Rev.*, **59**, 278–292.

Olakanmi, O., Schlesinger, L.S., Ahmed, A. and Britigan, B.E. (2002) Intraphagosomal *Mycobacterium tuberculosis* acquires iron from both extracellular transferrin and intracellular iron pools. Impact of interferon-gamma and hemochromatosis. *J. Biol. Chem.*, **277**, 49727–49734.

Olakanmi, O., Schlesinger, L.S. and Britigan, B.E. (2007) Hereditary hemochromatosis results in decreased iron acquisition and growth by *Mycobacterium tuberculosis* within human macrophages. *J. Leukoc. Biol.*, **81**, 195–204.

Oliveira-Junior, E.B., Bustamante, J., Newburger, P.E. and Condino-Neto, A. (2011) The human NADPH oxidase: primary and secondary defects impairing the respiratory burst function and the microbicidal ability of phagocytes. *Scand. J. Immunol.*, **73**, 420–427.

Onabanjo, O.O., Jerling, J.C., Covic, N., *et al.* (2012) Association between iron status and white blood cell counts in African schoolchildren of the North-West Province, *South Africa. J. Epidemiol. Glob. Health*, **2**, 103–110.

Oppenheimer, S.J. (2001) Iron and its relation to immunity and infectious disease. *J. Nutr.*, **131** (2S-2), 616S–633S.

Pae, H.O. and Chung, H.T. (2009) Haem oxygenase-1: its therapeutic roles in inflammatory diseases. *Immune Network*, **9**, 12–19.

Pan, X., Tamilselvam, B., Hansen, E.J. and Daefler, S. (2010) Modulation of iron homeostasis in macrophages by bacterial intracellular pathogens. *BMC Microbiol.*, **25**, 10–64.

Parkhurst, C.N. and Gan, W.B. (2010) Microglia dynamics and function in the CNS. *Curr. Opin. Neurobiol.*, **20**, 595–600.

Peyssonaux, C. and Johnson, R.S. (2004) An unexpected role for hypoxic response: oxygenation and inflammation. *Cell Cycle*, **3**, 168–171.

Peyssonnaux, C., Zinkernagel, A.S., Datta, V., *et al.* (2006) TLR4-dependent hepcidin expression by myeloid cells in response to bacterial pathogens. *Blood*, **107**, 3727–3732.

Porter, J.B. (2009) Pathophysiology of transfusional iron overload: contrasting patterns in thalassemia major and sickle cell disease. *Hemoglobin*, **33** (Suppl. 1), S37–S45.

Porto, G. and De Sousa, M. (2007) Iron overload and immunity. *World J. Gastroenterol.*, **13**, 4707–4715.

Ray, S., Britschgi, M., Herbert, C., *et al.* (2007) Classification and prediction of clinical Alzheimer's diagnosis based on plasma signaling proteins. *Nat. Med.*, **13**, 1359–1362.

Recalcati, S., Locati, M., Marini, A., *et al.* (2010) Differential regulation of iron homeostasis during human macrophage polarized activation. *Eur. J. Immunol.*, **40**, 824–835.

Roy, C.N., Custodio, A.O., de Graaf, J., *et al.* (2004) An Hfe-dependent pathway mediates hyposideremia in response to lipopolysaccharide-induced inflammation in mice. *Nat. Genet.*, **36**, 481–485.

Ruland, J. (2011) Return to homeostasis: downregulation of NF-κB responses. *Nat. Immunol.*, **12**, 709–714.

Silvestri, L., Pagani, A., Fazi, C., *et al.* (2007) Defective targeting of hemojuvelin to plasma membrane is a common pathogenetic mechanism in juvenile hemochromatosis. *Blood*, **109**, 4503–4510.

Silvestri, L., Pagani, A. and Camaschella, C. (2008) Furin-mediated release of soluble hemojuvelin: a new link between hypoxia and iron homeostasis. *Blood*, **111**, 924–931.

Simpson, R.J. and McKie, A.T. (2015) Iron and oxygen sensing: a tale of 2 interacting elements? *Metallomics*, **7**, 223–231.

Soe-Lin, S., Apte, S.S., Andriopoulos, B., Jr, *et al.* (2009) Nramp1 promotes efficient macrophage recycling of iron following erythrophagocytosis in vivo. *Proc. Natl Acad. Sci. USA*, **106**, 5960–5965.

Sow, F.B., Florence, W.C., Satoskar, A.R., *et al.* (2007) Expression and localization of hepcidin in macrophages: a role in host defense against tuberculosis. *J. Leukoc. Biol.*, **82**, 934–945.

Tacchini, L., Gammella, E., De Ponti, C., Recalcati, S. and Cairo, G. (2008) Role of HIF-1 and NF-kappaB transcription factors in the modulation of transferrin receptor by inflammatory and anti-inflammatory signals. *J. Biol. Chem.*, **283**, 20674–2086.

Techau, M.E., Valdez-Taubas, J., Popoff, J.F., *et al.* (2007) Evolution of differences in transport function in Slc11a family members. *J. Biol. Chem.*, **282**, 35646–35656.

Theurl, I., Theurl, M., Seifert, M., *et al.* (2008) Autocrine formation of hepcidin induces iron retention in human monocytes. *Blood*, **111**, 2392–2399.

van Asbeck, B.S., Marx, J.J., Struyvenberg, A. and Verhoef, J. (1984) Functional defects in phagocytic cells from patients with iron overload. *J. Infect.*, **8**, 232–240.

Vidal, S., Gros, P. and Skamene, E. (1995) Natural resistance to infection with intracellular parasites: molecular genetics identifies Nramp1 as the Bcg/Ity/Lsh locus. *J. Leukoc. Biol.*, **58**, 382–390.

Wang, L. and Cherayil, B.J. (2009) Ironing out the wrinkles in host defense: interactions between iron homeostasis and innate immunity. *J. Innate Immun.*, **1**, 455–464.

Wang, L., Harrington, L., Trebicka, E., *et al.* (2009) Selective modulation of TLR4-activated inflammatory responses by altered iron homeostasis in mice. *J. Clin. Invest.*, **119**, 3322–3328.

Ward, D.M. and Kaplan, J. (2012) Ferroportin-mediated iron transport: expression and regulation. *Biochim. Biophys. Acta*, **1823**, 1426–1433.

Ward, R.J., Wilmet, S., Legssyer, R., *et al.* (2009) Effects of marginal iron overload on iron homeostasis and immune function in alveolar macrophages isolated from pregnant and normal rats. *Biometals*, **22**, 211–223.

Ward, R.J., Crichton, R.R., Taylor, D.L., *et al.* (2011) Iron and the immune system. *J. Neural Transm.*, **118**, 315–328.

Wessling-Resnick, M. (2010) Iron homeostasis and the inflammatory response. *Annu. Rev. Nutr.*, **30**, 105–122.

Yang, F., Wang, X., Haile, D.J., Piantadosi, C.A. and Ghio, A.J. (2002) Iron increases expression of iron-export protein MTP1 in lung cells. *Am. J. Physiol. Lung Cell. Mol. Physiol.*, **283**, L932–L939.

Zhang, Y., Crichton, R.R., Boelaert, J.R., *et al.* (1998) Decreased release of nitric oxide (NO) by alveolar macrophages after in vivo loading of rats with either iron or ethanol. *Biochem. Pharmacol.*, **55**, 21–25.

13

Iron and Oxidative Stress

13.1 Oxidative Stress

13.1.1 Introduction – Milestones in the History of Life

The Belgian astronomer and cosmologist, Monsignor Georges Lemaître, professor of physics at the Université Catholique de Louvain, formulated the modern 'big bang theory' (Lemaître, 1927, 1931a, b; Berger, 1984), which holds that the universe began at least 10 billion years ago in the cataclysmic explosion of a small primeval 'super-atom'. The universe then expanded very rapidly from this state of high temperature and density, with a significant decrease in density and temperature, and about 4.5 billion years ago the Earth began to form when some of the rocks from the cloud of dust surrounding the young Sun collided. During the early stages of its formation, the Earth was subjected to bombardment by enormous rocks that were attracted by its gravitational pull. In these early stages of Earth's formation, melting would have caused denser substances to sink toward the centre of the Earth, with the consequence that the inner core of the Earth is essentially composed of iron (80%) and nickel. Indeed, as was seen in Chapter 2, iron is the most abundant element in planet Earth, and the fourth most abundant element in the Earth's crust. The first clear traces of life in the fossil record date from 3.4 billion years ago, and include microorganisms which were able to use solar energy to make sugars out of simpler molecules. Of course, what is required to convert these simpler molecules such as CO_2 into carbohydrates are electrons, together with a few protons to balance the charges. Whereas photosynthesis is classically thought of as being described by the reaction:

$$CO_2 + H_2O + h\nu \rightarrow (CH_2O) + O_2 \qquad (13.1)$$

Iron Metabolism – From Molecular Mechanisms to Clinical Consequences, Fourth Edition. Robert Crichton.
© 2016 John Wiley & Sons, Ltd. Published 2016 by John Wiley & Sons, Ltd.

these first photosynthesising organisms used sources of electrons such as H_2S, and therefore produced sulphur rather than oxygen:

$$CO_2 + 2H_2S + hv \rightarrow (CH_2O) + 2S + H_2O \tag{13.2}$$

Indeed, as Cornelis van Niel demonstrated in 1931 (van Niel, 1931, 1935), the general reaction of photosynthesis is:

$$CO_2 + 2H_2A + hv \rightarrow (CH_2O) + 2A + H_2O \tag{13.3}$$

where in the light-dependent reaction hydrogen was transferred from H_2S in green sulphur bacteria or H_2O in green plants to an unknown acceptor (called A), which was reduced to H_2A. Then, in the dark reaction, the reduced acceptor H_2A reacted with CO_2 to form carbohydrate (CH_2O) and the oxidised form of the acceptor, A. Accordingly, the equation for green plant photosynthesis [Eq. (13.1)], should be rewritten, correctly, as Eq. (13.4):

$$CO_2 + 2H_2O + hv \rightarrow (CH_2O) + O_2 + H_2O \tag{13.4}$$

This clearly contradicted the then popular (but incorrect) view that oxygen was derived from CO_2, but rather predicted that it came from H_2O. This was confirmed in 1941 in one of the very first studies with $H_2^{18}O$, by the classic experiment of Ruben *et al.* (1941). Thus, for the first half of its history, the Earth's atmosphere was essentially anaerobic.

The course of evolution was dramatically altered by the appearance of light-driven water oxidation by Photosystem II (PSII), the water-oxidising enzyme, which gradually filled the atmosphere with oxygen. PSII evolved only once in an ancestor of the phylum Cyanobacteria. However, the exact timing for the origin of oxygenic photosynthesis is debated, from shortly before the Great Oxygenation Event, which occurred 2.4 billion years ago (Kopp *et al.*, 2005; Kirschvink and Kopp, 2008; Rasmussen *et al.*, 2008) to several hundred million years prior to that (Waldbauer *et al.*, 2009; Flannery and Walter, 2012; Lyons *et al.*, 2014). Oxygenic photosynthesis involves the light-driven oxidation of water at a complex tetramanganese cluster (Mn_4CaO_5) within Photosystem II. In this reaction, four electrons are extracted from two water molecules, with the release of four protons into the thylakoid lumen and O_2 as a byproduct. All cyanobacteria discovered and studied until now have descended from a common ancestor with a photosynthetic apparatus that is already highly specialised for oxygenic photosynthesis.

Recently, the origin and evolution of water oxidation has been reconstructed at an unprecedented level of detail by studying the phylogeny of all D1 subunits, the main protein coordinating the water-oxidising cluster (Mn_4CaO_5) of PSII. The first D1 forms with a full set of ligands to the Mn_4CaO_5 cluster are grouped with D1 proteins expressed only under low oxygen concentrations, and the latest evolving form is the dominant type of D1 found in all cyanobacteria and plastids (Figure 13.1) (Cardona *et al.*, 2015).

Thus, in the space of a relatively short time – at least, as measured on a geological time scale – the previously essentially reducing atmosphere of Earth was transformed into an oxidising atmosphere, as oxygen became a dominant chemical entity. One of the consequences, clearly visible in the Precambrian deposits of red ferric Fe(III) oxides laid down in the geological strata at that time, was that iron, which was freely available in its reduced Fe^{2+} form, became much less so as the product of its oxidation, Fe^{3+}, was hydrolysed, polymerised and precipitated. At the same time, copper, which was poorly available in its reduced Cu^+ form, became much more accessible as the more water-soluble Cu^{2+}.

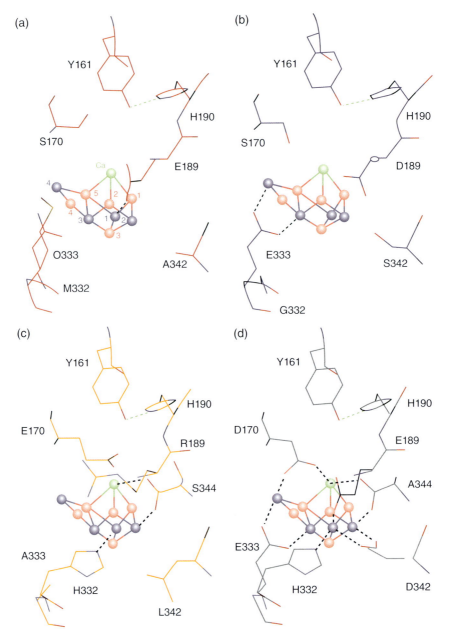

Figure 13.1 *Molecular models of the ligand sphere of the Mn_4CaO_5 cluster in the atypical D1 forms. (a) A model of the atypical D1 from G. kilaueensis, assuming that the C terminus could fold in a D1-like manner. (b) A model from a Group 1 D1 and (c) a Group 2 D1 from Synechococcus sp. PCC 7335. (d) The water-oxidising complex of Photosystem II from Thermosynechococcus vulcanus at 1.9 Å resolution. Numbers in purple and red represent the numeration for Mn and O atoms, respectively. Reprinted from Cardona, T., Murray, J.W. and Rutherford, A.W. (2015) Origin and evolution of water oxidation before the last common ancestor of the Cyanobacteria. Mol. Biol. Evol., 32, 1310–1328. This is an open access article distributed under the Creative Commons Attribution License*

13.1.2 Reactive Oxygen Species (ROS) and Reactive Nitrogen Species (RNS)

The positive side of the arrival of oxygen was that organisms which developed respiratory chains were able to extract almost 20 times more energy from metabolism than was available when using redox-balanced fermentations. However, the downside was that molecular oxygen proved to be toxic, particularly in the presence of redox active metal ions like iron and copper. Since humans live in an oxygen-rich environment, the consequence is that there is a continuous production of oxygen-derived free radicals, so-called reactive oxygen species (ROS). The interactions of iron with dioxygen and the chemistry of oxygen free radicals was discussed in detail in Chapter 1. In addition to ROS, reactive nitrogen species (RNS) are also generated. The most physiologically relevant of these include superoxide ($O_2 .^-$), nitric oxide (NO.), hydroxyl radical (HO.), carbonate radical ($CO_3 .^-$), nitrogen dioxide ($NO_2 .$), hydrogen peroxide (H_2O_2), peroxynitrite ($ONOO^-$), and hypochlorite (OCl^-) (Koskenkorva-Frank *et al.*, 2013) (Figure 13.2). Under normal conditions, the concentrations of these species are kept within a narrow range, as we will see shortly, by balancing the rate of production with the rate of removal by a cascade of enzymatic antioxidants, such as superoxide dismutase (SOD), glutathione peroxidase (GPx) and catalase, and nonenzymatic anti-oxidants such as ascorbic acid (asc; vitamin C), α-tocopherol (vitamin E), glutathione (GSH), urate, carotenoids, cysteine, bilirubin and flavonoids. However, under certain circumstances greater amounts of ROS and RNS may be produced, which may not be effectively scavenged by the cellular defence mechanisms. This is the so-called oxygen paradox – oxygen is an absolute necessity for an energy-economical anaerobic life style, yet it is a potential toxin.

Since transition metals, like iron and copper, can accept and donate single electrons they greatly facilitate the reduction of dioxygen. The first oxyradical, or ROS, to be formed from dioxygen, is the superoxide radical, O_2^-. Superoxide is not itself particularly reactive but it is the precursor of much more reactive radicals. However, it can react rapidly with nitric oxide, leading to the diffusion-controlled formation of the potent oxidising and nitrating agent peroxynitrite ($ONOO^-$). Nitric oxide (NO), a relatively stable, mildly reactive free radical, is itself generated from L-arginine,

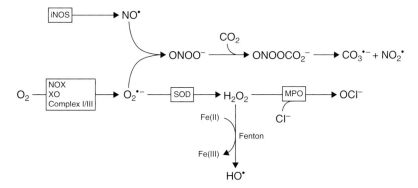

Figure 13.2 *Pathways leading to the formation of physiologically and pathologically relevant oxidants. Complex I, NADH dehydrogenase; Complex III, ubiquinol–cytochrome c reductase; iNOS, inducible nitric oxide synthase; MPO, myeloperoxidase; NOX, nicotine adenine dinucleotide phosphate oxidase; SOD, superoxide dismutase; XO, xanthine oxidase. Reprinted with permission from Elsevier from Koskenkorva-Frank, T.S., Weiss, G., Koppenol, W.H. and Burckhardt, S. (2013) The complex interplay of iron metabolism, reactive oxygen species, and reactive nitrogen species: insights into the potential of various iron therapies to induce oxidative and nitrosative stress. Free Radic. Biol. Med., **65**, 1174–1194*

NADPH and oxygen by NO synthase (NOS). The addition of a second electron to O_2^- gives the peroxide ion O_2^{2-}, which is not a free radical. At neutral pH values, O_2^{2-} will be protonated to give hydrogen peroxide, H_2O_2. The one-electron reduction of H_2O_2, the well known Fenton reaction (Fenton, 1894), gives the hydroxyl radical, OH^- [Eq. (13.5)], one of the most reactive free radical species known, which can react with a wide number of cellular constituents:

$$Fe^{2+} + H_2O_2 \rightarrow Fe^{3+} + \bullet OH + OH^- \tag{13.5}$$

It has been suggested that superoxide can then reduce Fe^{3+} to molecular oxygen and Fe^{2+}. The sum of the reaction in Eq. (13.6) plus the Fenton reaction [Eq. (13.5)] leads to the production of molecular oxygen plus hydroxyl radical and hydroxyl anion from superoxide and hydrogen peroxide [Eq. (13.3)] in the presence of catalytic amounts of iron; this is the Haber–Weiss reaction, as described by Haber and Weiss (1934), but which cannot function in the absence of trace amounts of iron.

$$Fe^{3+} + O_2^- \rightarrow Fe^{2+} + O_2 \tag{13.6}$$

$$O_2^- + H_2O_2 \rightarrow O_2 + \bullet OH + OH^- \tag{13.7}$$

However, care must be taken to avoid the pitfall of using standard redox potentials determined under equilibrium conditions, which are certainly not found within cells (Pierre *et al.*, 2002). Under physiological conditions, it may not be so easy to carry out the reaction in Eq. (13.6), particularly in competition with the rapid dismutase reaction.

ROS are produced in the course of normal metabolism by some enzyme-catalysed reactions such as xanthine oxidase and cyclooxygenases. However, the most important cellular source of free radicals (including ROS) is the electron transport chain in the mitochondria (Cadenas, 2004; Mailloux and Harper, 2011). It is generally agreed that the two major sites of mitochondrial ROS production are complexes I and III of the respiratory chain. Current methods to study and evaluate ROS have been recently reviewed (Winterbourn, 2014, and articles therein).

ROS play an important role in signal transduction and gene expression, through the activation of nuclear transcription factors. However, there are some cells in the body which use the cytotoxicity of ROS to attack and kill invading microorganisms. When macrophages and neutrophils encounter a bacterium or other foreign particle, they ingest it and internalise it within an intracellular compartment known as a *phagosome* (Figure 13.3). The multicomponent enzyme, NADPH oxidase, is then assembled within the membrane of the phagosome. Two of the subunits, p22[phox] (phox for phagocyte oxidase) and gp91[phox] (the subunit also known as NOX2), form a membrane-bound, heterodimeric flavohaemoprotein referred to as cytochrome *b* (cytochrome b_{558}). Cytochrome *b*, which was already encountered at the apical pole of the enterocyte (see Chapter 7), constitutes the catalytic part of the NADPH-oxidase (Bylund *et al.*, 2010).

Whereas NADPH oxidase (NOX) was originally thought to be associated essentially with inflammatory cells, it is currently recognised as an important enzyme system in many cell types, with a wide array of functional properties ranging from antimicrobial host defence to immune regulation and cell proliferation, differentiation and apoptosis. NOX then generates superoxide inside the phagosome, which undergoes dismutation to hydrogen peroxide, and leads to Fe^{2+}-catalysed hydroxyl radical formation. In neutrophils, the presence of myeloperoxidase allows the production of very reactive hypochlorous acid from the reaction between hydrogen peroxide and choride ions:

$$H_2O_2 + Cl^- \rightarrow HOCl + OH^- \tag{13.8}$$

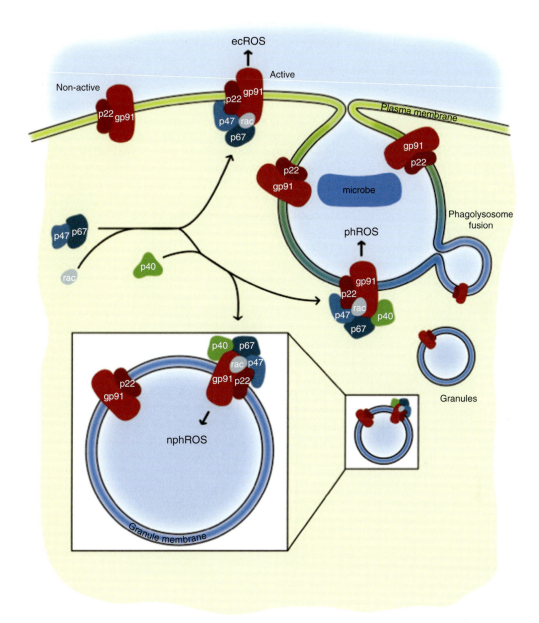

Figure 13.3 *Structure and assembly of the NADPH oxidase. Cytochrome* b *(red), consisting of gp91^{phox} (NOX2; gene name* CYBB*) and p22^{phox} (*CYBA*), resides in the plasma membrane as well as in membranes of intracellular granules. Upon activation, the cytosolic components (blue and green) p47^{phox} (NOXO2; NCF1), p67^{phox} (NOXA2; NCF2), p40^{phox} (NCF4) and Rac2 (Rac2) translocate to cytochrome* b *and form a functional NADPH oxidase. Activation of the NADPH oxidase at the plasma membrane results in extracellular release of ROS (ecROS), whereas phagosomal ROS (phROS) and nonphagosomal intracellular ROS (nphROS) are retained in the cells. The cytosolic component p40^{phox} (green) is necessary for activation of the NADPH oxidase at intracellular membranes, but dispensable at the plasma membrane. Reprinted with permission from Elsevier from Bylund, J., Brown, K.L., Movitz, C., Dahlgren, C. and Karlsson, A. (2010) Intracellular generation of superoxide by the phagocyte NADPH oxidase: how, where, and what for?* Free Radic. Biol. Med., *49, 1834–1845*

In the presence of Fe^{2+}, hypochlorous acid can also generate hydroxyl radicals:

$$Fe^{2+} + HOCl \rightarrow OH\bullet + Cl^- + Fe^{3+} \tag{13.9}$$

These activated killer cells also produce RNS in response to infection and inflammation, as described below.

Since its initial identification as an endothelial-derived relaxing factor, $NO^\bullet$ has emerged as a fundamental signalling device, regulating virtually every critical cellular function, as well as a potent mediator of cellular damage in a wide range of conditions (Pacher *et al.*, 2007). However, $NO^\bullet$ itself is unlikely to kill intracellular pathogens and tumours directly, and it has become evident that most of the cytotoxicity attributed to $NO^\bullet$ is due to the much more powerful oxidant peroxynitrite ($ONOO^-$).

$NO^\bullet$ is produced by NOS, which generates $NO^\bullet$ and citrulline from arginine in a five-electron oxidation reaction. Several different tissue-specific $NO^\bullet$ synthases are known, namely nNOS (neuronal NOS), eNOS, (endothelial NOS) and iNOS (inducible NOS). As $NO^\bullet$ diffuses very rapidly through water and across cell membranes. $NO^\bullet$ can easily diffuse from one cell to the next, and is rapidly removed by diffusion through tissues into red blood cells, where it is converted to nitrate by a reaction with oxyhaemoglobin, which limits its biological half-life *in vivo* to less than one second. The first physiological action of $NO^\bullet$ to be observed, smooth muscle relaxation, is mediated through its binding to Fe^{2+} in haemoproteins, notably soluble guanylate cyclase which forms cyclic GMP (cGMP), an intracellular second messenger. When $NO^\bullet$ reacts with guanylate cyclase to form nitrosohaem, the eNOS activity is increased some 50-fold. $NO^\bullet$ can also cause vasodilation of the cerebral arteries, since nerve impulses cause an increase in $[Ca^{2+}]$ in nerve terminals, which stimulates nNOS. The $NO^\bullet$ generated diffuses to neighbouring smooth muscle cells and acts on guanylate cyclise, as described above.

Once it has been formed, $NO^\bullet$ can diffuse and exert its effects on other cells, but it can also react to form other RNS (Figure 13.2) such as peroxynitrite, $ONOO^-$, $NO_2^\bullet$ and nitrous anhydride, N_2O_3 (Pacher *et al.*, 2007; Koskenkorva-Frank *et al.*, 2013). The latter is formed by the autoxidation of $NO^\bullet$ by molecular oxygen, and is a powerful nitrosating agent, thought to be the principal RNS responsible for nitrosative deamination of nucleobases in DNA. Another nitrogen dioxide radical, $NO_2^\bullet$, is thought to be the agent responsible for the nitration of proteins and lipids. Neutrophils produce and secrete the enzyme myeloperoxidase, and it has been proposed that myeloperoxidase can convert nitrite and peroxides to a nitrating agent for lipids and proteins.

Activated macrophages not only generate large fluxes of $NO^\bullet$ by induction of iNOS, they also concurrently produce $O_2^{\bullet-}$. While neither of these is particularly reactive, they will rapidly combine to form the much more reactive peroxynitrite, $ONOO^-$, which is a strong biological oxidant and nitrating compound:

$$NO^\bullet + O_2^{\bullet-} \rightarrow ONOO^-$$

Peroxynitrite undergoes a particularly rapid reaction with carbon dioxide (CO_2), giving rise to an unstable product (nitrosoperoxycarbonate, $ONOOCO_2^-$), which is rapidly converted into the carbonate radical ($CO_3^{\bullet-}$) and $NO_2\bullet$. The carbonate radical is probably more toxic than the hydroxyl radical and yields many of the same types of oxidation products as the hydroxyl radical (Pacher *et al.*, 2007).

13.1.3 Cellular Defence Mechanisms Against Oxidative Stress

Because of the oxidative stress caused by ROS and RNS, aerobic organisms from microbes to humans have developed systems of cytoprotection. These include cytoprotective enzymes which react directly with some of the reactive oxidants, as well as a number of low-molecular-weight antioxidant molecules present within the cell which function in a cooperative manner to scavenge ROS and RNS. The first point is to consider the enzymes (and proteins) which can react either with ROS and RNS directly, or with their products, after which the antioxidant molecules which are involved in protection against oxidative damage can briefly be considered.

The major endogenous antioxidant pathways which scavenge oxygen-derived reactive species are illustrated in Figure 13.4. Superoxide ($O^{\bullet-}$) is scavenged by superoxide dismutase (SOD), and the hydrogen peroxide (H_2O_2) product can be scavenged by the haem enzyme catalase or by one of two thiol-based systems. The glutathione (GSH) system utilises glutathione peroxidase (GPx) and GSH, and the glutathione disulphide (GSSG) is recycled by the NADPH-dependent glutathione reductase (GR). The thioredoxin (Trx) system uses peroxiredoxins (Prx) and Trx, and the oxidised Trx is recycled by the NADPH-dependent thioredoxin reductase (TR).

In the very first step of the oxygen reduction pathway, SODs intervene to transform two molecules of superoxide anion into one each of hydrogen peroxide and oxygen:

$$O_2^- + O_2^- + 2H^+ \;\rightarrow\; H_2O_2 + O_2$$

Three distinct SODs have been identified and characterised in mammalian cells (for reviews, see Zelko *et al.*, 2002; Johnson and Guilivi, 2005; Miao and St Clair, 2009; Perry *et al.*, 2010), each of which are unique and highly compartmentalised.

The first, SOD1, commonly known as Cu/Zn-SOD, is found in the cytosol in all eukaryotic species as a homodimer containing one Cu and one Zn ion per subunit. The overall fold in each subunit is described (Figure 13.5a) as an eight-stranded antiparallel β-barrel connected by three

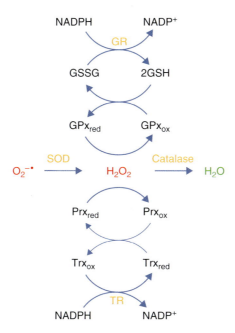

Figure 13.4 *The major endogenous antioxidant pathways which scavenge oxygen-derived reactive species. Reprinted with permission from Elsevier from Day, B.R. (2014) Antioxidant therapeutics: Pandora's box. Free Radic. Biol. Med.,* **66**, *58–64*

(a) (b)

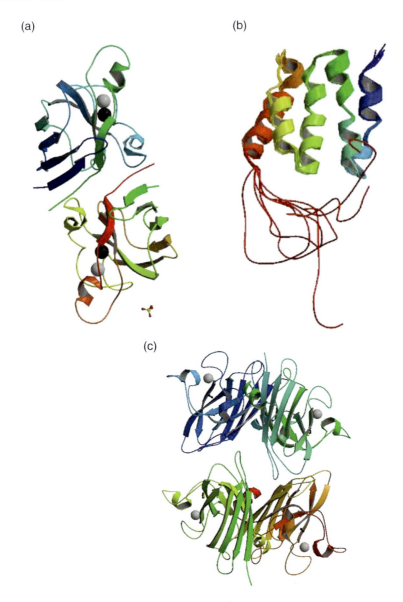

(c)

Figure 13.5 *Structures of SODs. (a) Human homodimeric SOD1 (PDB 1PU0) (DiDonato* et al.*, 2003). (b)* Saccharomyces cerevisiae *homotetrameric SOD2 (PDP 2LSU) (Sheng* et al.*, 2011). (c) Human homotetrameric SOD3 (PDP 2JLP) (Antonyuk* et al.*, 2009)*

external loops (Tainer *et al.*, 1982). The metal ions in SOD1 (Figure 13.6) are bridged by the imidazole ring of residue His63, which acts as a ligand to both metals. The Cu(II) is further coordinated to three histidine residues (46, 48 and 120) and a water molecule to form a distorted square-pyramidal geometry, while the Zn coordination is completed by a further two histidine residues (71 and 80) and an aspartate residue (83) in a distorted tetrahedral geometry (Tainer *et al.*, 1982). The synthesis of SOD1 is increased by metal ions through a metal responsive element on the *SOD1* gene (Yoo *et al.*, 1999), and the *SOD1* gene is subjected to extensive transcriptional and post- transcriptional regulation (Milani *et al.*, 2011). Dominantly inherited mutations in the human

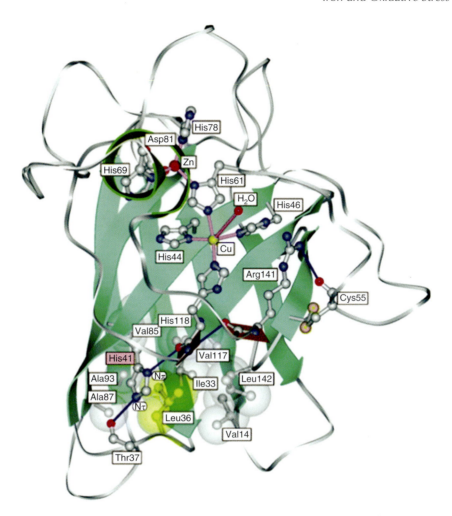

Figure 13.6 *Subunit structure of bovine superoxide dismutase (SOD) (Tainer et al., 1982). The atomic coordinates were taken from those of subunit B in the X-ray crystal structure of bovine SOD (Protein Data Bank entry 2SOD). The side chains are shown for the residues in the active site, on the rim of the active site pocket, and at an opening of the β-barrel near His41. For the hydrophobic residues closing off the β-barrel opening, transparent balls with van der Waals radii are superimposed on the ball-and-stick model. The central hydrophobic plug Leu38 is coloured yellow. Blue thin sticks represent hydrogen bonds, and brown plates represent amide planes. Reprinted with permission from Toyama, A., Takahashi, Y. and Takeuchi, H. (2004) Catalytic and structural role of a metal-free histidine residue in bovine Cu-Zn superoxide dismutase. Biochemistry,* **43***, 4670–4679; © 2004, American Chemical Society*

SOD1 gene give rise to familial forms of the fatal neurodegenerative disease amyotrophic lateral sclerosis (ALS) (Deng *et al.*, 1993; Rosen *et al.*, 1993).

The second, SOD2, or Mn-SOD, is a tetrameric manganese-containing enzyme, synthesised with a leader peptide which targets it exclusively to the mitochondria (Wispé *et al.*, 1992; Sutton *et al.*, 2003). SOD2 belongs to the highly conserved Mn/Fe-SOD family which adopts the α/β-fold (Figure 13.5b) and have either manganese or iron incorporated at the active site. The manganese or iron is invariably coordinated with a distorted trigonal bipyramidal geometry by three histidines, one aspartate and a solvent molecule (Miller, 2012). Human MnSOD is significantly more product-inhibited than bacterial MnSODs at high concentrations of superoxide (O_2^-). This behaviour limits the amount of H_2O_2 produced at high [(O_2^-)]; its desirability can be explained by the multiple roles of H_2O_2 in mammalian cells, particularly its role in signalling (*vide infra*). Transcription of the *SOD2* gene is induced by a large number of compounds, including cytokines, lipopolysaccharides and interferon-γ (Zelko *et al.*, 2002).

SOD3 is a copper- and zinc-containing tetramer, synthesised with a signal peptide which directs it exclusively to extracellular spaces, including the cerebrospinal fluid. SOD3 is highly expressed in airways and lung parenchyma, it seems to play an important protective role in blood vessel walls, and its level is markedly increased by factors which increase blood pressure. The enzyme has multiple roles including protection of the lungs against hyperoxia and the preservation of NO. The common mutation R213G, which reduces the affinity of SOD3 for heparin, is associated with an increased risk of myocardial infarction and stroke. The crystal structure of human SOD3 at 1.7 Å resolution (Antonyuk *et al.*, 2009) reveals (Figure 13.5c) that the overall subunit fold and the subunit–subunit interface of the SOD3 dimer are similar to the corresponding structures in Cu/Zn-SOD (SOD1). The core structural element containing the Cu and Zn sites is very similar to SOD1, providing a structural explanation of the almost identical turnover rates of SOD1 and SOD3 for superoxide dismutation.

The overall structures of these three families of SODs are presented in Figure 13.6. While the overall subunit fold and the active site configurations of SOD1 and SOD3 are very similar, they are quite different from SOD2. Nevertheless, despite their structural differences there are two striking mechanistic similarities (Sheng *et al.*, 2014). The first, and most obvious, is that they all contain redox-active metal ions at their active sites: $Mn^{2+/3+}$ in MnSOD, and $Cu^{1+/2+}$ in Cu/Zn-SOD1 and 3. Second, they all catalyse $O_2^{\cdot-}$ disproportionation by a very similar ping-pong mechanism, with $O_2^{\cdot-}$ acting alternately to reduce the oxidised metal ion and then to oxidise the reduced metal ion (Sheng *et al.*, 2014).

The product of the two-electron reduction of molecular oxygen, and of superoxide dismutation, hydrogen peroxide, can be metabolised to nontoxic products by catalases and by glutathione peroxidases and peroxiredoxins (Figure 13.4). Catalase, a haem enzyme which is localised within the intracellular compartment known as the peroxisome, uses H_2O_2 both as an electron donor and as an electron acceptor:

$$H_2O_2 + H_2O_2 \quad \rightarrow \quad 2H_2O + O_2$$

Gpxs are ubiquitiously expressed with particularly high levels in erythrocytes, liver and kidney (Esposito *et al.*, 2000), and mammalian cells express six human Prxs distributed in various subcellular organelles (Rhee *et al.*, 2012). In contrast, catalase is mainly found in the peroxisomes (together with Prdx1, GPX, MnSOD, Cu, ZnSOD and other ROS-decomposing enzymes) (Schrader and Fahimi, 2006), which implies that cytosolic H_2O_2 can only be scavenged by catalase after diffusing into the peroxisomes. In transgenic catalase-overexpressing mice, catalase can also be found in the cytosol and nucleus but not in the mitochondria (Zhou and Kang, 2000). An extensive analysis of tumour cell lines *in vitro* has shown that they are regularly characterised by: (i) extracellular superoxide anion generation; and (ii) the expression of membrane-associated catalase that protects the cells against intercellular ROS signaling and apoptosis (Bauer, 2014).

Whereas catalase only catalyses the dismutation of H_2O_2, both glutathione peroxidase and peroxiredoxin can also catalyse the reduction of organic hydroperoxides and of peroxynitrite (Bryk *et al.*, 2000; Sies and Arteel, 2000). Catalases and glutathione peroxidases have either a haem (catalase) or a seleno-cysteine residue (Gpx) as cofactor, and are very effective catalysts of peroxide degradation, with second-order rate constant k_{cat}/K_M values of near 10^8 and 10^7 M^{-1} s^{-1}, respectively

(Karplus, 2015). The more recently discovered peroxiredoxins have no special cofactor, but simply use cysteine residues for catalysis. Initially, their importance was underestimated because they appeared to be less efficient catalysts than catalases and glutathione peroxidases, but later studies yielded a k_{cat}/K_M value in excess of 10^7 M^{-1} s^{-1} (Peskin *et al.*, 2007; Parsonage *et al.*, 2008), a range now seen to be typical for Prxs, making it clear that their efficiencies are equivalent to catalases and Gpxs. Prxs also tend to be much more highly expressed than catalase and Gpxs. For instance in yeast, the most abundant Prx was expressed at 50-fold higher levels than the most abundant Gpx, and 500-fold higher than the most abundant catalase (Ghaemmaghami *et al.*, 2003). It has been estimated that in human cells, over 99% of the peroxide in the cytosol and over 90% of the peroxide in the mitochondria will react with peroxiredoxins rather than other enzymes or small-molecule thiols (Winterbourn and Hampton, 2008; Cox *et al.*, 2010).

The peroxiredoxins (Prxs) constitute an ancient family of enzymes which are the predominant peroxidases for nearly all organisms from archae to humans, and play an essential role in reducing hydrogen peroxide, organic hydroperoxides, and peroxynitrite (Lu and Holmgren, 2014). Prxs are single-domain proteins with a thioredoxin fold which have evolved from a thioredoxin-like ancestor (Copley *et al.*, 2004), with a common structural core containing seven central β-strands surrounded by five α-helices. The six human Prxs can be classified as 2-Cys Prx isoforms (Prx1–4), atypical 2-Cys Prx isoform (Prx5) and one 1-Cys Prx isoform (Prx6). Figure 13.7a presents the sequence alignment of human Prxs (Lu and Holmgren, 2014). As will be seen, the thioredoxin (Txr) system can transfer electrons to 2-Cys Prx isoforms and atypical 2-Cys Prx to remove hydrogen peroxide, organic hydroperoxides, and peroxynitrite (Wood *et al.*, 2003a; Rhee *et al.*, 2012). These Pxrs have two Cys residues in their active site, the N-terminal 'peroxidatic' Cys$_p$, and the C-terminal 'resolving' Cys$_R$ (Figure 13.7a).

Only four positions are highly conserved among all Prxs, and of these three are located in an eight-residue PxxxTxxC motif which makes up the loop preceding helix α2 and the first turn of the helix. The Cys in this segment is the peroxidatic Cys$_p$, and the loop is called the C$_p$-loop. The Pro and Cys are fully conserved and the Thr is occasionally placed by Ser. The fourth conserved position is an Arg, located near the beginning of strand β6. All four residues are close to one another in the fully folded peroxidatic active site (Figure 13.8a).

The catalytic mechanism involves two steps. Within the active site (Figure 13.8a) the pK_a of the Cys$_p$ is lowered to around 6 or even lower, maintaining it in the nucleophilic, thiolate state. The conformation of the enzyme which has an active site pocket ready for substrate binding is termed 'fully folded' (FF). In the first step, the thiolate Cys$_p$ attacks the peroxide substrate (Figure 13.8b) in a S_N2 nucleophilic reaction, forming a Cys-sulphenic acid (Prx-S$_p$OH) and releasing water or alcohol. Subsequently, the active site unfolds locally, which may involve as many as 35 residues (Perkins *et al.*, 2013), as illustrated in the centre of Figure 13.8b. For typical 2-Cys Prxs, this enables the C-terminal resolving Cys$_R$ in the other subunit to react with the Cys$_p$ sulphenic acid to form an intermolecular disulphide bond (Figure 13.8b). To complete the catalytic cycle, these disulphide bonds are reduced by thioredoxin (Trx) or a thioredoxin-like protein (Wood *et al.*, 2003a; Rhee *et al.*, 2005; Rhee and Woo, 2011; Jönsson *et al.*, 2007), and the Pxr is returned to the FF conformation. Whereas H_2O_2 scavenging by Prxs is very fast, with reaction rates up to 10^7–10^8 M^{-1} s^{-1}, comparable with glutathione peroxidases, haem peroxidases and catalases (Cox *et al.*, 2009; Manta *et al.*, 2009; Ogusucu *et al.*, 2007), the reaction rate between H_2O_2 and normal thiolate groups in small molecules or proteins ranges between 0.89 and 500 M^{-1} s^{-1}, even when the pK_a values of the thiol in some proteins such as thioredoxin (Trx) or protein tyrosine phosphatase 1B (PTP1B) are lower or similar to those in Prx (Winterbourn and Metodiewa, 1999; Winterbourn and Hampton, 2008). It is thought that the Arg, Pro and Thr in the active site stabilise the transition

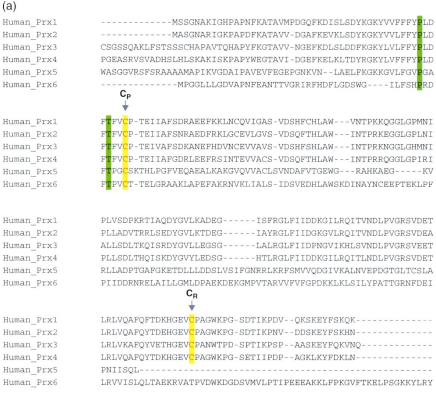

(a)

```
Human_Prx1    ------------MSSGNAKIGHPAPNFKATAVMPDGQFKDISLSDYKGKYVVFFFYPLD
Human_Prx2    ------------MASGNARIGKPAPDFKATAVV-DGAFKEVKLSDYKGKYVVLFFYPLD
Human_Prx3    CSGSSQAKLFSTSSSCHAPAVTQHAPYFKGTAVV-NGEFKDLSLDDFKGKYLVLFFYPLD
Human_Prx4    PGEASRVSVADHSLHLSKAKISKPAPYWEGTAVI-DGEFKELKLTDYRGKYLVFFFYPLD
Human_Prx5    WASGGVRSFSRAAAAMAPIKVGDAIPAVEVFEGEPGNKVN--LAELFKGKKGVLFGVPGA
Human_Prx6    --------------MPGGLLLGDVAPNFEANTTVGRIRFHDFLGDSWG----ILFSHPRD
```

C$_P$ ↓

```
Human_Prx1    FTFVCP-TEIIAFSDRAEEFKKLNCQVIGAS-VDSHFCHLAW---VNTPKKQGGLGPMNI
Human_Prx2    FTFVCP-TEIIAFSNRAEDFRKLGCEVLGVS-VDSQFTHLAW---INTPRKEGGLGPLNI
Human_Prx3    FTFVCP-TEIVAFSDKANEFHDVNCEVVAVS-VDSHFSHLAW---INTPRKNGGLGHMNI
Human_Prx4    FTFVCP-TEIIAFGDRLEEFRSINTEVVACS-VDSQFTHLAW---INTPRRQGGLGPIRI
Human_Prx5    FTPGCSKTHLPGFVEQAEALKAKGVQVVACLSVNDAFVTGEWG---RAHKAEG-----KV
Human_Prx6    FTPVCT-TELGRAAKLAPEFAKRNVKLIALS-IDSVEDHLAWSKDINAYNCEEPTEKLPF
```

```
Human_Prx1    PLVSDPKRTIAQDYGVLKADEG------ISFRGLFIIDDKGILRQITVNDLPVGRSVDET
Human_Prx2    PLLADVTRRLSEDYGVLKTDEG------IAYRGLFIIDGKGVLRQITVNDLPVGRSVDEA
Human_Prx3    ALLSDLTKQISRDYGVLLEGSG------LALRGLFIIDPNGVIKHLSVNDLPVGRSVEET
Human_Prx4    PLLSDLTHQISKDYGVYLEDSG------HTLRGLFIIDDKGILRQITLNDLPVGRSVDET
Human_Prx5    RLLADPTGAFGKETDLLLDDSLVSIFGNRRLKRFSMVVQDGIVKALNVEPDGTGLTCSLA
Human_Prx6    PIIDDRNRELAILLGMLDPAEKDEKGMPVTARVVFVFGPDKKLKLSILYPATTGRNFDEI
```

C$_R$ ↓

```
Human_Prx1    LRLVQAFQFTDKHGEVCPAGWKPG-SDTIKPDV--QKSKEYFSKQK--------------
Human_Prx2    LRLVQAFQYTDEHGEVCPAGWKPG-SDTIKPNV--DDSKEYFSKHN--------------
Human_Prx3    LRLVKAFQYVETHGEVCPANWTPD-SPTIKPSP--AASKEYFQKVNQ-------------
Human_Prx4    LRLVQAFQYTDKHGEVCPAGWKPG-SETIIPDP--AGKLKYFDKLN-------------
Human_Prx5    PNIISQL-----------------------------------------------------
Human_Prx6    LRVVISLQLTAEKRVATPVDWKDGDSVMVLPTIPEEEAKKLFPKGVFTKELPSGKKYLRY
```

(b)

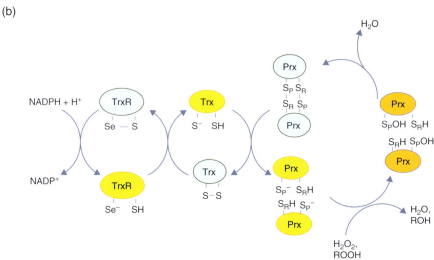

Figure 13.7 *Multiple sequence alignment of human Prxs and the reaction mechanism of typical 2-Cys peroxidase. (a) Multiple sequence alignment of six human Prxs. Protein sequences of human Prx1 (gi:13937907), Prx2 (gi:12804327), Prx3 (gi:12803699), Prx4 (gi:119619402), Prx5 (gi:109731385) and Prx6 (gi:4758638) were obtained from the PubMed Protein Database and the multiple sequence alignments were performed by ClustalW2. The conserved active site PXXXTXXC and resolving Cys$_R$ in typical 2-Cys Prxs are highlighted. (b) Scheme of reaction mechanism of typical 2-Cys peroxidase. Under neutral pH conditions, deprotonated Cys$_P$ reacts with H$_2$O$_2$ or ROOH via a nucleophilic attack to form Cys$_P$ sulphenic acid with the release of water or ROH. Then, the C-terminal resolving Cys$_R$ in the other subunit will react with Cys$_P$ sulphenic acid and form intermolecular disulphide bonds. These disulphide bonds are reduced by the Trx system to obtain the active form again. Reprinted with permission from Elsevier from Lu, J. and Holmgren, A. (2014) The thioredoxin antioxidant system.* Free Radic. Biol. Med., **66**, 75–87

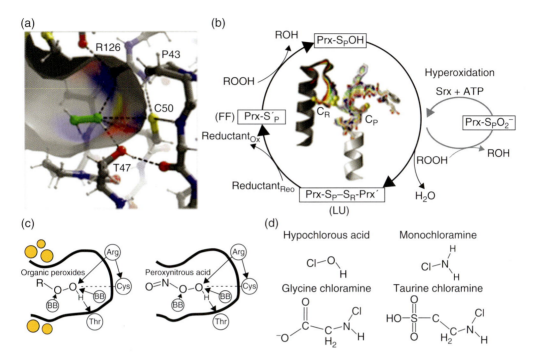

Figure 13.8 *Catalysis by peroxiredoxins. (a) Michaelis complex of peroxide (green) bound to the FF active site of ApTpx (PDB entry 3a2v) with atom colouring (grey carbons, bound to the FF active site of ApTpx (PDB entry 3a2v) with atom colouring (grey carbons, white hydrogens, yellow sulphurs, red oxygens, and blue nitrogens) showing key hydrogen bonds (dashed lines). (b) The normal Prx catalytic cycle (black) is shown along with the hyperoxidation shunt (grey). To illustrate the change in conformation necessary for Prx catalysis, the centre shows a morph between FF and LU conformations for the Prx1 subfamily member St AhpC; the C_P- and C_R-containing chains are coloured white and dark grey, respectively, and the C-terminal region beyond C_R is not shown. (c) An organic peroxide and peroxynitrous acid are shown bound to the active site in ways that mimic the interactions made by peroxide in panel (a). 'BB' refers to a backbone NH hydrogen bond donor. Placement of the hydrophobic collar seen in some organic peroxide-selective Prxs is noted by orange circles. (d) Chemical structures of some other molecules recently reported to react with Prxs (see text for details). Reprinted with permission from Perkins A., Poole, L.B. and Karplus, P.A. (2014) Tuning of peroxiredoxin catalysis for various physiological roles. Biochemistry,* **53***, 7693–7705; © 2014, American Chemical Society*

state of the reaction by forming hydrogen bonds, which explains the remarkably high catalytic efficiency of Prx (Hall *et al.*, 2010, 2011). Organic hydroperoxides and peroxynitrous acid bind to the active site in ways which mimic the interactions with peroxide (Figure 13.8c), while hypochlorous acid and chloramines can also target the thiolate of Pxrs (Figure 13.8d) (Stacey *et al.*, 2012).

The tripeptide glutathione (γ-glutamylcysteinylglycine, GSH) plays a critical role in protecting cells from oxidative damage and the toxicity of xenobiotic electrophiles, as well as in maintaining cellular redox homeostasis (Forman *et al.*, 2009). Reduced GSH is the biologically active form which is oxidised to the disulphide (GSSG) during oxidative stress, and therefore the ratio of GSH-to-GSSG is often used as a simple and convenient expression of cellular oxidative stress. GSH is present within cells at millimolar concentrations, although absolute concentrations vary considerably from tissue to tissue (Ward *et al.*, 1994). Typically, cells exhibit a high ratio of GSH-to-GSSG, with more than 90% of total GSH in the reduced form through the joint actions of cytosolic *de novo* GSH synthesis, the enzymatic reduction of GSSG (by glutathione reductase), and exogenous GSH uptake.

As seen earlier (Figure 13.4), there are two major thiol-dependent antioxidant systems in mammalian cells, the GSH and the thioredoxin (Trx) antioxidant systems. GSH is the most abundant nonprotein thiol in mammalian cells, while thioredoxins are ubiquitous 12-kDa reductases distributed from archae and bacteria to humans, which catalyse protein disulphide/dithiol-exchange. The structure of Txrs consists of a central core of five β-strands surrounded by α-helices, with the active site disulphide located after β-sheet 2, forming the N-terminal portion of α-helix 2 (Eklund *et al.*, 1991). Many of the enzymes involved in the thiol-dependent antioxidant systems have the thioredoxin fold, including glutathione peroxidase (Epp *et al.*, 1983), peroxiredoxin (Wood *et al.*, 2003b) and glutaredoxin (Fernandes and Holmgren, 2004).

Mammalian cells have two Trx systems, the cytosolic/nuclear Trx1 and the mitochondrial Trx2 (Figure 13.9). The GSH and Trx systems probably evolved very early in aerobic organisms, and both systems are based on common sulphur biochemistry. They therefore require: (i) an electron relay, linking the universal reducing agent NADPH to thiol/disulphide-metabolism; and (ii) a thiol-containing adapter molecule to transfer electrons to a set of different acceptors (Deponte, 2013). Flavoproteins are widely used as electron relays, and reducing equivalents from NADPH enter the GSH/Txr systems via the homodimeric flavoprotein enzymes glutathione reductase (GR) (Schultz *et al.*, 1978; Karplus and Schultz, 1989) and thioredoxin reductase (TrxR) (Muller, 1996; Kanzok *et al.*, 2001; Marty *et al.*, 2009; Buchholz *et al.*, 2010; Tan *et al.*, 2010). While the overall structures of mammalian Txrs are similar to GR (Zhong *et al.*, 2000; Cheng *et al.*, 2009), they have in addition a C-terminal extension sequence containing a selenocysteine (Cheng *et al.*, 2009).

In the cytosol and the nucleus (Figure 13.9a), Trx1 provides electrons to thioredoxin-dependent peroxiredoxins (Prx1 and 2), and GSH provides electrons to glutathione peroxidase, both of which can efficiently remove ROS/RNS. Both, Trx1 and glutaredoxin (Grx1) can reduce ribonucleotide reductase (RNR), while GSH and Grx1 can reduce glutathionated proteins (P-SSG). In addition, Trx1 reduces methionine sulphoxide reductases, is involved in the repair of oxidised proteins, and regulates the activities of many oxidative-sensitive transcription factors such as NF-κB, Nrf-2, and P53 (Txr1 is thus involved in redox signaling; see next section). The GSH system can serve as a backup system to reduce thioredoxin when the electron transfer pathway from TrxR1 is blocked.

In the mitochondrion (Figure 13.9b), Trx2 and Grx2 supply electrons to Prx3, GSH does likewise to GPx1 and 4, which remove H_2O_2, ROOH and ONOO⁻, and both GSH and Grx2 reduce glutathionated proteins (P-SSG). Mitochondrial Grx2 can be reduced by mitochondrial TrxR2 and GSH. The rapid removal of ROS by Prxs and GPxs are represented by thick black lines in Figure 13.9.

A steady supply of NADPH is necessary to protect cells against oxidative stress, and in mammalian cells the source of NADPH is the pentose phosphate pathway. The first enzyme of this pathway is glucose-6-phosphate dehydrogenase (G6PD), and congenital defects in G6PD, the most common genetic disease in humans, result in an increased sensitivity to oxidative stress. Both, the synthesis of intracellular GSH and of pentose phosphate pathway enzymes are increased under conditions of oxidative stress, and the effectiveness of this response will, to a large extent, determine the capacity of the cell to protect itself from ROS toxicity.

Haem oxygenase (HO; as seen in Chapter 8) catalyses the oxygenation of haem to Fe^{2+}, carbon monoxide and biliverdin, which is converted into bilirubin, requiring large amounts of reducing equivalents, in the form of NADPH, and O_2. Its activation reduces oxidative stress in cells and inhibits inflammation (Barañano and Snyder, 2001), due to the removal of haem and because of the biological activity of the bilirubin and biliverdin products, despite the concomitant production of Fe^{2+}, potentially capable of participating in Fenton chemistry to produce hydroxyl radicals. In

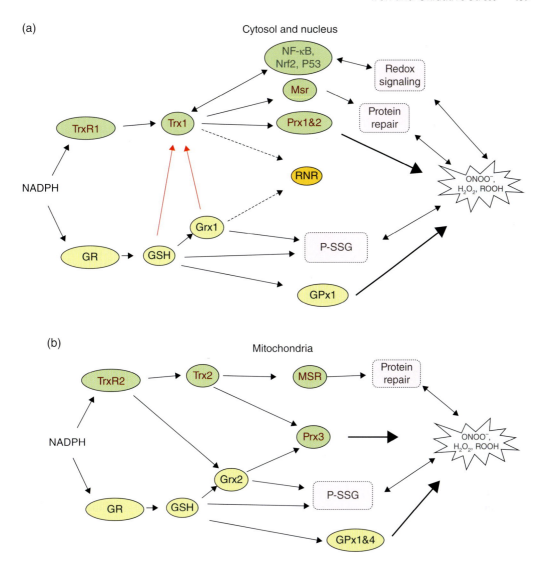

Figure 13.9 *Thioredoxin (Trx) and glutathione (GSH) systems are the two major thiol-dependent antioxidant systems in mammalian cells. (a) Mammalian thiol-dependent redox system in cytosol, nucleus. The Trx system provides the electrons to Trx-dependent peroxireductases (Prx1&2), which can efficiently remove ROS as glutathione peroxidase (GPx1). Moreover, Trx reduces methionine sulphoxide reductases and is involved in the repair of oxidised proteins. Trx regulates the activities of many oxidative-sensitive transcription factors such as NF-κB, Nrf-2 and P53, and thus is involved in the redox signalling. The GSH system can serve as a backup to reduce Trx when the electron transfer pathway from TrxR1 is blocked. (b) Mammalian mitochondria thiol-dependent redox systems. Mitochondrial Grx2 can be reduced by mitochondria TrxR2 and GSH. Mitochondrial Prx3 can be reduced by both mitochondrial Trx2 and Grx2. The thick black lines represent the direct reaction between the protein and ROS in a fast reaction rate. Reprinted with permission from Elsevier from Lu, J. and Holmgren, A. (2014) The thioredoxin antioxidant system. Free Radic. Biol. Med.,* **66**, *75–87*

addition, CO may act similarly to NO, activating soluble guanylate cyclase (Grochot-Przeczek *et al.*, 2012) and elevating cGMP production, causing smooth muscle relaxation. There are two haem oxygenases in humans, both of which are thought to be cytoprotective (Barañano and Snyder, 2001). HO1 is found at high levels in spleen, where senescent and abnormal red blood cells are destroyed in the liver. Its transcription can be induced by transition metal ions and by oxidative stress. In contrast, HO2 is constitutively expressed at high levels in some regions of the brain, where the bilirubin and biliverdin so formed could exert a neuroprotective effect. Like NO, the CO produced by neuronal HO2 can stimulate guanylate cyclase and cause smooth muscle relaxation. CO is a neurotransmitter in the brain and in the peripheral autonomic nervous system (Barañano and Snyder, 2001). In order to function as a gaseous neurotransmitter, CO must be synthesised rapidly following neuronal depolarisation. It has been shown that this can be achieved by the activation of HO2 during neuronal stimulation by Ca^{2+}-dependent phosphorylation by CK2 (formerly casein kinase 2) in several model systems (Boehning *et al.*, 2003).

While it is likely that the major role in antioxidant defence is fulfilled by antioxidant enzymes (Sies, 2015), there are a number of low-molecular-weight antioxidants which can react directly with some of the products of oxidative damage (Chaudiere and Ferrari-Iliou, 1999). The hydrophobic scavengers β-carotene (a precursor of vitamin A) and α-tocopherol (vitamin E) are found in lipoproteins and membranes, where they either interrupt the propagation step of lipid peroxidation (Halliwell and Chirico, 1993) by destroying peroxyl radicals ROO·, or block the formation of hydroperoxides from singlet oxygen $^1O_2$. Vitamin E (α-tocopherol) is the most efficient scavenger of peroxyl radicals in phospholipid bilayers, its antioxidant advantage being reinforced by the fact that it is preferentially incorporated by means of specific transport proteins (Murphy and Mavis, 1981; Sato *et al.*, 1991). α-tocopherol scavenges lipid peroxyl radicals LOO· through hydrogen atom transfer (Burton and Ingold, 1981).

In contrast to these two hydrophobic vitamins, which are found in proximity to membranes, ascorbate (vitamin C) is water-soluble and is thought to be capable of regenerating α-tocopherol (McCay, 1985) from its radical form. Figure 13.10 illustrates the cooperative interactions between vitamin E, vitamin C, GSH and glutathione peroxidase(s), and their metabolic coupling to NADPH-generating pathways. There are a number of other molecules which have been reported to have antioxidant properties including, as seen above, bilirubin and biliverdin derived from haem breakdown, uric acid, the end product of the degradation of nucleic acid purine bases, and many more.

13.1.4 Role of ROS and RNS in Cell Signalling

There are a large number of intracellular signalling pathways, responsible for transmitting information within the cell. The majority respond to external stimuli which arrive at the cell membrane, often in the form of a chemical signal (growth factor, hormone, neurotransmitter) which, upon binding to a receptor, transfers the information across the membrane via a variety of transducers and amplification cascades to trigger the activation/deactivation of diverse intracellular pathways. There are also a number of signalling pathways which are activated by signals generated within the cell to initiate a variety of signalling pathways. GTP-binding proteins often play a central role in the transduction process responsible for initiating many of these signalling pathways (Berridge, 2014), as do conformational changes induced by altering the charge of proteins, either by phosphorylation/dephosphorylation via kinases/phosphatases, or by Ca^{2+}- binding.

As will be seen shortly, most living organisms have a system of defences which is both elaborate and redundant to protect them from the potential damage that can be inflicted by both ROS and RNS. However, during the past few decades it has become clear that, whereas high levels of ROS

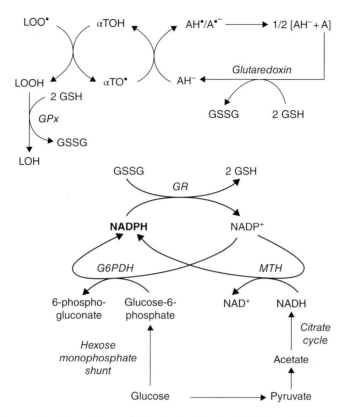

Figure 13.10 *Cooperative interactions of vitamin E, vitamin C, GSH and glutathione peroxidase(s), and their metabolic coupling to NADPH-generating pathways. The phenoxyl radical (αTO•) produced upon scavenging of lipid peroxyl radicals (LOO•) is reduced back to α-tocopherol (αTOH) by ascorbate (AH⁻) at the membrane/water interface. This mechanism of free radical translocation takes advantage of the spontaneous dismutation of the ascorbyl radical (AH•/A•⁻) into non-radical species. Hydroperoxide degradation by PHGPx or another glutathione peroxidase, and ascorbate regeneration by glutaredoxin, both produce GSSG, which is reduced back to GSH by NADPH-dependent glutathione reductase. There are other possible cooperative schemes, but the antioxidant protection generally relies on cytosolic and mitochondrial pathways of NADPH production. Reprinted with permission from Elsevier from Chaudiere, J. and Ferrari-Iliou, R. (1999). Intracellular antioxidants: from chemical to biochemical mechanisms.* Food Chem. Toxicol., **37**, 949–962

and RNS have deleterious effects (catalysing pathways which result in essentially irreversible modifications of amino acid residues in proteins), at low concentrations they can play an important signalling role in the control of cellular function by responding to changes in the intracellular redox potential. Research conducted during the past two decades has provided evidence for the existence of an extensive intracellular redox signalling, control and feedback network based on different cysteine-containing proteins and enzymes (Janssen-Heininger *et al.*, 2008: Klomsiri *et al.*, 2011; Holmstrom and Finkel, 2014). Together, these proteins enable the living cell to sense and respond towards external and internal redox changes in a measured, gradual, and reversible manner. The chemical basis of this crucial regulatory 'thiolstat' is the post-translational modification of protein cysteine residues.

These signalling oxidants can function as second messengers in intracellular signalling, sensing redox changes through reversible covalent modifications of the cysteine residues of proteins by ROS and RNS, notably hydrogen peroxide (H_2O_2) and nitric oxide (NO•). Modification of redox-sensitive amino acid residues as a means of regulating protein function is comparable to other posttranslational modifications, such as the phosphorylation and Ca^{2+} binding referred to above.

Known cysteine modifications (Figure 13.11) include the formation/reduction of disulphide bonds, S-nitrosylation, S-glutathionylation, as well as sulphenic acid or sulphinic acid formation.

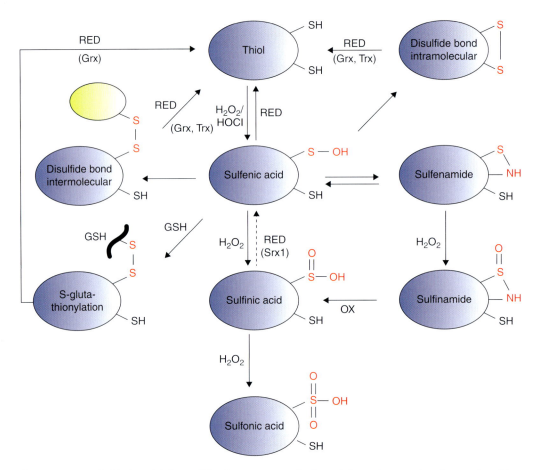

Figure 13.11 *Oxidative thiol modifications commonly found in redox-regulated proteins. Upon reaction with peroxide (H_2O_2) or hypochlorous acid (HOCl), redox-sensitive thiol groups (RSH) rapidly form sulphenic acids (RSOH). These sulphenates are highly reactive and tend to quickly react with nearby cysteine thiols to form inter- or intramolecular disulphide bonds (RSSR). Alternatively, they form mixed disulphides with the small tripeptide glutathione (GSH) (RSSG), or undergo cyclic sulphenamide formation (RSNHR). These oxidative thiol modifications are fully reversible, and reduction (RED) is catalysed by members of the glutaredoxin (Grx) or thioredoxin (Trx) system. Further oxidation of sulphenic acid to sulphinic acid (RSO_2H), sulphinamide (RSONHR) or sulphonic acid (RSO_3H) is irreversible. One exception is the active site sulphinic acid in peroxiredoxin, whose reduction is mediated by the highly specialised ATP-dependent sulphiredoxin Srx1. Reprinted with permission from Elsevier from Groitl, B. and Jakob, U. (2014) Thiol-based redox switches. Biochim. Biophys. Acta, **1844**, 1335–1343*

Upon reaction with peroxide (H_2O_2) or hypochlorous acid (HOCl), redox-sensitive thiol groups rapidly form sulphenic acids. These sulphenates are highly reactive and tend to quickly react with nearby cysteine thiols to form inter- or intramolecular disulphide bonds. Alternatively, they form mixed disulphides with the small tripeptide GSH, or undergo cyclic sulphenamide formation. These oxidative thiol modifications are fully reversible, and reduction can be catalyzed by members of the glutaredoxin or thioredoxin system. Further oxidation of sulphenic acid to sulphinic acid, sulphinamide or sulphonic acid is irreversible. One exception is the active site sulphinic acid in peroxiredoxin, whose reduction is mediated by the highly specialised ATP-dependent sulphiredoxin Srx1 (Rhee *et al.*, 2007).

Thus, physiological levels of ROS and RNS production can lead to alterations in cellular and extracellular redox state, and such subtle changes in redox balance can signal changes in numerous cellular processes, including gene expression (activation of certain nuclear transcription factors), and even determine the ultimate death of the cell by apoptosis or necrosis. As awareness of this dual character of ROS and RNS has grown, from uniquely causing oxidative damage towards involvement in metabolic responses to oxidative stress, the view has developed that whereas signalling mechanisms involve hydrogen peroxide (H_2O_2), or other two-electron electron oxidants (Forman *et al.*, 2010), free radicals are responsible for oxidative damage. It has been recently suggested that free radicals may also be involved in redox signalling (Winterbourn, 2015).

Redox signalling can be defined as a cellular response to an oxidant or to an alteration in redox status which leads to a variety of downstream effects on cell function, and can be broadly classified into two types: (i) a stress response to excessive production of or exposure to an oxidant; or (ii) a response to a receptor agonist such as a growth factor, hormone, or cytokine, that activates the cells to produce one or more ROS (Winterbourn, 2015).

In the case of thiol-based redox signalling, the consensus (Janssen-Heininger *et al.*, 2008; Winterbourn and Hampton, 2008; Forman *et al.*, 2010; Holmstrom and Finkel, 2014; Marinho *et al.*, 2014; Winterbourn, 2015) is that, regardless of the initiating event, the ultimate oxidant in receptor-mediated signalling is H_2O_2, which acts as a second messenger to transmit the signal. Signal transmission occurs by the reversible oxidation of selected thiol proteins, impacting on phosphorylation pathways and, depending on the signal, altering gene transcription, cytoskeletal organisation, ion channel activity and other cell functions. In order to achieve specificity, oxidant production is localised in the cell, and transmission of the signal occurs locally.

Before considering the reactivity of thiol groups in proteins towards H_2O_2, it must be emphasised that the peroxide-metabolising enzymes (catalase, glutathione peroxidase) and the peroxiredoxins maintain endogenous concentrations of H_2O_2 in the submicromolar range. This is the range within which redox signalling must operate, whereas at higher concentrations, oxidative stress responses intervene (Winterbourn and Hampton, 2008). However, while H_2O_2 is a strong oxidising agent on account of its high redox potential, most of its reactions have high activation energy and are slow. The most favourable reactions of H_2O_2 are with transition metals, such as iron or copper, while metalloproteins such as haem catalases and peroxidases, cytochromes, Fe–S clusters and other non-haem iron proteins (Jang and Imlay, 2007; Imlay, 2008; Davies *et al.*, 2008; Landry and Ding, 2014) react faster than most thiol proteins (Winterbourn, 2015). Furthermore, H_2O_2 reacts exclusively with the thiolate anion, and therefore the pK_a of the cysteine thiol determines to a large degree its reactivity towards H_2O_2, although it is not the sole determinant of H_2O_2 reactivity.

Thus, only proteins with very high reactivity (Winterbourn and Hampton, 2008; Hall *et al.*, 2009; Rhee *et al.*, 2012) are likely to be direct targets for H_2O_2, whereas other more modestly reactive thiol proteins are more likely to be oxidised by an indirect mechanism (Winterbourn and Hampton, 2008). The most straightforward mechanism for activating a redox signalling pathway would be for the oxidant (H_2O_2) to react directly with the regulatory protein to switch its activity on or off. However, as pointed out above, the redox-active thiol proteins in signalling pathways, including tyrosine phosphatases and transcription factors, are up to a million times less reactive with H_2O_2 than the Prxs and glutathione peroxidases that are abundantly present in cells. An alternative would be to utilise the highly reactive thiol peroxidases as sensors which could react with H_2O_2 and subsequently transfer oxidising equivalents to the less-reactive regulatory proteins (Winterbourn and Hampton, 2008; Winterbourn, 2008). A very recent study (Sobotta *et al.*, 2015) describes a relay system involving Prx 2 as a peroxide sensor which oxidises the mammalian transcription factor STAT3 via a mixed disulphide intermediate. This provides an attractive mechanism for overcoming the need for highly reactive targets while ensuring specificity through protein–protein interactions with individual thiol peroxidases, and a search for other interacting proteins may now reveal whether redox relays have a major role in signal transduction.

Some examples of non-oxidative-stress-related peroxide signalling are illustrated in Figure 13.12 (Perkins *et al.*, 2014). The binding of growth factors to their cognate receptors leads to the activation of oxidases which produces superoxide, and this is subsequently converted to peroxide. Certain aquaporins have been shown to facilitate the entry of peroxide into the cell (Sies, 2014) where kinases, phosphatases and transcription factors (Giorgio *et al.*, 2007; Wood *et al.*, 2003a) can be oxidatively activated or inactivated (Sies, 2014). Active peroxiredoxin (Prxs) degrades these peroxides; it can also be inactivated by hyperperoxidation, and the hyperperoxidised Prxs can be reactivated by sulphiredoxin (Srx). Two other examples of peroxide signalling are illustrated in Figure 13.12, LPA-mediated signalling (Klomsiri *et al.*, 2014) and murine adrenal corticosteroid production (Kil *et al.*, 2012).

Lysophosphatidic acid (LPA) is a growth factor for many cells which stimulates the H_2O_2 production required for growth, and the widespread expression of LPA receptors and their coupling to several classes of G-proteins enables LPA-dependent regulation of numerous processes, such as vascular development, neurogenesis, wound healing, immunity and cancerogenesis. These include many of the hallmarks of cancer, including cellular processes such as proliferation, survival, migration, invasion and neovascularisation. LPA (Figure 13.12) stimulation results in the binding of LPA to the extracellular portion of the LPA receptor (LPA1), leading to the recruitment of G-proteins to the receptor and costimulation of NADPH oxidase (NOX) through association of cytosolic organiser and activator proteins (step 1 in Figure 13.12). Together, activated LPA receptor and Nox complexes are internalised (step 2), and superoxide is produced by Nox inside the endosome (step 3). H_2O_2 generated by the spontaneous or enzyme-catalysed dismutation of superoxide can diffuse out of the endosome and then oxidise thiolate (R-S^-)-containing proteins within or near the endosomes to sulphenic acid (R-SOH).

In murine adrenal corticosteroid production (Kil *et al.*, 2012), the binding of ACTH to its receptor leads to activation of the cAMP-PKA pathway, and then to phosphorylation and activation of steriodogenic acute regulatory protein (StAR). StAR makes cholesterol available for conversion via 11-deoxy corticosterone to corticosterone (CS). H_2O_2 is generated during CS production, and since PrxIII is by far the most important H_2O_2-eliminating enzyme in the mitochondria of the adrenal cortex, the H_2O_2 is eliminated. During the course of the reaction two reduced PrxIII subunits (PrxIII-SH) are converted to a disulphide-linked dimer (PrxIII-S–S-PrxIII), which is then reduced back to PrxIII-SH by thioredoxin 2 (Trx2). However, during catalysis PrxIII is occasionally hyperoxidised to sulphinic PrxIII (PrxIII-SO$_2$), and becomes inactivated. This hyperoxidation is reversed by Srx. The fraction of PrxIII molecules that undergo hyperoxidation is low, but proportional to the number of H_2O_2 molecules reduced by the enzyme. In the early stages of ACTH stimulation, the level of sulphinic PrxIII does not increase substantially above the basal level because the activity of Srx in mitochondria is sufficient to counteract the low level of hyperoxidation. At a later stage

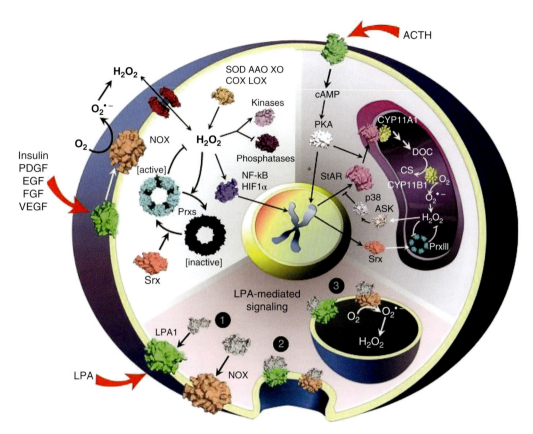

Figure 13.12 *Examples of peroxide signalling. The white panel (left) shows a general scheme of growth factor-triggered signalling. Binding of growth factors to receptors (green) leads to the activation of oxidases (orange) producing superoxide, which is subsequently converted to peroxide. Certain aquaporins (dark red) facilitate the entry of peroxide into the cell (Sies, 2014) where kinases (light purple), phosphatases (dark purple) and transcription factors (Giorgio et al., 2007; Wood et al., 2003a) (dark blue) can be oxidatively activated or inactivated (Sies, 2014). Active peroxiredoxin (Prxs) (cyan toroid) degrades these peroxides; it can also be inactivated by hyperperoxidation (dark toroid), and the hyperperoxidised Prxs can be reactivated by sulphiredoxin (Srx). The magenta and purple panels illustrate other examples of peroxide signalling. In LPA-mediated signalling (Klomsiri et al., 2014) (magenta, bottom), binding of LPA to its receptor (green) activates NADPH oxidase (NOX, orange), and through endocytosis, a 'reductosome' is formed. Superoxide/peroxide accumulates in the reductosome, and it serves as a hub for modifying regulatory factors. In murine adrenal corticosteroid production (Angelucci et al., 2013) (purple, top right), binding of ACTH to its receptor (green) leads to activation of the cAMP-PKA pathway (the transcription factor cAMP response element-binding protein is denoted by *) and then to phosphorylation and activation of steriodogenic acute regulatory protein (StAR). StAR makes cholesterol available for conversion via 11-deoxy corticosterone to corticosterone (CS), in the process producing superoxide which is converted to peroxide by SOD, which inactivates PrxIII. After further build-up of peroxide, a negative feedback loop activates p38, which in turn suppresses the synthesis of StAR. Reprinted with permission from Perkins A., Poole, L.B. and Karplus, P.A. (2014) Tuning of peroxiredoxin catalysis for various physiological roles. Biochemistry,* **53***, 7693–7705; © 2014, American Chemical Society*

of such stimulation, when CS synthesis is increased, H_2O_2 production also increases and is followed by an increase in the level of PrxIII hyperoxidation. The capacity of Srx in mitochondria is now no longer sufficient to counteract this increased hyperoxidation, and this results in an accumulation of inactive PrxIII and the consequent build-up of H_2O_2 in mitochondria and its overflow into the cytosol, where it triggers the phosphorylation of p38 by activating ASK1. Phosphorylated (activated) p38 inhibits StAR synthesis through an unknown mechanism, resulting in a downregulation of the production of CS.

The initial biological effect of NO• was thought to be mediated by the binding of NO• to the haem moiety of guanylate cyclase, thereby activating the enzyme and releasing cyclic GMP to induce vasodilation (Nakamura *et al.*, 2013; Hess *et al.*, 2005). The resulting activation of cGMP-dependent kinases was then found to trigger a multitude of other signalling events through protein phosphorylation (Murad, 2006). Subsequently, it was found that S-nitrosylation, the post-translational modification of cysteines by species derived from NO•, affects protein activity and stability, protein–protein interactions, and protein trafficking and location in bacteria, plants and mammals (Nakamura *et al.*, 2013, Seth *et al.*, 2012; Yun *et al.*, 2011). In many ways, S-nitrosylation serves as a post-translational modification reminiscent of phosphorylation or acetylation and, in fact, may be even more ubiquitous (Gould *et al.*, 2013; Jia *et al.*, 2014), and S-nitrosylation has emerged as a major mechanism for the signalling actions of NO. The chemistry involved in the formation of *S*-nitrosocysteine *in vivo* remains uncertain (Gould *et al.*, 2013). Although the source of NO is primarily enzymatic, the formation of *S*-nitrosocysteine includes cysteine oxidation, metal catalysis, exchange reactions with low-molecular-weight thiols such as *S*-nitrosoglutathione (GSNO), or transnitrosation reactions between proteins, principally by *S*-nitrosothioredoxin (Mitchell and Marletta, 2005; Mitchell *et al.*, 2007). For reviews on the chemistry of *S*-nitrosocysteine formation, see Hess *et al.* (2005), Zhang and Hogg (2005), Seth and Stamler (2011) and Smith and Marletta (2012).

Peroxynitrite also behaves as a potent modulator of a number of cell signal transduction pathways (Liaudet *et al.*, 2009). Because both peroxynitrite and its downstream products have the capacity to nitrate tyrosine residues, peroxynitrite particularly affects cellular processes involving tyrosine phosphorylation. By modulating the activity of various kinases and phosphatases, this affects the regulation of key signalling pathways for cardiovascular homeostasis, including protein kinases B and C, MAP (mitogen-activated protein) kinases, nuclear factor kappa B (NF-κB), as well as signalling dependent on insulin and the sympatho-adrenergic system (Pacher *et al.*, 2007).

13.1.5   ROS, RNS and Oxidative Damage

Reactive oxygen species are constantly generated inside cells, and as has been seen, there are several cellular systems that lead to their elimination. Nonetheless, endogenous and exogenous triggers can cause the overproduction of ROS or impairment of the antioxidant defence systems, leading to a deleterious condition known as 'oxidative stress' which is associated with the oxidative modification of DNA, carbohydrates, proteins and lipids, This concept of 'oxidative stress' in redox biology and medicine, which was first formulated in 1985, generated approximately 138 000 PubMed entries at the beginning of 2015 (Sies, 2015). While the adaptive upregulation of defence systems can protect against damage, either completely or partially, oxidative-stress-mediated damage to all types of biological macromolecules often leads to tissue injury, and eventually to cell death by necrosis or apoptosis (Dalle-Donne *et al.*, 2003) (Figure 13.13). There is growing evidence (as will be seen in Chapter 15) that both ROS and RNS are involved in a great number of neurodegenerative pathologies.

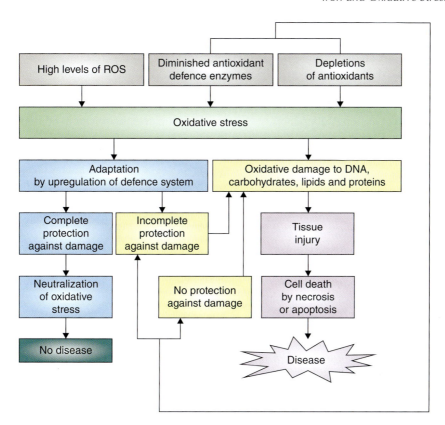

Figure 13.13 *Origins and consequences of oxidative stress in disease. Reactive oxygen species (ROS) are constantly generated inside cells by oxidase enzymes and by dismutation of the superoxide anion, and their intended functions range from host defence to signal transduction. There are several cellular systems that eliminate ROS, thereby balancing the ratio between generation and detoxification of ROS, including antioxidant enzymes such as catalases, superoxide dismutases, peroxiredoxins and glutathione peroxidases, and low-molecular-weight compounds such as vitamin E (α-tocopherol), vitamin C (ascorbic acid) and glutathione. However, endogenous and exogenous triggers can cause the overproduction of ROS or the impairment of antioxidant defence systems, leading to a deleterious condition known as 'oxidative stress'. Adaptive upregulation of defence systems can protect against damage, either completely or partially, but oxidative-stress-mediated damage to all types of biological macromolecules often leads to tissue injury, and eventually to cell death by necrosis or apoptosis. Reprinted with permission from Elsevier from Dalle-Donne, I., Giustarini, D., Colombo, R., Rossi, R. and Milzani, A. (2003) Protein carbonylation in human diseases.* Trends Mol. Med., **9**, *169–176*

Proteins are major targets of ROS and RNS, and numerous reversible or irreversible modifications have been characterised which may lead to changes in the structure and/or function of the oxidised protein. The oxidation of methionine to its sulphoxide, and of cysteine to sulphenic, sulphinic and sulphonic acids, can often be reversed (with the exception of sulphonic acids) by enzymatic reduction. The oxidative modification of proteins can result either from a direct oxidation of amino acid residues or through the formation of reactive intermediates derived from the oxidation of other cellular components. A significant portion of ROS-induced post-translational modifications result in the addition of reactive carbonyl functional groups on proteins, generically termed 'protein carbonylation' (Dalle-Donne *et al.*, 2003; Nyström, 2005; Aldini *et al.*, 2006; Grimsrud *et al.*, 2008).

Carbonyl groups are generated during lipid peroxidation, and can react with the sulphydryl group of cysteine, the ε-amino group of lysine or the imidazole group of histidine residues, forming advanced lipoxidation end products (ALEs). They can also be produced by the reaction of reducing sugars or their oxidation products with lysine residues of proteins, leading to the formation of advanced glycation end products (AGEs) or from oxidative modification of amino acids in proteins. ALEs and AGEs have a pathogenetic role in the development and progression of different oxidative-based diseases including diabetes, atherosclerosis and neurological disorders (Vistoli *et al.*, 2013). The various ways in which protein carbonyls can be generated are outlined schematically in Figure 13.14. Protein carbonylation ultimately results in protein conformational changes, misfolding and the formation of aggregates, often with amyloid-like extended β-sheet structures.

ROS production by redox metals such as iron and copper in proximity to membrane phospholipids initiates the peroxidation of polyunsaturated fatty acids (PUFAs) and of less-susceptible monounsaturated fatty acids (MUFAs). This oxidative event is reversible through reduction by peroxiredoxin and glutathione peroxidase, as noted earlier. Lipid-derived aldehyde derivatives are then formed during the propagation phase of lipid peroxidation in the presence of reducing metal ions such as Fe^{2+} and Cu^+. The lipid hydroperoxides (PUFA-OOH) generated initially are unstable and highly susceptible to breakdown through non-enzymatic Hock cleavage, forming a variety of reactive aldehydes (Figure 13.15), which can be classified into five main groups (Kawai *et al.*, 2007) according to their structure and reactivity: alkanals (and hydroxyalkanals); 2-alkenals; 4-hydroxy-2-alkenals; keto-alkenals; and alkanedials (dialdehydes) (Figure 13.16). The main aldehyde formed during lipid peroxidation of n-6 PUFAs, such as linoleic acid C18:2 n-6 and arachidonic acid C20:4 n-6 is the 4-hydroxy-2-alkenal-4-hydroxynonenal (HNE) (Uchida, 2003), whereas the peroxidation of n-3 PUFAs such as α-linolenic acid C18:3 n-3 and docosahexaenoic acid C22:6 n-3 generates the closely related compound, 4-hydroxy-2-hexenal (HHE) (Figure 13.15). Other lipid peroxidation products generated include the α,β-unsaturated aldehydes crotonaldehyde, and acrolein and the dialdehydes glyoxal and malondialdehyde (MDA). For reviews on the mechanisms by which these 4-hydroxyalkenals might be formed from membrane phospholipid PUFAs, see Guéraud *et al.* (2010) and Domingues *et al.* (2013).

The highly reactive α,β-unsaturated aldehydes can be conjugated to GSH by glutathione *S*-transferase alpha 4 (GSTA4), leading to their efflux from the cell by the GSH conjugate transporter RLIP76. In addition, oxidation by aldehyde dehydrogenase or reduction by alcohol dehydrogenase, aldehyde reductase or aldose reductase converts free aldehydes into less-toxic molecules. The α,β-unsaturated aldehydes that escape cellular metabolism serve as electrophiles in the covalent modification of proteins.

4-Hydroxy-2-alkenals are very reactive aldehydes and can form Schiff and Michael adducts. 4-Hydroxy-2-nonenal (HNE) is by far the most investigated, reacting with a wide variety of substrates (Zarkovic, 2003). The carbonyl group yields a Schiff base, while the β-carbon of the α,β-unsaturated aldehyde group acts as an electrophilic centre and thus as a potential target for the nucleophilic amino acid residues of proteins, allowing the formation of Michael adducts (Figure 13.17). These adducts can be stabilised by the formation of intermolecular pyrroles and hemiacetal (Figure 13.18). HHE, the reactive aldehyde generated by lipid peroxidation of n-3 PUFAs can also form adducts with similar structures to those from HNE (Long and Piklo, 2010; Riahha *et al.*, 2010; Pillon *et al.*, 2011).

The bifunctional nature of HNE enables it to crosslink proteins via the Michael addition of amino acid nucleophiles (Cys, His, Arg or Lys) at the C3 position, and Schiff base formation at the

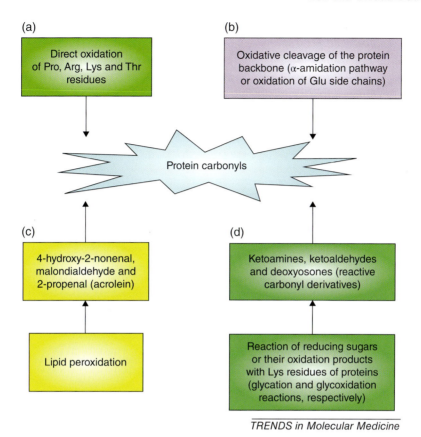

(a) Direct oxidation of Pro, Arg, Lys and Thr residues

(b) Oxidative cleavage of the protein backbone (α-amidation pathway or oxidation of Glu side chains)

Protein carbonyls

(c) 4-hydroxy-2-nonenal, malondialdehyde and 2-propenal (acrolein)

Lipid peroxidation

(d) Ketoamines, ketoaldehydes and deoxyosones (reactive carbonyl derivatives)

Reaction of reducing sugars or their oxidation products with Lys residues of proteins (glycation and glycoxidation reactions, respectively)

TRENDS in Molecular Medicine

Figure 13.14   *The production of protein carbonyls (aldehydes and ketones). (a) This can arise from direct oxidation of amino acid side chains (Pro, Arg, Lys and Thr), resulting in the formation of 2-pyrrolidone from proline, glutamic semialdehyde from arginine and proline, α-aminoadipic semialdehyde from lysine, and 2-amino-3-ketobutyric acid from threonine residues. (b) Protein carbonyl derivatives can also be generated through oxidative cleavage of proteins, via the α-amidation pathway or through oxidation of glutamine side chains, leading to the formation of a peptide in which the N-terminal amino acid is blocked by an α-ketoacyl derivative. (c) The introduction of carbonyl groups into proteins can occur by Michael addition reactions of α,β-unsaturated aldehydes, such as 4-hydroxy-2-nonenal, malondialdehyde and 2-propenal (acrolein), derived from lipid peroxidation, with either the amino group of lysine, the imidazole moiety of histidine, or the sulphydryl group of cysteine (advanced lipoxidation end products). (d) Carbonyl groups can also be introduced into proteins by addition of reactive carbonyl derivatives (ketoamines, ketoaldehydes and deoxyosones), produced by the reaction of reducing sugars or their oxidation products, to the amino group of lysine residues, by mechanisms referred to as glycation and glycoxidation. This eventually yields advanced glycation end products, such as carboxymethyllysine and pentosidine. Reprinted with permission from Elsevier from Dalle-Donne, I., Giustarini, D., Colombo, R., Rossi, R. and Milzani, A. (2003) Protein carbonylation in human diseases. Trends Mol. Med.,* **9***, 169–176*

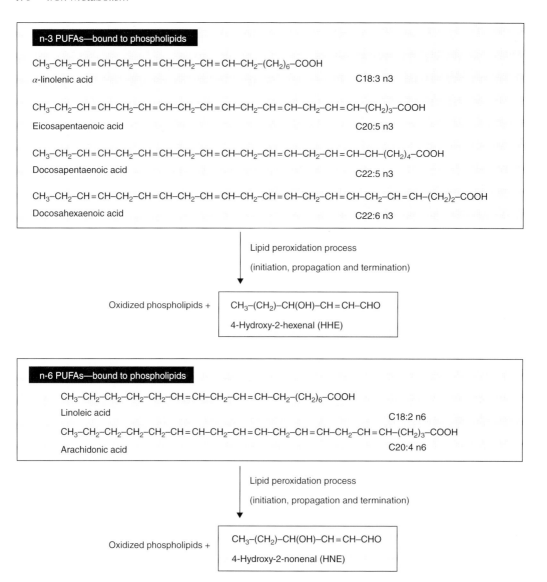

Figure 13.15 *Schematic diagram of reactive hydroxy-alkenals generated during lipid peroxidation of n-3 and n-6 polyunsaturated fatty acids. Reprinted from Catala, A. (2013) Five decades with polyunsaturated Fatty acids: chemical synthesis, enzymatic formation, lipid peroxidation and its biological effects. J. Lipids, 710290. doi: 10.1155/2013/710290. This is an open access article distributed under the Creative Commons Attribution License*

C1 carbonyl with the ε-amino group of Lys or Arg (Uchida and Stadtman, 1991; Friguet *et al.*, 1994; Cohn *et al.*, 1996; Stewart *et al.*, 2007). It has recently been proposed that, whereas oxidised proteins are degraded after ubiquitination by the 20S proteasome, oxidised, crosslinked proteins inhibit the proteasome and the oxidised, crosslinked protein aggregates are taken up by macrophagy into lysosomes (Höhn *et al.*, 2013).

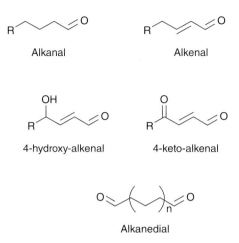

Alkanal

Alkenal

4-hydroxy-alkenal

4-keto-alkenal

Alkanedial

Figure 13.16 *Structures of the main fatty acid-derived aldehydes formed due to cleavage of the oxidised fatty acyl chain during lipid peroxidation. According to their structure and reactivity, they can be classified into five main groups: alkanals (and hydroxyalkanals); 2-alkenals; 4-hydroxy-2-alkenal; keto-alkenals; and alkanedial (dialdehydes). Reprinted with permission from Elsevier from Domingues, R.M., Domingues, P., Melo, T., et al. (2013) Lipoxidation adducts with peptides and proteins: deleterious modifications or signaling mechanisms? J. Proteomics, **92**, 110–131*

Nucleic acids are also targets for oxidative stress. Surprisingly, the characterisation and quantification of spontaneous, endogenously produced DNA damage indicates that main events, such as hydrolytic depurination, deamination of cytosine residues, oxidation of guanine and pyrimidine residues and methylation of adenine residues to 3-methyladenine, amount to 10 000 potentially mutagenic and cytotoxic changes per day in a human genome (Lindahl, 2013). These results strongly indicate that special DNA repair enzymes and mechanisms must exist to counteract endogenous DNA damage. And indeed they do.

ROS possess the ability to damage both the DNA nucleobases and the sugar phosphate backbone, leading to a wide spectrum of lesions, including non-bulky (8-oxoguanine and formamidopyrimidine) and bulky (cyclopurine and etheno adducts) base modifications, abasic sites, nonconventional single-strand breaks, protein–DNA adducts, and intrastrand/interstrand DNA crosslinks (Berquist and Wilson, 2012). Figure 13.19 illustrates the classic and atypical forms of oxidative DNA damage and associated DNA repair pathways.

Oxidative damage to DNA is thought mainly to involve modification of the nucleobases, generating primarily non-helix-distorting (or non-bulky) lesions. All four nucleobases are susceptible to reaction with ROS, in particular the hydroxyl radical. Guanine is the most easily oxidised base (Kovacic and Wakelin, 2001) and produces principally 8-oxo-7,8-dihydro-2′-deoxyguanosine (8-oxoG) (Wood *et al.*, 1990) and 2,6-diamino-4-hydroxy-5-formamidopyrimidine (fapyG) (Gajewski *et al.*, 1990). The modification of nucleobases to yield helix-distorting (or bulky) modified bases can occur via reactions with the hydroxyl radical or breakdown products of lipid peroxides. For example, tandem base lesions can arise through free radical attack of the C5 or C6 atoms of pyrimidine nucleobases, generating pyrimidine radicals that can attack a neighbouring purine nucleobase to yield intrastrand nucleobase–nucleobase crosslinks (Bellon *et al.*, 2002). 4-Hydroxy-nonenal interacts with nucleobases to form etheno adducts, including N3-(3-oxypropyl)-guanine, as well as the cyclic adducts 1,N^2-ethenoguanine (1,N^2-ethenoG), 1,N^6-ethanoadenine

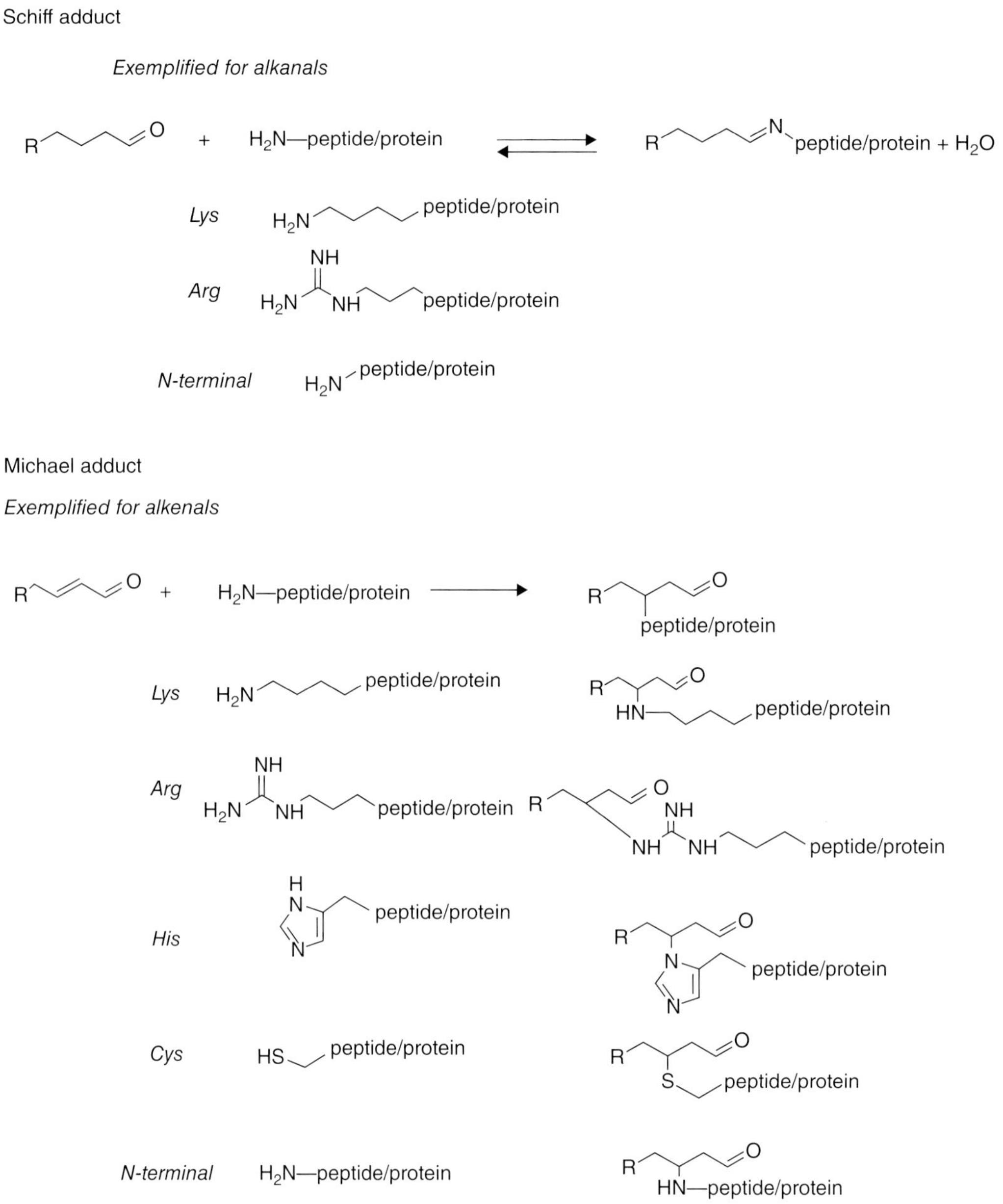

Schiff adduct

Exemplified for alkanals

Michael adduct

Exemplified for alkenals

Figure 13.17 *Formation of Schiff and Michael adducts between α,β-unsaturated carbonyl compounds derived from lipid peroxidation products and Lys, His, Cys and N-terminal amines of peptides. Reprinted with permission from Elsevier from Domingues, R.M., Domingues, P., Melo, T., et al. (2013) Lipoxidation adducts with peptides and proteins: deleterious modifications or signaling mechanisms?* J. Proteomics, **92***, 110–131*

(a) Schiff adducts: stabilization to pyrrole

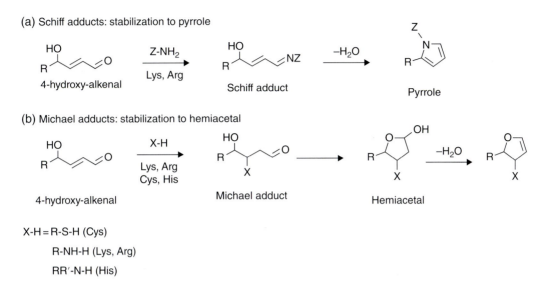

(b) Michael adducts: stabilization to hemiacetal

X-H = R-S-H (Cys)

     R-NH-H (Lys, Arg)

     RR′-N-H (His)

Figure 13.18 *Stabilisation of peptide/protein lipoxidation adducts via cyclisation of Schiff base (a) and Michael adducts (b) to form pyrroles and hemiacetals, respectively. Reprinted with permission from Elsevier from Domingues, R.M., Domingues, P., Melo, T., et al. (2013) Lipoxidation adducts with peptides and proteins: deleterious modifications or signaling mechanisms?* J. Proteomics, **92**, *110–131*

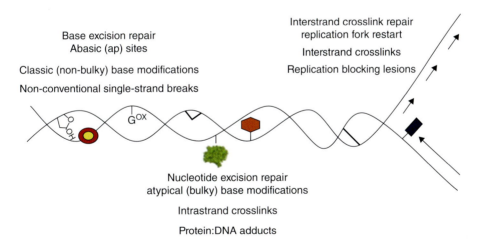

Figure 13.19 *Classic and atypical forms of oxidative DNA damage and associated DNA repair pathway(s). G^{ox}, 8-oxoG; red/yellow circle, 5′ or 3′ terminal blocking group; green protein, protein–DNA adduct; red hexagon, bulky base modification; thick lines, intra- or inter-strand crosslink; blue rectangle, replication blocking lesion. Reprinted with permission from Elsevier from Berquist, B.R. and Wilson, D.M., III (2012) Pathways for repairing and tolerating the spectrum of oxidative DNA lesions.* Cancer Lett., **327**, *61–72*

(1,N^6-ethanoA), and 3,N^4-ethenocytidine (Minko *et al.*, 2009). Three DNA polymerases, all members of the B-family, are thought to act as the main mammalian replicative DNA polymerases for genome duplication during cell division (Polα, Polδ, and Polε). When DNA or RNA polymerases encounter interstrand crosslinks or a replication blocking lesion, the replicative polymerases are ineffective. The remainder of the eukaryotic DNA polymerases, members of the A, B, Y and X families, are thought to be principally involved in translesion synthesis and/or DNA repair, and intervene when there are problems in replication.

Base-excision repair (BER), nucleotide-excision repair (NER), strand break (single- and double-stranded) repair, homologous recombination (HR) and interstrand crosslink (ICL) repair pathways all act to remedy ROS-induced DNA damage, maintain genetic information and provide genomic stability. Three of these DNA repair strategies – BER, NER and ICL – are presented schematically in Figure 13.20 (Berquist and Wilson, 2012).

BER (Figure 13.20a), is the primary pathway for coping with non-bulky base modifications (e.g. 8-oxoG), and consists of five major enzymatic steps: (i) removal of the damaged base by a DNA glycosylase; (ii) incision at the resulting abasic site by an APE1 endonuclease or lyase, leaving a 3′-hydroxyl (OH) and a 5′-deoxyphosphate (dRP); (iii) clean-up of the 5′ and/or 3′ terminal strand break ends by a lyase or phosphodiesterase, respectively; (iv) gap-filling by a DNA polymerase; and (v) nick sealing by a DNA ligase.

The major steps in the NER pathway are shown in Figure 13.20b. Helix-distorting DNA damage (e.g. an oxidatively damaged DNA base) can be recognised by the XPC–HR23B protein complex (global genome-NER) or by an elongating RNA polymerase in concert with the CSA and CSB proteins (transcription-coupled-NER). XPA, RPA, TFIIH (including the XPB and XPD ATPases/helicases) are recruited to the site of the damage, and the DNA surrounding the damage is unwound. XPG and XPF/ERCC1 nucleases are recruited and cleave the DNA phosphodiester backbone on the 3′ and 5′ sides of the damage, respectively, releasing the damage-containing DNA section. A DNA polymerase is then enlisted to fill the gap, leaving a nick in the phosphodiester backbone that is sealed by a DNA ligase, producing intact, undamaged duplex DNA.

A model for the major steps in the repair of ICLs is shown in Figure 13.20c. In the G_1 phase of the cell cycle, an ICL can be recognised by the XPC–HR23B protein complex, the MutSβ (MSH2–MSH3) protein complex, or by an elongating RNA polymerase in concert with the CSA and CSB proteins. Once the ICL has been recognised, it is unhooked from one strand by the action of the classic NER pathway, which involves the XPG and XPF/ERCC1 nucleases, or potentially through the endonuclease activity of the MLH1–PMS2 protein complex. The ICL remnant is then bypassed through the action of translesion DNA polymerases: REV1 then POLκ, and/or POLζ, POLν, and possibly additional DNA polymerases. At this point, a second round of DNA repair is initiated to remove the covalently linked ICL remnant from the second DNA strand. NER, involving the nuclease actions of XPG and XPF/ERCC1, likely acts to remove a DNA segment containing the physically linked ICL remnant, or the ICL remnant can be removed through the action of the NEIL1 DNA glycosylase. DNA can then be restored to the native duplex form through the activity of DNA polymerase(s), to fill in the gap, and a DNA ligase, to seal the nick in the phosphodiester backbone.

During the S-phase of the cell cycle (Figure 13.20c), an ICL is detected by stalling of a single replication fork (left) or two converging replication forks (right). FANCM is initially recruited to the stalled replication fork complex and probably acts either to regress or to stabilise the fork. The FA core complex, comprised of FANCA, B, C, E, F, G and L, recognises the FANCM bound/stabilised replication fork and ubiquitinates the FANCD2/I protein complex, with FANCL acting as the E3 ubiquitin ligase. Ubiquitinated FANCD2/I then associates with chromatin. For simplicity, action at a single replication fork is shown further. FANCP coordinates endonucleolytic cleavage

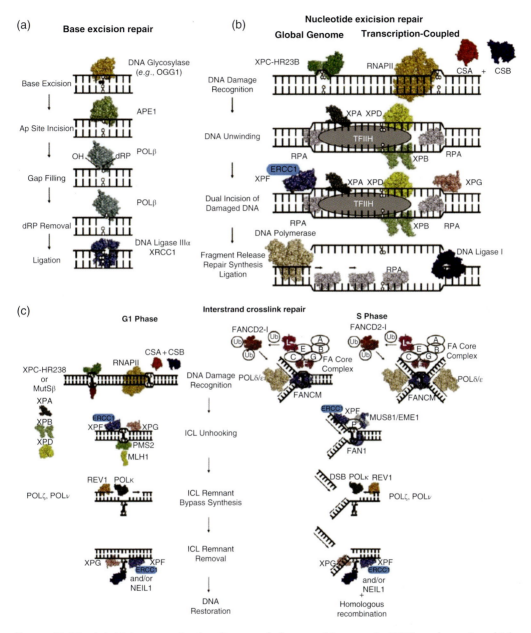

Figure 13.20 *(a) Major steps in the short-patch base-excision repair (BER) pathway in which a damaged base is detected, excised and replaced. (b) Major steps in the nucleotide-excision repair (NER) pathway in which helix-distorting DNA damage can be recognised, excised and the resulting gap replaced, producing intact, undamaged duplex DNA. (c) Model of major steps in the repair of interstrand crosslinks (ICLs) in the G_1 phase of the cell cycle (left) and in the S phase of the cell cycle. Reprinted with permission from Elsevier from Berquist, B.R. and Wilson, D.M., III (2012) Pathways for repairing and tolerating the spectrum of oxidative DNA lesions.* Cancer Lett., **327**, *61–72*

of the ICL stalled replication fork by XPF/ERCC1, MUS81/EME1, and FAN1. Cleavage by these nucleases unhooks the ICL from one DNA strand and generates a double-strand break (DSB). DNA polymerisation past the unhooked ICL remnant by translesion DNA polymerases, REV1 then POLκ, and/or POLζ, POLν, and possibly additional DNA polymerases, ensues. A second round of repair is initiated to remove the unhooked ICL remnant by NER and/or NEIL1. Homologous recombination is then used to reform the replication fork.

References

Aldini, G., Dalle-Donne, I., Colombo, R., *et al.* (2006) Lipoxidation-derived reactive carbonyl species as potential drug targets in preventing protein carbonylation and related cellular dysfunction. *ChemMedChem.*, **1**, 1045–1058.

Angelucci F., Saccoccia F., Ardini M., *et al.* (2013) Switching between the alternative structures and functions of a 2-Cys peroxiredoxin, by site-directed mutagenesis. *J. Mol. Biol.*, **425**, 4556–4568.

Antonyuk, S.V., Strange, R.W., Marklund, S.L. and Hasnain, S.S. (2009) The structure of human extracellular copper-zinc superoxide dismutase at 1.7 Å resolution: insights into heparin and collagen binding. *J. Mol. Biol.*, **388**, 310–326.

Barañano, D.E. and Snyder, S.H. (2001) Neural roles for heme oxygenase: contrasts to nitric oxide synthase. *Proc. Natl Acad. Sci. USA*, **98**, 10996–11002.

Bauer, G. (2014) Targeting extracellular ROS signaling of tumor cells. *Anticancer Res.*, **34**, 1467–1482.

Bellon, S., Ravanat, J.L., Gasparutto, D. and Cadet, J. (2002) Cross-linked thymine-purine base tandem lesions: synthesis, characterization, and measurement in gamma-irradiated isolated DNA. *Chem. Res. Toxicol.*, **15**, 598–606.

Berger, A. (ed.) (1984) *The Big Bang and Georges Lemaître, 1984*. D. Reidel Publ. Co., Dordrecht, Holland, pp. 420.

Berquist, B.R. and Wilson, D.M., III (2012) Pathways for repairing and tolerating the spectrum of oxidative DNA lesions. *Cancer Lett.*, **327**, 61–72.

Boehning, D., Moon, C., Sharma, S., *et al.* (2003) Carbon monoxide neurotransmission activated by CK2 phosphorylation of heme oxygenase-2. *Neuron*, **40**, 129–137.

Bryk, R., Griffin, P. and Nathan, C. (2000) Peroxynitrite reductase activity of bacterial peroxiredoxins. *Nature*, **407**, 211–215.

Buchholz, K., Putrianti, E.., Rahlfs, S., *et al.* (2010) Molecular genetics evidence for the in vivo roles of the two major NADPH-dependent disulfide reductases in the malaria parasite. *J. Biol. Chem.*, **285**, 37388–37395.

Burton, G.W. and Ingold, K.U. (1981) Autoxidation of biological molecules. 1. The antioxidant activity of vitamin E and related chain-breaking phenolic antioxidants in vitro. *J. Am. Chem. Soc.*, **103**, 6472–6477.

Bylund, J., Brown, K.L., Movitz, C., Dahlgren, C. and Karlsson, A. (2010) Intracellular generation of superoxide by the phagocyte NADPH oxidase: how, where, and what for? *Free Radic. Biol. Med.*, **49**, 1834–1845.

Cadenas, E. (2004) Mitochondrial free radical production and cell signaling. *Mol. Aspects Med.*, **25**, 17–26.

Cardona, T., Murray, J.W. and Rutherford, A.W. (2015) Origin and evolution of water oxidation before the last common ancestor of the Cyanobacteria. *Mol. Biol. Evol.*, **32**, 1310–1328.

Catala, A. (2013) Five decades with polyunsaturated fatty acids: chemical synthesis, enzymatic formation, lipid peroxidation and its biological effects. *J. Lipids*, **710290**. doi: 10.1155/2013/710290.

Chaudiere, J. and Ferrari-Iliou, R. (1999) Intracellular antioxidants: from chemical to biochemical mechanisms. *Food Chem. Toxicol.*, **37**, 949–962.

Cheng, Q., Sandalova, T., Lindqvist, Y. and Arnér, E.S. (2009) Crystal structure and catalysis of the selenoprotein thioredoxin reductase 1. *J. Biol. Chem.*, **284**, 3998–4008.

Cohn, J.A., Tsai, L., Friguet, B. and Szweda, L.I. (1996) Chemical characterization of a protein-4-hydroxy-2-nonenal cross-link: immunochemical detection in mitochondria exposed to oxidative stress. *Arch. Biochem. Biophys.*, **328**, 158–164.

Copley, S.D., Novak, W.R. and Babbitt, P.C. (2004) Divergence of function in the thioredoxin fold suprafamily: evidence for evolution of peroxiredoxins from a thioredoxin-like ancestor. *Biochemistry*, **43**, 13981–13995.

Cox, A.G., Peskin, A.V., Paton, L.N., Winterbourn, C. and Hampton, M.B. (2009) Redox potential and peroxide reactivity of human peroxiredoxin 3. *Biochemistry*, **48**, 6495–6501.

Cox, A.G., Winterbourn, C. and Hampton, M.B. (2010) Mitochondrial peroxiredoxin involvement in antioxidant defence and redox signalling. *Biochem. J.*, **425**, 313–325.

Dalle-Donne, I., Giustarini, D., Colombo, R., Rossi, R. and Milzani, A. (2003) Protein carbonylation in human diseases. *Trends Mol. Med.*, **9**, 169–176.

Davies, M.J., Hawkins, C.L., Pattison, D.I. and Rees, M.D. (2008) Mammalian heme peroxidases: from molecular mechanisms to health implications. *Antioxid. Redox Signal.*, **10**, 1199–1234.

Day, B.R. (2014) Antioxidant therapeutics: Pandora's box. *Free Radic. Biol. Med.*, **66**, 58–64.

Deng, H.X., Hentati, A., Tainer, J.A., *et al.* (1993) Amyotrophic lateral sclerosis and structural defects in Cu,Zn superoxide dismutase. *Science*, **261**, 1047–1051.

Deponte, M. (2013) Glutathione catalysis and the reaction mechanisms of glutathione-dependent enzymes. *Biochim. Biophys. Acta*, **1830**, 3217–3266.

DiDonato, M., Craig, L., Huff, M.E., *et al.* (2003) ALS mutants of superoxide dismutase form aggregates via framework destabilization. *J. Mol. Biol.*, **332**, 601–615.

Domingues, R.M., Domingues, P., Melo, T., *et al.* (2013) Lipoxidation adducts with peptides and proteins: deleterious modifications or signaling mechanisms? *J. Proteomics*, **92**, 110–131.

Eklund, H., Gleason, A.K. and Holmgren, A. (1991) Structural and functional relations among thioredoxins of different species. *Proteins*, **11**, 13–28.

Epp, G., Ladenstein, R. and Wendel, A. (1983) The refined structure of the selenoenzyme glutathione peroxidase at 0.2-nm resolution. *Eur. J. Biochem.*, **133**, 51–69.

Esposito, L.A., Kokoszka, J.E., Waymire, K.G., Cottrell, B., *et al.* (2000) Mitochondrial oxidative stress in mice lacking the glutathione peroxidase-1 gene. *Free Radic. Biol. Med.*, **28**, 754–766.

Fenton, H.J.H. (1894) The oxidation of tartaric acid in presence of iron. *J. Chem. Soc. Trans.*, **10**, 157–158.

Fernandes, A.P. and Holmgren, A. (2004) Glutaredoxins: glutathione-dependent redox enzymes with functions far beyond a simple thioredoxin backup system. *Antioxid. Redox Signal.*, **6**, 63–74.

Flannery, D.T. and Walter, M.R. (2012) Archean tufted microbial mats and the Great Oxidation Event: new insights into an ancient problem. *Aust. J. Earth Sci.*, **59**, 1–11.

Forman, H.J., Zhang, H. and Rinna, A. (2009) Glutathione: overview of its protective roles, measurement, and biosynthesis. *Mol. Aspects Med.*, **30**, 1–12.

Forman, H.J., Maiorino, M. and Ursini, F. (2010) Signaling functions of reactive oxygen species. *Biochemistry*, **49**, 835–842.

Friguet, B., Stadtman, E.R. and Szweda, L.I. (1994) Modification of glucose-6-phosphate dehydrogenase by 4-hydroxy-2-nonenal. Formation of cross-linked protein that inhibits the multicatalytic protease. *J. Biol. Chem.*, **269**, 21639–21643.

Gajewski, E., Rao, G., Nackerdien, Z. and Dizdaroglu, M. (1990) Modification of DNA bases in mammalian chromatin by radiation-generated free radicals. *Biochemistry*, **29**, 7876–7882.

Ghaemmaghami, S., Huh, W.K., Bower, K., *et al.* (2003) Global analysis of protein expression in yeast. *Nature*, **425**, 737–741.

Giorgio, M., Trinei, M., Migliaccio, E. and Pelicci, P.G. (2007) Hydrogen peroxide: a metabolic by-product or a common mediator of ageing signals? *Nat. Rev. Mol. Cell Biol.*, **8**, 722–728.

Gould, N., Doulias, P.T., Tenopoulou, M., Raju, K. and Ischiropoulos, H. (2013) Regulation of protein function and signaling by reversible cysteine S-nitrosylation. *J. Biol. Chem.*, **288**, 26473–26479.

Grimsrud, P.A., Xie, H., Griffin, T.J. and Bernlohr, D.A. (2008) Oxidative stress and covalent modification of protein with bioactive aldehydes. *J. Biol. Chem.*, **283**, 21837–21841.

Grochot-Przeczek, A., Dulak, J. and Jozkowicz, A. (2012) Haem oxygenase-1: non-canonical roles in physiology and pathology. *Clin. Sci. (Lond)*, **122**, 93–103.

Groitl, B. and Jakob, U. (2014) Thiol-based redox switches. *Biochim. Biophys. Acta*, **1844**, 1335–1343.

Guéraud, F., Atalay, M., Bresgen, N., *et al.* (2010) Chemistry and biochemistry of lipid peroxidation products. *Free Radic. Res.*, **44**, 1098–1124.

Haber, F. and Weiss, J. (1934) The catalytic decomposition of hydrogen peroxide by iron salts. *Proc. Roy. Soc. Ser. A*, **147**, 332–351.

Hall, A., Karplus, P.A. and Poole, L.B. (2009) Typical 2-Cys peroxiredoxins – structures, mechanisms and functions. *FEBS J.*, **276**, 2469–2477.

Hall, A., Parsonage, D., Poole, L.B. and Karplus, P.A. (2010) Structural evidence that peroxiredoxin catalytic power is based on transition-state stabilization. *J. Mol. Biol.*, **402**, 194–209.

Hall, A., Nelson, K., Poole, L.B. and Karplus, P.A. (2011) Structure-based insights into the catalytic power and conformational dexterity of peroxiredoxins. *Antioxid. Redox Signal.*, **15**, 795–815.

Halliwell, B. and Chirico, S. (1993) Lipid peroxidation: its mechanism, measurement and significance. *Am. J. Clin. Nutr.*, **57**, 715S–725S.

Hess, D.T., Matsumoto, A., Kim, S.O., Marshall, H.E. and Stamler, J.S. (2005) Protein S-nitrosylation: purview and parameters. *Nat. Rev. Mol. Cell Biol.*, **6**, 150–166.

Höhn, A., König, J. and Grune, T. (2013) Protein oxidation in aging and the removal of oxidized proteins. *J. Proteomics*, **92**, 132–159.

Holmstrom, K.M. and Finkel, T. (2014) Cellular mechanisms and physiological consequences of redox-dependent signalling. *Nat. Rev. Mol. Cell Biol.*, **15**, 411–421.

Imlay, J.A. (2008) Cellular defenses against superoxide and hydrogen peroxide. *Annu. Rev. Biochem.*, **77**, 755–776.

Jang, S. and Imlay, J.A. (2007) Micromolar intracellular hydrogen peroxide disrupts metabolism by damaging iron-sulfur enzymes. *J. Biol. Chem.*, **282**, 929–937.

Janssen-Heininger, Y.M., Mossman, B.T., Heintz, N.H., Forman, H.J., *et al.* (2008) Redox-based regulation of signal transduction: principles, pitfalls, and promises. *Free Radic. Biol. Med.*, **45**, 1–17.

Jia, J., Arif, A., Terenzi, F., *et al.* (2014) Target-selective protein S-nitrosylation by sequence motif recognition. *Cell*, **159**, 623–634.

Johnson, F. and Giulivi, C. (2005) Superoxide dismutases and their impact upon human health. *Mol. Aspects Med.*, **26**, 340–352.

Jönsson, T.J., Ellis, H.R. and Poole, L.B. (2007) Cysteine reactivity and thiol-disulfide interchange pathways in AhpF and AhpC of the bacterial alkyl hydroperoxide reductase system. *Biochemistry*, **46**, 5709–5721.

Kanzok, S.M., Schirmer, R.H., Turbachova, I., Iozef, R. and Becker, K. (2001) The thioredoxin system of the malaria parasite *Plasmodium falciparum*. Glutathione reduction revisited. *J. Biol. Chem.*, **275**, 40180–40186.

Karplus, P.A. (2015) A primer on peroxiredoxin biochemistry. *Free Radic. Biol. Med.*, **80**, 183–190.

Karplus, P.A. and Schultz, G.E. (1989) Substrate binding and catalysis by glutathione reductase as derived from refined enzyme: substrate crystal structures at 2 Å resolution. *J. Mol. Biol.*, **210**, 163–180.

Kil, I.S., Lee, S.K., Ryu, K.W., *et al.* (2012) Feedback control of adrenal steroidogenesis via H_2O_2-dependent, reversible inactivation of peroxiredoxin III in mitochondria. *Mol. Cell*, **46**, 584–594.

Kirschvink, J.L. and Kopp, R.E. (2008) Palaeoproterozoic ice houses and the evolution of oxygen-mediating enzymes: the case for a late origin of photosystem II. *Philos. Trans. R. Soc. Lond. B Biol. Sci.*, **363**, 2755–2765.

Klomsiri, C., Karplus, P.A. and Poole, L.B. (2011) Cysteine-based redox switches in enzymes. *Antioxid. Redox Signal.*, **14**, 1065–1077.

Klomsiri, C., Rogers, L.C., Soito, L., *et al.* (2014) Endosomal H_2O_2 production leads to localized cysteine sulfenic acid formation on proteins during lysophosphatidic acid-mediated cell signaling. *Free Radic. Biol. Med.*, **71**, 49–60.

Kopp, R.E., Kirschvink, J.L., Hilburn, I.A. and Nash, C.Z. (2005) The Paleoproterozoic snowball Earth: a climate disaster triggered by the evolution of oxygenic photosynthesis. *Proc. Natl Acad. Sci. USA*, **102**, 11131–11136.

Koskenkorva-Frank, T.S., Weiss, G., Koppenol, W.H. and Burckhardt, S. (2013) The complex interplay of iron metabolism, reactive oxygen species, and reactive nitrogen species: insights into the potential of various iron therapies to induce oxidative and nitrosative stress. *Free Radic. Biol. Med.*, **65**, 1174–1194.

Kovacic, P. and Wakelin, L.P. (2001) Review: DNA molecular electrostatic potential: novel perspectives for the mechanism of action of anticancer drugs involving electron transfer and oxidative stress. *Anticancer Drug Des.*, **16**, 175–184.

Landry, A.P. and Ding, H. (2014) Redox control of human mitochondrial outer membrane protein MitoNEET [2Fe-2S] clusters by biological thiols and hydrogen peroxide. *J. Biol. Chem.*, **289**, 4307–4315.

Lemaître, G. (1927) Un univers homogène de masse constante et de rayon croissant, rendant compte de la vitesse radiale des nébuleuses extra-galactiques. *Ann. Soc. Scient. de Bruxelles*, **47A**, 49–59.

Lemaître, G. (1931) The beginning of the world from the point of view of quantum theory. *Nature*, **127**, 709.

Lemaître, G. (1931) Contributions to a British Association Discussion on the Evolution of the Universe. *Nature*, **128**, 704–706.

Liaudet, L., Vassalli, G. and Pacher, P. (2009) Role of peroxynitrite in the redox regulation of cell signal transduction pathways. *Front. Biosci. (Landmark Ed.)*, **14**, 4809–4814.

Lindahl, T. (2013) My Journey to DNA Repair. *Genom. Proteom. Bioinform.*, **11**, 2–7.

Long, E.K. and Picklo, M.J. (2010) Trans-4-hydroxy-2-hexenal, a product of n-3 fatty acid peroxidation: make some room HNE. *Free Radic. Biol. Med.*, **49**, 1–8.

Lu, J. and Holmgren, A. (2014) The thioredoxin superfamily in oxidative protein folding. *Free Radic. Biol. Med.*, **66**, 75–87.

Lyons, T.W., Reinhard, C.T. and Planavsky, N.J. (2014) The rise of oxygen in Earth's early ocean and atmosphere. *Nature*, **506**, 307–315.

Mailloux, R.J. and Harper, M.-E. (2011) Uncoupling proteins and the control of mitochondrial reactive oxygen species production. *Free Radic. Biol. Med.*, **51**, 1106–1115.

Manta, B., Hugo, M., Ortiz, C., *et al.* (2009) The peroxidase and peroxynitrite reductase activity of human erythrocyte peroxiredoxin 2. *Arch. Biochem. Biophys.*, **484**, 146–154.

Marinho, H.S., Real, C., Cyrne, L., Soares, H. and Antunes, F. (2014) Hydrogen peroxide sensing, signaling and regulation of transcription factors. *Redox Biol.*, **2**, 535–562.

Marty, L., Siala, W., Schwartzlander, M., *et al.* (2009) The NADPH-dependent thioredoxin system constitutes a functional backup for cytosolic glutathione reductase in *Arabidopsis*. *Proc. Natl Acad. Sci. USA*, **106**, 9109–9114.

McCay, P. (1985) Vitamin E: Interactions with free radicals and ascorbate. *Annu. Rev. Nutr.*, **5**, 323–340.

Miao, L. and St Clair, D.K. (2009) Regulation of superoxide dismutase genes: implications in disease. *Free Radic. Biol. Med.*, **47**, 344–356.

Milani, P., Gagliardi, S., Cova, E. and Cereda, C. (2011) SOD1 transcriptional and posttranscriptional regulation and its potential implications in ALS. *Neurol. Res. Int.*, **60**, 51–60.

Miller, A.F. (2012) Superoxide dismutases: ancient enzymes and new insights. *FEBS Lett.*, **586**, 585–595.

Minko, I.G., Kozekov, I.D., Harris, T.M., *et al.*, (2009) Chemistry and biology of DNA containing 1,N(2)-deoxyguanosine adducts of the alpha,beta-unsaturated aldehydes acrolein, crotonaldehyde, and 4-hydroxynonenal. *Chem. Res. Toxicol.*, **22**, 759–778.

Mitchell, D.A. and Marletta, M.A. (2005) Thioredoxin catalyzes the S-nitrosation of the caspase-3 active site cysteine. *Nat. Chem. Biol.*, **1**, 154–158.

Mitchell, D.A., Morton, S.U., Fernhoff, N.B. and Marletta, M.A. (2007) Thioredoxin is required for S-nitrosation of procaspase-3 and the inhibition of apoptosis in Jurkat cells. *Proc. Natl Acad. Sci. USA*, **104**, 11609–11614.

Muller, E.G. (1996) A glutathione reductase mutant of yeast accumulates high levels of oxidized glutathione and requires thioredoxin for growth. *Mol. Biol. Cell*, **7** (11), 1805–1813.

Murad, F. (2006) Shattuck Lecture. Nitric oxide and cyclic GMP in cell signaling and drug development. *N. Engl. J. Med.*, **355**, 2003–2011.

Murphy, D.J. and Mavis, R.D. (1981) A comparison of the in vitro binding of alpha-tocopherol to microsomes of lung, liver, heart and brain of the rat. *J. Biol. Chem.*, **256**, 10464–10468.

Nakamura, T., Tu, S., Akhtar, M.W., *et al.* (2013) Aberrant protein S-nitrosylation in neurodegenerative diseases. *Neuron*, **78**, 596–614.

Nyström, T. (2005) Role of oxidative carbonylation in protein quality control and senescence. *EMBO J.*, **24**, 1311–1317.

Ogusucu, R., Rettori, D., Munhoz, D.C., Netto, L.E. and Augusto, O. (2007) Reactions of yeast thioredoxin peroxidases I and II with hydrogen peroxide and peroxynitrite: rate constants by competitive kinetics. *Free Radic. Biol. Med.*, **42**, 326–334.

Pacher, P., Beckman, J.S. and Liaudet, L. (2007) Nitric oxide and peroxynitrite in health and disease. *Physiol. Rev.*, **87**, 315–424.

Parsonage, D., Karplus, P.A. and Poole, L.B. (2008) Substrate specificity and redox potential of AhpC, a bacterial peroxiredoxin. *Proc. Natl Acad. Sci. USA*, **105**, 8209–8214.

Perkins A., Nelson, K.J., Williams, J.R., *et al.* (2013) The sensitive balance between the fully folded and locally unfolded conformations of a model peroxiredoxin. *Biochemistry*, **52**, 8708–8721.

Perkins, A., Poole, L.B. and Karplus, P.A. (2014) Tuning of peroxiredoxin catalysis for various physiological roles. *Biochemistry*, **53**, 7693–7705.

Perry, J.J., Shin, D.S., Getzoff, E.D. and Tainer, J.A. (2010) The structural biochemistry of the superoxide dismutases. *Biochim. Biophys. Acta*, **1804**, 245–262.

Peskin, A.V., Low, F.M., Paton, L.N., *et al.* (2007) The high reactivity of peroxiredoxin 2 with H_2O_2 is not reflected in its reaction with other oxidants and thiol reagents. *J. Biol. Chem.*, **282**, 11885–11892.

Pierre, J.L., Fontecave, M. and Crichton, R.R. (2002) Chemistry for an essential biological process: the reduction of ferric iron. *Biometals*, **15**, 341–346.

Pillon, N.J., Vella, R.E., Soulère, L., *et al.* (2011) Structural and functional changes in human insulin induced by the lipid peroxidation byproducts 4-hydroxy-2-nonenal and 4-hydroxy-2-hexenal. *Chem. Res. Toxicol.*, **24**, 752–762.

Rasmussen, B., Fletcher, I.R., Brooks, J.J. and Kilburn, M.R. (2008) Reassessing the first appearance of eukaryotes and cyanobacteria. *Nature*, **455**, 1101–1104.

Rhee, S.G. and Woo, H.A. (2011) Multiple functions of peroxiredoxins: peroxidases, sensors and regulators of the intracellular messenger H_2O_2, and protein chaperones. *Antioxid. Redox Signal.*, **15**, 781–794.

Rhee, S.G., Chae, H.Z. and Kim, K. (2005) Peroxiredoxins: a historical overview and speculative preview of novel mechanisms and emerging concepts in cell signaling. *Free Radic. Biol. Med.*, **38**, 1543–1552.

Rhee, S.G., Jeong, W., Chang, T.S. and Woo, H.A. (2007) Sulfiredoxin, the cysteine sulfinic acid reductase specific to 2-Cys peroxiredoxin: its discovery, mechanism of action, and biological significance. *Kidney Int. Suppl.*, **72**, S3–S8.

Rhee, S.G., Woo, H.A., Kil, I.S. and Bae, S.A. (2012) Peroxiredoxin functions as a peroxidase and a regulator and sensor of local peroxides. *J. Biol. Chem.*, **287**, 4403–4410.

Riahha, Y., Cohen, G., Shamni, O. and Sasson, S. (2010) Signaling and cytotoxic functions of 4-hydroxyalkenals. *Am. J. Physiol. Endocrinol. Metab.*, **299**, E879–E886.

Rosen, D.R., Siddique, T., Patterson, D., *et al.* (1993) Mutations in Cu/Zn superoxide dismutase gene are associated with familial amyotrophic lateral sclerosis. *Nature*, **362**, 59–62.

Ruben, S., Randall, M., Kamen, M. and Hyde, J.L. (1941) Heavy Oxygen (O^{18}) as a tracer in the study of photosynthesis. *J. Am. Chem. Soc.*, **63**, 877–879.

Sato, Y., Hagiwara, K., Akai, H. and Inoue, K. (1991) Purification and characterization of α-tocopherol transfer protein from rat liver. *FEBS Lett.*, **288**, 41–45.

Schrader, M. and Fahimi, H.D. (2006) Peroxisomes and oxidative stress. *Biochim. Biophys. Acta*, **1763**, 1755–1766.

Schultz, G.E., Schirmer, R.H., Sachsenheimer, W. and Pai, E.F. (1978) The structure of the flavoenzyme glutathione reductase. *Nature*, **273**, 120–124.

Seth, D. and Stamler, J.S. (2011) The SNO-proteome: causation and classifications. *Curr. Opin. Chem. Biol.*, **15**, 129–136.

Seth, D., Hausladen, A., Wang, Y.J. and Stamler, J.S. (2012) Endogenous protein S-nitrosylation in *E. coli*: regulation by OxyR. *Science*, **336**, 470–473.

Sheng, Y., Stich, T.A., Barnese, K., *et al.* (2011) Comparison of two yeast MnSODs: mitochondrial *Saccharomyces cerevisiae* versus cytosolic *Candida albicans*. *J. Am. Chem. Soc.*, **133**, 20878–20889.

Sheng, Y., Abreu, I.A., Cabelli, D.E., *et al.* (2014) Superoxide dismutases and superoxide reductases. *Chem. Rev.*, **114**, 3854–3918.

Sies, H. (2014) Role of metabolic H_2O_2 generation: redox signaling and oxidative stress. *J. Biol. Chem.*, **289**, 8735–8741.

Sies, H. (2015) Oxidative stress: a concept in redox biology and medicine. *Redox Biol.*, **4**, 180–183.

Sies, H. and Arteel, G.E. (2000) Interaction of peroxynitrite with selenoproteins and glutathione peroxidase mimics. *Free Radic. Biol. Med.*, **28**, 1451–1455.

Smith, B.C. and Marletta, M.A. (2012) Mechanisms of S-nitrosothiol formation and selectivity in nitric oxide signaling. *Curr. Opin. Chem. Biol.*, **16**, 498–506.

Sobotta, M.C., Liou, W., Stöcker, S., *et al.* (2015) Peroxiredoxin-2 and STAT3 form a redox relay for H_2O_2 signaling. *Nat. Chem. Biol.*, **11**, 64–70.

Stacey, M.M., Vissers, M.C. and Winterbourn, C.C. (2012) Oxidation of 2-cys peroxiredoxins in human endothelial cells by hydrogen peroxide, hypochlorous acid, and chloramines. *Antioxid. Redox Signal.*, **17**, 411–421.

Stewart, B.J., Doorn, J.A. and Petersen, D.R. (2007) Residue-specific adduction of tubulin by 4-hydroxynonenal and 4-oxononenal causes cross-linking and inhibits polymerization. *Chem. Res. Toxicol.*, **20**, 1111–1119.

Sutton, A., Khoury, H., Prip-Buus, C., *et al.* (2003) The Ala16Val genetic dimorphism modulates the import of human manganese superoxide dismutase into rat liver mitochondria. *Pharmacogenetics*, **13**, 145–157.

Tainer, J.A., Getzoff, E.D., Beem, K.M., Richardson, J.S. and Richardson, D.C. (1982) Determination and analysis of the 2 Å structure of copper, zinc superoxide dismutase. *J. Mol. Biol.*, **160**, 181–217.

Tan, S.X., Greetham, D., Raeth, S., *et al.* (2010) The thioredoxin-thioredoxin reductase system can function in vivo as an alternative system to reduce oxidized glutathione in *Saccharomyces cerevisiae*. *J. Biol. Chem.*, **285**, 6118–6126.

Toyama, A., Takahashi, Y. and Takeuchi, H. (2004) Catalytic and structural role of a metal-free histidine residue in bovine Cu-Zn superoxide dismutase. *Biochemistry*, **43**, 4670–4679.

Uchida, K. (2003) 4-Hydroxy-2-nonenal: a product and mediator of oxidative stress. *Prog. Lipid Res.*, **42**, 318–343.

Uchida, K. and Stadtman, E.R. (1991) Covalent attachment of 4-hydroxynonenal to glyceraldehyde-3-phosphate dehydrogenase. A possible involvement of intra- and intermolecular cross-linking reaction. *J. Biol. Chem.*, **268**, 6388–6393.

van Niel, C.B. (1931) On the morphology and physiology of the purple and green sulfur bacteria. *Arch. Mikrobiol.*, **3**, 1–112.

van Niel, C.B. (1935) Photosynthesis of bacteria. *Cold Spring Harbor Symp. Quant. Biol.*, **3**, 138–150.

Vistoli, G., De Maddis, D., Cipak, A., *et al.* (2013) Advanced glycoxidation and lipoxidation end products (AGEs and ALEs): an overview of their mechanisms of formation. *Free Radic. Res.*, **47** (Suppl. 1), 3–27.

Waldbauer, J.R., Sherman, L.S., Sumner, D.Y. and Summons, R.E. (2009) Late Archean molecular fossils from the Transvaal Supergroup record the antiquity of microbial diversity and aerobiosis. *Precambrian Res.*, **169**, 28–47.

Ward, R.J., Abiaka, C. and Peters, T.J. (1994) Inflammation and tissue injury: the world of free radicals. *J. Nephrol.*, **7**, 89–96.

Winterbourn, C.C. (2008) Reconciling the chemistry and biology of reactive oxygen species. *Nat. Chem. Biol.*, **4**, 278–286.

Winterbourn, C. (2014) Current methods to study reactive oxygen species – pros and cons. *Biochim. Biophys. Acta*, **1840**, 707.

Winterbourn, C.C. (2015) Are free radicals involved in thiol-based redox signaling? *Free Radic. Biol. Med.*, **80**, 164–170.

Winterbourn, C.C. and Metodiewa, D. (1999) Reactivity of biologically important thiol compounds with superoxide and hydrogen peroxide. *Free Radic. Biol. Med.*, **27**, 322–328.

Winterbourn, C. and Hampton, M.B. (2008) Thiol chemistry and specificity in redox signaling. *Free Radic. Biol. Med.*, **45**, 549–561.

Wispé, J.R., Warner, B.B., Clark, J.C., *et al.* (1992) Human Mn-superoxide dismutase in pulmonary epithelial cells of transgenic mice confers protection from oxygen injury. *J. Biol. Chem.*, **267**, 23937–23941.

Wood, M.L., Dizdaroglu, M., Gajewski, E. and Essigmann, J.M. (1990) Mechanistic studies of ionizing radiation and oxidative mutagenesis: genetic effects of a single 8-hydroxyguanine (7-hydro-8-oxoguanine) residue inserted at a unique site in a viral genome. *Biochemistry*, **29**, 7024–7032.

Wood, Z.A., Poole, L.B. and Karplus, P.A. (2003a) Peroxiredoxin evolution and the regulation of hydrogen peroxide signaling. *Science*, **300**, 650–653.

Wood, Z.A., Schroder, E., Robin Harris, J. and Poole, L.B. (2003b) Structure, mechanism and regulation of peroxiredoxins. *Trends Biochem. Sci.*, **28** (1), 32–40.

Yoo, H.Y., Chang, M.S. and Rho, H.M. (1999) Heavy metal-mediated activation of the rat Cu/Zn superoxide dismutase gene via a metal-responsive element. *Mol. Gen. Genet.*, **262**, 310–313.

Yun, B.W., Feechan, A., Yin, M., *et al.* (2011) S-nitrosylation of NADPH oxidase regulates cell death in plant immunity. *Nature*, **478**, 264–268.

Zarkovic, N. (2003) 4-Hydroxynonenal as a bioactive marker of pathophysiological processes. *Mol. Aspects Med.*, **24**, 281–291.

Zelko, I.N., Mariani, T.J. and Folz, R.J. (2002) Superoxide dismutase multigene family: a comparison of the CuZn-SOD (SOD1), Mn-SOD (SOD2), and EC-SOD (SOD3) gene structures, evolution, and expression. *Free Radic. Biol. Med.*, **33**, 337–349.

Zhang, Y. and Hogg, N. (2005) S-Nitrosothiols: cellular formation and transport. *Free Radic. Biol. Med.*, **38**, 831–838.

Zhong, L., Arnér, E.S. and Holmgren, A. (2000) Structure and mechanism of mammalian thioredoxin reductase: the active site is a redox-active selenolthiol/selenenylsulfide formed from the conserved cysteine-selenocysteine sequence. *Proc. Natl Acad. Sci. USA*, **97**, 5854–5859.

Zhou, Z. and Kang, Y.J. (2000) Cellular and subcellular localization of catalase in the heart of transgenic mice. *J. Histochem. Cytochem.*, **48**, 585–594.

14

Interactions between Iron and other Metals

14.1 Introduction

Over the past 30 to 40 years the extraordinarily important role that metals play in biology, the environment and medicine has become increasingly evident. Na^+ and K^+ (together with H^+ and Cl^-), which bind weakly to organic ligands and are highly mobile, are ideally suited to generate ionic gradients across biological membranes and to ensure the maintenance of osmotic balance, and this is precisely what these two essential alkali metal ions do in biological systems. In contrast, Mg^{2+} and Ca^{2+} with intermediate binding strengths to organic ligands, can play important structural roles and, in the particular case of Ca^{2+}, serve as a charge carrier and a trigger for signal transmission within the cell. The six transition metal ions – Co, Cu, Fe, Mn, Mo and Zn – are essential trace elements for humans. Zn^{2+} has ligand-binding constants intermediate between those of Mg^{2+} and Ca^{2+} and the other five transition metal ions. However, unlike these other metals, zinc effectively does not have access to any other oxidation state than Zn^{2+}. It is found in a large number of enzymes, where it not only plays a structural role, but can also fulfil a very important function in catalysis as a Lewis acid. The other five transition metal ions bind tightly to organic ligands, and participate in innumerable redox reactions.

Before the arrival of oxygenic photosynthesis, when there was no oxygen, elements such as Fe, Ni and W would have been relatively available and important, whereas Cu and Mo, for reasons of solubility, would have been poorly accessible. However, as the environment became increasingly oxidising in nature, Ni and W became increasingly scarce and were replaced by Co and Mo, while Cu became bioavailable. Although Fe was now poorly available on solubility grounds, it had become so fundamentally important for biology that specific systems were developed to ensure its uptake from the environment.

Iron Metabolism – From Molecular Mechanisms to Clinical Consequences, Fourth Edition. Robert Crichton.
© 2016 John Wiley & Sons, Ltd. Published 2016 by John Wiley & Sons, Ltd.

There are also metals such as aluminium, cadmium and lead in the environment which represent a serious toxic hazard. In contrast to such toxic metals, other metals are used as drugs, such as cisplatin and related metal-based drugs to treat cancer, and lithium (as lithium carbonate) in the treatment of manic depression. The use of noninvasive techniques such as magnetic resonance imaging (MRI) in modern medicine depends heavily on the use of paramagnetic metal complexes as contrast agents in diagnosis, and also of a number of metals such as cobalt, gallium and technetium as radiopharmaceuticals to deliver sterilising radiation to targets within the body.

14.2 Iron Interactions with Essential Metals

As was seen in earlier chapters, the unique coordination chemistry of Fe(III) allows microorganisms and Strategy II plants to take up iron selectively from the environment using siderophores, while mammals transport Fe(III) in extracellular fluids bound to transferrin. In contrast, when iron must move across membranes from one compartment to another, the preferred form is Fe(II). The difficulty of selectively coordinating Fe(II) is reflected by the observation that the mammalian divalent metal transporter DMT1 transports not only Fe^{2+} but also Zn^{2+}, Mn^{2+}, Co^{2+}, Cu^{2+}, Cd^{2+}, Ni^{2+} and Pb^{2+} (Gunshin *et al.*, 1997). Both experimental data and clinical findings have indicated that diseases of iron metabolism can be associated with alterations in the metabolism of other metals, particularly divalent cations (Figure 14.1) (reviewed in Loréal *et al.*, 2014). Thus, an increased absorption of Co^{2+}, Mn^{2+} and Zn^{2+} was observed in iron-deficient rats, whereas the absorption of Ca^{2+}, Mg^{2+} and Cu^{2+} was not affected (Pollack *et al.*, 1965). Iron deficiency increases the expression of the Zn^{2+} transporter ZIP 5, whereas the hepatic expression of three others – ZIPs 6, 7 and 10 – decreases (Nam and Knutson, 2012). These Fe-deficient rats also had higher liver copper concentrations. Several studies have shown increased concentrations of divalent metals in specific brain regions in iron-deficient animals, including copper, manganese and zinc (Shukla *et al.*, 1989; Chua and Morgan, 1996; Erikson *et al.*, 2004), which could be due to increased DMT1 expression. Iron loading resulting from inflammatory processes or from systemic iron overload has also been shown to affect other metals, whereas alterations in the metabolism of other divalent metal ions have been shown to affect iron metabolism (Loréal *et al.*, 2014).

In the following, we consider first the interactions between iron and other essential metal ions, and the interactions with metal ions that are potentially toxic. The survey has been limited to iron–metal interactions in mammals.

14.2.1 Copper

14.2.1.1 Introduction

Both, iron and copper have played a key role in human evolution. However, between 1200 and 1000 BC the ability to heat and forge iron led to the rapid and widespread export of knowledge of iron metallurgy and of iron objects, and the Iron Age supplanted the copper-based Bronze Age. With the large-scale production of iron implements came new patterns of more permanent settlement. On the other hand, the utilisation of iron for weapons put arms in the hands of the masses for the first time and set off a series of large-scale movements of peoples that did not end for 2000 years, in the process dramatically changing the face of Europe and Asia.

Given their similar physico-chemical properties, it is no surprise that iron and copper metabolism are intertwined, and important physiological interactions between iron and copper were

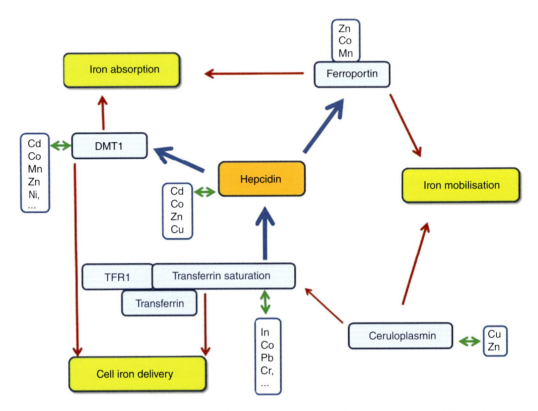

Figure 14.1 *Schematic representation of potential connections between iron, hepcidin and non-iron metals. Special focus has been made on three major processes in iron metabolism: digestive iron absorption, iron mobilisation and cell iron delivery (yellow boxes); and some major proteins and parameters directly involved in iron metabolism (blue boxes). White boxes indicate non-iron metals for which relationships have been reported with adjacent iron metabolism protein. Red arrows represent an involvement of the protein in the targeted biological process. Blue arrows indicate an impact of the protein on the expression/activity of the targeted protein. Reprinted from Loréal, O., Cavey, T., Bardou-Jacquet, E., et al. (2014) Iron, hepcidin and the metal connection.* Front. Pharmacol., *5, 128. This is an open-access article distributed under the terms of the Creative Commons Attribution License (CC BY)*

established in humans many years ago (Fox, 2003; Collins *et al.*, 2010; Gulec and Collins, 2014a). The landmark 1928 paper of Hart, Elvehjem and coworkers (Hart *et al.*, 1928) is generally given credit for the initial identification of the copper/iron link, specifically for their discovery of the role of copper in forming haemoglobin and in overcoming anaemia. However, as Paul Fox (Fox, 2003) has pointed out in his elegant review, metabolic links between copper and iron were first documented over a century-and-a-half ago by clinicians in France and Italy. To date, the homeostatic effects of one on the other has not been elucidated at the molecular level, although recently mechanistic insights into how copper influences iron metabolism have begun to be unravelled. In iron deficiency, elevated copper levels are observed in the intestinal mucosa, liver and blood. As will be described in the following, copper accumulation and/or redistribution within enterocytes may influence iron transport, and high levels of hepatic copper may enhance the biosynthesis of circulating ferroxidase ceruloplasmin, which potentiates iron release from stores.

14.2.1.2   Copper Acquisition and Metabolism

Many of the initial studies on Cu metabolism were made in the model eukaryote, the yeast *Saccharomyces cerevisiae* (Nevitt *et al.*, 2012), and proved helpful in identifying the orthologous proteins which operate in a similar manner in mammalian cells (Figure 14.2). As will be seen, mutations in many of these proteins lead to human disease. However, it is clear that despite the high degree of structural and functional conservation of proteins of Cu metabolism between yeast and mammals, both their expression and their regulation differ. In yeast, mechanisms of high-affinity Cu acquisition are activated only under conditions where environmental levels of Cu availability fall below a critical level; otherwise, low-affinity uptake systems are used. In contrast, the high-affinity system is the only one operational in mammalian cells, and is regulated post-transcriptionally, whereas the regulation of copper uptake in yeast is drastically different.

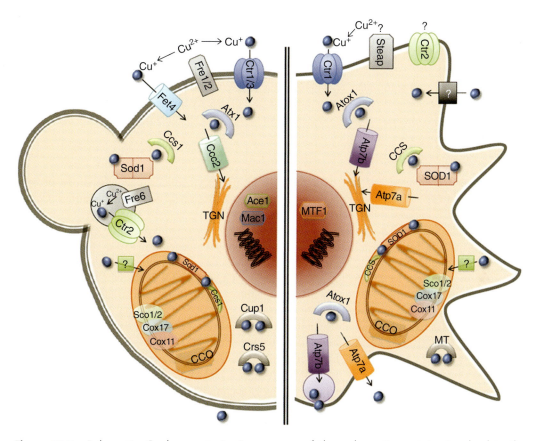

Figure 14.2 *Eukaryotic Cu homeostasis. A summary of the eukaryotic proteins involved in the sensing, acquisition, intracellular distribution and mobilisation of copper (Cu). Each protein, and its function and mode of action, are discussed in the text. The model to the left depicts the copper homeostasis machinery in S. cerevisiae, whereas the model on the right depicts these components in a generic mammalian cell. Reprinted with permission from Elsevier from Nevitt, T., Öhrvik, H. and Thiele, D.J. (2012) Charting the travels of copper in eukaryotes from yeast to mammals. Biochim. Biophys. Acta,* **1823***, 1580–1593*

When Cu concentrations are adequate the cellular requirements of *S. cerevisiae* for Fe, Cu, Mn and Zn are met by the Fe^{2+} transporter Fet4 and the Smf (Suppressor of mitochondrial function) family of divalent metal transporters orthologous to the NRAMP (Natural Resistance-Associated Macrophage Protein) family of mammalian metal permeases (Dix *et al.*, 1997; Liu *et al.*, 1997). However, when Cu concentrations fall below the K_m for transport by Smf transporters (approximately 25–50 µM Cu), the expression of cell-surface metalloreductases, required to reduce Cu^{2+}, and high-affinity Cu^+ transporters (K_m for Cu approximately 1–5 µM) is activated by the Mac1 and Cuf1 transcription factors, leading to the accumulation of Ctr (Cu transporter) and Fre (ferri-reductase) proteins at the plasma and vacuolar membranes. Together, these drive the concerted mobilisation of this metal from environmental sources as well as intracellular stores.

Mammalian cells acquire Cu (Figure 14.2) via the high-affinity Cu^+ importer, Ctr1, a homologue of the yeast Ctr family. As in yeast, mammalian Ctr1 requires prior reduction of Cu^{2+} to Cu^+ and it seems that members of the Steap family of metalloreductases (Steap2, Steap3 and Steap4) can function as both cupric and ferric reductases (Ohgami *et al.*, 2006). The regulation of Ctr1 activity occurs predominantly at the level of transporter localisation and abundance. Ctr1 is present at the plasma membrane at times of cellular demand for Cu and, following Ctr1 endocytosis in response to elevated exogenous Cu, on the membrane of intracellular vesicles (Petris *et al.*, 2003; Guo *et al.*, 2004). A structurally related Ctr protein designated Ctr2 (Zhou and Gitschier, 1997) has been identified in mice and mammals, although its function in mammalian Cu transport *in vivo* is still uncertain (Nevitt *et al.*, 2012). A role for the transport of dietary copper as Cu-chloride complexes by an intestinal apical anion exchanger (Zimnicka *et al.*, 2011) has been proposed.

14.2.1.3 Copper Chaperones

Once copper has entered the cell it binds to specialised cytosolic copper chaperone proteins (Figure 14.2), CCS and Atox1, which then transfer copper to specific cellular destinations. Copper chaperones are found not only in the cytosol but also in numerous cell organelles, and bind Cu^+ at coordination sites which are stable enough to sequester the metal yet labile enough to allow efficient metal transfer between protein partners. The copper is transferred from the chaperone to its specific partner, which has a higher copper-binding activity, through specific metal-mediated protein–protein interactions (Banci *et al.*, 2006, 2010). CCS activates cytosolic Cu, Zn-dependent superoxide dismutase (SOD1), while Atox1 transfers copper to the Cu^+-transporting ATPases Atp7a and Atp7b in the secretory pathway. The active form of SOD1 is a stable homodimer with an intramolecular disulphide bond, and both copper transfer and disulphide bond formation are catalysed by CCS (Rae *et al.*, 1999, 2004; Furukawa *et al.*, 2004; Proescher *et al.*, 2008; Banci *et al.*, 2013). Mutations in the Cu^+-transporting ATPases Atp7a and Atp7b are responsible for the two classic disorders of Cu metabolism, Wilson's disease and Menkes disease. In Wilson's disease a lack of functional Atp7b results in excessive copper accumulation in hepatic and neuronal tissues, whereas Menkes disease mutations in the *ATP7A* gene result in a massive peripheral copper deficiency due to the blockade of intestinal Cu absorption. Atp7b is involved in the transport of copper into the post-Golgi network and mediates copper efflux for biliary excretion (Roelofsen *et al.*, 2000). Early studies showed that the small, ubiquitously expressed protein MURR1, now known as copper metabolism Murr1 domain-containing (Commd1) protein, is defective in canine copper toxicosis (van den Sluis *et al.*, 2002; Klomp *et al.*, 2003), and liver-specific Commd1 knockout mice have also been shown to be susceptible to hepatic copper accumulation (Vonk *et al.*, 2011). Knockdown experiments using siRNA have confirmed that COMMD1 plays a role in biliary copper excretion (Miyayama *et al.*, 2010), although it may not be via a copper-induced modulation of Atp7b (Weiss *et al.*, 2008). More recently, it has been proposed that COMMD1 regulates the endosomal sorting of Atp7b (Phillips-Krawczak *et al.*, 2015).

The terminal oxidase of the respiratory chain, cytochrome *c* oxidase (CCO), as we saw in Chapter 2, is a haem-copper oxidase, and the insertion of Cu into the two mitochondrially encoded subunits Cox1 and Cox2 is mediated by the concerted action of several Cu-chaperones, Cox17, Cox 11, Sco1 and Sco2.

14.2.1.4 Iron–Copper Interactions

As outlined earlier, important interactions between iron and copper have been described in mammals (Fox, 2003; Collins *et al.*, 2010; Gulec and Collins, 2014a), and in the following the aim was to identify the nature of these interactions at the molecular level. The best established Cu–Fe interaction is that involving the multicopper oxidases (MCOs) which have ferroxidase activity (Vashchenko and MacGillivray, 2013), and their role in the mobilisation of intracellular iron (Chapter 6). There are some 12 cuproenzymes known in mammals, of which four are MCOs, all with ferroxidase activity.

MCOs are unique among copper proteins in that they contain at least one each of the three types of biological copper sites – type 1, type 2, and the binuclear type 3. MCOs are descended from the family of small blue copper proteins (cupredoxins) which probably arose as a complement to the haem-iron-based cytochromes involved in electron transport; this event corresponded to the aerobiosis of the biosphere that resulted in the conversion of Fe(II) to Fe(III) as the predominant redox state of this essential metal and the solubilisation of copper from Cu_2S to $Cu(H_2O)n^{2+}$ (Kosman, 2010). MCOs are widely distributed throughout Nature and play essential roles in the physiology of essentially all aerobes. Together with the terminal copper-haem oxidases of the respiratory chain, MCOs share the ability to catalyse the four-electron reduction of O_2 to two molecules of water. A subset of MCO proteins exhibit specificity for Fe^{2+}, Cu^+ and/or Mn^{2+} as reducing substrates, and have been designated as metallooxidases. These enzymes, in particular the ferroxidases found in all fungi and metazoans, play critical roles in the metabolism of these metals. Ferroxidases catalyse the reactions (14.1) and (14.2):

$$4Fe^{2+} + 4Cu^{2+} - MCO \rightarrow 4Fe^{3+} + 4Cu^+ - MCO \tag{14.1}$$

$$4Cu^+ - MCO + 4H^+ + O_2 \rightarrow 4Cu^{2+} - MCO + 2H_2O \tag{14.2}$$

to give the global reaction (14.3)

$$4Fe^{2+} + 4H^+ + O_2 \rightarrow 4Fe^{3+} + 2H_2O \tag{14.3}$$

MCOs are derived from 100- to 150-residue mononuclear blue copper proteins, exemplified by rusticyanin, azurin and plastocyanin. The cupredoxin protein fold consists of a mixture of antiparallel and parallel β-strands; connected by a mixture of β-turns and relatively large loops resulting in a Greek-key β-barrel folding motif (Murphy *et al.*, 1997). This is a unique fold distinguishable from the Greek-key motif characteristic of the immunoglobulin fold found in Cu,Zn superoxide dismutase, for example. MCOs contain two, three or six of these cupredoxin domains assembled into a single polypeptide chain by cycles of gene duplication and loss (Figure 14.3).

The ancestral 'blue copper' type 1 Cu-coordination site has the sequence –His–50–70 residues– Cys–four residues–His–five residues–Met or Leu–, as illustrated for rusticyanin in Figure 14.3. Although 'shielded' from solvent by the coordinating amino acid side chains, the T1 Cu atom is strikingly redox active. Its characteristic intrinsic electronic properties are due to the highly efficient

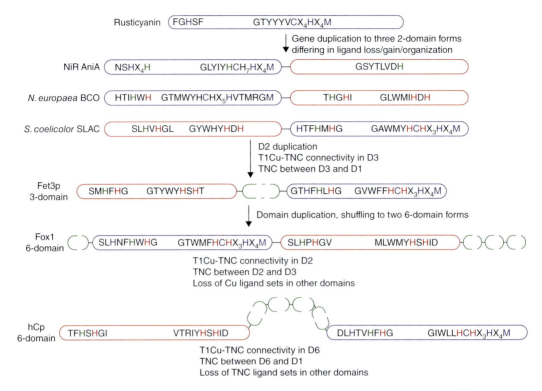

Figure 14.3 *Evolutionary trajectory from a cupredoxin to six-domain multicopper oxidase (MCO) proteins. The initial gene duplication event producing a two-domain cupredoxin from the ancestral small, blue Cu protein (e.g., rusticyanin) is not archived; the presumed progeny of this event are represented by nitrite reductase (NiR) proteins and the small 'laccases' (SLAC). The former are not true MCOs since they possess only type 1 (T1; ligands shown in blue) and type 2 (T2; ligands shown in green) Cu sites while lacking the type 3 (T3) binuclear pair that is the core of the trinuclear cluster (TNC) found in true MCOs (ligands shown in orange). These two-domain species assemble their T2 sites (NiRs) and TNCs [blue copper oxidase (BCO), SLAC] between adjacent subunits, e.g., they are active as trimers of these two-domain monomeric units. Subsequent gene duplication and shuffling gave rise to three- and six-domain MCOs, represented here by the ferroxidases Fet3p, human ceruloplasmin (hCp), and Fox1. Note that the TNC in the former two proteins assembles between the N- and C-terminal cupredoxin domains, whereas in Fox1 it assembles between D2 and D3. This difference reflects a different sequence of evolutionary domain shuffling. Note also how the GN_n C or GN_nH motif in essentially all ligand-containing domains traces back to the ancestral cupredoxin. Reprinted with kind permission from Springer Science and Media from Kosman, D.J. (2010) Multicopper oxidases: a workshop on copper coordination chemistry, electron transfer, and metallophysiology.* J. Biol. Inorg. Chem., **15**, 15–28*

charge transfer from an Spπ orbital into the Cu3$dx2-y2$ orbital, resulting in a highly covalent Cu–S bond, which dominates the spectroscopic properties of MCOs. The three-dimensional structures of the sequence motif characteristic of the TI Cu cupredoxin loop is reflected in the almost perfect superposition of the $\beta\alpha\beta$-fold which wraps around the T1 Cu in six proteins of the MCO family (Figure 14.4). The nature of the axial ligand in the type 1 copper centre is a strong modulator of the copper reduction potential (Xu *et al.*, 1999; Palmer *et al.*, 2003; Solomon *et al.*, 2004).

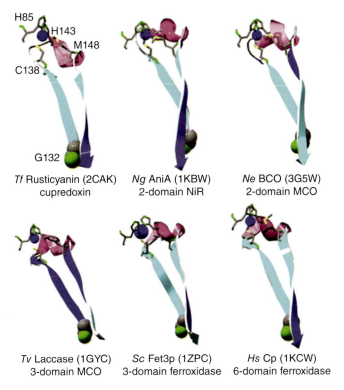

H85
H143
M148
C138
G132

Tf Rusticyanin (2CAK)   *Ng* AniA (1KBW)   *Ne* BCO (3G5W)
cupredoxin   2-domain NiR   2-domain MCO

Tv Laccase (1GYC)   *Sc* Fet3p (1ZPC)   *Hs* Cp (1KCW)
3-domain MCO   3-domain ferroxidase   6-domain ferroxidase

Figure 14.4   *The T1 Cu cupredoxin loop. The sequence motif characteristic of the cupredoxin T1 Cu site is reflected in the near superimposition of the βαβ-fold that wraps around the T1 Cu in these six proteins. The Met ligand, if present, is found at the end of the short helical connectivity. The His ligand at this site not within this antiparallel motif is found approximately 50 residues N-terminal to it (e.g., H85 in rusticyanin). Note that this structural motif is seen in all cupredoxin descendants, irrespective of domain number, number of Cu sites overall, or function. Tf, Thiobacillus ferrooxidans; Ng, Neisseria gonorrhoeae; Ne, Nitrosomonas europaea; Tv, Trametes versicolor; Sc, Saccharomyces cerevisiae; Hs, Homo sapiens. Reprinted with kind permission from Springer Science and Media from Kosman, D.J. (2010) Multicopper oxidases: a workshop on copper coordination chemistry, electron transfer, and metallophysiology. J. Biol. Inorg. Chem., **15**, 15–28*

Most MCOs are composed of three domains with type I copper in domain 3, and a trinuclear cluster at the interface of domains 1 and 3, whereas six-domain MCOs, such as ceruloplasmin (and most probably hephaestin) contain type 1 copper in domains 2, 4 and 6, and a trinuclear cluster comprising one type 2 copper and a dinuclear type 3 centre at the interface of domains 1 and 6 (Nakamura and Go, 2005). Electrons are transferred from the type I copper centres to the trinuclear centre, where oxygen binds and is reduced to water. The structure of human Cp is shown in Figure 14.5. Whereas in most MCOs the reducing substrate binds via a hydrogen bond to at least one of the T1 His ligands (illustrated for *T. versicolor* laccase in Figure 14.6a), in the metallooxidase Fet3p the corresponding His is shielded from solvent by the carboxylate side chains. Structurally, homologous carboxylates shield the redox active T1 Cu sites in ceruloplasmin (Lindley *et al.*, 1997). It is proposed that in ferroxidases like Fet3p and Cp, the Fe(II) binds to these carboxylates. In Fet3p, the substrate does not contact the coordinating His imidazoles, but binds to the protein via two carboxylate groups, which themselves are in H-bond contact with the two His

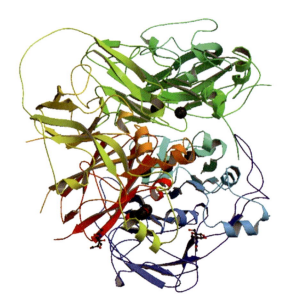

Figure 14.5 *Structure of human ceruloplasmin (PDB 1KCW)*

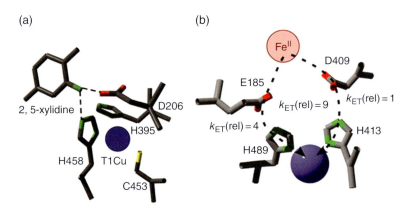

Figure 14.6 *Substrate binding modes and electron transfer pathways. (a) In laccases, phenolic and aromatic amine substrates bind via an H-bond to at least one of the T1 His ligands, e.g., H458 in T. versicolor Lac. This could provide the electron transfer pathway to the T1 Cu(II) (1KYA). (b) In ferroxidases (Fet3p, 1ZPU), these His ligands are shielded from solvent by carboxylate side chains that are themselves H-bonded to the Nε2–NH groups on these imidazoles; the Fe(II) binds to these carboxylate groups. Reprinted with kind permission from Springer Science and Media from Kosman, D.J. (2010) Multicopper oxidases: a workshop on copper coordination chemistry, electron transfer, and metallophysiology.* J. Biol. Inorg. Chem., **15**, *15–28*

ligands (H413 and H489) at the T1 Cu. This H-bonding network provides the outer sphere electron transfer pathway in Fet3p, and presumably also in Cp (Kosman, 2010).

Ceruloplasmin, which binds 70–90% of plasma copper, was the first MCO to be discovered. Its primary function, together with ferroportin, is to mediate the release of Fe^{2+} from cells and the transfer of Fe^{3+} to apotransferrin (see Chapter 6). Aceruloplasminaemia (Chapter 15), the human disease caused by the absence or mutation of Cp, results in an accumulation of iron, notably in the liver and brain, underlining this role. Cp is mostly synthesised by hepatocytes, where the P-type ATPase Atp7B inserts copper into ApoCp during its transit through the trans-Golgi network (Lutsenko *et al.*, 2007) and is secreted into the plasma. A splice-variant of Cp which was originally characterised in brain (Patel and David, 1997; Patel *et al.*, 2000), linked by a glycosylphosphati-dylinositol (GPI) anchor to membranes (GPI-Cp), has also been found in several other tissues including macrophages and hepatocytes (De Domenica *et al.*, 2007; Mostad and Prohaska, 2011; Marques *et al.*, 2012). The intestinal enriched MCO named hephaestin (Vulpe *et al.*, 1999) plays the same role as Cp at the basolateral membrane of intestinal epithelial cells (Chapter 7), while the recently described zyklopen is proposed to mediate iron transfer between mother and foetus in placenta and mammary gland (Chen *et al.*, 2012).

In the intestine, the copper status may affect iron uptake at the apical membrane of enterocytes, and iron efflux at the basolateral face (Figure 14.7). The ferrireductase Dcyb1 can reduce both iron and copper, and since Dcyb1 is induced by copper deprivation (Matak *et al.*, 2013) it has been proposed that the hypoxia resulting from copper-deficiency anaemia leads to an increased transcription of Dcyb1 mediated by the hypoxia-inducible transcription factor HIF2α. It was previously thought that the iron transporter DMT1 could be involved in the transport of Cu^+ across the apical border of the intestinal epithelium. There is some evidence that DMT1 can transport Cu in cell cultures (Arredonda *et al.*, 2003, 2014; Espinoza *et al.*, 2012), and the overexpression of DMTI leads to specific Cu transport in iron deficiency (Jiang *et al.*, 2013). However, data for human DMT1 expressed in RNA-injected *Xenopus* oocytes, using radiotracer assays and the continuous measurement of transport by fluorescence, do not support previous reports that copper is a substrate of DMT1 (Illing *et al.*, 2012). The data show that, whereas DMT1 clearly selects Fe^{2+} over its other physiological substrates, it is a likely route of entry for Cd^{2+} and may serve in the transport of Co^{2+}, Mn^{2+} and Vo^{2+}. The authors predicted that DMT1 should contribute little, if at all, to the absorption or uptake of Zn^{2+}. Clearly, the physiological role of DMT1 in copper transport across the apical membrane of enterocytes remains to be established unequivocally.

It has been established that Cu is absorbed at the apical membrane of the intestinal lumen by the human copper transporter hCtr1 (Nose *et al.*, 2010). hCtr1 transports Cu in its reduced form, Cu^+, and therefore requires the assistance of the ferrireductase Dcyb, which also functions as a cupric reductase (Wyman *et al.*, 2008). In this manner, Cu^+ and Fe^{2+} availability is linked on the lumenal level in addition to the systemic level, further strengthening the coregulation of these two micronutrients, as outlined in Figure 14.7.

Cellular iron efflux by FPN1 may also be modulated by copper, although whereas copper deficiency in mice was shown to increase FPN1 mRNA expression, (Matak *et al.*, 2013), contradictory results were observed in another study (Prohaska and Broderius, 2012). Perturbation of intracellular copper homeostasis by knockdown of the ATP7A copper transporter (Gulec and Collins, 2014b) enhanced FPN1 expression and increased cellular iron efflux.

Clearly, since the MCOs require copper, their activity could be influenced by copper levels. In the intestine of copper-deficient mice the ferroxidase activity attributed to hephaestin (HEPH) decreased, possibly contributing to the development of systemic iron deficiency (Chen *et al.*, 2006). Iron absorption was also decreased in copper-deficient rats (Reeves and DeMars, 2004), perhaps due to impaired HEPH activity (Reeves *et al.*, 2005). When copper-deficient rats were re-fed a copper-containing diet, HEPH protein levels increased and iron absorption was restored (Reeves and DeMars, 2005), confirming earlier studies of impaired iron absorption in copper-deficient swine (Lee *et al.*, 1968). HEPH interacts directly with FPN1 in rat enterocytes, and this interaction was reduced on iron feeding (Yeh *et al.*, 2009). Thus, copper restriction, via its

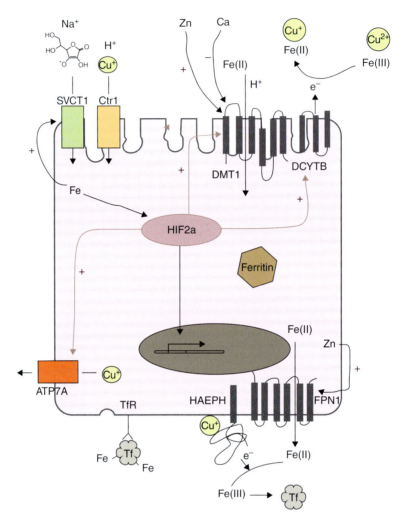

Figure 14.7 *Overview of interactions between Fe, Cu and ascorbate transporters with the hypoxia transcription factor HIF-2α, Fe, Cu, Zn and Ca in enterocytes. Cu transport and the control of transcription by HIF-2α is central for regulation of iron absorption. Reprinted from Scheers, N. (2013) Regulatory effects of Cu, Zn, and Ca on Fe absorption: the intricate play between nutrient transporters. Nutrients, **5**, 957–970. This is an open-access article distributed under the terms of the Creative Commons Attribution License (CC BY)*

influence on HEPH biosynthesis, could indirectly affect FPN1 protein levels on the basolateral surface of enterocytes and influence transepithelial iron flux.

Iron deficiency would be expected to modify copper homeostasis in duodenal enterocytes, and the intracellular copper-binding proteins metallothionein I/II (MTI/MTII) (Collins, 2006; Collins *et al.*, 2005; Gulec and Collins, 2013) and the copper exporter Atp7a (Ravia *et al.*, 2005; Collins *et al.*, 2005; Gulec and Collins, 2013) are upregulated in duodenal enterocytes from iron-deficient rats, consistent with copper accumulation in the intestinal mucosa. How copper enters enterocytes during iron deficiency is not clear, although Dmt1 expression is also upregulated by iron deprivation and it is proposed that Dmt1 transports copper during iron deficiency (Jiang *et al.*, 2013). These copper-related events occur in the setting of increased iron transport, suggesting that alterations in copper homeostasis may be functionally linked to iron metabolism. The increased MT, DMT1 and Atp7A expression in duodenal enterocytes during iron deficiency was associated with not only copper accumulation in the intestinal mucosa but also in the liver (Collins *et al.*, 2005; Ravia *et al.*, 2005). Since copper homeostasis in duodenal enterocytes and in the liver is altered during iron deficiency, it was postulated that the Atp7A copper transporter influenced iron transport. Atp7A knockdown increased transepithelial iron flux, supporting this hypothesis (Gulec and Collins, 2014b), and this increase was associated with transcriptional induction of FPN1 expression, consistent with enhanced basolateral iron transfer in the knockdown cells. Collectively, this provides further evidence of the importance of copper in the regulation of intestinal iron absorption (Gulec and Collins, 2014a).

The role of hypoxia inducible factor-2α (HIF-2α) in regulating the expression of genes involved in iron absorption was discussed in Chapter 10. Both, iron and copper deficiency can upregulate HIF-2α, and several HIF-target genes are involved in the homeostasis of these metals. Under conditions of iron deficiency, decreased haemoglobin levels cause hypoxia and stimulate erythropoiesis. In conditions of iron deficiency, hypoxia or increased erythropoietic drive, HIF-2 is stabilised in the duodenal enterocyte and transcriptionally upregulates the expression of DMT1, DcytB, and FPN. This leads to an increased expression of DMT1 and DcytB at the apical brush border membrane and of FPN at the basal membrane (Taylor *et al.*, 2011; Mastrogiannaki *et al.*, 2009; Shah *et al.*, 2009; Anderson *et al.*, 2011). The direct binding of HIF-2 to consensus HRE elements in the regulatory regions of the promoters has been shown for DcytB and DMT1. At the systemic level, the same three factors repress hepatic hepcidin production, preventing its inhibitory action on duodenal iron absorption (Mastrogiannaki *et al.*, 2013).

Copper deficiency leads to anaemia, duodenal hypoxia, upregulation of HIF-2α and altered expression of iron absorption genes in mice (Matak *et al.*, 2013). Copper has been shown to be required for transactivation of gene expression by the HIF transcriptional complex (which contains a hypoxia-responsive HIFα subunit and a constitutively expressed HIFβ subunit) (Martin *et al.*, 2005; Feng *et al.*, 2009). The HIFα subunits are also stabilised by iron deprivation *in vivo* and *in vitro* (Pan *et al.*, 2007). Consistent with this, a recent study in Caco-2 cells demonstrated that iron chelation led to a preferential induction of HIF-responsive genes (Hu *et al.*, 2010). HIF-related regulation of gene expression is thus likely influenced by iron and copper levels, and importantly, several HIF-target genes are involved in the homeostasis of these metals. The intestinal copper transporter Atp7A is also regulated by HIF2α (Xie and Collins, 2011, 2013), while the gene encoding another intestinal copper transporter, CTR1, has also been shown to be basally regulated by HIF2α (Pourvali *et al.*, 2012).

As we saw in Chapter 7, ascorbate is an important regulator of iron transport, assisting DcytB in the intestinal lumen by reducing ferric iron to the ferrous form. In addition, cellular ascorbate status influences enterocyte protein levels of DMT1 and DcytB in the absence of iron (Scheers and Sandberg, 2008). HIF-2α, which regulates DMT1, DcytB and FPN1 transcription, is degraded by ascorbate-, iron- and oxygen-dependent prolyl hydroxylases. Thus, low ascorbate, iron and oxygen levels stabilise HIF-2α, providing a possible mechanism for the effects of ascorbate on DMT1 and DcytB expression. Ascorbate is absorbed in the intestinal lumen by means of the ascorbate/sodium transporter SVCT1 (Figure 14.7). The SVCT1 expression is regulated by ascorbate (MacDonald *et al.*, 2002) and also by iron (Scheers and Sandberg, 2011). Increased cellular iron levels upregulate ascorbate uptake, after which increased ascorbate levels downregulate DCYTB and DMT1 in response to the iron load, closing the feedback loop. It has recently been shown that iron transport across the basal border via FPN1 is influenced by the intracellular status of ascorbate and that IRP2 and HIF-2α are involved (Scheers and Sandberg, 2014).

The liver represents a major focus for iron–copper interactions, as the site of biosynthesis, the insertion of its complement of six copper atoms and secretion into the circulation of the multicopper ferroxidase, Cp. As we saw in Chapter 6, Cp mediates the oxidation of ferrous iron released from some tissues (including the liver) by ferroportin and its incorporation into transferrin. Iron-deficient rats load copper into the liver and, conversely, copper-deficient rats and mice have increased hepatic iron levels (Sourkes *et al.*, 1968; Owen, 1973; Williams *et al.*, 1983; Singh and Medeiros, 1984; Ravia *et al.*, 2005). While the molecular mechanisms underlying liver copper loading during iron deficiency are not understood, the latter observation is most likely due to reduced Cp activity (Broderius *et al.*, 2010). The liver is also the site of biosynthesis of hepcidin, the key regulator of systemic iron homeostasis, and direct effects of copper on the expression and activity of hepcidin have been reported. Decreased hepcidin expression is observed in both copper-deficient mice (Chen *et al.*, 2006) and rats (Jenkitkasemwong *et al.*, 2010; Broderius *et al.*, 2012). Although the earliest link between iron and copper was the role of the latter in overcoming anaemia, thereby establishing the importance of copper in haemoglobin formation (Hart *et al.*, 1928), nearly a century later we are still none the wiser as to how copper intervenes in haemoglobin synthesis in erythroid cells. Signs of iron deficiency in copper-deficient rats are not affected by iron supplements administered either by diet or by injection (Reeves and DeMars, 2006), and copper-deficiency anaemia in mice can occur even when plasma iron concentrations are normal (Pyatskowit and Prohaska, 2008). So, if a lack of iron is not the cause of the anaemia, the logical conclusion is that copper deficiency in some as-yet to be established way impairs iron utilisation by erythroid cells (Gulec and Collins, 2014b). Finally, it is evident that since the ferroportin/ceruloplasmin tandem is required for cellular iron mobilisation, copper deficiency, reflected by lower levels of Cp, will result in a decreased iron availability for haem synthesis from the reticuloendothelial stores of iron from effete red blood cells.

14.2.2 Zinc

14.2.2.1 Introduction

Zinc is a trace element nutrient which is essential for life as it plays a vital role in many cellular processes. After iron, Zn^{2+} is the second most abundant trace element in the human body. The average adult human contains about 3 g of Zn^{2+}, most of it (95%) intracellular. Zn^{2+} binds to around 10% of proteins in the human proteome, is required for the function of over 2000 transcription factors, and is a cofactor for over 300 enzymes. Indeed, it is the only metal to have representatives in each of the six classes of enzymes (oxidoreductases, transferases, hydrolases, lyases, isomerases and ligases). Zinc deficiency causes growth retardation, immune dysfunction, cognitive impairment, metabolic disorders and infertility, whereas excess zinc is toxic. Thus, despite the high demand for zinc in cells, free or labile zinc must be kept at very low levels. In humans, two major zinc transporter families, the SLC30 (ZnT) and SLC39 (ZIP), function to maintain cellular zinc homeostasis. Essentially, the two families of zinc transporters work in opposite directions to control zinc trafficking in and out of the cell or in and out of intracellular compartments such as the endoplasmic reticulum, Golgi, mitochondria, and vesicles.

The SLC30 family, also known as the ZnT family, comprises 10 members which are involved in: (i) moving zinc from the cytoplasm into intracellular compartments to supply zinc for zinc-containing proteins and to store zinc intracellularly; and (ii) shuffling cytoplasmic zinc out to the extracellular space to avoid zinc toxicity (Palmiter and Huang, 2004; Huang and Tepaamorndech, 2013).

The localisation of ZnT transporters in a generalised mammalian cell is shown in Figure 14.8a. Their localisation in an intestinal epithelial cell, a secreting mammary epithelial cell, and of ZnT3 in a synaptic vesicle of an axon terminals are shown respectively in the other three panels of Figure 14.8. The absence of ZnT10 in the figure reflects the lack of publications to date on its properties.

The SLC39 family, also called the ZIP (derived from the yeast Zrt1 protein and the *Arabidopsis thaliana* Irt1 protein) family has 14 members, and their cellular localisation is shown in Figure 14.9. They all have eight predicted transmembrane (TM) domains with their N and C termini facing the extracytoplasmic space (Figure 14.9, inset), and function in the uptake of zinc into the cytoplasm from the extracellular space of the cell or from the intracellular storage compartment when the cytoplasmic zinc level is low (Eide, 2004; Jeong and Eide, 2013). The two zinc transporter families work together to maintain zinc homeostasis in the cell.

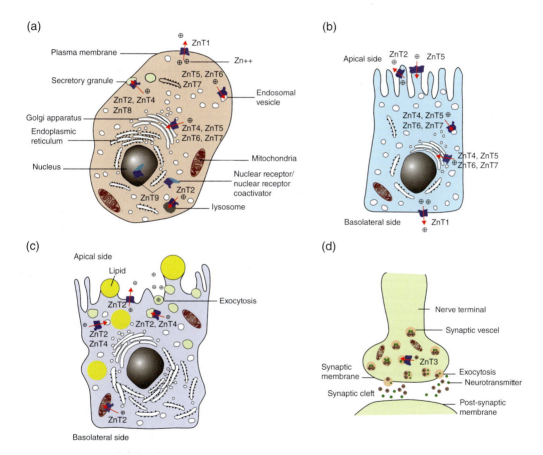

Figure 14.8 *Cellular localisation of ZnT transporters. (a) Localisation of ZnT transporters in a generalised mammalian cell. (b) Localisation of ZnT transporters in an intestinal epithelial cell. (c) Localisation of ZnT transporters in a secreting mammary epithelial cell. (d) Localisation of ZnT3 in an axon terminal. Organelles of the cell are labelled in panel (a). Arrows indicate the direction of translocation of zinc ions (⊕) across the membrane by ZnT transporters (𝗪). Reprinted with permission from Elsevier from Huang, L. and Tepaamorndech, S. (2013) The SLC30 family of zinc transporters – a review of current understanding of their biological and pathophysiological roles. Mol. Aspects Med., **34**, 548–560*

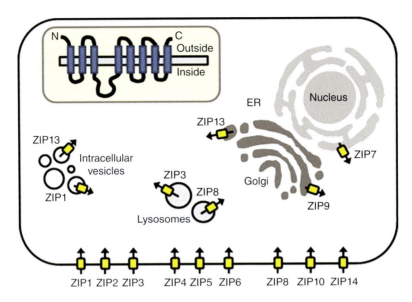

Figure 14.9 *Subcellular localisation of human ZIP transporters. Directions of zinc transport are shown as arrows. Note that this figure only provides a very simplified view, as the expression of some ZIP proteins are tissue- or cell type-specific, and regulated by zinc status or other signals. The inset shaded in yellow depicts the predicted topology of a ZIP transporter. Reprinted with permission from Elsevier from Jeong, J. and Eide, D.J. (2014) The SLC39 family of zinc transporters. Mol. Aspects Med., 34, 612–619*

14.2.2.2   Iron–Zinc Interactions

While ferroportin1 (*FPN1*) expression can be transcriptionally regulated by iron (Knutson *et al.*, 2003; Delaby *et al.*, 2008), it can also be regulated by other transition metals, such as zinc, manganese, cadmium, cobalt and copper (Troadec *et al.*, 2010). Zinc and cadmium induce FPN1 transcription in murine macrophages through the action of Metal Transcription Factor-1 (*MTF-1*). MTF-1 targets genes coping with heavy metal loading such as metallothionein 1 (MT-1) or the zinc efflux transporter Znt1. *MTF-1* can also mediate the induction of MT genes in response to other stress situations, such as oxidative stress and hypoxia (Laity and Andrews, 2007). MTF-1 binds to the *FPN1* promoter in the presence of zinc, but not in response to iron, and mutagenesis of the two Metal Responsive Elements (MREs) in the *FPN1* promoter abolishes the MTF-1 zinc responsiveness. Cadmium also induces FPN1 transcription in an MRE-dependent manner. It was also shown that Fpn can transport zinc and can protect zinc sensitive cells from high zinc toxicity. More recently (Mitchell *et al.*, 2014), the expression of human FPN in *Xenopus* oocytes was shown to stimulate not only Fe efflux but also the efflux of Zn and Co, but not of Cu, Cd or Mn. Hepcidin treatment of oocytes inhibited the efflux of Fe, Zn and Co.

Zn upregulates the apical uptake of iron by increasing the level of DMT1 in human CaCo-2 cells (Yamaji *et al.*, 2001) while increasing both the expression of FPN1 mRNA and the basolateral efflux of iron (Figure 14.7). The systemic acute phase response to infection and inflammation include hypoferraemia, involving regulation of the iron transporter ferroportin 1 by hepcidin, and hypozincaemia. The mechanism whereby plasma zinc is reduced is thought to involve the Zn transporter Zip14, which is upregulated by interleukin (IL)-6 in primary hepatocyte cultures and localises to the plasma membrane (Liuzzi *et al.*, 2005). Subsequently, it has been suggested that

Zip14 mediates non-transferrin-bound iron uptake by hepatocytes, thereby contributing to the hepatic iron loading that characterises haemochromatosis and transfusional iron overload (Liuzzi *et al.*, 2006). Zip14 seems to be a broad-scope metal ion transporter which, under normal conditions, mediates cellular Zn uptake but which in iron overload can also transport NTBI (Pinilla-Tenas *et al.*, 2011).

Mutations in the human *Zip4* gene cause acrodermatitis enteropathica, a rare, pseudo-dominant, lethal genetic disorder. An enterocyte-specific knockout of this gene in mice which mimics this human disorder was created, and established that Zip4 is expressed throughout the intestine, is required for intestinal integrity, and is crucial for zinc absorption (Geiser *et al.*, 2012). Whether Zip4 plays a role in iron absorption remains to be established.

14.2.3 Cobalt

14.2.3.1 Introduction

Although its concentration in human serum is less than 1% that of iron, copper or zinc, the primary function of cobalt in humans involves its role as the cofactor of a number of important vitamin B_{12}-dependent enzymes. Co has the particularity, simillar to Ni, that in lower oxidation states some of their 3d electrons are forced into exposed σ- (or π-) orbitals: the outcome is that the tetragonal low spin d^7 Co(II) ion is a reactive free radical, and this property is exploited in vitamin B_{12}-dependent enzymatic transformations which require a source of free radicals, like the Class II ribonucleotide reductases of *Lactobacillus* sp. (see Chapter 2).

Vitamin B_{12} (a generic term for all cobalamines biologically active in humans) is a water-soluble tetrapyrrole vitamin (for reviews, see Krautler, 2012; Kozyraki and Cases, 2013; Gerasim *et al.*, 2013). It comprises a central cobalt atom which is the functional part of vitamin B_{12}, coordinated to four equatorial nitrogen ligands of the planar corrin ring (Figure 14.10a). The fifth Co ligand is a nitrogen atom from a 5.6-dimethylbenzimidazole nucleotide covalently linked to the corrin ring, while the sixth ligand can be either a cyanide-, methyl- or deoxyadenosyl- group. Cyanocobalamine is the vitamin itself, whereas methylcobalamine and adenosylcobalamine are the metabolically active derivatives of vitamin B_{12} representing respectively 75–90% and 10–25% of the endogenous vitamin B_{12} pool. Vitamin B_{12} is essential for carbohydrate, fat and protein metabolism, the formation and regeneration of red blood cells, and maintenance of the central nervous system.

Vitamin B_{12} was first identified in 1925 as the antipernicious anaemia factor. However, unlike other water-soluble vitamins there is a unique absorption, delivery, and activation system for vitamin B_{12} in mammals. The selective absorption of vitamin B_{12} is a multistep process, involving the stomach, pancreas and small intestine (Figure 14.10b). It is mediated by two carriers, haptocorrin (HC) and intrinsic factor (IF); these two homologous proteins each carry a single vitamin B_{12} molecule (Greibe *et al.*, 2012). The malabsorption of vitamin B_{12} due to a dysfunction of any of these steps can lead to vitamin B_{12} deficiency. Dietary vitamin B_{12} is released in the upper gastrointestinal tract with the help of gastric acid and pepsin, and subsequently binds to HC, a glycoprotein present in the saliva and gastric fluids. In the duodenum, HC is degraded by pancreatic proteases releasing vitamin B_{12} and allowing its binding to IF; the IF–vitamin B_{12} complex is then taken up into the mucosal cells of the distal ileum by receptor-mediated endocytosis. The initial steps of vitamin B_{12} absorption then involve binding of the IF–vitamin B_{12} complex to cubililn (CUBN), a peripheral membrane protein expressed at the apical pole of the enterocyte, and also in the kidney (Kozyraki *et al.*, 1998; Moestrup *et al.*, 1998; Kristiansen *et al.*, 1999). As CUBN lacks both transmembrane and cytoplasmic domains its internalisation is dependent on two other transmembrane proteins, Amnionless (AMN) and Megalin/LRP2. These proteins

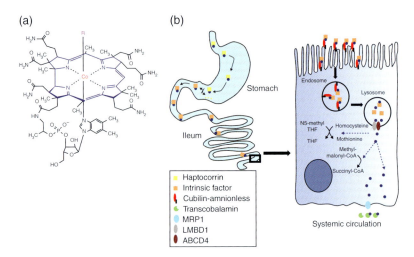

Figure 14.10 *Structure and cellular metabolism of vitamin B$_{12}$. (a) Structure of vitamin B$_{12}$; R may be methyl, deoxyadenosine, cyanide or hydroxyl. (b) In the upper gastrointestinal tract dietary vitamin B$_{12}$ (in blue) binds to haptocorrin. After degradation of haptocorrin in the duodenum, B$_{12}$ binds to the intrinsic factor and reaches the terminal ileum. Cubilin expressed at the apical pole of the enterocyte together with Amnionless binds and internalises the intrinsic factor–vitamin B$_{12}$ complex. Subsequent endocytic transport results in the recycling of Cubilin and Amnionless to the plasma membrane and the lysosomal degradation of the intrinsic factor. Vitamin B$_{12}$ exits the lysosome via LMBD1 and ABCD4. Vitamin B$_{12}$ is released to the bloodstream most likely through the basolateral transporter MRP1. The enzymatic processes which require vitamin B$_{12}$ as a cofactor are shown. Reprinted with permission from Elsevier from Kozyraki, R. and Cases, O. (2013) Vitamin B$_{12}$ absorption: mammalian physiology and acquired and inherited disorders.* Biochimie, **95**, 1002–1007

need to be coexpressed/colocalised with CUBN and to interact physically with CUBN and/or CUBN–ligand complexes (Kozyraki *et al.*, 2001; Strope *et al.*, 2004). Subsequent endocytic transport results in the recycling of Cubilin and Amnionless to the plasma membrane and the lysosomal degradation of the intrinsic factor. Vitamin B$_{12}$ exits the lysosome via LMBD1 and ABCD4, and is released into the bloodstream most likely through the basolateral transporter MRP1 (Kozyraki and Cases, 2013). Once in the bloodstream, cobalamine is associated with two carriers, transcobalamine and HC. Approximately 20% of the circulating cobalamine is bound to transcobalamine, a homologue of HC and IF (Li *et al.*, 1995), while the remainder is bound to HC (Hall *et al.*, 1977; Seetharam and Yammani, 2003). Whereas cobalamine bound to HC is unavailable for uptake by cells outside of the liver, cobalamine bound to transcobalamine is taken up by endocytosis mediated by the cell-surface transcobalamine receptor (TCblR). Transcobalamine is broken down in the lysosomes, releasing free cobalamine, which is transferred across the lysosomal membrane into the cytoplasm by a poorly understood process.

14.2.3.2 Iron–Cobalt Interactions

There are only two known B$_{12}$ enzymes in mammals (Kolhouse and Allen, 1977; Mellman *et al.*, 1977): (i) methionine synthase, a cytoplasmic enzyme which catalyses the transfer of a methyl group from methyltetrahydrofolate to homocysteine to yield tetrahydrofolate and methionine (Ludwig and Matthews, 1997); and (ii) methylmalonyl-CoA mutase, a mitochondrial enzyme that catalyses the isomerisation of methylmalonyl-CoA to succinyl-CoA (Banerjee and Ragsdale, 2003). A functional deficiency in methionine synthase or methylmalonyl-CoA mutase leads to homocystinuria and methylmalonic aciduria, respectively (Shevell and Rosenblatt, 1992; Chandler and Venditti, 2005).

In seeking to explain the interactions between cobalt and iron in humans, it is the methionine synthase reaction which holds the key. Pernicious anaemia, one of many types of the larger family of megaloblastic anaemias which is an often fatal condition in the elderly, is the disease most frequently associated with cobalt and vitamin B_{12}. However, long before the discovery of vitamin B_{12} there were many reports of very varied nervous-system complications associated with megaloblastic anaemia, and it was found that in the absence of treatment nearly all patients with megaloblastic anaemia eventually developed some nervous system involvement before death. From 1945 onwards, folic acid was used in the treatment of pernicious anaemia as the possibly deficient dietary factor. The introduction of vitamin B_{12} treatment, with its beneficial effects on both blood and nervous system, led to the erroneous assumption that the neuropsychiatric symptoms of megaloblastic anaemia were solely due to a deficiency of vitamin B_{12} and not of folic acid (Reynolds, 1979).

Pernicious anaemia is not due to dietary insufficiency of vitamin B_{12}, but to lack of adequate secretion of IF. A more common cause of mild preclinical B_{12} deficiency is the malabsorption of B_{12} from food, which may be linked to *Helicbacter pylori* infections and the long-term use of antacids and biguanides (Andrès *et al.*, 2007). The megaloblastic anaemia found in patients with congenital absence or defective synthesis of IF or transcobalamine is morphologically indistinguishable from the megaloblastic anaemia observed in folic acid deficiency. The neuropsychiatric syndromes and neuropathology observed in both B_{12} and folic acid deficiencies are also virtually identical (Reynolds, 2006).

Vitamin B_{12} and folate play crucial roles in erythropoiesis. Erythroblasts require both folate and vitamin B_{12} for proliferation during their differentiation. A deficiency of folate or vitamin B_{12} inhibits purine and thymidylate syntheses, impairs DNA synthesis, and causes erythroblast apoptosis, resulting in anaemia from ineffective erythropoiesis (Koury and Ponka, 2004). What links folate and vitamin B_{12} in intermediary metabolism is their interconnected role in one-carbon metabolism (Figure 14.11). A key interaction is that between vitamin B_{12} and folate in the synthesis of methionine from homocysteine catalysed by methionine synthase, in which both 5-methyl-tetrahydrofolate and methyl-vitamin-B_{12} are cofactors (Figure 14.11). The one-carbon cycle, which synthesises methyl groups, is essential for many genomic and nongenomic methylation reactions, via *S*-adenosylmethionine and, indirectly, for the synthesis of purines and thymidine and, therefore, of nucleotides, DNA and RNA.

The physiological regulation of red blood cell mass depends on the enhanced transcription in response to hypoxia of the gene for erythropoietin, which is secreted by the kidney and the liver. The regulation of feedback mechanisms which sense levels of tissue oxygenation is mediated by HIFs. HIF-1α is a transcription factor which, during hypoxia, binds with HIF-1β in the nucleus to promoter elements in hypoxia-responsive target genes causing the upregulation of HIF target genes, including erythropoietin. It has been reported that cobalt stabilises HIF-1α by inhibiting the interaction between the von Hippel–Landau protein and hydroxylated HIF-1 (Yuan *et al.*, 2003; Samelko *et al.*, 2013), thereby stimulating erythropoietin synthesis (Zhang *et al.*, 2014). Pre-exposure to hypoxia for 3 h protects rat brain against combined hypoxia/ischaemia 24 h later by causing an upregulation of HIF target genes, and this hypoxia preconditioning can be mimicked by iron chelators such as desferrioxamine and transition metals such as Co^{2+} which inhibit prolyl hydroxylases and increase HIF-1α levels in the brain (Ran *et al.*, 2005).

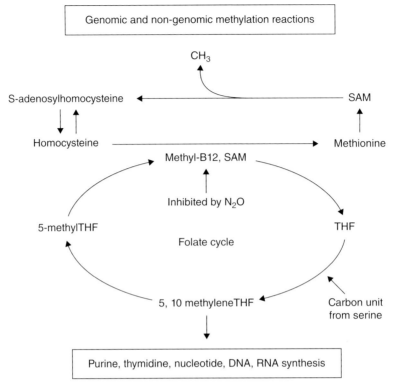

Figure 14.11 *Associations between the folate cycle, vitamin B$_{12}$, methylation, and nucleotide synthesis. SAM, S-adenosylmethionine; THF, tetrahydrofolate. Reprinted with permission of Elsevier from Reynolds, E. (2006) Vitamin B$_{12}$, folic acid, and the nervous system. Lancet Neurol., **5**, 949–960*

14.2.4 Manganese

14.2.4.1 Iron–Manganese Interactions

Manganese is an essential element of the human diet and has many roles in the human body, including the key antioxidant enzyme superoxide dismutase and enzymes involved in neurotransmitter synthesis and metabolism. Nevertheless, elevated Mn levels can cause neurotoxicity, resulting in motor deficits (Parkinson-like syndrome) or psychiatric damage ('manganese madness'), while developmental Mn exposure can adversely affect childhood neurological development (Neal and Guilarte, 2013). Mn deposition in the brain results in a disruption of the basal ganglia circuitry, with globus pallidus, substantia nigra, pars reticulata and striatum being the primary targets (Aschner *et al.*, 2007). A plethora of evidence suggests that Mn directly affects neurons by impairing energy metabolism and increasing the formation of ROS, but Mn may also indirectly enhance neurotoxicity through the activation of glial cells (astrocytes and microglia), inducing the release of non-neuronal-derived ROS and inflammatory mediators (Filipov and Dodd, 2011). Excessive exposure to Mn can occur in the workplace (Gorell *et al.*, 1999), in the environment, such as in populations living near manganese mines (Rodríguez-Agudelo *et al.*, 2006), or in patients receiving long-term parenteral nutrition (Fell *et al.*, 1996). Environmental concerns have been raised by the continuing use of a Mn-containing fuel additive, methylcyclopentadienyl manganese tricarbonyl (MMT), and the increased environmental burdens resulting from its combustion (Pfeifer *et al.*, 2004).

The possibility that ferroportin 1 (Fpn1) could transport transition metal ions other than iron (Troadec *et al.*, 2010) is supported by a growing body of evidence that Fpn1 may also be involved in Mn efflux from cells and in Mn homeostasis (Yin *et al.*, 2010; Madejczyk and Ballatori, 2012; Li *et al.*, 2013; Chakraborty *et al.*, 2015; Seo and Wessling-Resnick, 2015). Another potential Mn transporter has been identified in patients with a mutation in SLC30A10 (Tuschl *et al.*, 2012; Quadri *et al.*, 2012; Stamelou *et al.*, 2012). SLC30A10 belongs to the cation diffusion facilitator superfamily of metal transporters responsible for transport of Fe, Cu, Zn and Mn, and although it was originally thought to be a zinc (Zn) transporter, but upon closer examination SLC30A10 was identified as a Mn efflux protein. Mn has long been considered a risk factor for Parkinson's disease, and patients with the SLC30A10 mutation display Parkinsonian-like gate disturbances and hypermanganesaemia, possibly reflecting the role of the SLC30A10 in Mn efflux from specific brain regions (DeWitt *et al.*, 2013).

There are many similarities between Mn and Pb neurotoxicity, and they share an important similarity in that they both disrupt presynaptic dysfunction. Mn appears to interfere with dopaminergic synaptic transmission, possibly by impairing presynaptic dopamine release (Guilarte *et al.*, 2006, 2008; Burton and Guilarte, 2009; Chen *et al.*, 2008). The developmental effects of either metal on cognition and behaviour in children may be linked to their effects on synaptic development. The development of synapses depends critically on feedback signalling between neurons (Fitzsimonds and Poo, 1998; Cohen-Cory *et al.*, 2010), and the developing brain is particularly sensitive to agents which disrupt synaptic activity (Rodier, 1995; Rice and Barone, 2000; Connors *et al.*, 2008). Presynaptic dysfunction has been identified in many neurological disorders and diseases, including dementia, autism, bipolar disorder, Down syndrome and schizophrenia (reviewed in Waites and Garner, 2011). Mn and/or Pb exposure has been linked to schizophrenia, dementia, Parkinson disease, autism and hyperactivity disorders (Landrigan *et al.*, 2005; Landrigan, 2010; Bouchard *et al.*, 2007; Froehlich *et al.*, 2009; Gitler *et al.*, 2009; Williams *et al.*, 2010; Brown, 2011).

Iron deficiency is a risk factor for Mn accumulation. As we saw earlier, in intestinal enterocytes the Fe^{2+} transporter DMT1 can transport Mn^{2+}. DMT1 also mediates uptake of Mn^{2+} across the olfactory epithelium into the brain (Thompson *et al.*, 2007). During iron deficiency, DMT1 expression is upregulated in both olfactory and intestinal epithelia (Gunshin *et al.*, 1997; Fleming *et al.*, 1998; Thompson *et al.*, 2007). Thus, changes in dietary iron exacerbate the accumulation and toxicity of Mn^{2+} in brain (Fitsanakis *et al.*, 2011; Kim *et al.*, 2012; Seo *et al.*, 2013). It has been suggested that Mn induces neuronal cell death through endoplasmic reticulum stress and the unfolded protein response pathway, and that this apoptotic effect is potentiated by iron deficiency most likely through an upregulation of DMT1 (Seo *et al.*, 2013).

Fe-deficient diets in humans can result in increased metal uptake through increased DMT1 levels, resulting in elevated blood Mn and Pb levels and increased susceptibility for toxicity. This is particularly significant in developing countries, which tend not only to have much higher rates of Fe deficiency than developed countries but also to have higher environmental levels of Pb and Mn. Thus, children in the developing world are at particular risk of experiencing metal toxicity, due to combined dietary deficits and elevated metal exposure (Neal and Guilarte, 2013).

14.2.5   Calcium

14.2.5.1   *Iron–Calcium Interactions*

Although Ca^{2+} has a quite different coordination chemistry from Fe^{2+}, not forgetting its properties as an alkaline earth Group 2 element, Ca^{2+} is generally believed to interfere with iron absorption. This effect requires a high Ca intake and occurs at the level of the intestinal lumen, via the noncompetitive, low-affinity inhibition of the iron transporter DMT1 by Ca^{2+} (Shawki and MacKenzie, 2010). Exactly how Ca^{2+} interferes with iron transport is not clear, although voltage dependence or intracellular Ca^{2+} signalling seems to be ruled out (Shawki and MacKenzie, 2010). Iron uptake, as indirectly estimated by intracellular ferritin content in Caco-2 cells, is only decreased with high concentrations (1.25–2.5 mM) of Ca^{2+} after a long exposure time (16–24 h) (Thompson *et al.*, 2010). The membrane expression of DMT1 was decreased accordingly, which suggests that the inhibition may involve the regulation of transporter abundance. It has also been reported that a short-term incubation (1.5 h) of human intestinal Caco-2 cells with Ca^{2+} down-regulated ferroportin levels at the basal membrane and the associated iron efflux (Lönnerdal, 2010), but these were restored after 4 h. Several studies in humans have shown a correlation between Ca^{2+} and decreased Fe absorption. However, it was concluded that prolonged high Ca^{2+} intake does not correlate with impaired iron status (Lönnerdal, 2010).

14.3 Iron Interactions with Toxic Metals

14.3.1 Lead

Chronic lead poisoning (saturnism) is a major cause of environmental concern. Pb toxicity affects several organ systems including the nervous, haematopoietic, renal, endocrine and skeletal systems. A major reason why Pb exposure has received worldwide attention is due to its ability to cause behavioural and cognitive deficits during nervous system development in infants and young children, and the growing body of evidence that exposure to Pb in early life may predispose to neurodegeneration later in life. Despite numerous global initiatives to reduce the use of Pb, exposure to it remains a widespread problem (Meyer *et al.*, 2008; Callan and Hinwood, 2011).

Low-level exposure to Pb can result from exposure to various environmental sources including lead-based paint and household dust from surfaces covered with such paints (Pb was removed from paint in Europe in 1922 and in the United States in 1978; Gibson, 2005; Gilbert and Weiss, 2006) as well as Pb in air, food and water. The main routes of exposure for Pb are inhalation and ingestion, with inhalation exposure the much more efficient route of absorption than ingestion. Since Pb can adsorb onto particulate matter and thus be inhaled, the removal of the Pb^{4+}-derived anti-knock agent (tetraethyl Pb), which was commonly added to petrol-based fuel to improve engine efficiency, has greatly reduced blood Pb levels in the urban population.

The intestinal absorption of Pb^{2+} is thought to involve carrier-mediated transport (Barton *et al.*, 1978; Fullmer, 1990), although the identity of the transporter or transporters is still a matter of debate. There is some evidence that DMT1 is responsible for transporting both Pb^{2+} and Cd^{2+} in addition to its physiological substrate, iron (Fe) (Bannon *et al.*, 2003). About 94% of the human Pb body burden is found in bone in adults, due to the displacement of Ca^{2+} in the bone matrix by Pb^{2+} via a cation-exchange process (Pounds *et al.*, 1991).

Anaemia is one of the best-known toxic effects of lead. A main target for lead poisoning is δ-aminolaevulinate dehydratase, also known as porphobilinogen synthase (PBGS), the enzyme which catalyses the second step of the haem biosynthetic pathway, condensing two molecules of δ-aminolaevulinate to form the pyrrole, porphobilinogen. Human δ-aminolaevulinate dehydratase, like the yeast enzyme, is a Zn^{2+} oligomeric enzyme with eight Zn/homo-octamers, of which only four Zn(II) are required for activity The X-ray structures of the Pb^{2+}-substituted *Saccharomyces cerevisiae* octamer and the subunit are shown in Figure 14.12 (PDB: 1QNV, Erskine *et al.*, 2000). The catalytic Zn site is unusual, with three Cys ligands all on the same side of the metal ion,

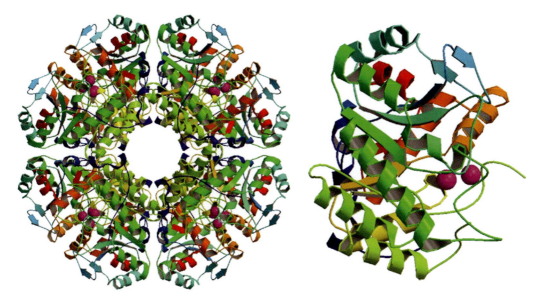

Figure 14.12 *Structures of the Pb²⁺-substituted δ-aminolaevulinate dehydratase PDB: 1QNV from the* yeast Saccharomyces cerevisiae *(left panel) and the homo 8-mer subunit (right panel)*

which makes it a primary target for inhibition by Pb (Jaffe *et al.*, 2001). It has been suggested that Pb²⁺-induced anaemia may be explained at least in part by increased phosphatidylserine exposure on erythrocytes, erythrophagocytosis, and the splenic sequestration of lead could affect the destruction of erythrocytes (Jang *et al.*, 2011).

It was emphasised earlier that one of the common links between Pb and Mn neurotoxicity is presynaptic dysfunction. In contrast to Mn²⁺, which affects the dopaminergic system, Pb²⁺ appears to interfere with glutamatergic neurotransmission and may disrupt the *trans*-synaptic signalling that is critical to synaptic development (Lasley and Gilbert, 1996, 2002; Neal *et al.*, 2010; Neal and Guilarte, 2010; Cohen-Cory *et al.*, 2010; Stansfield *et al.*, 2012). It is possible that presynaptic dysfunction may account for many of the chronic effects of Pb and Mn exposure, and increase the susceptibility to neurological diseases which have an environmental aetiology (Neal and Guilarte, 2013).

14.3.2 Cadmium

Low levels of chronic exposure to cadmium result in diverse symptoms, affecting many tissues. Many of the toxic effects of Cd²⁺ in animal cells are due to its interference with other essential metal ions. The Cd²⁺ ion is large and easily polarised, a soft Lewis acid with a preference for easily oxidised soft ligands (particularly sulphur), and can displace Zn²⁺ from proteins where the Zn coordination environment is sulphur-dominated. Like Zn²⁺, it has its full complement of *d* electrons and so Cd²⁺ does not change oxidation state. Because of the similarity of its ionic radius with that of Ca²⁺ it can exchange with Ca²⁺ in calcium-binding proteins.

A schematic representation of the interaction of cadmium with iron in mammalian cells is presented in Figure 14.13 (Moulis, 2010). Transporters and receptors for free and complexed forms of essential metals such as Ca²⁺, Fe²⁺, Zn²⁺ or Cu²⁺ may mediate the uptake of Cd²⁺ (Bressler *et al.*, 2004; Thévenod, 2010). The most likely transporter of Cd²⁺ across the intestinal barrier is

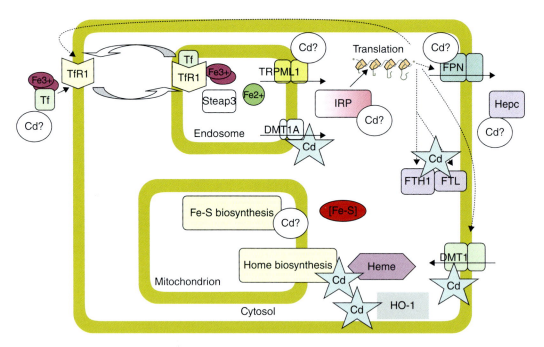

Figure 14.13 *Schematic representation of iron homeostasis in relation to Cd toxicity. The arrows indicate the direction of iron flow. Targets of Cd are shown with a Cd symbol within a blue star for those which have been established, and within a circle for those without* in vivo *experimental evidence. Dotted arrows point to the proteins for which the corresponding mRNAs are regulated by iron regulatory proteins (IRPs). Abbreviations: FPN, ferroportin; FTH1 and FTL, ferritin subunits; Tf, transferrin; TfR1, transferrin receptor; Hepc, hepcidin. Reprinted with kind permission from Springer Science and Media from Moulis, J.-M. (2010) Cellular mechanisms of cadmium toxicity related to the homeostasis of essential metals.* Biometals, **23**, *877–896*

DMTI (Gunshin *et al.*, 1997; Bressler *et al.*, 2004; Kim *et al.*, 2007; Mackenzie *et al.*, 2007). DMT1 repression in a human enterocyte model decreases cadmium transport, whereas its over-expression strongly increases cadmium uptake (Bressler *et al.*, 2004). Since there is an IRE-containing form of DMT1, which is targeted to the apical membrane of the enterocyte, dietary Cd^{2+} uptake – and, in parallel, its toxicity – will be influenced by the iron status of the host. Endosomal DMT1 may also transport internalised Cd^{2+} from endosomes, but since Cd^{2+} is only weakly bound by transferrin (Harris and Madsen, 1988) it is unlikely that it ever gets there in the first place. It has been proposed that Ca(V)3.1 channels represent a likely non-transferrin-dependent pathway for Fe^{2+} entry into cells with clinically relevant concentrations of extracellular Fe^{2+} (Lopin *et al.*, 2012a). Ca(v)3.1 channels have also been shown to be a candidate pathway for Cd^{2+} entry into cells during Cd^{2+} exposure. Incubation with radiolabelled $^{109}Cd^{2+}$ confirmed the uptake of Cd^{2+} into cells with Ca(v)3.1 channels (Lopin *et al.*, 2012b). Cd^{2+} bound to metallothionein can be released from the liver and internalised by cubulin in cells of the kidney proximal tubules (Abouhamed *et al.*, 2007; Nordberg *et al.*, 2009), contributing to the accumulation of Cd^{2+} in the kidneys.

Because the ionic radii of Ca^{2+} and Cd^{2+} are similar, Cd^{2+} can possibly be taken up by voltage- or receptor-operated Ca^{2+} channels, and the inhibition of Ca^{2+} channels can sometimes protect against Cd^{2+} toxicity. Even in the presence of external calcium, cadmium penetrates into neurons via voltage-gated calcium channels (Hinkle *et al.*, 1987; Gavazzo *et al.*, 2005).

Cadmium export through the basolateral membrane may not be as efficient as uptake, since high-cadmium diets result in an accumulation of the toxic metal in enterocytes. The reversibility of cadmium accumulation in enterocytes upon iron replenishment of the diet (Ryu *et al.*, 2004) suggests that there must be some export mechanism, and it has been proposed that FPN1 may be involved in the transport of Cd^{2+} into the bloodstream, Like zinc, cadmium can upregulate the expression of FPN1 (Troadec *et al.*, 2010) through the action of metal transcription factor-1 (*MTF-1*). However, more recently the expression of human FPN in *Xenopus* oocytes was shown to stimulate Fe, Zn and Co efflux, but not that of Cu, Cd or Mn (Mitchell *et al.*, 2014). Alternative efflux pathways may involve calcium-ATPases and Zn^{2+} exporters (Bridges and Zalups, 2005).

Cellular iron metabolism may also be influenced by Cd^{2+}. Ferrochelatase, the enzyme which inserts iron into protoporphyrin IX to form haem is inhibited by Cd^{2+} (Fadigan and Dailey, 1987), and the Zn-enzyme δ-aminolaevulinate synthase may also be influenced by Cd^{2+}.

14.3.3 Aluminium

Despite comprising 8% of the Earth's crust, the most abundant metal and the third most abundant element after oxygen and silicon, aluminium, is not used in biology. The reasons for this remain obscure, but may be related to the metal's chemical properties and toxicity. The neurotoxicity of aluminium was recognised a long time ago, but it did not represent any cause for concern until quite recently, since Al had little or no access to the human population. Despite its abundance in the Earth's crust, most natural waters contained insignificant amounts of Al, with most of the Al disappearing into sediment as insoluble hydroxides. However, this all changed when Al insidiously was given a means of entry through a series of events, all of them man-made (see Figure 14.15). One major contributor was the acidification of soils by a number of human activities, including the use of ammonium-based fertilisers and the generation of 'acid rain'. The precursors of acid rain formation are increased emissions of SO_2 and nitrogen oxides, produced by the combustion of fossil fuels and resulting in higher than normal amounts of sulphuric and nitric acids. The consequence of soil acidification is the progressive leaching of Al from mineral deposits in the soil, leading to increased Al concentrations in ground water. Al concentrations in fresh water lakes at pH <6 can be in the micromolar range, close to the toxic levels for many aquatic plants and animals.

Al was also used for many years as a phosphate binder in the dialysis fluids of haemodialysis patients; many orally active antacids are aluminium-based; and tobacco also contains appreciable amounts of Al (500–2000 μg per cigarette, although only <0.02–0.075 μg are in the smoke from one cigarette).

It is likely that, whereas much of the toxicity of aluminium is related to its interference with Ca^{2+} signalling pathways, its access to tissues is a function of the similarity of Al^{3+} to Fe^{3+} (Ward *et al.*, 2001). Nonetheless, the inability of Al^{3+} to undergo a change of oxidation state prevents Al^{3+} from following the well established pathways of iron transport and storage. Clearly, in the intestinal tract neither of the two pathways for iron uptake – the haem uptake system or the non-haem route, involving reduction followed by transport of the divalent Fe^{2+} – could be used by Al^{3+}. Two possibilities can be envisaged: (i) the existence of a distinct ferric iron uptake pathway involving β(3)-integrin and mobilferrin (Conrad *et al.*, 2000; Conrad and Umbreit, 2002); or (ii) the passage of Al^{3+} through the gap junctions between the enterocytes.

Once in the circulation aluminium can bind to transferrin, since in the extracellular fluids of mammals transferrin usually has 70% of its binding capacity free, and also to albumin and

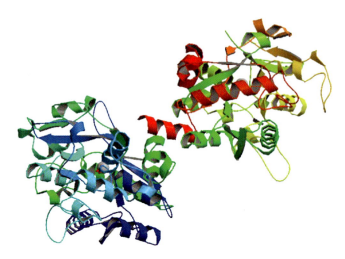

Figure 14.14   *Structure of Al^{3+}-bound ovotransferrin (PDB 2D3I)*

low-molecular-weight ligands such as citrate. The transferrin–aluminium complex is illustrated in Figure 14.14 (Mizutani *et al.*, 2005), and will be able to enter cells via the transferrin-transferrin receptor pathway. Within the acidic environment of the endosome, it is assumed that Al^{3+} will be released, although how it exits from this compartment is unknown. In the cytosol, Al^{3+} is unlikely to be incorporated into ferritin, which requires redox cycling between Fe^{2+} and Fe^{3+}. It seems likely that most aluminium accumulates in the mitochondria, where it can interfere with Ca^{2+} homeostasis. There is little doubt that aluminium, once in the circulation, can cross the blood–brain barrier.

The toxicity of Al^{3+} is implicated in anaemia, osteomalacia, hepatic disorders and neurological disorders (Figure 14.15) (Mailloux *et al.*, 2011), disorders which arise for example from long-term chronic exposure in dialysis patients (Verstraeten *et al.*, 2008). The anaemia seems to result from an accelerated clearance of circulating erythrocytes. Suicidal erythrocyte death or eryptosis (Lang and Lang, 2015) is characterised by erythrocyte shrinkage, cell membrane blebbing, and cell membrane scrambling with phosphatidylserine (PS) translocation to the erythrocyte surface. Macrophages are equipped with PS receptors, and they then bind, engulf and degrade PS-exposing cells. Al^{3+} was found to decrease the life span of circulating erythrocytes by inducing eryptosis (Niemoeller *et al.*, 2006). The second is consistent with interference with Ca^{2+} deposition in bone, and the accumulation of Al^{3+} in the bone matrix. It has been suggested that Al^{3+} induces osteoblast apoptosis by activating the oxidative stress-mediated JNK pathway, which causes cell injuries and reduces the number and function of osteoblasts, thereby inhibiting bone formation (Li *et al.*, 2012).

Al has been shown to exert its effects by disrupting lipid membrane fluidity, perturbing iron homeostasis, and causing oxidative stress (Zatta *et al.*, 2002; Becaria *et al.*, 2006). Not surprisingly, a systems biology approach in cultured hepatoblastoma cells (HepG2) has identified mitochondrial metabolism as the main site of the Fe-dependent toxicological effects of Al (Mailloux *et al.*, 2011). In an effort to compensate for diminished mitochondrial function and increase ATP production by glycolysis, Al-treated cells stabilise HIF-1α. Additionally, Al toxicity leads to an increase in intracellular lipid accumulation due to enhanced lipogenesis and a decrease in the β-oxidation of fatty acids.

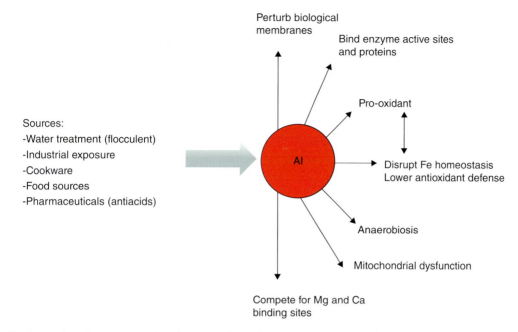

Figure 14.15 *Exposure to Al and its toxicological impacts. Dietary uptake represents the major route of Al uptake. Due to the chemical properties of Al, this trivalent metal disrupts multiple cellular processes. The ability of Al to exert these negative effects on cells has been linked to a number of pathologies. Reprinted with permission from Elsevier from Mailloux, R.J., Lemire, J. and Appanna, V.D. (2011) Hepatic response to aluminum toxicity: dyslipidemia and liver diseases.* Exp. Cell Res., *317, 2231–2238*

References

Abouhamed, M., Wolff, N.A., Lee, W.K., Smith, C.P. and Thévenod F. (2007) Knockdown of endosomal/lysosomal divalent metal transporter 1 by RNA interference prevents cadmium-metallothionein-1 cytotoxicity in renal proximal tubule cells. *Am. J. Physiol. Renal Physiol.*, **293**, F705–F712.

Anderson, E.R., Xue, X. and Shah, Y.M. (2011) Intestinal hypoxia-inducible factor-2alpha (HIF-2alpha) is critical for efficient erythropoiesis. *J. Biol. Chem.*, **286**, 19533–19540.

Andrès, E., Vidal-Alaball, J., Federici, L., *et al.*, (2007) Clinical aspects of cobalamin deficiency in elderly patients. Epidemiology, causes, clinical manifestations, and treatment with special focus on oral cobalamin therapy. *Eur. J. Intern. Med.*, **18**, 456–462.

Arredonda, M., Muñoz, P., Mura, C.V. and Nùñez, M.T. (2003) DMT1, a physiologically relevant apical Cu1+ transporter of intestinal cells. *Am. J. Physiol. Cell Physiol.*, **284**, C1525–C1530.

Arredonda, M., Mendiburo, M.J., Flores, S., Singleton, S.T. and Garrick, M.D. (2014) Mouse divalent metal transporter 1 is a copper transporter in HEK293 cells. *Biometals*, **27**, 115–123.

Aschner, M., Guilarte, T.R., Schneider, J.S. and Zheng, W. (2007) Manganese: recent advances in understanding its transport and neurotoxicity. *Toxicol. Appl. Pharmacol.*, **221**, 131–147.

Banci, L., Bertini, I., Cantini, F., *et al.* (2006) The Atx1-Ccc2 complex is a metal-mediated protein–protein interaction. *Nat. Chem. Biol.*, **2**, 367–368.

Banci, L., Bertini, I., Ciofi-Baffoni, S., *et al.* (2010) Affinity gradients drive copper to cellular destinations. *Nature*, **465**, 645–648.

Banci, L., Cantini, F., Kozyreva, T. and Rubino, J.T. (2013) Mechanistic aspects of hSOD1 maturation from the solution structure of Cu(I)-loaded hCCS domain 1 and analysis of disulfide-free hSOD1 mutants. *ChemBioChem*, **14**, 1839–1844.

Banerjee, R. and Ragsdale, S.W. (2003) The many faces of vitamin B_{12}: Catalysis by cobalamin-dependent enzymes. *Annu. Rev. Biochem.*, **72**, 209–247.

Bannon, D.I., Abounader, R., Lees, P.S. and Bressler, J.P. (2003) Effect of DMT1 knockdown on iron, cadmium, and lead uptake in Caco-2 cells. *Am. J. Physiol. Cell Physiol.*, **284**, C44–C50.

Barton, J.C., Conrad, M.E., Nuby, S. and Harridon, I. (1978) Effects of iron on the absorption and retention of lead. *J. Lab. Clin. Med.*, **92**, 536–547.

Becaria, A., Lahiri, D.K., Bondy, S.C., *et al.* (2006) Aluminum and copper in drinking water enhance inflammatory or oxidative events specifically in the brain. *J. Neuroimmunol.*, **176**, 16–23.

Bouchard, M., Laforest, F., Vandelac, L., Bellinger, D. and Mergler, D. (2007) Hair manganese and hyperactive behaviors: pilot study of school-age children exposed through tap water. *Environ. Health Perspect.*, **115**, 122–127.

Bressler, J.P., Olivi, L., Cheong, J.H., Kim, Y. and Bannona, D. (2004) Divalent metal transporter 1 in lead and cadmium transport. *Ann. N. Y. Acad. Sci.*, **1012**, 142–152.

Bridges, C.C. and Zalups, R.K. (2005) Molecular and ionic mimicry and the transport of toxic metals. *Toxicol. Appl. Pharmacol.*, **204**, 274–308.

Broderius, M., Mostad, E., Wendroth, K. and Prohaska, J.R. (2010) Levels of plasma ceruloplasmin protein are markedly lower following dietary copper deficiency in rodents. *Comp. Biochem. Physiol. C Toxicol. Pharmacol.*, **151**, 473–479.

Broderius, M., Mostad, E. and Prohaska, J.R. (2012) Suppressed hepcidin expression correlates with hypotransferrinemia in copper-deficient rat pups but not dams. *Genes Nutr.*, **7**, 405–414.

Brown, A.S. (2011) The environment and susceptibility to schizophrenia. *Prog. Neurobiol.*, **93**, 23–58.

Burton, N.C. and Guilarte, T.R. (2009) Manganese neurotoxicity: lessons learned from longitudinal studies in nonhuman primates. *Environ. Health Perspect.*, **117**, 325–332.

Callan, A.C. and Hinwood, A.L. (2011) Exposures to lead. *Rev. Environ. Health*, **26**, 13–15.

Chakraborty, S., Chen, P., Bornhorst, J., *et al.* (2015) Loss of pdr-1/parkin influences Mn homeostasis through altered ferroportin expression in *C. elegans*. *Metallomics*, **7**, 847–856.

Chandler, R.J. and Venditti, C.P. (2005) Genetic and genomic systems to study methylmalonic acidemia *Mol. Genet. Metab.*, **86**, 34–43.

Chen, H., Huang, G., Su, T., *et al.* (2006) Decreased hephaestin activity in the intestine of copper-deficient mice causes systemic iron deficiency. *J. Nutr.*, **136**, 1236–1241.

Chen, H., Attieh, Z.K., Syed, B.A., *et al.* (2012) Identification of zyklopen, a new member of the vertebrate multicopper ferroxidase family, and characterization in rodents and human cells. *J. Nutr.*, **140**, 1728–1735.

Chen, M.K., Kuwabara, H., Zhou, Y., *et al.* (2008) VMAT2 and dopamine neuron loss in a primate model of Parkinson's disease. *J. Neurochem.*, **105**, 78–90.

Chua, A.C. and Morgan, E.H. (1996) Effects of iron deficiency and iron overload on manganese uptake and deposition in the brain and other organs of the rat. *Biol. Trace Elem. Res.*, **55**, 39–54.

Cohen-Cory, S., Kidane, A.H., Shirkey, N.J. and Marshak, S. (2010) Brain-derived neurotrophic factor and the development of structural neuronal connectivity. *Dev. Neurobiol.*, **70**, 271–288.

Collins, J.F. (2006) Gene chip analyses reveal differential genetic responses to iron deficiency in rat duodenum and jejunum. *Biol. Res.*, **39**, 25–37.

Collins, J.F., Franck, C.A., Kowdley, K.V. and Ghishan, F.K. (2005) Identification of differentially expressed genes in response to dietary iron deprivation in rat duodenum. *Am. J. Physiol. Gastrointest. Liver Physiol.*, **288**, G964–G971.

Collins, J.F., Prohaska, J.R. and Knutson, M.D. (2010) Metabolic crossroads of iron and copper. *Nutr. Rev.*, **68**, 133–147.

Connors, S.I., Levitt, P., Matthews, S.G., *et al.* (2008) Fetal mechanisms in neurodevelopmental disorders. *Pediatr. Neurol.*, **38**, 163–176.

Conrad, M.E. and Umbreit, J.N. (2002) Pathways of iron absorption. *Blood Cells Mol. Dis.*, **29**, 336–355.

Conrad, M.E., Umbreit, J.N., Moore, E.G., *et al.* (2000) Separate pathways for cellular uptake of ferric and ferrous iron. *Am. J. Physiol. Gastrointest. Liver Physiol.*, **279**, G767–G774.

De Domenica, I., Ward, D.M., di Patti, M.C., *et al.* (2007) Ferroxidase activity is required for the stability of cell surface ferroportin in cells expressing GPI-ceruloplasmin. *EMBO J.*, **26**, 2823–2831.

Delaby, C., Pilard, N., Puy, H. and Canonne-Hergaux, F. (2008) Sequential regulation of ferroportin expression after erythrophagocytosis in murine macrophages: early mRNA induction by haem, followed by iron-dependent protein expression. *Biochem. J.*, **411**, 123–131.

DeWitt, M.R., Chen, P. and Aschner, M. (2013) Manganese efflux in Parkinsonism: insights from newly characterized SLC30A10 mutations. *Biochem. Biophys. Res. Commun.*, **432**, 1–4.

Dix, D., Bridgham, J., Broderius, M. and Eide, D. (1997) Characterization of the FET4 protein of yeast. Evidence for a direct role in the transport of iron. *J. Biol. Chem.*, **272**, 11770–11777.

Eide, D.J. (2004) The SLC39 family of metal ion transporters. *Pflugers Arch.*, **447**, 796–800.

Erikson, K.M., Syversen, T., Steinnes, E. and Aschner, M. (2004). Globus pallidus: a target brain region for divalent metal accumulation associated with dietary iron deficiency. *J. Nutr. Biochem.*, **15**, 335–341.

Erskine, P.T., Duke, E.M., Tickle, U., *et al.* (2000) MAD analyses of yeast 5-aminolaevulinate dehydratase: their use in structure determination and in defining the metal-binding sites. *Acta Crystallogr. D Biol. Crystallogr.*, **56**, 421–430.

Espinoza, A., Le Blanc, S., Olivares, M., *et al.* (2012) Iron, copper, and zinc transport. Inhibition of divalent metal transporter 1 (DMT1) and human copper transporter 1 (hCTR1) by shRNA. *Biol. Trace Elem. Res.*, **146**, 281–286.

Fadigan, A. and Dailey, H.A. (1987) Inhibition of ferrochelatase during differentiation of murine erythroleu-kaemia cells. *Biochem. J.*, **243**, 419–424.

Fell, J.M., Reynolds, A.P., Meadows, N., *et al.* (1996) Manganese toxicity in children receiving long-term parenteral nutrition. *Lancet*, **347**, 1218–1221.

Feng, W., Ye, F., Xue, W., Zhou, Z. and Kang, Y.J. (2009) Copper regulation of hypoxia-inducible factor-1 activity. *Mol. Pharmacol.*, **75**, 174–182.

Filipov, M.N. and Dodd, C.A. (2011) Role of glial cells in manganese neurotoxicity. *J. Appl. Toxicol.*, **32**, 310–317.

Fitsanakis, V.A., Zhang, N., Avison, M.J., *et al.*, (2011) Changes in dietary iron exacerbate regional brain manganese accumulation as determined by magnetic resonance imaging. *Toxicol. Sci.*, **120**, 146–153.

Fitzsimonds, R.M. and Poo, M.M. (1998) Retrograde signaling in the development and modification of synapses. *Physiol. Rev.*, **78**, 143–170.

Fleming, M.D., Romano, M.A., Su, M.A., *et al.* (1998) Nramp2 is mutated in the anemic Belgrade (b) rat: evidence of a role for Nramp2 in endosomal iron transport. *Proc. Natl Acad. Sci. USA*, **95**, 1148–1153.

Fox, P.L. (2003) The copper-iron chronicles: the story of an intimate relationship. *Biometals*, **16**, 9–40.

Froehlich, T.E., Lanphear, B.P., Auinger, P., *et al.*, (2009) Association of tobacco and lead exposures with attention-deficit/hyperactivity disorder. *Pediatrics*, **124** (6), e1054–e1063.

Fullmer, C.S. (1990) Intestinal lead and calcium absorption: effect of 1,25-dihydroxycholecalciferol and lead status. *Proc. Soc. Exp. Biol. Med.*, **194**, 258–264.

Furukawa, Y., Torres, A.S. and O'Halloran, T.V. (2004) Oxygen-induced maturation of SOD1: a key role for disulfide formation by the copper chaperone CCS. *EMBO J.*, **23**, 2872–2881.

Gavazzo, P., Morelli, E. and Marchetti, C. (2005) Susceptibility of insulinoma cells to cadmium and modulation by L-type calcium channels. *Biometals*, **18**, 131–142.

Geiser, J., Venken, K.J., De Lisle, R.C. and Andrews, G.K. (2012) A mouse model of acrodermatitis enteropathica: loss of intestine zinc transporter ZIP4 (Slc39a4) disrupts the stem cell niche and intestine integrity. *PLoS Genet.*, **8**, e1002766.

Gerasim, C., Lofgren, M. and Banerjee, R. (2013) Navigating the B_{12} road: assimilation, delivery, and disorders of cobalamin. *J. Biol. Chem.*, **288**, 33917–33925.

Gibson, J.L. (2005) A plea for painted railings and painted walls of rooms as the source of lead poisoning amongst Queensland children. *Public Health Rep.*, **120**, 301–304.

Gilbert, S.G. and Weiss, B. (2006) A rationale for lowering the blood lead action level from 10 to 2 microg/dL. *Neurotoxicology*, **27**, 693–701.

Gitler, A.D., Chesi, A., Geddie, M.L., *et al.* (2009) Alpha-synuclein is part of a diverse and highly conserved interaction network that includes PARK9 and manganese toxicity. *Nat. Genet.*, **41**, 308–315.

Gorell, J.M., Johnson, C.C., Rybicki, B.A., *et al.* (1999) Occupational exposure to manganese, copper, lead, iron, mercury and zinc and the risk of Parkinson's disease. *Neurotoxicology*, **20**, 239–247.

Greibe, E., Fedosov, S., Sorensen, B.S., *et al.* (2012) A single rainbow trout cobalamine-binding protein stands in for three human binders. *J. Biol. Chem.*, **287**, 13186–13193.

Guilarte, T.R., Chen, M.K., McGlothan, J.L., *et al.*, (2006) Nigrostriatal dopamine system dysfunction and subtle motor deficits in manganese-exposed non-human primates. *Exp. Neurol.*, **202**, 381–390.

Guilarte, T.R., Burton, N.C., McGlothan, J.L., *et al.* (2008) Impairment of nigrostriatal dopamine neurotransmission by manganese is mediated by pre-synaptic mechanism(s): implications to manganese-induced parkinsonism. *J. Neurochem.*, **107**, 1236–1247.

Gulec, S. and Collins, J.F. (2013) Investigation of iron metabolism in mice expressing a mutant Menke's copper transporting ATPase (Atp7a) protein with diminished activity. *PLoS ONE*, **8**, e6601.

Gulec, S. and Collins, J.F. (2014a) Molecular mediators governing iron-copper interactions. *Annu. Rev. Nutr.*, **34**, 95–116.

Gulec, S. and Collins, J.F. (2014b) Silencing the Menkes copper-transporting ATPase (Atp7a) gene in rat intestinal epithelial (IEC-6) cells increases iron flux via transcriptional induction of ferroportin 1 (Fpn1). *J. Nutr.*, **144**, 12–19.

Gunshin, H., Mackenzie, B., Berger, U.V., *et al.* (1997) Cloning and characterization of a mammalian proton-coupled metal-ion transporter. *Nature*, **388**, 482–488.

Guo, Y., Smith, K., Lee, J., Thiele, D.J. and Petris, M.J. (2004) Identification of methionine-rich clusters that regulate copper-stimulated endocytosis of the human Ctr1 copper transporter. *J. Biol. Chem.*, **279**, 17428–17433.

Hall, C.A. (1977) The carriers of native vitamin B_{12} in normal human serum. *Clin. Sci. Mol. Med.*, **53**, 453–457.

Harris, W.R. and Madsen, L.J. (1988) Equilibrium studies on the binding of Cd(II) to human serum transferrin. *Biochemistry*, **27**, 284–288.

Hart, E.B., Steenbock, H., Waddell, J. and Elvehjem, C.A. (1928) Iron in nutrition VII. Copper as a supplement to iron for hemoglobin building in the rat. *J. Biol. Chem.*, **77**, 797–833.

Hinkle, P.M., Kinsella, P.A. and Osterhoudt, K.C. (1987) Cadmium uptake and toxicity via voltage-sensitive calcium channels. *J. Biol. Chem.*, **262**, 16333–16337.

Hu, Z., Gulec, S. and Collins, J.F. (2010) Cross-species comparison of genomewide gene expression profiles reveals induction of hypoxia-inducible factor-responsive genes in iron-deprived intestinal epithelial cells. *Am. J. Physiol. Cell Physiol.*, **299**, C930–C938.

Huang, L. and Tepaamorndech, S. (2013) The SLC30 family of zinc transporters – a review of current understanding of their biological and pathophysiological roles. *Mol. Aspects Med.*, **34**, 548–560.

Illing, A.C., Shawki, A., Cunningham, C.L. and Mackenzie, B. (2012) Substrate profile and metal-ion selectivity of human divalent metal-ion transporter-1. *J. Biol. Chem.*, **287**, 30485–30496.

Jaffe, E.K., Martins, J., Li, J., Kervinen, J. and Dunbrack, R.L. Jr (2001) The molecular mechanism of lead inhibition of human porphobilinogen synthase. *J. Biol. Chem.*, **276**, 1531–1537.

Jang, W.H., Lim, K.M., Kim, K., *et al.*, (2011) Low level of lead can induce phosphatidylserine exposure and erythrophagocytosis: a new mechanism underlying lead-associated anemia. *Toxicol. Sci.*, **122**, 177–184.

Jenkitkasemwong, S., Broderius, M., Nam, H., Prohaska, J.R. and Knutson, M.D. (2010) Anemic copper-deficient rats, but not mice, display low hepcidin expression and high ferroportin levels. *J. Nutr.*, **140**, 723–730.

Jeong, J. and Eide, D.J. (2013) The SLC39 family of zinc transporters. *Mol. Aspects Med.*, **34**, 612–619.

Jiang, I., Garrick, M.D., Garrick, L.M., Zhao L. and Collins, J.F. (2013) Divalent metal transporter 1 (Dmt1) mediates copper transport in the duodenum of iron-deficient rats and when overexpressed in iron-deprived HEK-293 cells. *J. Nutr.*, **143**, 1927–1933.

Kim, D.W., Kim, K.Y., Choi, B.S., *et al.* (2007) Regulation of metal transporters by dietary iron, and the relationship between body iron levels and cadmium uptake. *Arch. Toxicol.*, **81**, 327–334.

Kim, J., Li, Y., Buckett, P.D., *et al.* (2012) Iron-responsive olfactory uptake of manganese improves motor function deficits associated with iron deficiency. *PLoS One*, **7**, e33533.

Klomp, A.E., van de Sluis, B., Klomp, L.W. and Wijmenga, C. (2003) The ubiquitously expressed MURR1 protein is absent in canine copper toxicosis. *J. Hepatol.*, **39**, 703–709.

Knutson, M.D., Vafa, M.R., Haile, D.J. and Wessling-Resnick, M. (2003) Iron loading and erythrophagocytosis increase ferroportin 1 (FPN1) expression in J774 macrophages. *Blood*, **102**, 4191–4197.

Kolhouse, J.F. and Allen, R.H. (1977) Recognition of two intracellular cobalmin binding proteins and their recognition as methylmalonyl-CoA mutase and methionine synthetase. *Proc. Natl Acad. Sci. USA*, **74**, 921–925.

Kosman, D.J. (2010) Multicopper oxidases: a workshop on copper coordination chemistry, electron transfer, and metallophysiology. *J. Biol. Inorg. Chem.*, **15**, 15–28.

Koury, M.J. and Ponka, P. (2004) New insights into erythropoiesis: the roles of folate, vitamin B12, and iron. *Annu. Rev. Nutr.*, **24**, 105–131.

Kozyraki, R. and Cases, O. (2013) Vitamin B_{12} absorption: mammalian physiology and acquired and inherited disorders. *Biochimie*, **95**, 1002–1007.

Kozyraki, R., Kristiansen, M., Silahtaroglu, A., *et al.* (1998) The human intrinsic factor-vitamin B12 receptor, cubilin: molecular characterization and chromosomal mapping of the gene to 10p within the autosomal recessive megaloblastic anemia (MGA1) region. *Blood*, **91**, 3593–3600.

Kozyraki, R., Fyfe, J., Verroust, P.J., *et al.* (2001) Megalin-dependent cubilin-mediated endocytosis is a major pathway for the apical uptake of transferrin in polarized epithelia. *Proc. Natl Acad. Sci. USA*, **98**, 12491–12496.

Krautler, B. (2012) Biochemistry of B$_{12}$-cofactors in human metabolism. *Subcell. Biochem.*, **56**, 323–346.

Kristiansen, M., Kozyraki, R., Jacobsen, C., *et al.* (1999) Molecular dissection of the intrinsic factor-vitamin B$_{12}$ receptor, cubilin, discloses regions important for membrane association and ligand binding. *J. Biol. Chem.*, **274**, 20540–20544.

Laity, J.H. and Andrews, G.K. (2007) Understanding the mechanisms of zinc-sensing by metal-response element binding transcription factor-1 (MTF-1). *Arch. Biochem. Biophys.*, **463**, 201–210.

Landrigan, P.J. (2010) What causes autism? Exploring the environmental contribution. *Curr. Opin. Pediatr.*, **22**, 219–225.

Landrigan, P.J., Sonawane, B., Butler, R.N., *et al.* (2005) Early environmental origins of neurodegenerative disease in later life. *Environ. Health Perspect.*, **113**, 1230–1233.

Lang, E. and Lang, F. (2015) Triggers, inhibitors, mechanisms, and significance of eryptosis: the suicidal erythrocyte death. *Biomed. Res. Int.*, **2015** 513518. doi: 10.1155/2015/513518.

Lasley, S.M. and Gilbert, M.E. (1996) Presynaptic glutamatergic function in dentate gyrus *in vivo* is diminished by chronic exposure to inorganic lead. *Brain Res.*, **736**, 125–134.

Lasley, S.M. and Gilbert, M.E. (2002) Rat hippocampal glutamate and GABA release exhibit biphasic effects as a function of chronic lead exposure level. *Toxicol. Sci.*, **66**, 139–147.

Lee, G.R., Nacht, S., Lukens, J.N. and Cartwright, G.E. (1968) Iron metabolism in copper-deficient swine. *J. Clin. Invest.*, **47**, 2058–2069.

Li, N., Seetharam, S. and Seetharam, B. (1995) Genomic structure of human transcobalamine II: comparison to human intrinsic factor and transcobalamine I. *Biochem. Biophys. Res. Commun.*, **208**, 756–764.

Li, X., Han, Y., Guan, Y., *et al.* (2012) Aluminum induces osteoblast apoptosis through the oxidative stress-mediated JNK signaling pathway. *Biol. Trace Elem. Res.*, **150**, 502–508.

Li, X., Xie, J., Lu, L., *et al.* (2013) Kinetics of manganese transport and gene expressions of manganese transport carriers in Caco-2 cell monolayers. *Biometals*, **26**, 941–953.

Lindley, P.F., Card, G., Zaitseva, I., *et al.* (1997) An X-ray structural study of human ceruloplasmin in relation to ferroxidase activity. *J. Biol. Inorg. Chem.*, **2**, 454-463.

Liu, X.F., Supek, F., Nelson, N. and Culotta, V.C. (1997) Negative control of heavy metal uptake by the *Saccharomyces cerevisiae* BSD2 gene. *J. Biol. Chem.*, **272**, 11763–11769.

Liuzzi, J.P., Lichten, L.A., Rivera, S., *et al.* (2005) Interleukin-6 regulates the zinc transporter Zip14 in liver and contributes to the hypozincemia of the acute-phase response. *Proc. Natl Acad. Sci. USA*, **102**, 6843–6848.

Liuzzi, J.P., Aydemir, F., Nam, H., Knutson, M.D. and Cousins, R.J. (2006) Zip14 (Slc39a14) mediates non-transferrin-bound iron uptake into cells. *Proc. Natl Acad. Sci. USA*, **103**, 13612–13617.

Lönnerdal, B. (2010) Calcium and iron absorption – Mechanisms and public health relevance. *Int. J. Vitamin Nutr. Res.*, **80**, 293–299.

Lopin, K.V., Gray, I.P., Obejero-Paz, C.A., Thévenod, F. and Jones, S.W. (2012a) Fe^{2+} block and permeation of CaV3.1 (α1G) T-type calcium channels: candidate mechanism for non-transferrin-mediated Fe^{2+} influx. *Mol. Pharmacol.*, **82**, 1194–1204.

Lopin, K.V., Thévenod, F., Page, J.C. and Jones, S.W. (2012b) Cd^{2+} block and permeation of CaV3.1 (α1G) T-type calcium channels: candidate mechanism for Cd^{2+} influx. *Mol. Pharmacol.*, **82,** 1183–1193.

Loréal, O., Cavey, T., Bardou-Jacquet, E., *et al.* (2014) Iron, hepcidin and the metal connection. *Front. Pharmacol.*, **5**, 128.

Ludwig, M.L. and Matthews, R.G. (1997) Structure-based perspectives on B$_{12}$-dependent enzymes. *Annu. Rev. Biochem.*, **66**, 269–313.

Lutsenko, S., Barnes, N.L., Bartee, M.Y. and Dmitriev, O.Y. (2007) Function and regulation of human copper-transporting ATPases. *Physiol. Rev.*, **87**, 1011–1046.

MacDonald, L., Thumser, A.E. and Sharp, P. (2002) Decreased expression of vitamin C transporter SVCT1 by ascorbic acid in a human intestinal epithelial cell line. *Br. J. Nutr.*, **87**, 97–100.

Mackenzie, B., Takanaga, H., Hubert, N., Rolfs, A. and Hediger, M.A. (2007) Functional properties of multiple isoforms of human divalent metal-ion transporter 1 (DMT1). *Biochem. J.*, **403**, 59–69.

Madejczyk, M.S. and Ballatori, N. (2012) The iron transporter ferroportin can also function as a manganese exporter. *Biochim. Biophys. Acta*, **1818**, 651–657.

Mailloux, R.J., Lemire, J. and Appanna VD. (2011) Hepatic response to aluminum toxicity: dyslipidemia and liver diseases. *Exp. Cell Res.*, **317**, 2231–2238.

Marques, L., Auriac, A., Willemetz, A., *et al.* (2012) Immune cells and hepatocytes express glycosylphosphatidylinositol-anchored ceruloplasmin at their cell surface. *Blood Cells Mol. Dis.*, **48**, 110–120.

Martin, F., Linden, T., Katschinski, D.M., *et al.* (2005) Copper-dependent activation of hypoxia-inducible factor (HIF)-1: implications for ceruloplasmin regulation. *Blood*, **105**, 4613–4619.

Mastrogiannaki, M., Matak, P., Keith, B., *et al.* (2009) HIF-2α, but not HIF-1α, promotes iron absorption in mice. *J. Clin. Invest.*, **119**, 1159–1166.

Mastrogiannaki, M., Matak, P. and Peyssonnaux, C. (2013) The gut in iron homeostasis: role of HIF-2 under normal and pathological conditions. *Blood*, **122**, 885–892.

Matak, P., Zumerle, S., Mastrogiannaki, M., *et al.*, (2013) Copper deficiency leads to anemia, duodenal hypoxia, upregulation of HIF-2α and altered expression of iron absorption genes in mice. *PLoS One*, **8**, e59538.

Mellman, I.S., Youngdahl-Turner, P., Huntington, F.W. and Rosenberg, L.E. (1977) Intracellular binding of radioactive hydroxocobalamin to cobalamin-dependent apoenzyme in rat liver. *Proc. Natl Acad. Sci. USA*, **74**, 916–920.

Meyer, P.A, Brown, M.J. and Falk, H. (2008) Global approach to reducing lead exposure and poisoning. *Mutat. Res.*, **659**, 166–175.

Mitchell, C.J., Shawki, A., Ganz, T., Nemeth, E. and Mackenzie, B. (2014) Functional properties of human ferroportin, a cellular iron exporter reactive also with cobalt and zinc. *Am. J. Physiol. Cell. Physiol.*, **306**, C450–C459.

Mizutani, K., Mikami, B., Aibara, S. and Hirose, M. (2005) Structure of aluminium-bound ovotransferrin at 2.15 Angstroms resolution. *Acta Crystallogr. D*, **61**, 1636–1642.

Miyayama, T., Hiraoka, D., Kawaji, F., *et al.* (2010) Roles of COMM-domain-containing 1 in stability and recruitment of the copper-transporting ATPase in a mouse hepatoma cell line. *Biochem. J.*, **429**, 53–61.

Moestrup, S.K., Kozyraki, R., Kristiansen, M., *et al.* (1998) The intrinsic factor-vitamin B_{12} receptor and target of teratogenic antibodies is a megalin-binding peripheral membrane protein with homology to developmental proteins. *J. Biol. Chem.*, **273** 5235–5242.

Mostad, E.J. and Prohaska, J.R. (2011) Glycosylphosphatidylinositol-linked ceruloplasmin is expressed in multiple rodent organs and is lower following dietary copper deficiency. *Exp. Biol. Med. (Maywood)*, **236**, 298–308.

Moulis, J.-M. (2010) Cellular mechanisms of cadmium toxicity related to the homeostasis of essential metals. *Biometals*, **23**, 877–896.

Murphy, M.E., Lindley, P.F. and Adman, E.T. (1997) Structural comparison of cupredoxin domains: domain recycling to construct proteins with novel functions. *Protein Sci.*, **6**, 761–770.

Nakamura, K. and Go, N. (2005) Function and molecular evolution of multicopper blue proteins. *Cell. Mol. Life Sci.*, **62**, 2050–2066.

Nam, H. and Knutson, M.D. (2012). Effect of dietary iron deficiency and overload on the expression of ZIP metal-ion transporters in rat liver. *Biometals*, **25**, 115–124.

Neal, A.P. and Guilarte, T.R. (2010) Molecular neurobiology of lead (Pb(2+)): effects on synaptic function. *Mol. Neurobiol.*, **42**, 151–160.

Neal, A.P. and Guilarte, T.R. (2013) Mechanisms of lead and manganese neurotoxicity. *Toxicol. Res. (Camb)*, **2**, 99–114.

Neal, A.P., Stansfield, K.H., Worley, P.F., Thompson, R.E. and Guilarte, T.R. (2010) Lead exposure during synaptogenesis alters vesicular proteins and impairs vesicular release: potential role of NMDA receptor-dependent BDNF signaling. *Toxicol. Sci.*, **116**, 249–263.

Nevitt, T., Öhrvik, H. and Thiele, D.J. (2012) Charting the travels of copper in eukaryotes from yeast to mammals. *Biochim. Biophys. Acta*, **1823**, 1580–1593.

Niemoeller, O.M., Kiedaisch, V., Dreischer, P., Wieder, T. and Lang, F. (2006) Stimulation of eryptosis by aluminium ions. *Toxicol. Appl. Pharmacol.*, **217**, 168–175.

Nordberg, G.F., Jin, T., Wu, X., *et al.* (2009) Prevalence of kidney dysfunction in humans – relationship to cadmium dose, metallothionein, immunological and metabolic factors. *Biochimie*, **91**, 1282–1285.

Nose, Y., Wood, L.K., Kim, B.E., *et al.* (2010) Ctr1 is an apical copper transporter in mammalian intestinal epithelial cells in vivo that is controlled at the level of protein stability. *J. Biol. Chem.*, **285**, 32385–32392.

Ohgami, R.S., Campagna, D.R., McDonald, A. and Fleming, M.D. (2006) The Steap proteins are metalloreductases. *Blood*, **15**, 1388–1394.

Owen, C.A. Jr (1973) Effects of iron on copper metabolism and copper on iron metabolism in rats. *Am. J. Physiol.*, **224**, 514–518.

Patel, B.N. and David, S. (1997) A novel glycosylphosphatidylinositol-anchored form of ceruloplasmin is expressed by mammalian astrocytes. *J. Biol. Chem.*, **272**, 20185–20190.

Patel, B.N., Dunn, R.J. and David, S. (2000) Alternative RNA splicing generates a glycosylphosphatidylinositol-anchored form of ceruloplasmin in mammalian brain. *J. Biol. Chem.*, **275**, 4305–4310.

Palmer, A.E., Szilagyi, R.K., Cherry, J.R., *et al.* (2003) Spectroscopic characterization of the Leu513His variant of fungal laccase: effect of increased axial ligand interaction on the geometric and electronic structure of the type 1 Cu site. *Inorg. Chem.*, **42**, 4006–4017.

Palmiter, R.D. and Huang, L. (2004) Efflux and compartmentalization of zinc by members of the SLC30 family of solute carriers. *Pflugers Arch.*, **447**, 744–751.

Pan, Y., Mansfield, K.D., Bertozzi, C.C., *et al.* (2007) Multiple factors affecting cellular redox status and energy metabolism modulate hypoxia-inducible factor prolyl hydroxylase activity in vivo and in vitro. *Mol. Cell. Biol.*, **27**, 912–925.

Petris, M.J., Smith, K., Lee, J. and Thiele, D.J. (2003) Copper-stimulated endocytosis and degradation of the human copper transporter, hCtr1. *J. Biol. Chem.*, **278**, 9639–9646.

Pfeifer, G.D., Roper, J.M., Dorman, D. and Lynam, D.R. (2004) Health and environmental testing of manganese exhaust products from use of methylcyclopentadienyl manganese tricarbonyl in gasoline. *Sci. Total Environ.*, **334–335**, 397–408.

Phillips-Krawczak, C.A., Singla, A., Starokadomskyy, P., *et al.* (2015) COMMD1 is linked to the WASH complex and regulates endosomal trafficking of the copper transporter ATP7A. *Mol. Biol. Cell*, **26**, 91–103.

Pinilla-Tenas, J.J., Sparkman, B.K., Shawki, A., *et al.* (2011) Zip14 is a complex broad-scope metal-ion transporter whose functional properties support roles in the cellular uptake of zinc and nontransferrin-bound iron. *Am. J. Physiol. Cell. Physiol.*, **301**, C862–C871.

Pollack, S., George, J.N., Reba, R.C., Kaufman, R.M. and Crosby, W.H. (1965) The absorption of nonferrous metals in iron deficiency. *J. Clin. Invest.*, **44**, 1470–1473.

Pounds, J.G., Long, G.J. and Rosen, J.F. (1991) Cellular and molecular toxicity of lead in bone. *Environ. Health Perspect.*, **91**, 17–32.

Pourvali, K., Matak, P., Latunde-Dada, G.O., *et al.* (2012) Basal expression of copper transporter 1 in intestinal epithelial cells is regulated by hypoxia-inducible factor 2α. *FEBS Lett.*, **586**, 2423–2427.

Proescher, J.B., Son, M., Elliott, J.L. and Culotta, V.C. (2008) Biological effects of CCS in the absence of SOD1 enzyme activation: implications for disease in a mouse model for ALS. *Hum. Mol. Genet.*, **17**, 1728–1737.

Prohaska, J.R. and Broderius, M. (2012) Copper deficiency has minimal impact on ferroportin expression or function. *Biometals*, **25**, 633–642.

Pyatskowit, J.W. and Prohaska, J.R. (2008) Copper deficient rats and mice both develop anemia but only rats have lower plasma and brain iron levels. *Comp. Biochem. Physiol. C Toxicol. Pharmacol.*, **147**, 316–323.

Quadri, M., Federico, A., Zhao, T., *et al.* (2012) Mutations in SLC30A10 cause Parkinsonism and dystonia with hypermanganesemia, polycythemia, and chronic liver disease. *Am. J. Hum. Genet.*, **90**, 467–477.

Rae, T.D., Schmidt, P.J., Pufahl, R.A., Culotta, V.C. and O'Halloran, T.V. (1999) Undetectable intracellular free copper: the requirement of a copper chaperone for superoxide dismutase. *Science*, **284**, 805–808.

Rae, T.D., Torres, A.S., Pufahl, R.A. and O'Halloran, T.V. (2004) Mechanism of Cu,Zn-superoxide dismutase activation by the human metallochaperone hCCS. *J. Biol. Chem.*, **276**, 5166–5176.

Ran, R., Xu, H., Lu, A., Bernaudin, M. and Sharp, F.R. (2005) Hypoxia preconditioning in the brain. *Dev. Neurosci.*, **27**, 87–92.

Ravia, J.J., Stephen, R.M., Ghishan, F.K. and Collins, J.F. (2005) Menkes copper ATPase (*Atp7a*) is a novel metal-responsive gene in rat duodenum, and immunoreactive protein is present on brush-border and basolateral membrane domains. *J. Biol. Chem.*, **280**, 36221–36227.

Reeves, P.G. and DeMars, L.C. (2004) Copper deficiency reduces iron absorption and biological half-life in male rats. *J. Nutr.*, **134**, 1953–1957.

Reeves, P.G. and DeMars, L.C. (2005) Repletion of copper-deficient rats with dietary copper restores duodenal hephaestin protein and iron absorption. *Exp. Biol. Med.*, **230**, 320–325.

Reeves, P.G. and DeMars, L.C. (2006) Signs of iron deficiency in copper-deficient rats are not affected by iron supplements administered by diet or by injection. *J. Nutr. Biochem.*, **17**, 635–642.

Reeves, P.G., DeMars, L.C., Johnson, W.T. and Lukaski, H.C. (2005) Dietary copper deficiency reduces iron absorption and duodenal enterocyte hephaestin protein in male and female rats. *J. Nutr.*, **135**, 92–98.

Reynolds, E.H. (1979) *Folic acid, vitamin B$_{12}$ and the nervous system: historical aspects, in Folic Acid in Neurology, Psychiatry, and Internal Medicine* (eds M.I. Botez and E.H. Reynolds), Raven Press, New York, pp. 1–5.

Reynolds, E. (2006) Vitamin B$_{12}$, folic acid, and the nervous system. *Lancet Neurol.*, **5**, 949–960.

Rice, D. and Baronne, S. Jr (2000) Critical periods of vulnerability for the developing nervous system: evidence from humans and animal models. *Environ. Health Perspect.*, **108** (Suppl. 3), 511–533.

Rodier, P.M. (1995) Developing brain as a target of toxicity. *Environ. Health Perspect.*, **103** (Suppl. 6), 73–76.

Rodríguez-Agudelo, Y., Riojas-Rodríguez, H., Ríos, C., *et al.* (2006) Motor alterations associated with exposure to manganese in the environment in Mexico. *Sci. Total Environ.*, **368**, 542–556.

Roelofsen, H., Wolters, H., Van Luyn, M.J., *et al.*, (2000) Copper-induced apical trafficking of ATP7B in polarized hepatoma cells provides a mechanism for biliary copper excretion. *Gastroenterology*, **119**, 782–793.

Ryu, D.Y., Lee, S.J., Park, D.W., *et al.* (2004) Dietary iron regulates intestinal cadmium absorption through iron transporters in rats. *Toxicol. Lett.*, **152**, 19–25.

Samelko, L., Caicedo, M.S., Lim, S.J., *et al.* (2013) Cobalt-alloy implant debris induce HIF-1α hypoxia associated responses: A mechanism for metal-specific orthopedic implant failure. *PLoS One*, **8**, e67127.

Scheers, N. (2013) Regulatory effects of Cu, Zn, and Ca on Fe absorption: the intricate play between nutrient transporters. *Nutrients*, **5**, 957–970.

Scheers, N. and Sandberg, A.-S. (2008) Ascorbic acid uptake affects ferritin, Dcytb and Nramp2 expression in Caco-2 cells. *Eur. J. Nutr.*, **47**, 401–408.

Scheers, N. and Sandberg, A.-S. (2011) Iron regulates the uptake of ascorbic acid and the expression of sodium-dependent vitamin C transporter 1 (SVCT1) in human intestinal Caco-2 cells. *Br. J. Nutr.*, **105**, 1734–1740.

Scheers, N. and Sandberg, A.-S. (2014) Iron transport through ferroportin is induced by intracellular ascorbate and involves IRP2 and HIF2α. *Nutrients*, **6**, 249–260.

Seetharam, B. and Yammani, R.R. (2003) Cobalamin transport proteins and their cell-surface receptors. *Expert Rev. Mol. Med.*, **5**, 1–18.

Seo, Y.A., Li, Y. and Wessling-Resnick, M. (2013) Iron depletion increases manganese uptake and potentiates apoptosis through ER stress. *Neurotoxicology*, **38**, 67–73.

Seo, Y.A. and Wessling-Resnick, M. (2015) Ferroportin deficiency impairs manganese metabolism in flatiron mice. *FASEB J.*, **29**, 2726–2733.

Shah, Y.M., Matsubara, T., Ito, S., Yim, S.H. and Gonzalez, F.J. (2009) Intestinal hypoxia-inducible transcription factors are essential for iron absorption following iron deficiency. *Cell Metab.*, **9**, 152–164.

Shawki, A. and Mackenzie, B. (2010) Interaction of calcium with the human divalent metal-ion transporter-1. *Biochem. Biophys. Res. Commun.*, **393**, 471–475.

Shevell, M.I. and Rosenblatt, D.S. (1992) The neurology of cobalamin. *Can. J. Neurol. Sci.*, **19**, 472–486.

Shukla, A., Agarwal, K.N. and Shukla, G.S. (1989) Effect of latent iron deficiency on metal levels of rat brain regions. *Biol. Trace Elem. Res.*, **22**, 141–152.

Singh, N.P. and Medeiros, D.M. (1984) Effect of copper deficiency and sodium intake upon liver lipid and mineral composition in the rat. *Biol. Trace Elem. Res.*, **6**, 423–429.

Solomon, E.I., Szilagyi, R.K., DeBeer, G.S. and Basumallick, L. (2004) Electronic structures of metal sites in proteins and models: contributions to function in blue copper proteins. *Chem. Rev.*, **104**, 419–458.

Sourkes, T.L., Lloyd, K. and Birnbaum, H. (1968) Inverse relationship of hepatic copper and iron concentrations in rats fed deficient diets. *Can. J. Biochem.*, **46**, 267–271.

Stamelou, M., Tuschl, K., Chong, W.K., *et al.* (2012) Dystonia with brain manganese accumulation resulting from SLC30A10mutations: a new treatable disorder. *Mov. Disord.*, **27**, 1317–1322.

Stansfield, K.H., Pilsner, J.R., Lu, Q., Wright, R.O. and Guilarte, T.R. (2012) Dysregulation of BDNF-TrkB signaling in developing hippocampal neurons by Pb(2+): implications for an environmental basis of neurodevelopmental disorders. *Toxicol. Sci.*, **127**, 277–295.

Strope, S., Rivi, R., Metzger, T., Manova, K. and Lacy, E. (2004) Mouse amnionless, which is required for primitive streak assembly, mediates cell-surface localization and endocytic function of cubilin on visceral endoderm and kidney proximal tubules. *Development*, **131**, 4787–4795.

Taylor, M., Qu, A., Anderson, E.R., *et al.* (2011) Hypoxia-inducible factor-2α mediates the adaptive increase of intestinal ferroportin during iron deficiency in mice. *Gastroenterology*, **140**, 2044–2055.

Thévenod, F. (2010) Catch me if you can! Novel aspects of cadmium transport in mammalian cells. *Biometals*, **23**, 857–875.

Thompson, B.A.V., Sharp, P.A., Elliott R. and Fairweather-Tait, S.J. (2010) Inhibitory effect of calcium on non-heme iron absorption may be related to translocation of DMT-1 at the apical membrane of enterocytes. *J. Agric. Food Chem.*, **58**, 8414–8417.

Thompson, K., Molina, R.M., Donaghey, T., *et al.* (2007) Olfactory uptake of manganese requires DMT1 and is enhanced by anemia. *FASEB J.*, **21**, 223–230.

Troadec, M.B., Ward, D.M., Lo, E., Kaplan, J. and De Domenico, I. (2010) Induction of FPN1 transcription by MTF-1 reveals a role for ferroportin in transition metal efflux. *Blood*, **116**, 4657–4664.

Tuschl, K., Clayton, P.T., Gospe, S.M. Jr, *et al.* (2012) Syndrome of hepatic cirrhosis, dystonia, polycythemia, and hypermanganesemia caused by mutations in SLC30A10, a manganese transporter in man. *Am. J. Hum. Genet.*, **90**, 457–466.

van den Sluis, B., Rothuizen, J., Pearson, P.L., van Oost, B.A. and Wijmenga, C. (2002) Identification of a new copper metabolism gene by positional cloning in a purebred dog population. *Hum Mol. Genet.*, **11**, 165–173.

Vashchenko, G. and MacGillivray, R.T. (2013) Multi-copper oxidases and human iron metabolism. *Nutrients*, **5**, 2289–2313.

Verstraeten, S.V., Aimo, L. and Oteiza, P.I. (2008) Aluminium and lead: molecular mechanisms of brain toxicity. *Arch. Toxicol.*, **82**, 789–802.

Vonk, W.I., Bartuzi, P., de Bie, P., *et al.* (2011) Liver-specific Commd1 knockout mice are susceptible to hepatic copper accumulation. *PLoS One*, **6**, e29183.

Vulpe, C.D., Kuo, Y.M., Murphy, T.L., *et al.* (1999) Hephaestin, a ceruloplasmin homologue implicated in intestinal iron transport, is defective in the sla mouse. *Nat. Genet.*, **21**, 195–199.

Waites, C.L. and Garner, C.C. (2011) Presynaptic function in health and disease. *Trends Neurosci.*, **34**, 326–337.

Ward, R.J., Zhang, Y. and Crichton, R.R. (2001) Aluminium toxicity and iron homeostasis. *J. Inorg. Biochem.*, **87**, 9–14.

Weiss, K.H., Lozoya, J.C., Tuma, S., *et al.* (2008) Copper-induced translocation of the Wilson disease protein ATP7B independent of Murr1/COMMD1 and Rab7. *Am. J. Pathol.*, **173**, 1783–1794.

Williams, B.B., Kwakye, G.F., Wegrzynowicz, M., *et al.* (2010) Altered manganese homeostasis and manganese toxicity in a Huntington's disease striatal cell model are not explained by defects in the iron transport system. *Toxicol. Sci.*, **117**, 169–179.

Williams, D.M., Kennedy, F.S. and Green, B.G. (1983) Hepatic iron accumulation in copper-deficient rats. *Br. J. Nutr.*, **50**, 653–660.

Wyman, S., Simpson, R.J., McKie, A.T. and Sharp, P.A. (2008) Dcytb (Cybrd1) functions as both a ferric and a cupric reductase in vitro. *FEBS Lett.*, **582**, 1901–1906.

Xie, L. and Collins, J.F. (2011) Transcriptional regulation of the Menkes copper ATPase (*Atp7a*) gene by hypoxia-inducible factor (HIF2α) in intestinal epithelial cells. *Am. J. Physiol. Cell Physiol.*, **300**, C1298–C1305.

Xie, L. and Collins, J.F. (2013) Transcription factors Sp1 and Hif2α mediate induction of the copper-transporting ATPase (*Atp7a*) gene in intestinal epithelial cells during hypoxia. *J. Biol. Chem.*, **288**, 23943–23952.

Xu, F., Palmer, A.E., Yaver, D.S., *et al.*, (1999) Targeted mutations in a *Trametes villosa* laccase. Axial perturbations of the T1 copper. *J. Biol. Chem.*, **274**, 12372–12375.

Yamaji, S., Tennant, J., Tandy, S., *et al.* (2001) Zinc regulates the function and expression of the iron transporters DMT1 and IREG1 in human intestinal Caco-2 cells. *FEBS Lett.*, **507**, 137–141.

Yeh, K.Y., Yeh, M., Mims, L. and Glass, J. (2009) Iron feeding induces ferroportin 1 and hephaestin migration and interaction in rat duodenal epithelium. *Am. J. Physiol. Gastrointest. Liver Physiol.*, **296**, G55–G65.

Yin, Z., Jiang, H., Lee, E.S., *et al.* (2010) Ferroportin is a manganese-responsive protein that decreases manganese cytotoxicity and accumulation. *J. Neurochem.*, **112**, 1190–1198.

Yuan, Y., Hilliard, G., Ferguson, T. and Millhorn, D.E. (2003) Cobalt inhibits the interaction between hypoxia-inducible factor-alpha and von Hippel-Lindau protein by direct binding to hypoxia-inducible factor-alpha. *J. Biol. Chem.*, **278**, 15911–15916.

Zatta, P., Kiss, T., Suwalsky, M. and Berthon, G. (2002) Aluminium (III) as a promoter of cellular oxidation. *Coord. Chem. Rev.*, **228**, 271–284.

Zhang, Y.B., Wang, X., Meister, E.A., *et al.* (2014) The effects of $CoCl_2$ on HIF-1α protein under experimental conditions of autoprogressive hypoxia using mouse models. *Int. J. Mol. Sci.*, **15**, 10999–11012.

Zhou, B. and Gitschier, A. (1997) hCTR1: a human gene for copper uptake identified by complementation in yeast. *Proc. Natl Acad. Sci. USA*, **94**, 7481–7486.

Zimnicka, A.M., Ivy, K. and Kaplan, J.H. (2011) Acquisition of dietary copper: a role for anion transporters in intestinal apical copper uptake. *Am. J. Physiol. Cell Physiol.*, **300**, C588–C599.

15

Iron Homeostasis and Neurodegeneration

15.1 Introduction

The brain, which constitutes just 2% of the human body mass, receives 15% of the cardiac output, consumes 20% of the total oxygen supply, and accounts for 25% of the total body glucose utilisation. Metal ions are absolutely essential and play important functions in these processes. However, in higher organisms they are also indispensible for brain function, for example, in nerve transmission and muscle contraction. The alkali metal ions Na^+ and K^+ play a crucial role in the transmission of nervous impulses, both within the brain and from the brain to other parts of the body. Within cells, including nerve cells, fluxes of Ca^{2+} ions play an important role in signal transduction. Ca^{2+} channels mediate Ca^{2+} influx into neurons in response to membrane depolarisation, mediating numerous intracellular processes, including neurotransmitter export. While 90% of brain Zn^{2+} is bound to proteins, about 10% is less tightly bound, much of it in synaptic vesicles, which is released together with glutamate when hippocampal nerve fibres are stimulated. Cu and Mn also play key roles in brain; the Cu enzyme, dopamine β-hydroxylase, transforms dopamine to noradrenaline, and both metals are essential components of the cytoplasmic and mitochondrial superoxide dismutatses (SODs) responsible for neuroprotection the O_2-rich brain.

Brain iron also plays a crucial role in neuronal function. Although brain iron only represents less than 2% of total body iron, homeostasis of iron is mandatory for normal physiological brain function. Iron is involved in a wide number of fundamental biological processes (see Chapter 2). Within the brain, iron plays an important role in various enzymes which are involved in neurotransmitter synthesis and myelination of the axons of motor neurons. Thus, tryptophan hydroxylase is required for serotonin synthesis, and tyrosine hydroxylase for the synthesis of dopamine, the precursor of adrenaline and noradrenaline; iron is also directly involved in myelin formation.

Iron Metabolism – From Molecular Mechanisms to Clinical Consequences, Fourth Edition. Robert Crichton.
© 2016 John Wiley & Sons, Ltd. Published 2016 by John Wiley & Sons, Ltd.

15.2   Brain Iron

15.2.1   Brain Iron Homeostasis

Peripheral cellular iron uptake and export has already been described in Chapter 6. The former involves endocytosis of the diferric transferrin (Tf-Fe$_2$)–transferrin receptor 1 (TfR1) complex, and iron transport into the cytoplasm via divalent metal ion transporter 1 (DMT1), where it can be incorporated into iron-containing proteins or stored in the soluble, nontoxic, bioavailable ferritin, Ft. The iron export protein ferroportin (Fpn) transports iron out of some cells and, together with the ferroxidases ceruloplasmin (Cp) and hephaestin, enables ferric iron loading onto apo-Tf. The translation of TfR, DMT1, Ft and Fpn mRNAs is regulated by iron regulatory proteins (IRPs). Circulating hepcidin orchestrates systemic iron homeostasis by interacting with Fpn when iron is abundant, resulting in the internalisation and degradation of Fpn, thereby blocking iron exportation. As circulating iron levels fall, hepcidin synthesis declines and iron exportation by Fpn resumes. Since most of these proteins have been identified in the brain, it has therefore been assumed that brain iron homeostasis might be comparable.

Figure 15.1 summarises the current understanding of iron homeostasis in the brain (Ward *et al.*, 2014). Iron bound to Tf could enter the endothelial cells of the blood–brain barrier (BBB) by the Tf/TfR system; TFR1 is highly expressed on the luminal side of endothelial cells (Jefferies *et al.*, 1984). Iron would then traverse the endothelial cell, to be released at the abluminal membrane by an unknown pathway which might involve ferroportin and/or other transporters and in an unknown form, possible as low-molecular-weight complexes (e.g. citrate, ATP, ascorbate). The iron released in the extracellular compartment could then be taken up by other cells, such as astrocytes and neurons. Transferrin is synthesised in the brain by the choroid plexus and oligodendrocytes, but only that in the choroid plexus is secreted (Leitner and Connor, 2012). It is thought that neurons acquire most of their iron using the Tf/TfR system, and it is likely that they can export iron via Fpn, since many neurons coexpress TfR and Fpn (Boserup *et al.*, 2011).

Because their perivascular end-foot processes ensheath the abluminal membrane of the BBB (Abbott *et al.*, 2006) and also form direct connections to neurons, astrocytes are thought to play a key role in regulating brain iron absorption (Dringen *et al.*, 2007). Astrocytes do not express TfR, but may take up iron at the BBB via DMT1, which is expressed at the end–foot processes associated with the BBB (Xu and Ling, 1994). Fpn together with glycophosphatidylinositol-anchored Cp constitutes the major efflux pathway in astrocytes (Jeong and David, 2003; Wu *et al.*, 2004). There is continuous signalling between neurons, microglia and astrocytes, thereby reflecting any changing environment within the brain such that appropriate action can be taken when required. Iron must also be transported down the axons of neurons to synapses, by unidentified mechanisms.

Oligodendrocytes contain large amounts of iron, required for axon myelination (Connor *et al.*, 1990; Badaracco *et al.*, 2010). Oligodendrocytes may extract iron from adjacent blood vessels (Connor and Menzies, 1996) or, less probably, from extracellular Ft (Leitner and Connor, 2012). Increasing information is now emerging of the role played by microglia in iron homeostasis. Most of the iron genes and proteins have been identified in glial cells (TfR1, DMT1, FPN1), and they are appropriately regulated during iron excess, depletion and inflammation (Ward *et al.*, 2009; Urrutia *et al.*, 2013); when they are activated microglia appear to upregulate iron uptake and downregulate iron exportation (Crichton and Ward, 2006; Rathore *et al.*, 2012). In oligodendrocytes, iron is present within Ft, while its form in astrocytes and microglia remains undefined (Badaracco *et al.*, 2010).

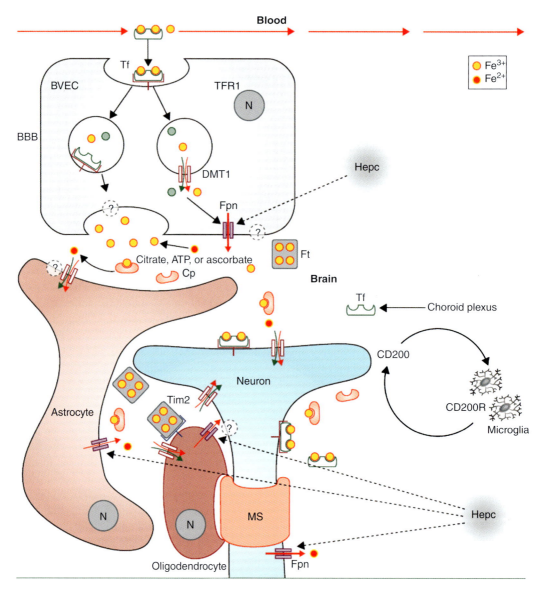

Figure 15.1 *The current understanding of iron homeostasis in the brain. Reproduced with permission from Elsevier from Ward, R.J., Zucca, F.A., Duyn, J.H., Crichton, R.R. and Zecca, L. (2014) The role of iron in brain ageing and neurodegenerative disorders.* Lancet Neurol., *13, 1045–1060*

15.2.2 Aging and Brain Iron Content

Aging is associated with low-grade chronic inflammation, termed inflammaging (Franceschi and Campisi, 2014). In older adults, a chronic subclinical inflammatory status exists, with proinflammatory cytokines increasing approximately twofold. Inflammaging results from several age-related factors, including increased numbers of dysfunctional cytokine-secreting senescent cells and an altered body composition. An increased body fat content and the redistribution of fat tissue with aging, which has as a consequence increased amounts of adipocytes that produce tumour necrosis factor alpha (TNF-α) and interleukin (IL)-6, hormonal deficiencies, increases in reactive oxygen species (ROS), multiple chronic diseases, environmental exposure to various stimulators of inflammation, a history and/or number of infections, a history of trauma, chronic stress, genetic factors, and lifestyle factors. There is a positive relationship between serum ferritin and this subclinical inflammatory state. The important consequence is a reorganisation of the control of iron homeostasis by the primary mediators of the acute-phase response, TNF-α and IL-1, thereby augmenting ferritin synthesis.

No extensive morphological changes have been identified in the brains of normally aging individuals; that is, there is no significant loss of cells within the hippocampus and neocortex, while the extensive dendritic branching in layer II of the parahippocampal gyrus is maintained. However, alterations in the mechanisms of plasticity that contribute to cognitive functions have been detected (Ward *et al.*, 2014). One functional alteration that could directly affect plasticity is a reduction in synapse numbers, which could make it more difficult to attain a sufficient amount of cooperatively active synapses which are necessary to lead to network modification. It is suggested, therefore, that most age-associated behavioural impairments result from region-specific changes in dendritic morphology, cellular connectivity, Ca^{2+} dysregulation, and gene expression.

In normal aging, beyond the age of 70 years, a selective accumulation of non-haem iron occurs in several brain regions, namely the putamen, globus pallidus, caudate and hippocampus, with iron present in fibres, glial cells and neuromelanin (NM)-free neurons (Figure 15.2). Neurons containing NM do not have detectable iron deposits. The levels of iron in cerebellum and premotor cortex are lower, with the majority of iron being bound within either ferritins or NM, with no pathological consequences. NM is a black-brownish pigment that accumulates in dopaminergic neurons during their life time, in the medulla oblongata, hypothalamus and cerebellum, but more specifically in dopaminergic neurons of the substantia nigra (SN) and in the noradrenergic neurons of the locus coerulus. The pigment is confined to cytoplasmic organelles and is surrounded by a double membrane (Zucca *et al.*, 2014). While the origin of NM organelles is unclear, it is proposed that NM synthesis results from an excess of cytosolic catecholamines that have not been incorporated into the synaptic vesicles (Zucca *et al.*, 2014). Dopamine oxidation occurs, involving a number of enzymes in this process, such as tyrosinase, peroxidase, prostaglandin H synthase, xanthine oxidase and tyrosine hydroxylase, which will oxidise dopamine to dopaminoquinone or to L-DOPA in the presence of cysteine to thioether derivatives, precursors of NM synthesis (reviewed by Zucca *et al.*, 2014). The function of NM is undefined, but it may be involved in iron homeostasis and neuronal protection against toxic agents, such as products of dopamine synthesis or in the removal of toxic metals such as iron, copper and zinc, which are sequestered by the melanic portion of the molecule.

NM has been implicated as having a potential role in intraneuronal iron homeostasis as it is able to bind a variety of metals, including iron. For example 7% (w/w) of isolated NM is reported to consist of iron, copper, zinc, manganese and chromium, while iron-binding studies using NM isolated from the human SN showed that NM contains high-affinity ($KD = 7.18 \pm 1.08$ nm) and low-affinity binding sites ($KD = 94.31 \pm 6.55$ nm) for Fe(III) (Double *et al.*, 2003). Mössbauer studies showed that iron is directly bound to NM granules in the SN, and that this signal is increased in Parkinson's disease (Tribl *et al.*, 2009). In addition, Mössbauer spectroscopy showed that iron-binding sites in NM isolated from the human SN are similar to those of human ferritin and haemosiderin (Tribl *et al.*, 2009). Physical techniques have suggested that

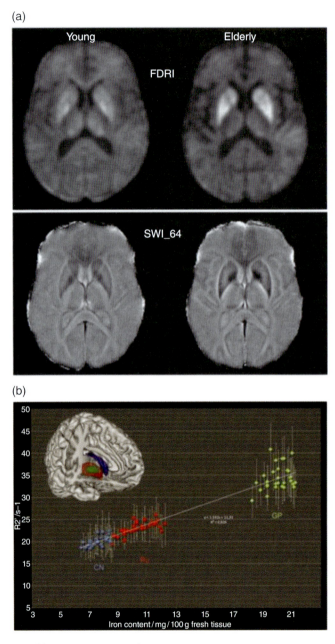

Figure 15.2 *Aging and brain iron accumulation. Magnetic resonance imaging (MRI) of iron in the human brain. (A) Young (left) and elderly (right) group means for FDRI images (acquired at 1.5 T and 3.0 T; top) and SWI images (1.5 T; bottom). Increasing iron concentrations engender higher (brighter) FDR. Reprinted with permission from Elsevier from Schipper, H.M. (2012) Neurodegeneration with brain iron accumulation – Clinical syndromes and neuroimaging.* Biochim. Biophys. Acta, *1822, 350–360*

NM has a protein component which forms the central core, around which there is an unstructured melanic polymer (Zucca *et al.*, 2014) which enlarges during pigment formation, with protein unfolding and aggregation induced by dopaminoquinone. This is supported by the hypothesis that the polymerisation of dopamine is initiated by the reaction of dopaminoquinone with proteins. The concentration of this iron-binding insoluble material increases with age in both the SN and locus coeruleus, as well as the premotor cortex, putamen and cerebellum. Detailed human studies on the effect of aging on the accumulation of NM and Ft in the SN and locus coeruleus show a linear increase of total iron content in the SN with age, whereas in the locus coeruleus the iron concentration is lower and remains stable throughout life. In contrast, the levels of iron in the locus coeruleus remain unchanged. The amount of intraneuronal iron bound to NM varies in different types of neurons, with dopaminergic neurons exhibiting the highest content.

Both H- and L- ferritins are present in brain, particularly within the microglia and astrocytes. In the aged brain there is a subpopulation of Ft-positive microglial cells, and the majority of these cells have an aberrant morphology of dystrophic type. Dystrophic and ferritin-positive microglia may contribute to the pathogenesis of neurodegenerative disorders due to altered microglial functioning (reviewed in Ward *et al.*, 2014). Women may have lower levels of brain ferritin than men (Bartzokis *et al.*, 2007). H-ferritin concentrations are low in the SN during the first year of life (29 ng mg^{-1}), but this increases to 200 ng mg^{-1} by the fourth decade, after which it remains stable (Zecca *et al.*, 2001). L-ferritin levels also increase during aging, but the concentration is 50% less than that of H-ferritin. It has been suggested that the higher levels of H-ferritin may be related to the proinflammatory state in the brain with aging (reviewed in Ward *et al.*, 2014). The cell protects itself against such events by upregulating ferritin approximately 80-fold through the antioxidant-response element, in part by binding to the transcription factor NF-E2-related factor 2. The resultant increase in ferritin leads to the sequestration of iron and minimises the generation of ROS in the cells (Singh *et al.*, 2014). Other regulators of ferritin include the inflammatory cytokines TNFα, IL-1 and IL-6. Since IL-6 receptors are present on the basolateral membrane of the choroid plexus epithelial cells, it is suggested that any increased levels of IL-6 in the blood could interact with these receptors (Marques *et al.*, 2009) to initiate changes in hepcidin expression. Indeed, animal studies suggest a correlation between the IL-6/STAT3 signalling pathway and hepcidin in the choroid plexus of aging rats, with mRNA hepcidin and protein expression remaining stable in young animals but increasing with age (Liu *et al.*, 2014). IL-6 may therefore regulate hepcidin expression in the choroid plexus upon interaction with the cognate cellular receptor and through the Stat3 signalling transduction pathway.

Oligodendrocytes, which represent the vast majority of cells (>85%) in the white matter of the brain, contain the largest amount of iron, stored mainly as ferritin. The levels of iron in these cells are reported to remain constant or to decrease with aging (Bartzokis *et al.*, 2007). This decrease may reflect changes in oligodendrocyte and myelin density with aging. It is estimated that up to 45% of myelinated fibre length is lost during aging, particularly from regions such as the frontal lobe.

The reason for such increases of iron in these different brain regions remains unclear. However, various hypotheses have been presented which include altered blood brain permeability, an inflammatory state (activated microglia cells altering the expression of ferroportin on their cell surface due to increased hepcidin production, thus retaining iron within the cells), or a redistribution of pools of iron within the brain, as well as alterations in iron homeostasis (reviewed in Ward *et al.*, 2014).

15.3 Iron and Neurodegeneration

15.3.1 Introduction

The association between iron accumulation in specific brain regions and neurodegenerative disorders has become increasingly obvious during the past decade (Crichton and Ward, 2006, 2014). There are at least seven genetically distinct disorders which are classified as 'Neurodegeneration with Brain Iron Accumulation (NBIA) (Keogh and Chinnery, 2011). While these represent a clinically and genetically heterogeneous group of conditions, neurodegeneration is clearly associated with elevated levels of brain iron. Two of them involve mutations in genes associated with iron homeostasis. Mutations in the ferritin light chain gene, *FTL*, cause neuroferritinopathy, an adult-onset autosomal-dominant movement disorder. and homozygous mutations in the ceruloplasmin gene. Mutations in the frataxin gene, *FRDA*, involved in the assembly of [4Fe–4S] clusters, causes an increased mitochondrial accumulation of iron in the brain, heart and liver. There are a growing number of other neurodegenerative diseases where secondary iron overload occurs, including Parkinson's disease, Alzheimer's disease, Huntington's disease and multiple sclerosis, where iron accumulation has been implicated as a primary cause.

Aging is the major risk factor for neurodegeneration, with the age-related accumulation of iron being an important contributing factor to the neurodegenerative processes. Recent studies have suggested that an accelerated trajectory of brain iron accumulation may be occurring during the transition from healthy aging into preclinical stages of neurodegenerative diseases such as Alzheimer's disease. Increases in iron content are discernible in many neurodegenerative diseases, but the comprehension of the role of iron in the development and progression of the disease is not clear. Furthermore, neurodegeneration is not necessarily due to defects in genes directly linked to iron metabolism, and there may also be other factors such as inflammation or enzyme deficiency. It remains unclear whether iron accumulation is a primary cause of the disorder or a consequence of a previous dysfunction. However, iron accumulation occurs in a particular area and becomes the hallmark of a specific neurodegenerative disorder.

Magnetic resonance imaging (MRI) has become the modality of choice for the investigation and differential diagnosis of neurodegenerative disorders associated with iron accumulation. Brain MRI is sensitive to the presence and concentration of non-haem iron, although at best it is only semi-quantitative. Iron deposits in brain cause local magnetic field inhomogeneities with decreased T2 relaxation times and appear hypointense on T2-weighted or T2* images. This technique has the ability to distinguish between the different iron-loading syndromes on the basis of the distribution of iron in the various brain regions.

15.3.2 Adverse Effects of Iron in Neurodegeneration

15.3.2.1 Toxicity of ROS and RNS

Increases in iron, particularly when the iron is present in a low-molecular-weight form, can induce many toxic effects which include the generation of ROS, notably the hydroxyl radical (Crichton and Ward, 2006, 2014), as this may damage DNA and mitochondrial DNA (mtDNA), affect DNA expression by epigenetic mechanisms (Kwok, 2010) as well as directly oxidising proteins and polyunsaturated fatty acids in membrane lipids (Catalá, 2009). ROS can also induce the release of iron from mitochondrial iron–sulphur cluster proteins of the respiratory chain, as well as from other storage proteins.

Inflammation, with the release of proinflammatory cytokines such as TNFα and IL-6 from activated microglia, induces the synthesis of DMT1 and promotes iron accumulation in neurons and microglia. The enzymes NADPH oxidase (NOX) and induced nitric oxide synthase (iNOS) will be activated in the microglia, with the formation of superoxide and hydroxyl radicals by the former, and of NO by the latter. The increased NO production, via the activation of transcription factors STAT1 and NF-κB, will increase the oxidative tone within the microglia. The expression of DMT1, TfR1 and of Fpt1 and cytosolic ferritin, which is transductionally regulated by the IRE/IRP system, will be altered by NO and ROS production. The proinflammatory cytokines TNFα, IL-6 and the TLR-4 agonist lipopolysaccharide (LPS) directly regulate DMT1 mRNA and protein levels and induce a transient decrease in ferroportin protein, thereby generating an increase in iron content both in neurons and microglia (Urrutia *et al.*, 2013). In other studies, primary cultures of mesencephalic neurons stimulated with TNFα or IL-1B induce an increase in DMT1 and TfR1 protein levels and a reduction in ferroportin levels, resulting in an increase in ferrous iron influx and decreased iron efflux in neurons (Wang *et al.*, 2013). It could therefore be suggested there is a circuit whereby the activation of microglia results in TNFα secretion and increases iron uptake by neurons via NF-κB-induced DMT1 expression. Inflammation may also promote hydroxyl radical production by the activation of two pathways: (i) DMT1-mediated release of iron; and (ii) increased hydrogen peroxide levels mediated by NOX activation. ROS induce intracellular signalling pathways resulting in the activation of various transcriptional factors such as NF-κB, Ap-1 and Nrf2 which can regulate the expression of proinflammatory mediators such as Cox-2, MCP-1, IL-6, TNFα, IL-1a and IL-1b. These can stimulate a cascade of events leading to increased oxidative stress via NOS and NOX activation.

15.3.2.2 Iron and Mitochondrial Function

Disruption of iron homeostasis can interfere with mitochondrial function with consequent progression of neurodegenerative mechanisms (Horowitz and Greenamyre, 2010). Mitochondrial dysfunction results in decreased ATP synthesis as well as decreased synthesis of iron–sulphur clusters and haem prosthetic groups. An association between mitochondrial dysfunction and mitochondrial iron accumulation has only been identified in Friedreich's ataxia, although there is evidence indicating that there is mitochondrial iron accumulation in experimental models of Parkinson's disease. There is a relationship between inflammation and mitochondrial activity. The production of ROS and RNS affects mitochondrial activity through the destabilisation of membranes. The free radical superoxide damages or oxidises [4Fe–4S] clusters, which results in the formation of the null [3Fe–4S] centre form. Additionally, NO reacts with [4Fe–4S] clusters to generate [(NO)$_2$Fe(SR)$_2$]-type complexes that inactivate several mitochondrial iron–sulphur enzymes and proteins which compose the electron transport chain (reviewed by Urrutia *et al.*, 2014). There is increasing evidence that mitochondrial dysfunction, iron accumulation and chronic inflammation play an important role in many neurodegenerative diseases, including Alzheimer's disease, Parkinson's disease, Huntington disease, amyotrophic lateral sclerosis and Friedrich's ataxia.

15.3.2.3 Protein Aggregation

The aggregation of some proteins involved in neurodegenerative disorders has been shown *in vitro* to be triggered by elevated iron levels; examples are α-synuclein (Li *et al.*, 2010) and hyperphosphorylated tau protein (Yamamoto *et al.*, 2002). Inclusion bodies containing damaged/aggregated proteins could cause endoplasmic reticulum stress, which is a common feature of several neurodegenerative diseases (Liu and Connor, 2012).

15.4 Neurodegeneration with Brain Iron Accumulation

The combination of MRI identification of causative genes has led to the recognition of a new group of neurodegenerative disorders. This set of degenerative extrapyramidal monogenic disorders with radiological evidence of focal accumulation of iron in the brain (usually in the basal ganglia) has been designated neurodegeneration with brain iron accumulation (NBIA) (Yoshida *et al.*, 1995; Gregory *et al.*, 2009; Gregory and Hayflick, 2011). They are characterised by an early or late onset nature, the main symptoms being associated with problems in movement, spasticity and cognitive impairment, and their diagnosis is made on the basis of the combination of representative clinical features along with MRI-based evidence of iron accumulation (Kruer and Boddaert, 2012). The specificity of the imaging details can orient the follow-up genetic analysis, such that the disease can be assigned to a genetically confirmed category or, in about 30% of all cases, to the idiopathic group (Dusek *et al.*, 2013).

The NBIA diseases identified to date include aceruloplasminaemia, neuroferritinopathy, pantothenate kinase-associated neurodegeneration (PKAN), phospholipase 2, group VI-associated neurodegeneration (PLAN), mitochondrial membrane protein-associated neurodegeneration (MPAN), fatty acid hydroxylase-associated neurodegeneration (FAHN), β-propeller protein-associated neurodegeneration (BPAN), and the recently discovered coenzyme A (CoA) synthase protein-associated neurodegeneration (CoPAN) (Dusi *et al.*, 2014). The NBIA diseases show variable incidence and from an epidemiological point of view are extremely rare (Dusek and Schneider, 2012; Dusek *et al.*, 2013).

15.4.1 Aceruloplasminaemia

As we saw in Chapter 14, on account of its ferroxidase activity (promoting the oxidation of Fe^{2+} to Fe^{3+} after efflux of iron from the cell via ferroportin), ceruloplasmin (Cp) plays a central role in cellular iron efflux and its transfer to apotransferrin. The essential role which Cp plays in iron metabolism was established unequivocally in 1995, with the identification of patients with aceruloplasminaemia (Harris *et al.*, 1995; Yoshida *et al.*, 1995), an autosomal recessive disorder where there is an absence of active CP, which results in the accumulation of iron within cells. It is thought that iron will initially accumulate in a non-toxic form within ferritin, which gradually becomes filled to capacity because of the reduced ability of the cell to efflux iron. Iron accumulates in the neurons and astrocytes of the brain, as well as in the retina, the liver and reticuloendothelial cells in the spleen and pancreatic cells. The cascade of events leading to neuronal death are not fully elucidated, but oxidative stress, exacerbated by heavy-metal accumulation, is the primary cellular toxic event.

Patients with aceruloplasminaemia usually present in their 40s or 50s, although it can present earlier, as young as16 years. Aceruloplasminaemia is characterised by a classic triad of neurologic symptoms that includes dementia, dysarthria and dystonia, together with insulin-dependent diabetes and retinal degeneration. These symptoms reflect iron accumulation in most parenchymal tissues, including the basal ganglia in the brain (a 10-fold increase, with iron accumulation in both neurons and microglia). Iron overload has been identified by MRI T2* in the basal ganglia, the red nuclei and deep cerebellar nuclei, as well as in the cortex as the disease progresses (Figure 15.3). In the central nervous system, under normal circumstances Cp is expressed as a

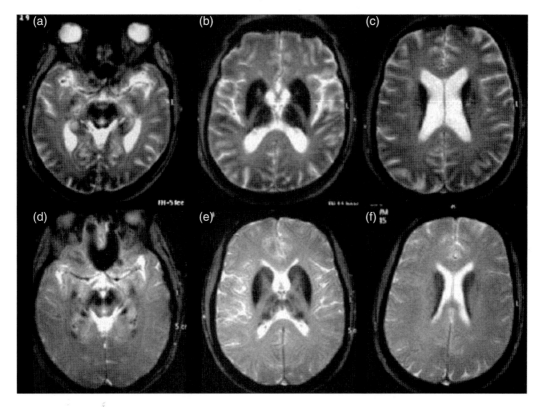

Figure 15.3 *Comparison of last available brain MRI of two siblings. Using the GRE (gradient echo) T2*-weighted images the overall brain iron deposition is clearly defined on the basis of hypointensity (due to paramagnetic effect). In the proband, hypointensity is more pronounced and more extensive, involving bilaterally the midbrain, the putamina, the globi pallidi, the caudate nuclei, the thalami, and the temporo-occipital cortex; moreover, iron deposition is associated with ventricular and subarachnoid spaces dilatation (a–c). In the proband's sister the degree of hypointensity is less pronounced, the cerebral cortex is almost completely spared, and the intracranial cerebrospinal fluid spaces appear normal in size (d,e). Reproduced with permission from John Wiley and Sons from Fasano, A., Colosimo, C., Miyajima, H., et al. (2008) Aceruloplasminemia: a novel mutation in a family with marked phenotypic variability. Mov. Disord., **23**, 751–755.*

glycophosphatidylinositol-anchored protein, in populations of astrocytes associated with micro-vasculature surrounding dopaminergic melanin-containing neurons in the SN and the inner cortex of the retina (Klomp and Gitlin, 1993).

Over 50 mutations have been reported in the Cp gene (Kono, 2013; Levi and Finazzi, 2014). For example, Cys-881 is essential for the trafficking and secretion of the truncated mutant Cp in aceruloplasminaemia (Kono *et al.*, 2007), a mutant protein without Cys-881 accumulates in the ER, inducing ER stress and eventually cell death. Analysis of Cp mutants shows that there are three different types of pathological mechanisms, which all result in loss of the ferroxidase activity of the protein: (i) retention of Cp in the endoplasmic reticulum, (ii) mis-incorporation of copper into apoceruloplasmin, and (iii) impaired ferroxidase activity (Hellman *et al.*, 2002; Kono *et al.*, 2007, 2010; di Patti *et al.*, 2009). All three block iron export from the cell, leading to cellular iron overload.

15.4.2 Neuroferritinopathy

The second neurodegenerative disease associated with mutations in proteins involved in iron homeostasis is neuroferritinopathy (Keogh *et al.*, 2012; Muhoberac and Vidal., 2013; Levi and Finazzi, 2014), a rare, adult-onset disorder in which patients present late in adulthood with a variety of extrapyramidal movement disorders. The disease was initially described in members of a large family from Cumbria in northwest England, resulting from the insertion of an adenine at position 460–461 in the ferritin light chain (*FTL1*) gene, which was predicted to alter the C terminus of the protein (Curtis *et al.*, 2001). Seven pathogenic mutations have been reported in exon 4 of the *FTL1* gene, six of which are frameshifts (Keogh *et al.*, 2012). They are all predicted to result in alterations of helix E, extending the ferritin light chain at the site of the fourfold channel (Figure 15.4). In addition, a missense mutation causing an A96T substitution on helix C may also be a causative agent of the disease (Maciel *et al.*, 2005).

These mutant FTL subunits can readily undergo assembly with wild-type FTH or FTL chains, forming dysfunctional ferritin shells (Vidal *et al.*, 2004) which exhibit iron loading-induced ferritin aggregation and decreased iron incorporation. The structural evaluation of one of these mutant proteins (p.Phe167SerfsX26) has shown that mutated L-chain overlap exactly with wild-type up to

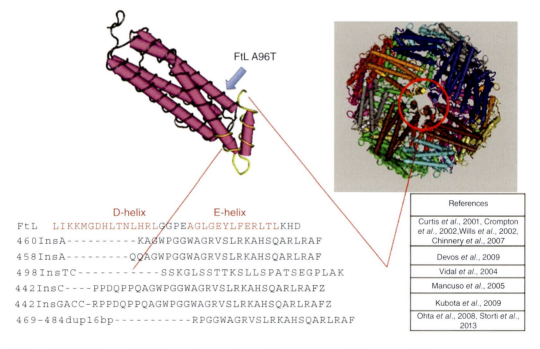

Figure 15.4 *Pile-up of the C terminus amino acid sequences of L-ferritin and the mutants causing neuroferritinopathy. All mutations, localised in exon 4 of FTL, are nucleotide insertions that cause large alterations of the C-terminal region of the subunit. This peptide portion forms the E-helix region, which is involved in the formation of the hydrophobic channel of the ferritin shell. The position of the A96T mutation is indicated by a blue arrow along the C-helix. Reprinted from Levi, S. and Finazzi, D. (2014). Neurodegeneration with brain iron accumulation: update on pathological mechanisms. Front. Pharmacol., **5**, 99. This is an open-access article distributed under the terms of the Creative Commons Attribution License (CC BY)*

Gly157, whereas the downstream portion of the amino acid sequence was not resolved, indicating that the final C-terminal extension is disordered/unstructured (Baraibar *et al.*, 2008, 2010; Luscieti *et al.*, 2010). Whereas the structure of the spherical shell is maintained in mutant ferritin homopolymers (Figure 15.5), close-up views of the fourfold pore from the interior of the wild-type and mutant FTL structures show a remarkable disruption in the mutant FTL, making the pores unstable and leaky. The disorganisation of the channel causes reduced physical stability of the protein due to the loss of stabilising interactions along the axis of symmetry and the formation of a wider and permeable quaternary channel. These alterations in the heteropolymer occur also when only one of four subunits making up the channel is changed (Luscieti *et al.*, 2010). Muhoberac *et al.* (2011) confirmed a greater propensity of ferritin to precipitation induced by iron and a lower functionality

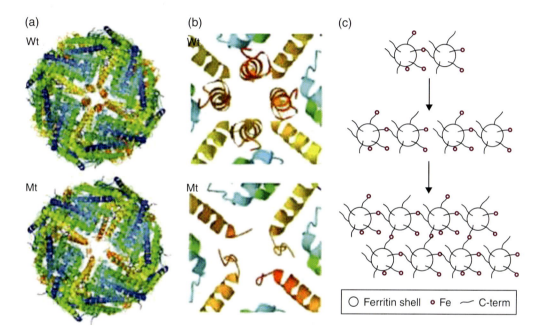

Figure 15.5 *Ferritin structural disruption and aggregation caused by Mt-FTL subunits. (a) The structure of the spherical shell is maintained in mutant ferritin as seen in the crystallographic structures of Wt- and Mt-FTL homopolymers viewed down one of their fourfold axes. (b) Close-up views of the fourfold pore from the interior of the Wt- and Mt-FTL structures, showing remarkable disruption in Mt-FTL, making the pores unstable and leaky. Note that since the last 26 amino acids of Mt-FTL remained unaccounted for crystallographically, mutant C termini are substantially longer than represented in (b), and if extended could reach as far as the diameter of the ferritin shell. (c) Iron loading-induced aggregation of Mt-FTL homopolymers is consistent with a model in which iron binds to the unravelled and extended portion of the mutant C termini on two different ferritin shells, bridging them and initiating a gradual accumulation of ferritin and iron into a precipitate. Bridging is not necessarily restricted to C termini, and may become more general, for example between a C-terminal group and a surface amino acid which both have affinity for iron. Structures were taken from RCSB (code 2FG8 for Wt-FTL and 3HX2 for Mt-FTL), and the precipitation model was modified from Baraibar et al. (2008). Reprinted with permission from Elsevier from Muhoberac, B.B., Baraibar, M.A. and Vidal, R. (2011) Iron loading-induced aggregation and reduction of iron incorporation in heteropolymeric ferritin containing a mutant light chain that causes neurodegeneration. Biochim. Biophys. Acta,* **1812**, *544–548*

of the heteropolymer containing variant chains. The mutated chains also have a greater propensity to oxidation, stressing that oxidative stress is a key component of the pathogenesis (Baraibar *et al.*, 2012).

It has been proposed that the disordered C-terminal extension can link up with other shells to form the ferritin aggregates (Muhoberac *et al.*, 2011), which explains the major neuropathological findings. Intracytoplasmic and intranuclear aggregates of ferritin are found in the glial cells and in some neuronal subtypes, together with deposits of iron, gliosis and neuronal death. Glial cells containing aggregates were mainly found in the caudate, putamen and globus pallidus, and these areas also showed the death of nerve cells and extracellular deposits of ferritin. In the cerebral cortex, aggregates were found in cells of the perineural and perivascular glia. The presence of aggregates in neurons was clearly visible in the putamen, the globus pallidus, thalamus, in cerebellar granules and in Purkinje cells (Curtis *et al.*, 2001; Vidal *et al.*, 2004; Mancuso *et al.*, 2005).

15.4.3 Other NBIAs

Mutations in genes such as *Pank2, Pla2G6, COASY, FA2H C19orf12, ATP13A2* and *WDR45* induce iron loading in the brain, although their protein functions are not related to iron metabolism (Levi and Finazzi, 2014). Of these genes the first four encode for proteins localised in mitochondria, which are directly or indirectly implicated in lipid metabolism and mitochondrial membrane remodelling (Figure 15.6).

Pantothenate kinase-associated neurodegeneration (PKAN or NBIA type I) is the most frequent syndrome among NBIA disorders, and was the first shown to be associated with mutations in a specific gene, namely pantothenate kinase 2 (*PanK2*; Zhou *et al.*, 2001). Under normal circumstances PANK2 generates phosphopantothenate, which then condenses with cysteine in the coenzyme A synthesis pathway (Figure 15.6). PKAN disease occurs in childhood or in atypical cases during adolescence. Iron overload in PKAN is thought to be secondary to cysteine accumulation, with cysteine binding iron to form a complex as a result of the underlying genetic enzymatic defect in the PKAN isoform, which is particularly present within the basal ganglia (PKAN2). MRI analysis of the brains of such patients shows a specific pattern 'the eye of the tiger' at $T2^*$-weighted MR images, which corresponds to bilateral areas of hypointensity in the medial globus pallidus with central spots of hyperintensity (Hayflick *et al.*, 2003) (Figure 15.7). The 'eye of the tiger' is characterised by a T_2 hyperintense core surrounded by T_2 hypointensity indicating pallidal iron deposition. A marked astrogliosis, microglial activation and overall parenchymal rarefaction was observed within the medial globus pallidus. The specific mechanism(s) by which defective Pank2 leads to neuronal degeneration, with the formation of neuroaxonal spheroids and iron deposition, are still unclear. Under normal circumstances, Pank2 localises to the mitochondria and catalyses a crucial step in the conversion of dietary pantothenate (vitamin B_5) into the cellular cofactor coenzyme A. The activity of Pank2 is negatively regulated by palmitoyl-CoA and acetyl-CoA, and stimulated by palmitoylcarnitine, which suggests a role in β-oxidation. Despite the degree of neurodegeneration that is present, little inflammatory response is evident apart from infiltrates of iron-containing macrophages and limited astrogliosis and microglial activation. A positive staining for ubiquitin was evident in degenerating neurons, and also in residual intact neurons in the globus pallidus, which could indicate that the accumulation of ubiquinated protein was an early event in the degenerative process.

A reduced level of Pank2 was associated with an increase in ferroportin expression. Increased levels of ROS have also been reported in the brains of patients with a Pank2 defect which could

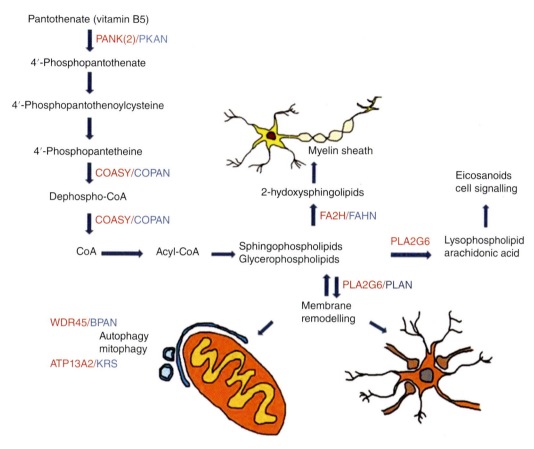

Figure 15.6 *Schematic description of genes and biochemical pathways involved in different types of neurodegeneration with brain iron accumulation (NBIA) disorder. The biochemical pathways of lipid metabolism and membrane/organelles (mitochondria) remodelling seem to play an important mechanistic role in many of the genetic NBIA disorders so far identified. Reprinted from Levi, S. and Finazzi, D. (2014) Neurodegeneration with brain iron accumulation: update on pathological mechanisms. Front Pharmacol., **5**, 99. This is an open-access article distributed under the terms of the Creative Commons Attribution License (CC BY)*

perturb IRP1 activity and the control of LIP, thereby inducing neuronal damage (reviewed in Levi and Finazzi, 2014).

COASY is a bifunctional enzyme with both 4′-PP adenyltransferase (PPAT) and dephospho-CoA kinase (DPCK) activities, which catalyses the last two steps in CoA biosynthesis. Mutations in COASY have recently been identified (Dusi *et al.*, 2014). However, the explanation for the accumulation of iron remains unknown. The PLAS2A protein is thought to be important in maintaining cell membrane homeostasis. Mutations in the *PLA2G6* gene, mostly missense mutations, induce cerebellar cortical atrophy that is often associated with gliosis. Iron accumulation is not a constant feature, but when it is detected it is present in the globus pallidus, SN and dentate nuclei, and increases with disease progression. In PLA2G6-associated degeneration, cerebral atrophy and sclerosis occurs with a loss of neurons and gliosis, an accumulation of lipids and degeneration of the optic nerve (reviewed by Levi and Finazzi, 2014). Numerous axonal swellings and spheroid

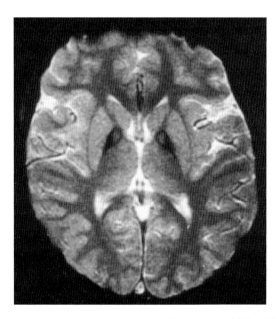

Figure 15.7 *Cranial magnetic resonance imaging using T*$_2$-weighted Echo-Planar sequences sensitive to ferric and ferrous deposits. This coronal section illustrates the typical 'eye of the tiger' sign in the globi pallidi of the Hallervorden–Spatz syndrome patient. Reprinted with permission from Elsevier from Castelnau, P., Zilbovicius, M., Ribeiro, M.J., et al. (2001) Striatal and pontocerebellar hypoperfusion in Hallervorden–Spatz syndrome.* Pediatr. Neurol., **25**, *170–174*

bodies containing a complex network of tubulovescicular membranes are detectable in the central nervous system. Diffuse synuclein-positive Lewy bodies were also identified possibly indicating a close relationship between PLAN and Parkinson's disease.

A distinct subgroup of childhood NBIA involves mutations in the gene encoding fatty acid hydroxylase, *FAH2* (Kruer *et al.*, 2010). FAH2 is involved in generating 2-hydroxylated fatty acids which are incorporated into ceramides, the essential lipid components of myelin. Kufor Rakeb disease (KRD, PARK9) is an autosomal recessive extrapyramidal–pyramidal syndrome with generalised brain atrophy due to ATP13A2 gene mutations, and bilateral putaminal and caudate iron accumulation (Schneider *et al.*, 2010). The absence of the orphan mitochondrial protein, c19orf12, has been implicated in a distinct clinical subtype of neurodegeneration with brain iron accumulation (Hartig *et al.*, 2011).

15.5 Other Monogenic Neurodegenerative Diseases

15.5.1 Huntington's Disease

An important class of genetic variation involves so-called 'tandem repeats' (TRs) (Gemayel *et al.*, 2010), and many eukaryotic genes and their promoters contain such an unstable repeat tract. A number of neurological diseases are caused by the expansion of unstable trinucleotide repeats within a single gene (Orr and Zoghbi, 2007), of which Huntington's disease (HD) and Friedreich's ataxia (FRDA) are perhaps the best known. HD is a genetic disorder caused by a defect on chromosome 4 in which the expansion of a CAG repeat in exon 1 of the gene for Huntingtin (Htt), coding for a poly-glutamine (polyQ) tract, is present many more times than in unaffected individuals (36–120 repeats versus 10–28 repeats, respectively).

Mutant Htt induces a selective loss of neurons in the basal ganglia, and the pathogenesis of HD is often associated with mitochondrial dysfunction (Figure 15.8; reviewed in Mena *et al.*, 2015), characterised by impaired mitochondrial ATP synthesis and deficits in the activity of complexes I, II and III, particularly in advanced stages of the disease. The exact nature and causes of mitochondrial dysfunction in HD remain unknown, although several studies have demonstrated that mutant Htt physically associates with mitochondria. Mutant Htt is found in the mitochondrial outer membrane in striatal cells obtained from patients with HD and from HD model transgenic mice. Postmortem brain tissue from HD patients shows an increase in the expression of mitochondrial

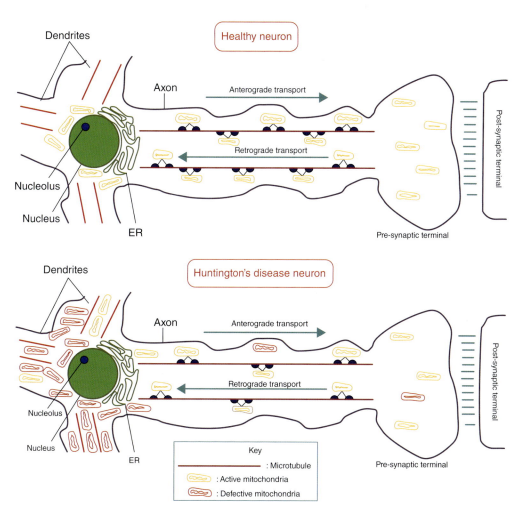

Figure 15.8 *Huntington's disease neuron showing excessive fragmentation of mitochondria, iron accumulation in cell soma, and abnormal distribution of mitochondria in neuronal processes and synapses. Reprinted with permission from Elsevier from Reddy, P.H. and Shirendeb, U.P. (2013). Mutant huntingtin, abnormal mitochondrial dynamics, defective axonal transport of mitochondria, and selective synaptic degeneration in Huntington's disease.* Biochim. Biophys. Acta, *1822, 101–110*

fission proteins Drp1 and Fis1 and a decreased expression of the fusion proteins mitofusin and OPA1. In addition, wild-type Htt interacts with Drp1, increasing its enzymatic activity. Mutant Htt can impair mitochondrial function via several mechanisms. First, by binding more tightly to Drp1 than wild-type Htt, it will disrupt the balance of mitochondrial fission–fusion dynamics in favour of fission. Second, it can act by decreasing anterograde and retrograde axonal transport of mitochondria. Finally, by binding to peroxisome proliferator-activated receptor coactivator-1α (PGC-1α) protein, its transcription factor activity is reduced. This will result in the reduced expression of PGC-1α target genes which are involved in mitochondrial biogenesis and antioxidant defences (Shirendeb et al., 2012; reviewed in Johri et al., 2013). The net result of these mitochondrial impairments is reduced ATP production, which may initially result in neuronal dysfunction followed by neuron death.

Iron accumulation does not seem to be a initial event in HD, but may be an early indicator of a pathological cascade. Iron accumulates in the basal ganglia of both HD patients and murine models of HD, particularly in myelinating oligodendrocytes and in microglia. The release of inflammatory cytokines by activated microglia will result in premature myelin breakdown and subsequent remyelination, as well as increasing iron levels which may contribute to HD pathogenesis. Htt appears to be required for transferrin receptor 1 (TfR1)-mediated iron uptake (Lumsden *et al.*, 2007). Because erythroid cells acquire iron via transferrin endocytosis, this might indicate a role for Htt in supporting iron uptake by transferrin-mediated endocytosis. Htt was upregulated by desferrioxamine treatment of embryonic stem cells, suggesting that Htt is involved in normal iron homeostasis (Hilditch-Maguire *et al.*, 2000). Thus, perturbation of the normal role of Htt in iron uptake by the polyQ tract expansion may contribute to the iron accumulation that is observed in HD pathology (reviewed by Mena *et al.*, 2015).

15.5.2 Friedreich's Ataxia

Friedreich's ataxia (FRDA) is also caused by anomalous expansion of unstable nucleotide repeats, but, unlike Huntington's disease, FRDA is unique among trinucleotide repeat neurological disorders because it is autosomal recessive, the repeat is intronic, and it is the only one known with a GAA expansion (Orr and Zoghbi, 2007). FRDA is the most common hereditary ataxia and is the most prevalent cerebellar ataxia among children and adults in Europe. FRDA is an exclusively mitochondrial disorder which is characterised by progressive cardiologic and neurological degeneration. The brain regions affected include the dorsal root ganglia, the spinal cord, and the cerebellum. The homozygous GAA repeat expansion mutation is in intron 1 of *FXN* gene, and its effect is to reduce the expression of frataxin, which, as we saw in Chapter 8, is a mitochondrial protein that acts as an iron chaperone in mitochondrial iron sulphur cluster, ISC, synthesis In normal circumstances frataxin delivers iron to the iron sulphur cluster assembly machinery. In addition to decreased ISC synthesis, frataxin insufficiency results in mitochondrial iron accumulation, which will induce extensive oxidative damage, loss of myelinated fibres, and subsequent cell death. Huang and collaborators identified four mitochondrial iron utilisation pathways which were reduced in frataxin knockout mice: ISC synthesis, mitochondrial iron storage, haem synthesis, and increased expression of the mitochondrial iron importer mitoferrin-2 (Huang *et al.*, 2009). Frataxin deficiency induces increased level of TfR1, ferritin, and haem oxygenase 1 and a decreased level of FPN1 (Huang et al., 2009), indicating increased iron uptake by the cell. Although the cause of these changes in protein levels is unknown, they may be mediated by a low cytosolic iron signal resulting from increased mitochondrial uptake (mitoferrin-2) and/or by increased IRP1 activity as the result of decreased ISC synthesis (reviewed by Mena et al., 2011). It was shown that frataxin mRNA expression is dependent on cytoplasmic iron levels, decreasing with iron depletion, and increasing with metal accumulation. Thus, the combination of mitochondrial iron overload and presumed cytosolic iron depletion potentially further compromise function in frataxin-deficient cells by decreasing frataxin expression (Li *et al.*, 2008).

15.6 Neurodegeneration Involving Multiple Genes

15.6.1 Parkinson's Disease (PD)

Early studies of postmortem material from PD patients showed an increase of total iron in the SN with moderate to advanced disease progression which was associated with disease severity (Dexter *et al.*, 1987, 1989). This was confirmed in other studies where MRI and transcranial ultrasound were utilised (Götz *et al.*, 2004; Jellinger, 1991). An increase of iron is observed also in the lateral globus pallidus which may be due to the retrograde degeneration of dopaminergic neurons in PD (Dexter *et al.*, 1987). The retrograde degenerative process is supported by the finding of an inverse relationship between dopamine concentration and iron concentrations in the putamen (Dexter *et al.*, 1991; Griffiths *et al.*, 1999). In PD patients, iron deposits are present in neurons and glia of the SN, putamen and globus pallidus, with an increase of Ft-loaded microglia cells in the SN (Figure 15.9) (Jellinger *et al.*, 1999). *In vitro*, such iron can catalyse the conversion of α-synuclein from α-helical to the β-sheet form present in Lewy bodies. Iron accumulates in Lewy bodies in the brains of PD subjects (Castellani *et al.*, 2000; El-Agnaf and Irvine, 2002).

Electron probe analysis confirmed that individual dopaminergic neurons in the SN of PD patients have raised iron levels (Oakley *et al.*, 2007), although no mention was made as to whether excessive amounts of iron were also present in glial cells. In the SN, iron is found in ferrritin, with increased levels of H-chain, and in NM, which also contains some iron and is present in dopaminergic neurons. Iron is also found within activated microglia in the SN, and may represent the main pool of iron present in the SN.

In addition to the iron contained within NM, iron deposits have also been found in microglia, oligodendrocytes and astrocytes, as well as on the rim of Lewy bodies and in pigmented neurons.

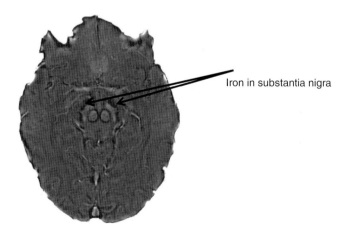

Iron in substantia nigra

Figure 15.9 *MRI scan of brain from Parkinson's disease patient. Image kindly supplied by Antonio Martin Bastida*

Both, L- and H-ferritin are present in the SN, with H-chain ferritin the predominant form present. The explanation for this remains unclear but may reflect the inflammatory milieu that exists within the PD brain. The presence of both NM and ferritins in the same organelle may provide a synergistic regulation of iron homeostasis, which guarantees effective neuroprotection from detrimental actions of iron via oxidative stress.

NM is of special interest because in PD, pallor of the SN pars compacta can be seen due to the depletion of dopaminergic neurons containing NM. The high concentration of NM in SN neurons seems to be linked to the presence of considerable amounts of cytosolic dopamine that has not been sequestered in synaptic vesicles. Intraneuronal NM can be a protective factor, shielding the cells from the toxic effects of redox-active metals, toxins and excesses of cytosolic catecholamines. In contrast, NM released by dying neurons may contribute to the activation of microglia, triggering the neuroinflammation that characterises PD. Furthermore, NM has been identified surrounding or contained within the activated microglia in the Parkinsonian brain postmortem, while the number of activated microglia in the aging SN is significantly and positively correlated with the amount of extracellular NM.

Immunohistochemistry studies identified a 60% decrease in iron-transferrin binding sites in the SN, the red nucleus and the oculomotor nucleus as well as a decrease in transferrin binding sites (Morris *et al.*, 1994), which could be due to cell loss. Several studies have investigated whether there are significant changes in the expression of various genes known to be involved in iron homeostasis. The elevated levels of iron in the SN may result from either an increased import or a decreased export (Qian and Shen, 2001). An elevated expression of DMT1 is found in the SN of animal models of PD (Jiang *et al.*, 2003), indicating that a disrupted expression of DMT1 might be involved in the nigral iron accumulation. Ferroportin1 (FP1) expression has been reported to be decreased in the SN (Wang *et al.*, 2007; Zhang *et al.*, 2014).

The source of the increased amount of iron in certain brain regions remains unknown, but could be caused by dysregulation of iron flux into the brain across the BBB, an overload in iron sequestration capacity due to malfunction of homeostatic control within the SN, or microglia activation with iron accumulation.

The BBB has been shown to be impaired in PD, particularly at late stages of the disease (Götz *et al.*, 2004). However, this does not account for the selectivity of iron accumulation in the SN region (Sian-Hülsmann *et al.*, 2011; Zecca *et al.*, 2004). The injection of iron directly into the SN of rats causes selective neuronal cell death of dopaminergic neurons and Parkinsonian behaviour (Sengstock *et al.*, 1997; Ben-Shachar and Youdim, 1991). Also, the amount of iron involved in this process exceeds the amount taken up into the brain, implying that the iron accumulated may be recycled from other parts of the brain rather than from the periphery (Crichton *et al.*, 2011). Therefore, changes in the BBB cannot be the sole cause of iron accumulation in PD.

Dysfunction of iron regulation within the SN may be another cause of iron accumulation. Cellular iron levels are controlled in three ways: iron uptake by the cell; iron storage within the cell; and iron export from the cell. Levels of TfR and DMT1 dictate iron import; the Tf/TfR system does not seem to be augmented in PD (Faucheux *et al.*, 1997), though this may be a compensatory mechanism (Sian-Hülsmann *et al.*, 2011). However, increased levels of DMT1 in the dopaminergic neurons of the SN have been observed (Hirsch, 2009), as well as a similar elevation in lactoferrin receptors (Sian-Hülsmann *et al.*, 2011), suggesting that iron uptake is increased. Mutations in the *HFE* gene are not a common cause for PD; in fact, there was a protective effect of C282Y heterozygosity, and no effect on the C282Y or H63D mutations or to a increased risk for PD in C282Y mutation carriers (Akbas *et al.*, 2006).

Though total iron levels are higher in PD, some findings show levels of ferritin do not increase correspondingly, suggesting that the iron storage capacity within SN neurons has been exceeded (Crichton *et al.*, 2011; Zecca *et al.*, 2004; Faucheux *et al.*, 2002). Phenotypically, the SN reacts as if it was iron-deficient. The downregulation of FPN results in cellular iron sequestration, similar to that seen following inflammation in the periphery with the mononuclear phagocyte system (Liu *et al.*, 2002). With blocked iron export, enhanced uptake and no corresponding increase in iron storage, oxidative stress by labile iron – and thus neuronal damage – will naturally ensue. Interestingly, certain Cp mutations have been identified in PD patients, which could alter Cp activity and increase iron deposition in the brain. In one study, the levels of Cp, iron transferrin and transferrin were analysed together with the ferroxidase activity in serum of patients with a diagnosis of PD who were carriers for Cp mutations I63T, D544E and R793H. *In vivo*, the I63T mutation resulted in half the normal Cp concentration and markedly reduced ferroxidase activity in serum from a heteroallelic PD patient. In cell culture, the I63T glycosylphosphatidylinositol (GPI)-linked Cp isoform was retained in the endoplasmic reticulum of human embryonic kidney cells. Furthermore, the D544E polymorphism resulted in significantly reduced serum Cp levels and ferroxidase activity in heteroallelic patients, and in the expression of mainly apo-Cp in cell culture. Such studies indicate that an altered activity of Cp may present a vulnerability factor for iron-induced oxidative stress in PD (Hochstrasser *et al.*, 2005).

Lastly, the influence of activated microglia on iron homeostasis could be a major factor in iron accumulation. *In-vitro* studies of primary cell cultures showed that inflammatory signals increase the expression of DMT1 and hepcidin in neurons and microglia, but only of DMT1 in astrocytes (Urrutia *et al.*, 2013). The release of hepcidin will decrease the expression of ferroportin in each if these cell types, which results in increases of iron in the neurons and microglia, but not in the astrocytes.

Recent studies have suggested that a deficiency of the microtubule-associated protein tau induces intracellular iron accumulation which results in the degeneration of dopaminergic neurons and parkinsonism with dementia (Lei *et al.*, 2012). This occurred as a result of the levels of soluble tau being reduced in the SN of PD patients, such that the ability of the amyloid precursor protein (AβPP) to combine with ferroportin was inhibited as a consequence of retention of AβPP within the endoplasmic reticulum. However, such findings have been challenged by other studies where tau-knockout mice had a normal life span and showed no neurological or behavioural effects (Morris *et al.*, 2011).

15.6.2 Alzheimer's Disease (AD)

Defective homeostasis of the redox-active metal iron is likely to contribute to the neuropathology of AD. High levels of iron are present in the amyloid plaques and neurofibrillary tangles that are characteristic of AD brains, and this focal accumulation may deprive other brain tissue of iron, leading to aberrant neuronal function (Roberts *et al.*, 2012). AD begins deep in the brain, in the entorhinal cortex, and slowly spreads over the course of about 20 years to other brain regions such as the hippocampus and cerebral cortex. An abnormal homeostasis of iron has also been implicated in the misfolding process associated with the amyloid-β (Aβ) peptide and the hyperphosphorylated tau found in the plaques and tangles, as well as contributing to neuronal oxidative stress (Sayre *et al.*, 2000). The accumulation of tau in neurofibrillary tangles is associated with the induction of haem oxygenase 1 (HO-1), a potent antioxidant which plays an important role in metabolising haem released from damaged mitochondria. Although the bilirubin that is generated in this process is an antioxidant (Perry *et al.*, 2002), ferrous iron is also released, which may participate in Fenton chemistry to produce hydroxyl radicals.

Iron may play an important role in the cleavage of the amyloid precursor protein, APP. The majority of the Aβ precursor protein (AβPP), is cleaved by the non-amyloidogenic pathway, involving first α-secretase followed by γ-secretase, to release p3 and leave the AβPP intracellular domain in the membrane. Alternatively, AβPP can first be cleaved by β-secretase and then γ-secretase to produce Aβ. This latter pathway is the neurodegenerative, amyloidogenic pathway (Altamura and Mückenthaler, 2009). Whether changes in iron homeostasis occur during this process remains unknown. Processing of the inactive pro-protein forms of both α- and β-secretases is modulated by furin, the proconvertase which activates hepcidin (Guillemot *et al.*, 2013). The transcription of furin is modulated by cellular levels of iron, and iron excess will decrease furin protein levels so as to favour π-secretase activity. In contrast, iron deficiency will have the opposite effect, altering both α-secretase and furin activities (Altamura and Mückenthaler, 2009; Silvestri and Camaschella, 2008). In addition, iron may modulate AβPP processing, by virtue of the presence of a putative IRE in the 5′-UTR of AβPP mRNA, located immediately upstream of an IL-1-responsive acute box domain (Rogers *et al.*, 2002). AβPP translation is thus responsive to cytoplasmic free iron levels, such that under conditions of iron excess the translation of AβPP is upregulated, increasing the amount of AβPP available to enter the amyloidogenic pathway that is already favoured by a decreased furin activity (Altamura and Mückenthaler, 2009). Increases in production of the cytokine IL-1 increases IRP binding to the AβPP 5′-UTR, thereby decreasing AβPP production (Rogers *et al.*, 2002). In addition, binding of the IRP to the IRE might interfere with AβPP translation and translocation across the endoplasmic reticulum membrane. This interference could be significant since α-secretase activity has been shown to require membrane-bound AβPP.

The AβPP molecule was recently reported to have ferroxidase activity (Duce *et al.*, 2010), although this observation has now been refuted in other studies with a peptide containing the REXXE motif and with the full-length protein (Ebrahimi *et al.*, 2012; Honarmand Ebrahimi *et al.*, 2013), and also by further biochemical evaluations of the results (Wong *et al.*, 2014). Subsequent investigations have suggested that APP modulates iron efflux from cells by stabilising the ferrous iron exporter ferroportin (McCarthy *et al.*, 2014; Wong *et al.*, 2014). However, if such results are correct, this would suggest that there should be a decrease of iron intracellularly, such that both ferritin and APP will be downregulated because of the IRP binding to the 5′ IRE. Clearly, further studies are needed of the role played by these various proteins in influencing iron homeostasis.

The increased iron levels that have been found to accompany Aβ aggregation in areas affected early on in the disease offer a potential opportunity for MRI-based diagnosis. Indeed, MRI studies of postmortem human brain tissue and a mouse model of the disease have demonstrated decreases in hippocampal T_2*, an MRI parameter sensitive to the magnetic properties of iron (Schenck, 2003; Haacke *et al.*, 2005) or its spatial variance, attributed in part to iron in Aβ plaques (Jack *et al.*, 2005; Nabuurs *et al.*, 2011; Antharam *et al.*, 2012). Although resolution constraints preclude the ability to detect individual plaques in patients, it may be possible to detect T_2* abnormalities resulting from plaque aggregates. When properly distinguished from potential confounds originating from haem iron, hippocampal T_2* changes may be a valuable complement to morphological measures in the development of a biomarker for early stages of the disease (Holland *et al.*, 2009).

Iron accumulation in the brains of animal models produces significant cognitive defects (Schroder *et al.*, 2013). In the presenilin/AβPP transgenic mice model of AD (Holcomb *et al.*, 1998), iron has been shown to colocalise with Aβ plaques (Falangola *et al.*, 2005), and increased brain iron was found to coincide with early plaque formation (Leskovjan *et al.*,

2011). The overexpression of HO-1 in mice leads to iron loading, and tau aggregation in brain, another characteristic of AD (Hui *et al.*, 2011).

15.6.3　Multiple Sclerosis (MS)

The origins of iron excess in MS remain unexplained, but may reflect inflammatory processes, disturbed axonal ion homeostasis combined with the aberrant expression of glutamate receptors and a number of ion channels, such as Na^+ channels and voltage-gated Ca^{2+} channels. MS is characterised by the infiltration of immune cells and subsequent loss of myelin, oligodendrocytes and axons. Abnormal iron deposits occur in both grey and white matter structures. The accumulation of iron begins early during the disease course in the grey matter, such as the caudate, globus pallidus, pulvinar, Rolandic cortex and putamen (reviewed by Weigel *et al.*, 2014). Since the caudate, globus pallidus thalamus and putamen are all interconnected, this might indicate that the disruption of one pathway or structure may result in neuronal degeneration and/or iron homeostasis. Typically, such increased iron deposition is bilaterally represented in matching grey matter structures across the hemispheres. The duration of the disease rather than its severity is a major contributing factor to iron accumulation. The pathological iron deposits in white matter are associated with cortical lesions at the sites of inflammation (Haacke *et al.*, 2009). Iron is present predominantly in non-phagocytosing macrophages/microglia at the edge of established demyelinated lesions. Iron precipitates are also present within and outside the white matter MS lesion, which could indicate microhaemorrhages. The varying distribution patterns of abnormal iron deposits between white matter and deep grey matter structures is suggestive of different mechanisms of iron accumulation.

Microglia express markers indicative of the proinflammatory M1 phenotype (e.g. iNOS), whereas myelin-loaded cells are typically strongly immunoreactive for CD206 and arginase, indicative of an anti-inflammatory M2 phenotype (Mehta *et al.*, 2013). Therefore, two macrophage/microglia populations are present: (i) iron-positive, myelin-negative non-phagocytosing proinflammatory microglia/macrophages at the edge of chronic active lesions; and (ii) iron-negative, myelin-loaded macrophages with an anti-inflammatory M2 phenotype, present in actively demyelinating lesions and at the lesion centre of the demyelinated lesions. Iron abnormally accumulates in mitochondria, microglia macrophages, neutrophils and, to a lesser extent, in neurons. Iron may promote disease activity in MS by amplifying the activated state of microglia (with increased production of proinflammatory mediators), inducing mitochondrial dysfunction and enhancing the production of ROS. Extensive lymphocyte cuffing, macrophage infiltration and fibrin deposits are localised around veins in active MS lesions. Abnormal iron deposits are present in perivenular locations in white matter (reviewed in Williams *et al.*, 2012). However, in the animal model of MS (experimental autoimmune encephalomyelitis; EAE), iron deposition around vessels occurred independently of inflammation, providing evidence against the hypothesis that iron deposits account for inflammatory cell infiltrates observed in MS (Williams *et al.*, 2012). Iron accumulation in MS may be related to active inflammation. The normal appearance of the white matter of the MS brain showed a low degree of inflammation, with microglia activation and acute axonal injury which decreased towards the edge of the lesion. A chronic inflammatory process with the release of proinflammatory cytokines (TNFα) and anti-inflammatory cytokines (TGFβ1) suggested that both cytokines induce iron uptake and retention in microglia (Hametner *et al.*, 2013). However, TNFα induced iron retention in astrocytes while TGFβ1 induced its release. It is suggested that iron-loaded oligodendrocytes are more vulnerable to TNFα and interferon gamma (IF-γ) *in vitro*, and that inflammatory cytokines could trigger iron release from these cells, comparable to the effect of TGFβ1 on astrocytes. The ferroxidase activity of both hephaestin and Cp was upregulated in oligodendrocytes and astrocytes particularly close to inflamed lesions, although no discernible changes in ferroportin were identified.

Recently, several studies have investigated whether genes involved in the import/export of iron are altered in the postmortem tissues of MS patients. Compared with age-matched control post-mortem tissue there was an upregulation of mRNA for mitochondrial ferritin and H- and L-ferritin, while the frataxin gene was downregulated in the initial lesion in white matter lesions (initial and active lesions) as well as periplaque white matter. Immunohistochemical studies identified a decrease in oligodendrocyte iron, with a corresponding increase in ferritin-positive microglia in the periplaque region of patients with active MS. Expression of the mRNA transferrin receptor is upregulated in normal-appearing white matter in MS patients in periplaque white matter and active lesions, which is somewhat surprising as inflammation would decrease its expression (reviewed by Williams *et al.*, 2012). However, MS lesions display hypoxia-like tissue injury, such that IRP1 and 2 would be upregulated with a subsequent upregulation of transferrin receptors and increased cellular iron storage.

In a further study of four MS patients, the expression of iron-related genes was investigated in white matter. There was upregulation of ferritin genes, H- and L-ferritin, as well as mitochondrial ferritin, but the latter only to a lesser extent. Frataxin was downregulated. Genes involved in iron import, *TfR*, *DMT1* and *ZIP14*, as well as hephaestin and amyloid-β precursor protein (APP) showed elevated transcription levels, particularly in the periplaque white matter. The authors (Hametner *et al.*, 2013) suggested that such data indicated an upregulation of cellular defence against iron toxicity and an upregulation of glial iron shuttling in the periplaque white matter around active lesions.

Lastly, there has been some debate as to the sources of iron in MS. It could be derived from damaged oligodendrocytes and myelin, perivascular inflammation, a breakdown of haem within the oligodendrocytes, a proinflammatory environment, or excitotoxic damage.

15.7 Intracerebral Haemorrhage

Intracerebral haemorrhage (ICH) is the primary event in approximately 10% of strokes, and has a higher rate of morbidity and mortality than ischaemic strokes. It is thought that the toxicity of haemoglobin and its degradation products contribute to the secondary injury. Extracellular haemoglobin is unstable at physiological conditions and spontaneously oxidises at its haem groups to ferric methaemoglobin, releasing superoxide. Haemin, the oxidised form of haem, accumulates on the intracranial hepatomas. Its breakdown is catalysed by haem oxygenases (i.e. inducible HO-1 and constitutively expressed HO-2) as well as haemopexin. However, the low concentration of haem/haemin-binding protein haemopexin in the brain will increase the possibility that haemin may be taken up by neurons and astrocytes. In addition, microglia will scavenge the haematoma in addition to intact erythrocytes, haemoglobin and haemoglobin–haptoglobin via the CD163 receptor, thereby possibly activating the microglia. Iron has been shown to play an important role in ICH-induced brain injury in experimental animals and patients (Xiong *et al.*, 2014). Brain injury after ICH shows several phases including: (i) an early phase involving the clotting cascade activations and thrombin production; and (ii) a phase involving erythrocyte lysis and iron toxicity, after which the iron content in the surrounding area is increased dramatically. High serum ferritin levels are associated with severe brain oedema and a poor outcome in ICH patients.

References

Abbott, N.J., Rönnbäck, L. and Hansson, E. (2006) Astrocyte-endothelial interactions at the blood-brain barrier. *Nat. Rev. Neurosci.*, **7**, 41–53.

Akbas, N., Hochstrasser, H., Deplazes, J., *et al.* (2006) Screening for mutations of the HFE gene in Parkinson's disease patients with hyperechogenicity of the substantia nigra. *Neurosci. Lett.*, **407**, 16–19.

Altamura, S. and Mückenthaler, M.U. (2009) Iron toxicity in diseases of aging: Alzheimer's disease, *Parkinson's disease and atherosclerosis. J. Alzheimer's Dis.*, **16**, 879–895.

Antharam, V., Collingwood, J.F., Bullivant, J.P., *et al.* (2012) High field magnetic resonance microscopy of the human hippocampus in Alzheimer's disease: quantitative imaging and correlation with iron. *Neuroimage*, **59**, 1249–1260.

Badaracco, M.E., Siri, M.V. and Pasquini, J.M. (2010) Oligodendrogenesis: the role of iron. *Biofactors*, **36**, 98–102.

Baraibar, M.A., Barbeito, A.G., Muhoberac, B.B. and Vidal R. (2008) Iron-mediated aggregation and a localized structural change characterize ferritin from a mutant light chain polypeptide that causes neurodegeneration. *J. Biol. Chem.*, **283**, 31679–31689.

Baraibar, M.A., Muhoberac, B.B., Garringer, H.J., Hurley, T.D. and Vidal R. (2010) Unraveling of the E-helices and disruption of 4-fold pores are associated with iron mishandling in a mutant ferritin causing neurodegeneration. *J. Biol. Chem.*, **285**, 1950–1956.

Baraibar, M.A., Barbeito, A.G., Muhoberac, B.B. and Vidal, R. (2012) A mutant light-chain ferritin that causes neurodegeneration has enhanced propensity toward oxidative damage. *Free Radic. Biol. Med.*, **52**, 1692–1697.

Bartzokis, G., Tishler, T.A.., Lu, P.H., *et al.* (2007) Brain ferritin iron may influence age- and gender-related risks of neurodegeneration. *Neurobiol. Aging*, **28**, 414–423.

Ben-Shachar, D. and Youdim, M.B. (1991) Intranigral iron injection induces behavioral and biochemical 'parkinsonism' in rats. *J. Neurochem.*, **57**, 2133–2135.

Boserup, M.W., Lichota, J., Haile, D. and Moos, T. (2011) Heterogenous distribution of ferroportin-containing neurons in mouse brain. *Biometals*, **24**, 357–375.

Castellani, R.J., Siedlak, S.L., Perry, G. and Smith, M.A. (2000) Sequestration of iron by Lewy bodies in Parkinson's disease. *Acta Neuropathol.*, **100**, 111–114.

Catalá, A. (2009) Lipid peroxidation of membrane phospholipids generates hydroxyl-alkenals and oxidized phospholipids active in physiological and/or pathological conditions. *Chem. Phys. Lipids*, **157**, 1–11.

Connor, J.R. and Menzies, S.L. (1996) Relationship of iron to oligodendrocytes and myelination. *Glia*, **17**, 83–93.

Connor, J.R., Menzies, S.L., St Martin, S.M. and Mufson, E.J. (1990) Cellular distribution of transferrin, ferritin and iron in normal and aged human brain. *J. Neurosci. Res.*, **27**, 595–611.

Crichton, R.R. and Ward, R.J. (2006) *Metal-based neurodegeneration. From Molecular Mechanisms to Therapeutic Strategies*. John Wiley & Sons, Chichester, UK, pp. 1–227.

Crichton, R.R. and Ward, R.J. (2014) *Metal-based neurodegeneration. From Molecular Mechanisms to Therapeutic Strategies*. John Wiley & Sons, Chichester, pp. 1–423.

Crichton, R.R., Dexter, D.T. and Ward, R.J. (2011) Brain iron metabolism and its perturbation in neurological diseases. *J. Neural. Transm.*, **118**, 301–314.

Curtis, A.R., Fey C., Morris C.M., *et al.* (2001). Mutation in the gene encoding ferritin light polypeptide causes dominant adult-onset basal ganglia disease. *Nat. Genet.*, **28**, 350–354.

Dexter, D.T., Wells, F.R., Agid, F., *et al.* (1987) Increased nigral iron content in postmortem parkinsonian brain *Lancet*, **2**, 1219–1220.

Dexter, D.T., Wells, F.R., Lees, A.J., *et al.* (1989) Increased nigral iron content and alterations in other metal ions occurring in brain in Parkinson's disease. *J. Neurochem.*, **52**, 1830–1836.

Dexter, D.T., Carayon, A., Javoy-Agid, F., *et al.* (1991) Alterations in the levels of iron, ferritin and other trace metals in Parkinson's disease and other neurodegenerative diseases affecting the basal ganglia. *Brain*, **114**, 1953–1975.

di Patti M.C., Maio, N., Rizzo, G., *et al.* (2009) Dominant mutants of ceruloplasmin impair the copper loading machinery in aceruloplasminemia. *J. Biol. Chem.*, **284**, 4545–4554.

Double, K.L., Gerlach, M., Schünemann, V., *et al.* (2003) Iron-binding characteristics of neuromelanin of the human substantia nigra. *Biochem. Pharmacol.*, **66**, 489–494.

Dringen, R., Bishop, G.M., Koeppe, M., Dang, T.N. and Robinson, S.R. (2007) The pivotal role of astrocytes in the metabolism of iron in the brain. *Neurochem. Res.*, **32**, 1884–1890.

Duce, J.A., Tsatsanis, A., Cater, M.A., *et al.* (2010) Iron-export ferroxidase activity of β-amyloid precursor protein is inhibited by zinc in Alzheimer's disease. *Cell*, **142**, 857–867.

Dusek, P. and Schneider, S.A. (2012) Neurodegeneration with brain iron accumulation. *Curr. Opin. Neurol.*, **25**, 499–506.

Dusek, P., Dezortova, M. and Wuerfel, J. (2013) Imaging of iron. *Int. Rev. Neurobiol.*, **110**, 195–239.

Dusi, S., Valletta, L., Haack, T.B., *et al.* (2014) Exome sequence reveals mutations in CoA synthase as a cause of neurodegeneration with brain iron accumulation. *Am. J. Hum. Genet.*, **94**, 11–22.

Ebrahimi, K.H., Hagedoorn, P.L. and Hagen, W.R. (2012) A synthetic peptide with the putative iron binding motif of amyloid precursor protein (APP) does not catalytically oxidize iron. *PLoS One*, **7**, e40287.

El-Agnaf, O.M. and Irvine, G.B. (2002) Aggregation and neurotoxicity of alpha-synuclein and related peptides. *Biochem Soc. Trans.*, **30**, 559–565.

Falangola, M.F., Lee, S.P., Nixon, R.A., Duff, K. and Helpern, J.A. (2005) Histological co-localization of iron in Abeta plaques of PS/APP transgenic mice. *Neurochem. Res.*, **30**, 201–205.

Faucheux, B.A, Hauw, J.J, Agid, Y. and Hirsch, E.C.(1997) The density of [125I]-transferrin binding sites on perikarya of melanized neurons of the substantia nigra is decreased in Parkinson's disease. *Brain Res.*, **749**, 170–174.

Faucheux, B.A., Martin, M.E., Beaumont, C., *et al.* (2002) Lack of up-regulation of ferritin is associated with sustained iron regulatory protein-1 binding activity in the substantia nigra of patients with Parkinson's disease. *J. Neurochem.*, **83**, 320–330.

Fasano, A., Colosimo, C., Miyajima, H., *et al.* (2008) Aceruloplasminemia: a novel mutation in a family with marked phenotypic variability. *Mov. Disord.*, **23**, 751–755.

Franceschi, C. and Campisi, J. (2014) Chronic inflammation (inflammaging) and its potential contribution to age-associated diseases. *J. Gerontol. A Biol. Sci. Med. Sci.*, **69** (Suppl. 1), S4–S9.

Gemayel, R., Vinces, M.D., Legendre, M. and Verstrepen, K.J. (2010) Variable tandem repeats accelerate evolution of coding and regulatory sequences. *Annu. Rev. Genet.*, **44**, 445–477.

Götz, M.E., Double, K., Gerlach, M., Youdim, M.B. and Riederer, P. (2004) The relevance of iron in the pathogenesis of Parkinson's disease. *Ann. N. Y. Acad. Sci.*, **1012**, 193–208.

Gregory, A. and Hayflick, S.J. (2011) Genetics of neurodegeneration with brain iron accumulation. *Curr. Neurol. Neurosci. Rep.*, **11**, 254–261.

Gregory, A., Polster, B.J. and Hayflick, S.J. (2009) Clinical and genetic delineation of neurodegeneration with brain iron accumulation. *J. Med. Genet.*, **46**, 73–80.

Griffiths, P.D., Dobson, B.R., Jones, G.R. and Clarke, D.T. (1999) Iron in the basal ganglia in Parkinson's disease. An in vitro study using extended X-ray absorption fine structure and cryo-electron microscopy. *Brain*, **122**, 667–673.

Guillemot, J., Canuel, M., Essalmani, R., Prat, A. and Seidah, N.G. (2013) Implication of the proprotein convertases in iron homeostasis: PC7 sheds human transferrin receptor 1 and furin activates hepcidin. *Hepatology*, **57**, 2514–2524.

Haacke, E.M., Cheng, N.Y., House, M.J., *et al.* (2005) Imaging iron stores in the brain using magnetic resonance imaging. *Magn. Reson. Imaging*, **23**, 1–25.

Haacke, E.M., Makki, M., Ge, Y., *et al.* (2009) Characterizing iron deposition in multiple sclerosis lesions using susceptibility weighted imaging. *J. Magn. Reson. Imaging*, **29**, 537–544.

Hametner, S., Wimmer, I., Haider, L., *et al.* (2013) Iron and neurodegeneration in the multiple sclerosis brain. *Ann. Neurol.*, **74**, 848–861.

Hartig, M.B., Iuso, A., Haack, T., *et al.* (2011) Absence of an orphan mitochondrial protein, c19orf12, causes a distinct clinical subtype of neurodegeneration with brain iron accumulation. *Am. J. Hum. Genet.*, **89**, 543–550.

Hayflick, S.J. (2003) Unraveling the Hallervorden–Spatz syndrome: pantothenate kinase-associated neurodegeneration is the name. *Curr. Opin. Pediatr.*, **15**, 572–577.

Hellman, N.E., Kono, S., Miyajima, H. and Gitlin, J.D. (2002) Biochemical analysis of a missense mutation in aceruloplasminemia. *J. Biol. Chem.*, **277**, 1375–1380.

Hilditch-Maguire, P., Trettel, F., Passani, L.A., *et al.* (2000) Huntingtin: an iron-regulated protein essential for normal nuclear and perinuclear organelles. *Hum. Mol. Genet.*, **9**, 2789–2797.

Hirsch, E.C. (2009) Iron transport in Parkinson's disease. *Parkinsonism Relat. Disord.*, **S3**, 209–211.

Hochstrasser, H., Tomiuk, J., Walter, U., *et al.* (2005) Functional relevance of ceruloplasmin mutations in Parkinson's disease. *FASEB J.*, **19**, 1851–1853.

Holcomb, L., Gordon, M.N., McGowan, E., *et al.* (1998) Accelerated Alzheimer-type phenotype in transgenic mice carrying both mutant amyloid precursor protein and presenilin 1 transgenes. *Nat. Med.*, **4**, 97–100.

Holland, D., Brewer, J.B., Hagler, D.J., Fennema-Notestine, C. and Dale, A.M. (2009) Subregional neuro-anatomical change as a biomarker for Alzheimer's disease. Alzheimer's Disease Neuroimaging Initiative. *Proc Natl Acad. Sci. USA*, **106**, 20954–20959.

Honarmand Ebrahimi, K., Dienemann, C., Hoefgen, S., *et al.* (2013) The amyloid precursor protein (APP) does not have a ferroxidase site in its E2 domain. *PLoS One*, **8**, e72177.

Horowitz, M.P. and Greenamyre, J.T. (2010) Mitochondrial iron metabolism and its role in neurodegeneration. *J. Alzheimer's Dis.*, **20**, S551–S568.

Huang, M.L., Becker, E.M., Whitnall, M., Suryo Rahmanto, Y., Ponka, P. and Richardson, D.R. (2009) Elucidation of the mechanism of mitochondrial iron loading in Friedreich's ataxia by analysis of a mouse mutant. *Proc. Natl Acad. Sci. USA*, **106**, 16381–16386.

Hui, Y., Wang, D., Li, W., *et al.* (2011) Long-term overexpression of heme oxygenase 1 promotes tau aggregation in mouse brain by inducing tau phosphorylation. *J. Alzheimer's Dis.*, **26**, 299–313.

Jack, C.R. Jr, Wengenack, T.M., Reyes, D.A., *et al.* (2005) In vivo magnetic resonance microimaging of individual amyloid plaques in Alzheimer's transgenic mice. *J. Neurosci.*, **25**, 10041–10048.

Jefferies, W.A., Brandon, M.R. and Hunt, S.V., *et al.* (1984) Transferrin receptor on endothelium of brain capillaries. *Nature*, **312**, 162–163.

Jellinger, K.A. (1991) Pathology of Parkinson's disease. Changes other than the nigrostriatal pathway. *Mol. Chem. Neuropathol.*, **14**, 153–197.

Jellinger, K., Paulus, W., Grundke-Iqbal, I., Riederer, P. and Youdim, M.B. (1999) Brain iron and ferritin in Parkinson's and Alzheimer's diseases. *J. Neural Transm. Park. Dis. Dement. Sect.*, **2**, 327–340.

Jeong, S.Y. and David, S. (2003) Glycosylphosphatidylinositol-anchored ceruloplasmin is required for iron efflux from cells in the central nervous system. *J. Biol. Chem.*, **278**, 27144–27148.

Jiang, H., Qian, Z.M. and Xie, J.X. (2003) Increased DMT1 expression and iron content in MPTP-treated C57BL/6 mice. *Sheng Li Xue Bao*, **55**, 571–576.

Johri, A., Chandra, A. and Beal, M.F. (2013) PGC-1α, mitochondrial dysfunction, and Huntington's disease. *Free Radic. Biol. Med.*, **62**, 37–46.

Keogh, M.J. and Chinnery, P.F. (2012) Current concepts and controversies in neurodegeneration with brain iron accumulation. *Semin. Pediatr. Neurol.*, **19**, 51–56.

Keogh, M.J., Jonas, P., Coulthard, A., *et al.* (2012) Neuroferritinopathy: a new inborn error of iron metabolism. *Neurogenetics*, **13**, 93–96.

Klomp, L.W.J. and Gitlin, J.D. (1993) Expression of the ceruloplasmin gene in the human retina and brain: implications for a pathogenic model in aceruloplasminemia. *Hum. Mol. Genet.*, **5**, 1989–1996.

Kono, S. (2013) Aceruloplasminemia: an update. *Int. Rev. Neurobiol.*, **110**, 125–151.

Kono, S., Suzuki, H., Oda, T., Shirakawa, K., Takahashi, Y., Kitagawa, M., *et al.* (2007) Cys-881 is essential for the trafficking and secretion of truncated mutant ceruloplasmin in aceruloplasminemia. *J. Hepatol.*, **47**, 844–850.

Kono, S., Yoshida, K., Tomosugi, N., *et al.* (2010) Biological effects of mutant ceruloplasmin on hepcidin-mediated internalization of ferroportin. *Biochim. Biophys. Acta*, **1802**, 968–975.

Kruer, M.C. and Boddaert, N. (2012) Neurodegeneration with brain iron accumulation: a diagnostic algorithm. *Semin. Pediatr. Neurol.*, **19**, 67–74.

Kruer, M.C., Paisán-Ruiz, C., Boddaert, N., *et al.* (2010) Defective FA2H leads to a novel form of neurodegeneration with brain iron accumulation (NBIA). *Ann. Neurol.*, **68**, 611–618.

Kwok, J.B. (2010) Role of epigenetics in Alzheimer's and Parkinson's disease. *Epigenomics*, **2**, 671–682.

Lei, P., Ayton, S., Finkelstein, D.I., *et al.* (2012) Tau deficiency induces parkinsonism with dementia by impairing APP-mediated iron export. *Nat. Med.*, **18**, 291–295.

Leitner, D.F. and Connor, J.R. (2012) Functional roles of transferrin in the brain. *Biochim. Biophys. Acta*, **1820**, 393–402.

Leskovjan, A.C., Kretlow, A., Lanzirotti, A. *et al.* (2011) Increased brain iron coincides with early plaque formation in a mouse model of Alzheimer's disease. *Neuroimage*, **55**, 32–38.

Levi, S. and Finazzi, D. (2014) Neurodegeneration with brain iron accumulation: update on pathological mechanisms. *Front Pharmacol.*, **5**, 99.

Li, K., Besse, E.K., Ha, D., Kovtunovych, G. and Rouault, T.A. (2008) Iron-dependent regulation of frataxin expression: implications for treatment of Friedreich ataxia. *Hum. Mol. Genet.*, **17**, 2265–2273.

Li, W.J., Jiang., H., Song, N. and Xie, J.X. (2010) Dose- and time-dependent alpha-synuclein aggregation induced by ferric iron in SK-N-SH cells. *Neurosci. Bull.*, **26**, 205–210.

Liu, C.B., Wang, R., Dong, M.W., Gao, X.R. and Yu, F. (2014) Expression of hepcidin at the choroid plexus in normal aging rats is associated with IL-6/Stat3 signaling pathway. *Sheng Li Xue*, **66**, 639–646.

Liu, X.B., Hill, P. and Haile, D.J. (2002) Role of the ferroportin iron-responsive element in iron and nitric oxide dependent gene regulation. *Blood Cells Mol. Dis.*, **29**, 315–326.

Liu, Y. and Connor, J.R. (2012) Iron and ER stress in neurodegenerative disease. *Biometals*, **25**, 837–845.

Lumsden, A.L., Henshall, T.L., Dayan, S., Lardelli, M.T. and Richards, R.I. (2007) Huntingtin-deficient zebrafish exhibit defects in iron utilization and development. *Hum. Mol. Genet.*, **16**, 1905–1920.

Luscieti, S., Santambrogio, P., Langlois d'Estaintot B., *et al.* (2010) Mutant ferritin L-chains that cause neurodegeneration act in a dominant-negative manner to reduce ferritin iron incorporation. *J. Biol. Chem.*, **285**, 11948–11957.

Maciel, P., Cruz, V.T., Constante, M., *et al.* (2005) Neuroferritinopathy: missense mutation in FTL causing early-onset bilateral pallidal involvement. *Neurology*, **65**, 603–605.

Mancuso, M., Davidzon, G., Kurlan, R.M., *et al.* (2005) Hereditary ferritinopathy: a novel mutation, its cellular pathology, and pathogenetic insights. *J. Neuropathol. Exp. Neurol.*, **64**, 280–294.

Marques, F., Falcao, A.M., Sousa, J.C., Coppola, G., Geschwind, D., Sousa, N., Correia-Neves, M. and Palha, J.A. (2009) Altered iron metabolism is part of the choroid plexus response to peripheral inflammation. *Endocrinology*, **150**, 2822–2828.

McCarthy, R.C., Park, Y.H. and Kosman, D.J. (2014) sAPP modulates iron efflux from brain microvascular endothelial cells by stabilizing the ferrous iron exporter ferroportin. *EMBO Rep.*, **15**, 809–815.

Mehta, A., Brewington, R., Chatterji, M., *et al.* (2013) Infection-induced modulation of m1 and m2 phenotypes in circulating monocytes: role in immune monitoring and early prognosis of sepsis. *Shock*, **22**, 423–430.

Mena, N.P., Bulteau, A.L., Salazar, J., Hirsch, E.C. and Núñez, M.T. (2011) Effect of mitochondrial complex I inhibition on Fe–S cluster protein activity. *Biochem. Biophys. Res. Commun.*, **409**, 241–246.

Mena, N.P., Urrutia, P.J., Lourido, F., Carrasco, C.M. and Nunez, M.T. (2015) Mitochondrial iron homeostasis and its dysfunctions in neurodegenerative disorders. *Mitochondrion*, **21**, 92–105.

Morris, C.M., Candy, J.M., Omar, S., Bloxham, C.A. and Edwardson, J.A. (1994) Transferrin receptors in the parkinsonian midbrain. *Neuropathol. Appl. Neurobiol.*, **20**, 468–472.

Morris, M., Maeda, S., Vossel, K. and Mucke, L. (2011) The many faces of tau. *Neuron*, **70**, 410–426.

Muhoberac, B.B. and Vidal, R. (2013) Abnormal iron homeostasis and neurodegeneration. *Front. Aging Neurosci.*, **5**, 32.

Muhoberac, B.B., Baraibar, M.A. and Vidal, R. (2011) Iron loading-induced aggregation and reduction of iron incorporation in heteropolymeric ferritin containing a mutant light chain that causes neurodegeneration. *Biochim. Biophys. Acta*, **1812**, 544–548.

Nabuurs, R.J., Hegeman, I., Natté, R., *et al.* (2011) High-field MRI of single histological slices using an inductively coupled, self-resonant microcoil: application to ex vivo samples of patients with Alzheimer's disease. *NMR Biomed.*, **24**, 351–357.

Oakley, A.E., Collingwood, J.F., Dobson, J., *et al.* (2007) Individual dopaminergic neurons show raised iron levels in Parkinson disease. *Neurology*, **68**, 1820–1825.

Orr, H.T. and Zoghbi, H.Y. (2007) Trinucleotide repeat disorders. *Annu. Rev. Neurosci.*, **30**, 575–621.

Perry, G., Nunomura, A., Hirai, K., *et al.* (2002) Is oxidative damage the fundamental pathogenic mechanism of Alzheimer's and other neurodegenerative diseases? *Free Radic. Biol. Med.*, **33**, 1475–1479.

Qian, Z.M. and Shen, X. (2001) Brain iron transport and neurodegeneration. *Trends Mol. Med.*, **7**, 103–108.

Rathore, K.I., Redensek, A. and David, S. (2012) Iron homeostasis in astrocytes and microglia is differentially regulated by TNFα and TGFβ1. *Glia*, **60**, 738–750.

Reddy, P.H. and Shirendeb, U.P. (2013) Mutant huntingtin, abnormal mitochondrial dynamics, defective axonal transport of mitochondria, and selective synaptic degeneration in Huntington's disease. *Biochim. Biophys. Acta*, **1822**, 101–110.

Roberts, B.R., Ryan, T.M., Bush, A.L., Masters, C.L. and Duce, J.A. (2012) The role of metallobiology and amyloid-β peptides in Alzheimer's disease. *J. Neurochem.*, **120** (Suppl. 1), 149–166.

Rogers, J.T., Randall, J.D., Cahill, C.M., *et al.* (2002) An iron-responsive element type II in the 5'-untranslated region of the Alzheimer's amyloid precursor protein transcript. *J. Biol. Chem.*, **277**, 45518–45528.

Sayre, L.M., Perry, G., Harris, P.L., *et al.* (2000) In situ oxidative catalysis by neurofibrillary tangles and senile plaques in Alzheimer's disease: a central role for bound transition metals. *J. Neurochem.*, **74**, 270–279.

Schneider, S.A., Paisan-Ruiz, C., Quinn, N.P., *et al.* (2010) ATP13A2 mutations (PARK9) cause neurodegeneration with brain iron accumulation. *Mov. Disord.*, **25**, 979–984.

Schipper, H.M. (2012) Neurodegeneration with brain iron accumulation – Clinical syndromes and neuroimaging. *Biochim. Biophys. Acta*, **1822**, 350–360.

Schroder, N., Figueiredo, L.S. and Martins de Lima, M. (2013) Role of brain iron accumulation in cognitive dysfunction: evidence from animal models and human studies. *J. Alzheimer's Dis.*, **34**, 797–812.

Sengstock, G.J., Zawia, N.H., Olanow, C.W., Dunn, A.J. and Arendash, G.W. (1997) Intranigral iron infusion in the rat. Acute elevations in nigral lipid peroxidation and striatal dopaminergic markers with ensuing nigral degeneration. *Biol. Trace Elem. Res.*, **58**, 177–195.

Shirendeb, U.P., Calkins, M.J., Manczak, M., *et al.* (2012) Mutant huntingtin's interaction with mitochondrial protein Drp1 impairs mitochondrial biogenesis and causes defective axonal transport and synaptic degeneration in Huntington's disease. *Hum. Mol. Genet.*, **21**, 406–420.

Sian-Hülsmann, J., Mandel, S., Youdim, M.B. and Riederer, P. (2011) The relevance of iron in the pathogenesis of Parkinson's disease. *J. Neurochem.*, **118**, 939–957.

Silvestri, L. and Camaschella, C. (2008) A potential pathogenetic role of iron in Alzheimer's disease. *J. Cell. Mol. Med.*, **12**, 1548–1550.

Singh, N., Haldar, S., Tripathi, A.K., *et al.* (2014) Brain iron homeostasis: from molecular mechanisms to clinical significance and therapeutic opportunities. *Antioxid. Redox Signal.*, **20**, 1324–1363.

Tribl, F., Asan, E., Arzberge, T.E., *et al.* (2009) Identification of L-ferritin in neuromelanin granules of the human substantia nigra. *Mol. Cell. Proteomics*, **8**, 1832–1838.

Urrutia, P., Aguirre, P., Esparza, A., *et al.* (2013) Inflammation alters the expression of DMT1, FPN1 and hepcidin, and it causes iron accumulation in central nervous system cells. *J. Neurochem.*, **126**, 541–549.

Urrutia, P.J., Mena, N.P. and Núñez, M.T. (2014) The interplay between iron accumulation, mitochondrial dysfunction, and inflammation during the execution step of neurodegenerative disorders. *Front. Pharmacol.*, **5**, 38.

Vidal, R., Ghetti, B., Takao, M., *et al.* (2004) Intracellular ferritin accumulation in neural and extraneural tissue characterizes a neurodegenerative disease associated with a mutation in the ferritin light polypeptide gene. *J. Neuropathol. Exp. Neurol.*, **63**, 363–380.

Wang, J., Jiang, H. and Xie, J.X. (2007) Ferroportin1 and hephaestin are involved in the nigral iron accumulation of 6-OHDA-lesioned rats. *Eur. J. Neurosci.*, **25**, 2766–2772.

Ward, R.J, Wilmet, S., Legssyer, R., *et al.* (2009) Effects of marginal iron overload on iron homeostasis and immune function in alveolar macrophages isolated from pregnant and normal rats. *Biometals*, **22**, 211–223.

Ward, R.J., Zucca, F.A., Duyn, J.H., Crichton, R.R. and Zecca, L. (2014) The role of iron in brain ageing and neurodegenerative disorders. *Lancet Neurol.*, **13**, 1045–1060.

Weigel, K.J., Lynch, S.G. and LeVine, S.M. (2014) Iron chelation and multiple sclerosis. *ASN Neuro.*, **6**, e00136.

Williams, R., Buchheit, C.L., Berman, N.E. and LeVine, S.M. (2012) Pathogenic implications of iron accumulation in multiple sclerosis. *J. Neurochem.*, **120**, 7–25.

Wong, B.X., Tsatsanis, A., Lim, L.Q., *et al.* (2014) β-Amyloid precursor protein does not possess ferroxidase activity but does stabilize the cell surface ferrous iron exporter ferroportin. *PLoS One*, **9**, e114174.

Wu, L.J., Leenders, A.G., Cooperman, S., *et al.* (2004) Expression of the iron transporter ferroportin in synaptic vesicles and the blood–brain barrier. *Brain Res.*, **1001**, 108–117.

Xiong, X.Y., Wang, J., Qian, Z.M. and Yang, Q.W. (2014) Iron and intracerebral hemorrhage: from mechanism to translation. *Transl. Stroke Res.*, **5**, 429–441.

Yamamoto, A., Shin, R.W., Hasegawa, K.H., *et al.* (2002) Iron (III) induces aggregation of hyperphosphorylated tau and its reduction to iron (II) reverses the aggregation: implications in the formation of neurofibrillary tangles of Alzheimer's disease. *J. Neurochem.*, **82**, 1137–1147.

Yoshida, K., Furihata, K., Takeda, S., Nakamura, A., Yamamoto, K., Morita, H., *et al.* (1995) A mutation in the ceruloplasmin gene is associated with systemic hemosiderosis in humans. *Nat. Genet.*, **9**, 267–272.

Zecca, L., Gallorini, M., Schünemann, V., *et al.* (2001) Iron, neuromelanin and ferritin content in the substantia nigra of normal subjects at different ages: consequences for iron storage and neurodegenerative processes. *J. Neurochem.*, **76**, 1766–1773.

Zecca, L., Youdim, M.B., Riederer, P., Connor, J.R. and Crichton, R.R. (2004) Iron, brain ageing and neurodegenerative disorders. *Nat. Rev. Neurosci.*, **5**, 863–873.

Zhang, Z., Hou, L., Song, J.L., *et al.* (2014) Pro-inflammatory cytokine-mediated ferroportin down-regulation contributes to the nigral iron accumulation in lipopolysaccharide-induced Parkinsonian models. *Neuroscience*, **257**, 20–30.

Zucca, F.A, Basso, E., Cupaioli, F.A, *et al.* (2014) Neuromelanin of the human substantia nigra: an update. *Neurotox. Res.*, **25**, 13–23.

Concluding Remarks

As we pass into 2016, it is fitting to remember that 2015 marked the centenary of the death of Paul Ehrlich, German physician and microbiologist, the founding father of chemotherapy, and recipient of the 1908 Nobel Prize for Medicine for his work on immunity. Ehrlich formulated the hypothesis that the injection of bacterial toxins into an animal induces the formation of toxin-neutralising antitoxins. Indeed, Ehrlich's first sketches illustrating the mechanism of neutralisation prefigure the way in which the reaction between an antigen and an antibody is represented, showing the union of two chemically complementary surfaces. However, Ehrlich also developed dyes that would specifically stain bacteria, such as fuchsin, which specifically stains the tuberculosis bacterium. Since he had observed that many of these dyes kill the bacterium to which they bind, he hypothesised that altering the dyes chemically and screening a vast number of such compounds could ultimately lead to a chemical 'magic bullet' (Zauberkugel) which would target the bacteria without harming the host. In 1907, Ehrlich and Alfred Bertheim made a derivative of the highly toxic pentavalent arsenic atoxyl, arsphenamine (Ehrlich 606) which, when tested in an animal model of syphilis (*Treponema pallidum*) by Sashiro Hata was found to kill the infectious agent while sparing the host. First marketed in 1910 by Hoechst as Salvarsan®, it was replaced a few years later by Neosalvarsam®, an easier-to-handle derivative of Salvarsan with improved water solubility. Ehrlich's methodical search for a specific cure for an identified disease can be regarded as the introduction of targeted chemotherapy (Ehrlich, 1910), and his postulate of creating 'magic bullets' for use in the fight against human diseases has inspired generations of scientists to devise powerful molecular therapeutics (Strebhardt and Ullrich, 2008).

The drug-screening approach pioneered by Ehrlich remains the basis for the discovery of new drugs for infectious diseases, as illustrated by the following examples. The 1939 Nobel Prize for Medicine was attributed to Gerhard Domagh, German bacteriologist and pathologist, for the

Iron Metabolism – From Molecular Mechanisms to Clinical Consequences, Fourth Edition. Robert Crichton.
© 2016 John Wiley & Sons, Ltd. Published 2016 by John Wiley & Sons, Ltd.

discovery of Prontosil, the first of the family of sulphonamide antibiotic drugs. He was able to save the life of his four-year-old daughter from a serious infection, and both Franklin D. Roosevelt and Winston Churchill also benefitted from treatment with Prontosil. The serendipitous discovery of penicillin by the Scottish microbiologist Alexander Fleming, due to the accidental contamination by *Penicillium notatum* of a poorly closed Petri dish, led to his receiving the 1945 Nobel Prize for Medicine together with Ernst Chain and Howard Florey (who developed its production), and the use of penicillin in World War II saved many lives. The Russian-American biochemist Selman Waksman used essentially the same drug-screening methods pioneered by Ehrlich to discover streptomycin and a number of other antibiotics, for which he received the 1952 Nobel Prize for Medicine. And so did the winners of the 2015 Nobel Prize for Medicine, the Japanese microbiologist Satoshi Omura (Burg *et al.*, 1979) and the Irish-American parasitologist William C. Campbell (Egerton *et al.*, 1979), who discovered a new drug, avermectin, the derivatives of which have radically lowered the incidence of river blindness and lymphatic filariasis, as well as showing efficacy against an expanding number of other parasitic diseases. The Chinese pharmacist Youyou Tu turned to traditional herbal medicine to tackle the challenge of developing novel malaria therapies, and discovered artemisinin, a drug that has significantly reduced the mortality rates for patients suffering from malaria by rapidly killing the malaria parasites at an early stage of their development (Tu, 2011).

Can we then hope to find 'magic bullets' for the numerous human diseases in which iron is involved? Iron uptake mechanisms are an obvious target for microbial and other infectious diseases, as well as for the treatment of cancers in which transferrin-mediated iron uptake is markedly upregulated. Antimicrobials directed to exploit siderophore uptake systems are obvious candidates for the former, and transferrin receptor 1 has been – and indeed continues to be – a prime target for anticancer therapeutics. At the other end of the scale, treating iron deficiency in the human population, which remains a major public health problem, could be greatly improved if we could increase the bioavailability of iron in the edible parts of basic crop plants (Briat *et al.*, 2015). The use of the conventional clinically approved chelators had until recently been essentially used in relieving the iron burden of patients with acquired iron overload. However, promising applications of deferiprone (Ferriprox®) in the treatment of Friedreich's ataxia (Pandolfo *et al.*, 2014) have raised hopes that chelation therapy could have multiple therapeutic applications in the many neurodegenerative diseases that afflict the increasingly ageing population. Recent clinical trials conducted in Lille, France (Devos *et al.*, 2014) and at Imperial College London (Bastida *et al.*, 2016) have established the potential of iron chelation therapy to at least slow disease progression in Parkinson's patients. There is, however, a need for more new targeted chelators as well as a better understanding of brain iron homeostasis to ensure that the use of chelators does not cause more harm than good with regard to the central nervous system. The other bright star in the iron firmament, hepcidin, has sparked the development of hepcidin analogues and other ways of targeting hepcidin production as an original approach to the potential therapy of iron deficiency as well as iron overload. However, homeostatic mechanisms function on a Ying–Yang principle, which decreases the production of the physiological 'hormone' in response to a stimulus, and overshoot, stimulating increased production of the hormone. Hence, the pharmacological agents need to used in a way which achieves overshoot, but not at the expense of long-term homeostasis.

The centenary of Paul Ehrlich's death in 1915 was commemorated by many parts of the scientific community across the world (Cabantchik and Drakesmith, 2015), including the International BioIron Society (IBIS) at its 2015 Biannual BioIron Meeting held in Hanzhou, China in September, 2015 (http://www.bioiron.org/). At the meeting, IBIS paid homage to Paul Ehrlich on the centennial of his death in 2015, by honouring "…a most distinguished scientist, prolific writer member

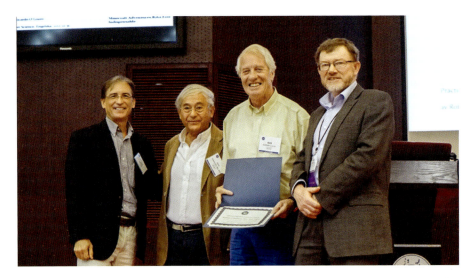

Figure C.1 *Presentation of the IBIS Paul Ehrlich Centenary Award in Hanzhou, China. Left to right: Robert Fleming, incoming President of IBIS; Ioav Cabantchik, who made the presentation; the recipient, Bob Crichton; and Greg Anderson, outgoing President of IBIS, who presented the award*

and founder of IBIS, who blended the chemistry and biology of iron in the tradition of Paul Ehrlich". I was totally surprised and deeply honoured to receive the IBIS Paul Ehrlich Centenary Award (Figure C.1), and would like to take this opportunity to thank all of my colleagues in the field for this. I will continue to try, through my writing if not through my no longer active research, to contribute to the greater community of iron researchers.

References

Bastida, A., Ward, R.J., Piccini, P., *et al.* (2016) Brain iron chelation in Parkinson's disease patients. *Nat. Comm.* (in press).

Briat, J.F., Dubos, C. and Gaymard, F. (2015) Iron nutrition, biomass production, and plant product quality. *Trends Plant Sci.*, **20**, 33–40.

Burg, R.W., Miller, B.M., Baker, E.E., *et al.* (1979) Avermectins, a new family of potent anthelmintic agents: producing organism and fermentation. *Antimicrob. Agents Chemother.*, **15**, 361–367.

Cabantchik, Z.I. and Drakesmith, H. (2015) From one Nobel Prize (P. Ehrlich) to another (Tu Youyou): 100 years of chemotherapy of infectious diseases. *Clin. Microbiol. Infect.* 2015 pii: S1198-743X(15)00993-3. doi: 10.1016/j.cmi.2015.11.011.

Devos, D., Moreau, C., Devedjian, J.C., *et al.* (2014) Targeting chelatable iron as a therapeutic modality in Parkinson's disease. *Antioxid. Redox Signal.*, **21**, 195–210.

Egerton, J.R., Ostlind, D.A., Blair, L.S., *et al.* (1979) Avermectins, a new family of potent anthelmintic agents: efficacy of the B1a component. *Antimicrob. Agents Chemother.*, **15** (3), 372–378.

Ehrlich, P. (1910) Die Behandlung der Syphilis mit dem Ehrlichschen Präparat 606. *Deutsche Med. Wochenschr.* 1893–1896.

Pandolfo, M., Arpa, J., Delatycki, M.B., *et al.* (2014) Deferiprone in Friedreich ataxia: a 6-month randomized controlled trial. *Ann. Neurol.*, **76**, 509–521.

Strebhardt, K. and Ullrich, A. (2008) Paul Ehrlich's magic bullet concept: 100 years of progress. *Nat. Rev. Cancer*, **8**, 473–480.

Tu, Y. (2011) The discovery of artemisinin (qinghaosu) and gifts from Chinese medicine. *Nat. Med.*, **17**, 1217–1220.

Index

Note: Page numbers in *italic* denote figures, when outside page ranges.

Iron Metabolism – From Molecular Mechanisms to Clinical Consequences, Fourth Edition. Robert Crichton.
© 2016 John Wiley & Sons, Ltd. Published 2016 by John Wiley & Sons, Ltd.